Health Information Management Technology

An Applied Approach

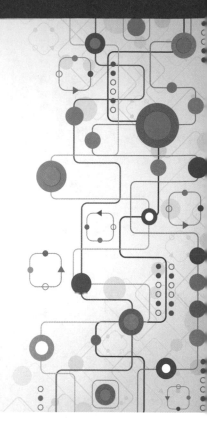

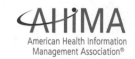

American Health Information
Management Association®

Health Information Management Technology

An Applied Approach

Fifth Edition

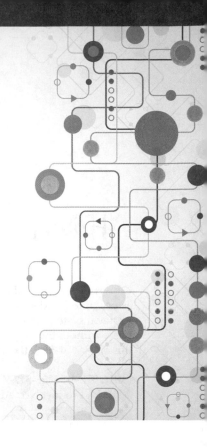

Volume Editors

Nanette B. Sayles, EdD, RHIA, CCS, CHDA, CHPS, CPHIMS, FAHIMA

Leslie L. Gordon, MS, RHIA, FAHIMA

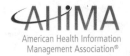

AHIMA
American Health Information
Management Association®

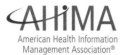

American Health Information
Management Association®

ISBN: 978-1-58426-517-7
AHIMA Product No.: AB103115

AHIMA Staff:
Caitlin Wilson, Assistant Editor
Megan Grennan, Senior Production Development Editor
Pamela Woolf, Director of Publications

For more information, including updates, about AHIMA Press publications, visit http://www.ahima.org/publications/updates.aspx.

American Health Information Management Association
233 North Michigan Avenue, 21st Floor
Chicago, Illinois 60601-5809
ahima.org

Brief Table of Contents

Table of Contents

Volume Editors

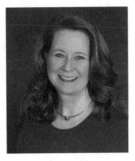

Nanette B. Sayles, EdD, RHIA, CCS, CHDA, CHPS, CPHIMS, FAHIMA, is an associate professor in the health information management program at East Central College in Union, MO, and has a BS in medical record administration, an MS in health information management, a master's degree in public administration, and a doctorate of education in adult education. Dr. Sayles has more than 10 years of experience as a health information management practitioner with experience in hospitals, a consulting firm, and a computer vendor. She was the 2005 American Health Information Management Association Triumph Educator award winner. She has held numerous volunteer roles for the American Health Information Management Association (AHIMA), the Georgia Health Information Management Association (GHIMA), the Alabama Association of Health Information Management (AAHIM), Middle Georgia Health Information Management Association (MGHIMA), and Birmingham Regional Health Information Management Association (BRHIMA). These positions include: AHIMA Educational Strategies Committee, AHIMA co-chair RHIA Workgroup, GHIMA director, and president of MGHIMA. Dr. Sayles has published two other books: *Professional Review Guide for the CHP, CHS, and CHPS Examinations* and *Case Studies for Health Information Management*. She is an editor for two chapters in the *PRG Professional Review Guide* for the RHIA and RHIT examinations.

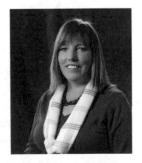

Leslie L. Gordon, MS, RHIA, FAHIMA, is an associate professor and the health information management program director at the University of Alaska Southeast (UAS), Sitka Campus. She earned a BA and an MS from the College of St. Scholastica and has been teaching at UAS since 2003. Before teaching she worked as a coder, reimbursement manager, and data analyst at a hospital in Sitka, AK, for many years. Ms. Gordon is an active member of the Alaska CSA (AKHIMA) and has served in several positions on the AKHIMA Board. She served on the Council for Education Excellence (CEE) as the Chair of the Curriculum Committee and was instrumental in the development of the updated AHIMA curriculum upon which this text is based. She is a Fellow of AHIMA and currently serves on the Board of Commissioners of the Council of Accreditation of Health Informatics and Information Management Education (CAHIIM).

Chapter Authors

Margret K. Amatayakul, MBA, RHIA, CHPS, CPHIT, CPEHR, FHIMSS, is president of Margret\A Consulting, LLC, in Schaumburg, IL, a consulting firm specializing in electronic health records (EHRs) and associated health information management (HIM) standards and regulations, such as HIPAA and ACA. She has more than 30 years of experience in national and international HIM. A leading authority on health IT strategies for healthcare organizations, she has extensive experience in EHR optimization and workflow redesign. She helped form and served as executive director of the Computer-based Patient Record Institute (CPRI), was associate executive director of AHIMA, associate professor at the University of Illinois at Chicago, and director of medical record services at the Illinois Eye and Ear Infirmary. She is a highly desired speaker, has published extensively, serves on several boards, and has earned numerous professional service awards.

Megan Brickner, MSA, RHIA, serves as the director of compliance programs and privacy officer for the Kettering Health Network in Dayton, OH. She is responsible for daily and strategic operations of the Kettering Health Network's information security and privacy program, titled PROTECT. Her PROTECT Program was highlighted at the 2012 Annual Ohio Hospital Association Meeting as a program of best practice and at the 2016 Ohio Health Information Management Association's 36th Annual Meeting and Trade Show. Ms. Brickner has nearly 20 years of experience in the area of healthcare compliance. She holds BS degrees in healthcare administration and health information management as well as a master's degree in healthcare administration. Ms. Brickner is a registered health information administrator (RHIA) and serves as an adjunct faculty member for the health information management department at Sinclair Community College in Dayton.

Danika Brinda, PhD, RHIA, CHPS, HCISPP, is an Assistant Professor in the Health Informatics and Information Management Department at the College of St. Scholastica in Duluth, MN. She teaches a variety of courses related to legal issues in healthcare, HIPAA privacy and security, compliance, and EHRs in healthcare. Dr. Brinda is also the CEO of TriPoint Healthcare Solutions, which focuses on helping organization understand, operationalize, and implement the complex healthcare privacy and security regulations. Dr. Brinda was an HIT consultant for the Regional Extension Center grant in Minnesota and North Dakota. She helped organizations of many different sizes navigate the EHR Incentive Program and prepare for successful attestation to the program. She also was a part of numerous EHR implementations in a large, integrated healthcare system in Minnesota. Dr. Brinda is both a state and national speaker on all aspects of privacy and security in healthcare. She enjoys making privacy and security regulations fun and understandable to all organizations and specialties in healthcare. She is a 2010 recipient of the AHIMA Rising Star Triumph Award.

Darcy Carter, DHSc, MHA, RHIA, earned her doctorate degree in health sciences with an emphasis in leadership and organizational behavior and a master's degree in healthcare administration. She is a faculty member of the health information management and technology programs and the master of healthcare administration program at Weber State University, where she teaches courses in coding, reimbursement, epidemiology, and quality improvement. Ms. Carter is the co-author of the sixth edition of the *Quality and Performance Improvement in Healthcare: Theory, Practice, and Management* textbook published by AHIMA. She is also the editor of the *Registered Health Information Technician (RHIT) Exam Preparation* and the *Registered Health Information Administrator (RHIA) Exam Preparation* books published by AHIMA. She currently serves as a board member for the Utah Health Information Management Association (UHIMA).

Kathy Giannangelo, MA, RHIA, CCS, CPHIMS, FAHIMA, is a medical informaticist with Language and Computing, Inc. (L&C). In this position, she supports the ontology, modeling, sales, and product development activities related to the creation and implementation of natural language-processing applications where clinical terminology and classification systems are utilized. Ms. Giannangelo has a comprehensive background in the field of clinical terminologies and classification, with more than 30 years of experience in the HIM field. Prior to joining L&C, she was director of practice leadership with AHIMA in Chicago. She has served as senior nosologist for a health information services company and worked in various HIM roles, including vice president of product development, education specialist, director of medical records, quality assurance coordinator, and manager of a Centers for Disease Control and Prevention research team. Ms. Giannangelo has developed classification, grouping, and reimbursement systems products for healthcare providers; conducted seminars; and provided consulting assessments throughout the United States as well as in Canada, Australia, Ireland, Bulgaria, and the United Kingdom. In addition, she has authored numerous articles and created online continuing education courses on clinical terminologies. As adjunct faculty at the College of St. Scholastica, she teaches clinical vocabularies and classification systems, a graduate-level course. In addition, she is actively involved as a volunteer in the HIM profession at the international, national, state, and local levels. Ms. Giannangelo holds a master's degree in HIM from the College of St. Scholastica.

Darline Foltz, RHIA, is a full-time assistant professor-educator in the online health information systems technology program at UC Clermont. She is in the process of working on her master of educational studies from the University of Cincinnati. Ms. Foltz has a BS in HIM from The Ohio State University and also has a bachelor's degree in information systems from the University of Cincinnati. Prior to joining UC Clermont in January, 2013, Ms. Foltz spent her career in many facets of HIM including owning her own consulting business; director of HIM at Deaconess Hospital, Cincinnati; director of HIM at the Drake Center; and director of IS and telecommunications at Deaconess Hospital, Cincinnati. Ms. Foltz has been a consultant for long-term and acute-care hospitals, nursing homes, dialysis clinics, physician offices, mental health agencies, drug and alcohol rehab centers, and rehab hospitals and she is the co-author of the textbook, *Exploring the EHR*. She obtained the AHIMA ICD-10 Coding Trainer certificate and, after working in the field for 35 years, is excited to teach the next generation of health information professionals.

Morley L. Gordon, RHIT, is an HIM analyst for Home Health and Hospice at Evergreen Hospital in Kirkland, WA. Previously she was the director of health information management at a long-term care facility in central Washington. She graduated from the University of Alaska HIT program and is continuing her education at Western Governors College. She credits her mom for introducing her to the field of HIM and for recommending she pursue HIM as a career. Ms. Gordon is grateful for the opportunities that she is afforded because of it.

Loretta A. Horton, MEd, RHIA, FAHIMA, received a medical record technician certificate from Research Hospital and Medical Center and a bachelor's degree in psychology from Rockhurst College, both in Kansas City, MO; a health information administration post-baccalaureate certificate from Stephens College in Columbia, MO; and a master's degree in education, with an emphasis in curriculum and instruction, from Wichita State University in Wichita, KS. She also has completed graduate work in sociology at the University of Nebraska in Omaha.

Horton has served as co-chair of the allied health department and coordinator of the health information technology program at Hutchinson Community College in Hutchinson, KS. Previously, she worked in a variety of health information settings, including acute care and mental health, and has consulted with long-term care, mental retardation, home health, hospice, and prison systems. Horton has been an instructor in the health information administration program at the College of St. Mary in Omaha, NE, and a marketing and training coordinator for 3M in Salt Lake City, UT.

Horton has been an active member of the Kansas Health Information Management Association receiving the Motivator award in 2002, the Achievement award in 2006, the Champion award in 2009, and the Outstanding Member award in 2015. She is an AHIMA Fellow and has served on the Item Writing Task Force for the Council on Certification, Council on Accreditation, Scholarship Committee, and Associate Education Consortium.

Donald W. Kellogg, PhD, RHIA, CPEHR, FAHIMA, is an assistant professor at University of Saint Mary in Leavenworth, KS, and is the coordinator of the bachelor of health science program as well as a faculty member in the health information technology program. He earned a bachelor's degree in health information management at the University of Kansas Medical Center and his doctorate in higher education administration at the University of Kansas. Dr. Kellogg has served the Kansas Health Information Management Association (KHIMA) as a director for three years; a delegate to the AHIMA House of Delegates for four years; and as president-elect, president, and past-president of KHIMA, in addition to chairing multiple committees. He is a recipient of KHIMA's Volunteer, Champion, and Achievement Awards. He was Kansas's first liaison to the AHIMA Foundation and Community Education Coordinator (CEC), a state association leadership position on personal health record public outreach and education efforts. Dr. Kellogg has also served on AHIMA's Educational Strategies Committee (ESC), for which he was chair in 2008; the Increasing the RHIA-Credentialed Workforce task force; and he is currently a commissioner with the Commission on Accreditation for Health Informatics and Information Management Education (CAHIIM).

Karen Lankisch, PhD, RHIA, is a Professor at the University of Cincinnati—Clermont College. She is the Program Director of the Online Health Information Systems Technology Program. She has a PhD in Education with a concentration in technology and adult learning, a Master's in Education, a Post-Bachelor Certificate in Health Information Management, and a Bachelor's in Business. She will graduate from the University of Cincinnati Health Informatics program in August 2016. She has over 10 years' experience in outpatient coding and practice management. Dr. Lankisch obtained the AHIMA ICD-10 Train-the-Trainer Certificate. She has co-authored two textbooks, *Our Digital World*, and *Exploring Electronic Health Records*. In 2013, she received the University of Cincinnati Faculty Award for Innovative Use of Technology in the Classroom.

Miland Palmer, MPH, RHIA, earned his master's degree in public health from the University of Utah and is currently working on his PhD in public health. Mr. Palmer is a full-time faculty member at Weber State University in the health administrative services department where he teaches courses in health administration, health information management, healthcare data governance, and epidemiology/biostatistics. Mr. Palmer has over 10 years' experience in public health, health administration, and health information management, spending time at the Utah Department of Health and the Department of Veterans Affairs Salt Lake City Healthcare System.

Valerie Prater, MBA, RHIT, FAHIMA, is a clinical assistant professor in the HIM program, department of biomedical and health information sciences, College of Applied Health Sciences, at the University of Illinois at Chicago (UIC). Prater was named 2015 Educator of the Year for the UIC College of Applied Health Sciences, and is the recipient of numerous citations for her commitment to teaching and student learning at UIC. She chairs the UIC Information Technology Governance Council Education Committee, is a member of the UIC faculty Collaborative for Excellence in Interprofessional Education, and served on the AHIMA Information Governance Tools and Resources Work Group.

Prater has extensive experience developing curricula for HIM programs, both in her current faculty role and in her previous position as program director, DeVry University, Corporate Academics. She has also served as adjunct instructor for the University of Connecticut's online health care information technology certificate program. Prior to entering education, Prater held healthcare management positions with responsibilities encompassing operations, strategic planning, quality management, business development, and health information management. She has delivered numerous presentations to local and national professional groups, including AHIMA's Assembly on Education.

Laurie A. Rinehart-Thompson, JD, RHIA, CHP, FAHIMA, is an associate professor and serves as the director of the health information management and systems program at The Ohio State University. She earned both her BS in medical record administration and her JD from The Ohio State University. In addition to education, her professional experiences span the behavioral health, home health, and acute care arenas. She has served as an expert witness in civil litigation, testifying as to the privacy and confidentiality of health information. She has served on numerous AHIMA committees including the Privacy and Security Practice Council, Council for Excellence in Education workgroups, and as chairperson of the AHIMA Professional Ethics Committee. Ms. Rinehart-Thompson is a member of the board of directors of the Ohio Health Information Management Association (OHIMA). She is a recipient of the AHIMA Triumph Award and the OHIMA Distinguished Member Award. A speaker on the HIPAA Privacy Rule, she is a co-editor and co-author of AHIMA's *Fundamentals of Law for Health Informatics and Information Management*; the author of AHIMA's *Introduction to Health Information Privacy and Security*; and a contributing author to *Health Information Management: Concepts, Principles and Practice* (AHIMA), *Documentation for Medical Practices* (AHIMA), and *Ethical Health Informatics: Challenges and Opportunities* (Jones & Bartlett). She has been published in the *Journal of AHIMA* and in AHIMA's *Perspectives in Health Information Management*.

Marcia Y. Sharp, EdD, MBA, RHIA, is associate professor and program director at the University of Tennessee Health Science Center in the department of health informatics and information management. She teaches leadership, information technology, and healthcare information systems. Prior to teaching, Dr. Sharp served in leadership roles in health information management for over 15 years. She also has human resource experience as an HR director, and has retired from the US Navy Reserve.

Dr. Sharp serves as member of AHIMA's Council for Excellence in Education. Previously she served on the CEE's faculty development workgroup and as a delegate for the Tennessee Health Information Management Association. In addition, Dr. Sharp is a reviewer for AHIMA's *Perspectives in Health Information Management*. She holds a doctoral degree in higher and adult education from the University of Memphis, an MBA from Webster University, and a BS in health information management from the University of Tennessee.

Valerie J.M. Watzlaf, PhD, RHIA, FAHIMA, is an associate professor within the department of health information management in the School of Health and Rehabilitation Sciences at the University of Pittsburgh. She also holds a secondary appointment in the Graduate School of Public Health. In those capacities, she teaches and performs research in the areas of HIM and epidemiology. She has worked and consulted in several healthcare organizations in health information management, long-term care, and epidemiology. She is very active in professional and scientific societies having served on several AHIMA committees, as a board member of AHIMA and the AHIMA Foundation, and as the chair of the Council for Excellence in Education of the AHIMA Foundation. She is currently serving on the IG Task Force of the CEE. She is also on the Editorial Advisory Board for the *Journal of AHIMA* and for *Perspectives in Health Information Management*. Dr. Watzlaf has published extensively in the field of HIM and is the recipient of numerous awards and professional accolades including AHIMA's Research Award and PHIMA's Distinguished Member Award. She is currently working as a partner with IOD/Healthport as part of the CareInnoLab conducting research in HIM applications.

Preface

Health information management (HIM) professionals are an integral part of the healthcare team. They serve the healthcare industry and the public by using best practices in managing healthcare information to support quality healthcare delivery. Whether stored on paper or in electronic file format, reliable health information is critical to high-quality healthcare. Enhancing individual patient care through timely and relevant information is one of the primary goals for the HIM profession.

The American Health Information Management Association (AHIMA) AHIMA represents more than 103,000 health information professionals who work throughout the healthcare industry. AHIMA has a long history of commitment to HIM education. Among other contributions, AHIMA has developed and maintained a rigorous accreditation process for academic programs, continuously developed up-to-date curriculum models, supported faculty development, and continued to research and study the needs and future directions of HIM education.

This text, specifically developed for associate degree programs in health information technology (HIT), is an outgrowth of AHIMA's ongoing effort to provide rich resources for the education and training of new HIM professionals. In addition, it offers a ready resource for current practitioners. Its subject matter is based on AHIMA's HIM Associate Degree Program Entry-Level Competencies and AHIMA's Registered Health Information Technician (RHIT) Certification Examination content domains. AHIMA made a significant change to the Entry-Level Competencies in 2014 and this curriculum change created the need for significant modifications to this edition. Following the prescribed curricular content found in the HIM Associate Degree Entry-Level Competencies, the text covers information and topics considered essential for every entry-level HIT practitioner. Although the text is directed primarily at students enrolled in two-year HIT programs, students in other HIM disciplines and allied health programs also will find its content highly useful.

The fundamental organization of the text is built on the curricular content of the HIM Associate Degree Entry-Level Competencies. Each of the content areas is represented in the book except those relating to the biomedical sciences and to technical aspects of classification systems such as the International Classification of Diseases. To provide maximum flexibility for instructional delivery, the content of each chapter is designed to stand on its own, providing maximum coverage of specific domains and competencies. Because of the interdependency of content areas that support knowledge and skills for performing many of the competencies, this approach has necessitated some duplication of material throughout the text. In these cases, the predominant content is covered in depth and is supplemented by a high-level overview of other supporting knowledge. Where appropriate, students are referred to other chapters for additional information or detail to round out necessary knowledge.

The organizing framework for content of the text is arranged in order by the six domains contained in the HIM Associate Degree Entry-Level Competencies. These domains are: Data Content Structure and Standards; Information Protection: Access, Disclosure, Archival, Privacy, and Security; Informatics, Analytics, and Data Use; Revenue Management; Compliance; and Leadership. This organization does not presuppose a pedagogical progression of presenting basic foundations and then progressing to advanced concepts. Therefore, given its student population, mission and goals, and other variables, each academic program must assess the appropriate sequence of presentation of the chapters within its curriculum. Additional information and models of chapter sequencing can be found in the instructor's manual.

The book's underlying structure is to translate basic theory into practice. A review of the cognitive and competency levels of the Entry-Level Competencies reveals that HIT programs are applied in nature. Outcome expectations are that students understand theory at a basic level with a major emphasis on skill building to perform day-to-day operational tasks in health information management.

Therefore, the features used throughout the book focus on translating basic theory into practice. To accomplish this, each chapter contains the following sections.

Check Your Understanding   These sections are content review exercises and the exercises are positioned throughout each chapter so that students can reinforce their understanding of the concepts they have just read before proceeding to the following concepts. Multiple-choice, matching, and true-and-false formats are used.

Real-World Cases   Located at the end of each chapter, this section presents two actual situations that HIM professionals may face.

The features in the accompanying student workbook include:

Real-World Case Discussion Questions   The questions in this section are designed to initiate discussion of and elaborate on the concepts presented in the Real-World Cases at the end of each chapter.

Application Exercises   The purpose of these exercises is to give students the opportunity to put theory into practice. Because skill building is an important part of the expected outcomes for HIT students, these exercises will bring the real world into their sphere.

Review Quizzes   The review quizzes are in multiple-choice format and test chapter content knowledge.

The text is divided into six parts that correspond with the domains from the 2014 AHIMA Associate Degree Entry-Level Competencies. Where appropriate, chapter content is expanded in the fifth edition to prepare students for transitional and changing roles in an electronic health information environment. All chapters in the fifth edition have been updated to reflect current trends, practices, standards, and legal issues.

Part I, Foundational Concepts   This part is not technically included in the 2014 AHIMA competencies; however is a vital foundational base to the understanding of HIM in general.

This part concentrates on the roles of the health information manager; the content, function, structure, and uses of health information; the healthcare delivery system; and how health information is managed. Chapter 1 Health Information Management Profession introduces the concept of health information management. The discussion focuses on the history of the HIM profession and the evolution of the roles and functions of HIM professionals over the years. Particular emphasis is placed on HIM future roles and their relationship to the movement toward an electronic health record (EHR). Chapter 2 Healthcare Delivery Systems introduces the history, organization, financing, and delivery of health services in the United States. Chapter 3 Health Information Functions, Purpose, and Users introduces the function and purpose of the health record function as well as who uses the record.

Part II, Data Content Structures and Standards   Part II reflects Domain I of the 2014 AHIMA competencies and explores the content related to diagnostic and procedural classification and terminologies, health record documentation requirements, data accuracy and integrity, data integration and interoperability, and the needs for data, information standards, and data management policies and procedures. Chapter 4 Health Record Content and Documentation introduces students to standards for the content of the health record and requirements for documentation. Chapter 5 Clinical Terminologies, Classifications, and Code Systems provides an introduction to clinical vocabularies and classification systems. Its purpose is to introduce the characteristics of prominent systems and help students understand how they are used throughout the healthcare system. Chapter 6 Data Management is an essential part of the day-to-day operations of a healthcare organization. It includes understanding data sources and where they exist, how they are transmitted, and where they are stored. Chapter 7 Secondary Data Sources explains the uses of the health record beyond patient care, such as registries and administrative functions.

Part III, Information Protection: Access, Disclosure, and Archival Privacy and Security This part contains healthcare law including theory of all healthcare law excluding what is covered by compliance, privacy, security, and confidentiality policies and procedures, in addition to the infrastructure and education of staff on information protection methods, risk assessment, access, and disclosure management and falls under Domain II of the 2014 AHIMA competencies. Chapter 8 Health Law discusses legal issues associated with health information and includes an overview of sources of law and legal system. Chapter 9 Data Privacy and Confidentiality are defined in terms of the legal rights of patients and the responsibility of healthcare organizations to protect those rights. Chapter 10 Data Security examines the concept of data security, which encompasses measures and tools to safeguard data and the information systems on which they reside from unauthorized access, use, disclosure, disruption, modification, or destruction.

Part IV, Informatics, Analytics and Data Use Part IV addresses the creation and use of business health intelligence, including the review of selection implementation, use and management of technology solutions, system and data architecture, interface consideration, information management planning, data modeling systems, testing technology, benefit realization analytics and decision support, data visualization techniques, trend analysis administrative reports, statistics, data quality and covers Domain III of the 2014 AHIMA competencies. Chapter 11 Health Information Technologies defines the scope of health information technology and how it has evolved into its current state in healthcare settings. The systems development life cycle is explored in terms of management of health IT. Chapter 12 Healthcare Information discusses the importance of healthcare information to the healthcare industry and the strategic uses of that information. Chapter 13 Research and Data Analysis provides methods to analyze and present healthcare data and information in an understandable and useful fashion. Chapter 14 Healthcare Statistics discusses common statistical measures and types of data used by organization in different healthcare settings.

Part V, Revenue Management and Compliance This part reflects Domains IV and V of the 2014 AHIMA competencies and includes healthcare reimbursement, as well as revenue cycle regulations and activities related to revenue management and compliance. Chapter 15 Revenue Cycle and Reimbursement explores the billing and payment methodologies. Chapter 16 Fraud and Abuse Compliance addresses federal laws that mandates all healthcare organizations comply with standards of quality care and proper billing practices.

Part VI, Leadership This part covers leadership models, theories and skills, change management, workflow analysis, design tools and techniques, human resources management training and development strategic planning, financial management, ethics and project management and reflects Domain VI of the 2014 AHIMA competencies. In Chapter 17 Leadership, leadership theories and styles are explored and the impact of change management on processes, people, and systems. Chapter 18 Performance Improvement is the continuous study and adaptation of a healthcare organization's functions and processes to increase the likelihood of achieving desired outcomes. Chapter 19 Management explores the process of planning, controlling, leading, and organizing the activities of a healthcare organization. Chapter 20 Human Resources Management and Professional Development help students understand the laws and regulations related to human resource management and the need for employee training and development. Chapter 21

Ethical Issues in Health Information Management discusses the ethical issues associated with health information management and presents the concepts of stewardship and the HIM professional's core ethical obligations.

A complete glossary of HIM terms is provided at the end of the book. **Boldface** type is used in the text chapters to indicate the first substantial reference to each glossary term. The bolded terms in a chapter are listed at the beginning of the chapter and are identified as key terms.

Appendices and a detailed content index complete the book.

AHIMA provides supplemental materials for educators who use this book in their classes. Instructor materials for this book include lesson plans, lesson slides, RHIT competency map, test bank, and other useful resources.

Acknowledgments

Many individuals contributed to the development of the fifth edition of this landmark textbook. First, the editors and AHIMA publications staff extend their sincere thanks to Merida L. Johns, PhD, RHIA, for pioneering this book through the first three editions and to all the chapter authors for sharing their expertise with new entrants into the HIM profession. Developing the rich content of this text along with searching for the best examples and resources was a time-consuming process for these very busy professionals.

Second, no text is ever complete without the diligent work of the content reviewers. Their careful review and insightful suggestions ensure the essential quality of any effort of this kind. We also would like to thank the following reviewers who lent a critical eye to this endeavor:

Darla D. Branda, MA, RHIA
Dana D. Carcamo, RHIA, CCS
Donna M Estes, RHIT, MPM, CPHQ
Judy A. Ferraro, RHIA
Karen Lankisch, PhD, RHIA
Charlotte J. McCuen, RHIA, MHA
Sharon McDonald, MSA, RHIT
Jody E. Scheller, MS, RHIA

Additionally, the editors would like to acknowledge authors who contributed chapters to each edition of this book. Their work served as the basis for several chapters that were revised by new authors:

Sandra Bailey, RHIA
Cathleen A. Barnes, RHIA, CCS
Mary Jo Bowie, MS, RHIA
Elizabeth D. Bowman, MPA, RHIA
Sheila Carlon, PhD, RHIA, CHPS, FAHIMA,
Bonnie S. Cassidy, MPA, RHIA, FHIMSS, FAHIMA
Lisa A. Cerrato, MS, RHIA
Michelle L. Dougherty, RHIA, CHP
Chris Elliott, MS, RHIA
Sandra R. Fuller, MA, RHIA
Michelle A. Green, MPS, RHIA, CMA, CHP
Laurinda B. Harman, PhD, RHIA, FAHIMA
Anita C. Hazelwood, MLS, RHIA, FAHIMA
Terrill Herzig, MSHI
Beth M. Hjort, RHIA
Joan Hicks, MSHI, RHIA
Cheryl V. Homan, MBA, RHIA
Merida L. Johns, PhD, RHIA
Kathleen M. LaTour, MA, RHIA, FAHIMA
Joan Ludwig, RHIA
Carol E. Osborn, PhD, RHIA
Bonnie Petterson, PhD, RHIA
Harry B. Rhodes, MBA, RHIA
Jane Roberts, MS, RHIA
Karen S. Scott, MEd, RHIA, CCS-P, CPC
Martin Smith, MEd, RHIT, CCA
Carol A. Venable, MPH, RHIA, FAHIMA
Karen A. Wager, DBA, RHIA
Frances Wickham Lee, DBA, RHIA
Susan B. Willner, RHIA
Andrea Weatherby White, PhD, RHIA

Foreword

With changes in technology infrastructure and systems, regulatory policies, and consumer involvement, shifts have followed in where health information professionals work, their daily work practices, and the method of delivery of health information. These changes have also resulted in new and expanded opportunities for graduates from health information management (HIM) programs. Most current studies from industry and the United States Department of Labor rank HIM as one of the top five professions for new graduates. For example, a recent study by Georgetown University noted that health information professions are expected to increase by almost 30 percent overall by 2020—the most dramatic growth of any labor sector of the United States (Georgetown University Center on Education and the Workforce 2012). Further, according to the United States Bureau of Labor and Statistics, the anticipated increase in employment for the health information field is much faster than average with a 22 percent increase in HIM-related technician jobs and a 23 percent increase in management jobs between 2012 and 2022 (United States Department of Labor 2016). This continued growth will provide new and exciting career pathway opportunities for those employed within the health information sector and those joining the profession.

Health information professionals are no longer relegated to single departments within a single healthcare entity, but rather cut across both departments and healthcare systems, filling innovative and shifting roles. Consequently, in addition to traditional knowledge required to manage a department, students joining the profession will be required to have knowledge of healthcare delivery systems, data management skills, and knowledge of new laws and practices regarding privacy and security. Furthermore, applied knowledge in statistics, research, and data analytics will be required for the HIM student of the future.

To meet the complexities and challenges of healthcare in the 21st century, students will need a resource that successfully combines theory and practice in a meaningful way. The book, *Health Information Management Technology: An Applied Approach*, fifth edition, edited by Nanette Sayles and Leslie Gordon, provides the requisite foundational knowledge to assist HIM professionals as they embark on their career journey. By bringing together an impressive array of health information leaders in academia and practice, this book bridges the gap between traditional health information education with new and exciting information on informatics, analytics, and leadership.

Information in this book will not only help you begin your career, but will serve as an excellent reference and guide for the health information professional as you continue your career in this exciting profession.

William J. Rudman, PHD, RHIA
Executive Director, AHIMA Foundation

References

Georgetown University Center on Education and the Workforce. 2012. Healthcare. http://www.healthreformgps.org/wp-content/uploads/Healthcare.FullReport.071812.pdf.

United States Department of Labor. 2016. National Bureau of Labor and Statistics. Occupational Outlook Handbook. http://www.bls.gov/ooh/healthcare/medical-records-and-health-information-technicians.htm.

Part I
Foundational
Concepts

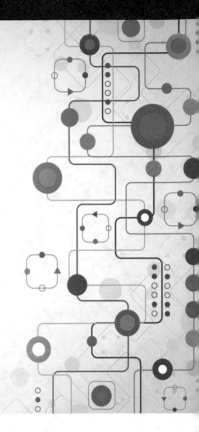

1

Health Information Management Profession

Nanette B. Sayles, EdD, RHIA, CCS, CHDA, CHPS, CPHIMS, FAHIMA

Learning Objectives

- Summarize the development of the health information management (HIM) profession from its beginnings to the present
- Discuss how professional practice must evolve to accommodate changes in the healthcare environment
- Identify the responsibilities of HIM professionals
- Describe the purpose and structure of the American Health Information Management Association (AHIMA)

- Explain AHIMA's certification processes
- Discuss the accreditation process of the Commission on Accreditation for Health Informatics and Information Management Education (CAHIIM)
- Identify the appropriate professional organizations for the various specializations of HIM

Key Terms

Accreditation
Active membership
American Academy of Professional Coders
American Association of Medical Record Librarians (AAMRL)
American College of Surgeons (ACS)
American Health Information Management Association (AHIMA)
American Medical Record Association (AMRA)
Association for Healthcare Documentation Integrity (AHDI)

Association of Record Librarians of North America (ARLNA)
Board of directors
Certification
Chief executive officer
Code of ethics
Commission on Accreditation for Health Informatics and Information Management Education (CAHIIM)
Commission on Certification for Health Informatics and Information Management (CCHIIM)

Component state associations (CSAs)
Continuing education units (CEUs)
Credential
Emeritus membership
Engage
Fellowship program
Group membership
Health information management (HIM)
Healthcare Information and Management Systems Society (HIMSS)
Hospital Standardization Program
House of Delegates

Information governance
National Cancer Registrars
   Association (NCRA)
New graduate membership

Registered Health Information
   Administrator (RHIA)
Registered Health Information
   Technician (RHIT)

Registration
Student membership

This chapter provides an introduction to the history of the **health information management (HIM)** profession and offers insights into the current and future roles and functions of those who manage health information. The role of HIM professionals is even more important now than it was when the **Association of Record Librarians of North America (ARLNA)** was created in 1928 due to the complexity of today's information- and technology-driven healthcare environment.

Early History of Health Information Management

The commitment, wisdom, and efforts of HIM pioneers are reflected in what we see today as the HIM profession. Four distinct steps influenced development of the HIM profession. These steps include the hospital standardization movement, the organization of records librarians, the approval of formal educational processes, and an educational curriculum for medical record (now known as health record) librarians.

Hospital Standardization

Before 1918, the creation and management of hospital health records were the sole responsibility of the attending physician. Physicians of that time, like many physicians today, often disliked doing paperwork. Unless the physician was interested in medical research, the health records in the early 20th century were "practically worthless and consisted principally of nurse's notes" (Huffman 1941, 101).

Health records of that time did not contain graphical records or laboratory reports. Because there was no general management of health record processes, incomplete records were often filed as received after the patient was discharged from the hospital. Hospitals made no effort to ensure that the missing or incomplete portions were completed. Furthermore, no standardized vocabulary was used to document why the patient was admitted to the hospital or the final diagnosis upon discharge.

In 1918, the hospital standardization movement was inaugurated by the **American College of Surgeons (ACS)**. The purpose of the resulting **Hospital Standardization Program** was to raise the standards of surgery by establishing minimum quality standards for hospitals. The ACS realized one of the most important items in the care of any patient was a complete and accurate report of the care and treatment provided during hospitalization. They identified that medical records must be collected on every patient seen in the healthcare facility. The medical record should contain test results, identification information, diagnoses, treatment, and more (Huffman 1941).

It was not long before hospitals realized that to comply with the hospital standards, new health record processes had to be implemented. In addition, staff had to be hired to ensure the new processes were appropriately carried out. Furthermore, hospitals recognized health records must be maintained and filed in an orderly manner and cross-indexes of disease, operations, and physicians must be compiled. Thus, the job position of health record clerk was established.

Organization of the Association of Record Librarians

A nucleus of 35 members of the Club of Record Clerks met at the Hospital Standardization Conference in Boston in 1928. Near the close of the meeting, ARLNA was formed. During its first year the association had a charter membership of 58 individuals. Members were admitted from 25 of the 48 states, the District of Columbia, and Canada (Huffman 1985). ARLNA was the original name of the American Health Information Management Association (AHIMA), which is discussed later in this chapter.

Approval of Formal Education and Certification Programs

Early HIM professionals understood that for an occupation to be recognized as a profession there must be preliminary training. They also understood such training needed to be distinguished from mere skill. That is, it needed to be intellectual in character, involving knowledge and learning. Therefore, work began on the formulation of a prescribed course of study as early as 1929. In 1932, the association adopted a formal curriculum for HIM education.

The first schools for medical record librarians were surveyed and approved by ARLNA in 1934. By 1941, 10 schools had been approved to provide training for medical record librarians. This formal approval program of academic programs was the precursor to the current accreditation program managed by Commission on Accreditation for Health Informatics and Information Management Education (CAHIIM). Accreditation is the following.

1. A voluntary process of institutional or organizational review in which a quasi-independent body created for this purpose periodically evaluates the quality of the entity's work against pre-established written criteria

2. A determination by an accrediting body that an eligible organization, network, program, group, or individual complies with applicable standards

3. The act of granting approval to a healthcare organization based on whether the organization has met a set of voluntary standards developed by an accreditation agency.

The Board of Registration, a certification board, was instituted in 1933 and developed the baseline by which to measure qualified health record librarians. They developed the eligibility criteria for registration and developed and administered a national qualifying examination. Today AHIMA's Commission on Certification for Health Informatics and Information Management (CCHIIM) functions as the Board of Registration. CCHIIM is discussed later in this chapter.

Development of the HIM profession coincided with the professionalization of other healthcare disciplines such as nursing, x-ray technology, and laboratory technology. All of these disciplines established registration or training programs around the same time.

The professional membership of the association of HIM professionals grew over the subsequent decades. Although the names of the association changed several times, the fundamental elements of the profession—formal training requirements and certification by examination—have remained the same.

Evolution of Practice

The various names given to the health record association and its associated credentials reveal a lot about the evolution of the profession and its practice. It was known as ARLNA until Canadian members formed their own organization in 1944. At that time, the name of the organization was changed to the American Association of Medical Record Librarians (AAMRL). In 1970, the organization changed its name again to eliminate the term *librarian*. The organization's name became the American Medical Record Association (AMRA). The organization underwent another name change in 1991 to become AHIMA.

The organization's title changes in 1970 and 1991 reflected the changing nature of the roles and functions of the association's professional membership. In 1970, the term *administrator* mirrored the work performed by members more accurately than the term *librarian*. Similarly, in 1991, association leaders believed that the management of *information*, rather than the management of *records*, would be the primary function of the profession in the future.

The names of the credentials conferred by the organization changed as the association's name changed. In 1999, AHIMA's House of Delegates (HOD) approved a credential name change. Registered Record Administrator (RRA) became **Registered Health Information Administrator (RHIA)**, and Accredited Record Technician (ART) became **Registered Health Information Technician (RHIT)**. This section will address the traditional practice of HIM, the current information-oriented management practice, as well as the future of HIM.

Traditional Practice

The original practice of HIM was based on the Hospital Standardization Program, initiated in 1918. The program emphasized the need to ensure complete and accurate health records were compiled and maintained for every patient. Accurate records were needed to support the care and treatment provided to the patient as well as to conduct various types of clinical research.

Traditional practices involved planning, developing, and implementing systems designed to control, monitor, and track the quantity of record content and the flow, storage, and retrieval of health records. In other words, activities centered primarily on the health record or reports within the record as a physical unit rather than on the data elements that make up the information within the health record.

In 1928, very few standards "addressed issues relating to determination of the completion, significance, organization, timeliness, or accuracy of information contained in the medical record or its usefulness to decision support" (Johns 1991, 57).

The HIM professional is employed in many different work settings. Traditionally HIM professionals worked in a hospital HIM department. Over time, HIM professionals have moved to settings like government agencies, consulting companies,

Table 1.1 HIM profession's job setting

Setting	Roles
Acute-care hospital	HIM director
	Cancer registrar
	Discharge analyst
	Privacy officer
Integrated healthcare delivery system	HIM director
	Privacy officer
	Coder
Other provider setting (such as long-term care and psychiatric)	HIM director
	Privacy officer
	Coder
Vendor	Sales
	Systems analyst
	Consultant
Insurance companies	Claims coordinator
Consulting	Consultant
Educational institution	Professor
Law firm	HIM director
Government agency	Reimbursement specialist
Pharmaceutical companies	Research assistant

and more. Some of the more common settings and some HIM roles are listed in table 1.1.

Information-Oriented Management Practice

The traditional model of practice roles would not be appropriate for today's information-intensive and automated healthcare environment. The traditional model of practice is department focused with an emphasis on tasks. These tasks include the processing and tracking of records rather than processing and tracking information.

In today's information age, information crosses departmental boundaries and is broadly disseminated throughout the organization and beyond. Because of the focus on information, **information governance** is critical. Information governance is the accountability framework and decision rights to achieve enterprise information management. In other words, the information must be controlled to ensure the needs of the organization are met. See chapter 6 for more on information governance.

Figure 1.1   Information-based roles in HIM

Standards developer
Chief privacy officer
Clinical documentation improvement coordinator
Compliance officer
Clinical vocabulary manager
Chief information officer
Corporate HIM director

©AHIMA

Information grows out of data manipulation from a variety of shared data sources, both internal and external to the organization. An information-oriented management model includes tasks associated with a broad range of information services. Therefore, the tasks performed as a health information manager—in contrast to tasks performed as a health record manager—are information-based, "emphasizing data manipulation and information management tasks and focusing on the provision of an extensive range of information services" (Johns 1991, 59). A sample of these information-based roles is listed in figure 1.1.

The Future of HIM

Research shows that the HIM profession is continuing to evolve from the traditional HIM roles to ones focused on information. Many of these changes result from the conversion to the electronic health record (EHR) but other factors including regulations, new technologies, and engaged consumers are all driving these changes (The Caviart Group 2015). The EHR is an electronic record of health-related information on an individual that conforms to nationally recognized interoperability standards and that can be created, managed, and consulted by authorized clinicians and staff across more than one healthcare organization. The EHR has dramatically increased the amount of information available and the ability to manipulate and interpret information. Changes have also come about because of changes in regulations as well as changes in technology. The 2015 Work Force Study, a research study on the roles and opportunities for HIM professions, identifies the top 10 skills required by HIM professionals both today and into the future (The Caviart Group 2015). Table 1.2 shows these skills in order of importance.

According to the Council for Excellence in Education, defined later in this chapter, the future of HIM will focus on:

- Coding skills including those related to clinical documentation improvement, the revenue cycle, and registries
- Data governance skills including those for data integrity, analytics, fraud, abuse, and privacy and security
- Leadership skills that support the roles of chief knowledge officer and chief learning officer (AHIMA Foundation 2012)

Table 1.2   Comparison of the most important present and future HIM skills

Today's most important skills	Future's most important skills
1. Medical record coding	1. Electronic health record (EHR) management
2. Managing information privacy and security	2. Managing information privacy and security
3. Analytical thinking	3. Analytical thinking
4. Ensuring data integrity	4. Critical thinking
5. Critical thinking	5. Ensuring data integrity
6. Clinical documentation improvement	6. Problem solving
7. Electronic health record (EHR) management	7. Communication (written, spoken, or presentation)
8. Communication (written, spoken, or presentation)	8. Clinical documentation improvement
9. Problem solving	9. Leadership
10. Developing and promoting HIM standards	10. Analyzing big data

Source: The Carviart Group 2015.

Check Your Understanding 1.1

Instructions: **Answer the following questions.**

1. The hospital standardization movement was inaugurated by the:
   A. American Health Information Management Association
   B. American College of Surgeons
   C. Record Librarians of North America
   D. American College of Physicians

2. HIM has been recognized as a profession since:
   A. 1910
   B. 1918
   C. 1928
   D. 2006

3. The HIM profession is changing due to:
   A. Changes in technology
   B. Demands of physicians
   C. Changes in medical staff bylaws
   D. Changes at AHIMA

4. The new model of HIM practice is:
   A. Information focused
   B. Record focused
   C. Department focused
   D. Traditional focused

5. The traditional model of HIM practice was:
   A. Department based
   B. Information based
   C. Electronically based
   D. Analytically based

6. The organization that accredits HIM education programs is:
   A. Joint Commission
   B. CAHIIM
   C. AHIMA
   D. CCHIIM

Today's Professional Organization

As previously described, AHIMA's name has changed several times over the years. The evolution of AHIMA was introduced earlier in the chapter. The following section will discuss the mission, membership, and organizational structure of the association.

AHIMA Mission

Before studying AHIMA's structure, it is important to understand why the organization exists and what contributions it makes to both its members and the healthcare system in general. The mission of an organization explains what the organization is and what it does. In other words, it describes

Figure 1.2 AHIMA mission, strategy, vision, and core values

Mission

AHIMA leads the health informatics and information management community to advance professional practice and standards.

Strategy

AHIMA is working to promote this mission through:
Informatics: Transforming data into health intelligence
Leadership: Developing HIM leaders across all healthcare sectors
Information governance: Being recognized as the health industry experts in information governance
Innovation: Increasing thought leadership and evidence-based HIM research
Public good: Empowering consumers to optimize their health through management of their personal health information

Vision

AHIMA ... leading the advancement and ethical use of quality health information to promote health and wellness worldwide.

Core Values

Quality: Demonstrated by an abiding commitment to innovation, relevance, and continuous improvement in programs, products, and services
Integrity: Demonstrated by openness in decision making, honesty in communication and activity, and ethical practices that command trust and support collaboration
Respect: Demonstrated by appreciation of the value of differing perspectives, enjoyable experiences, courteous interaction, and celebration of achievements that advance our common cause
Leadership: Demonstrated by visionary thinking, decisions responsive to membership and mission, and accountability for actions and outcomes

Source: AHIMA 2015a.

the organization's distinctive purpose. Figure 1.2 shows AHIMA's current mission, strategy, vision, and core values.

AHIMA is a membership organization that represents more than 103,000 health information professionals. The members work throughout the healthcare industry. These professionals serve the healthcare industry and the public by managing, analyzing, and utilizing information vital for patient care and making it accessible to healthcare providers when and where it is needed.

AHIMA strives to foster the professional development of its members through education, certification, lifelong learning, and to advocate for the HIM profession. By doing this, AHIMA promotes the development of high-quality information that benefits the public, healthcare consumers, healthcare providers, and other users of clinical data. The organization has certification programs that set high standards to ensure the minimum qualifications of the individuals who practice as health information managers and technicians. In addition, it supports numerous continuing education (CE) programs to help its credentialed members and others maintain their knowledge base and skills.

To accomplish its mission, AHIMA expects all its members to follow a code of professional ethics (a complete discussion of ethical principles and AHIMA's Code of Ethics is provided in chapter 21). As the code of ethics stipulates, all members of AHIMA are expected to act in an ethical manner and comply with all laws, regulations, and standards governing the practice of HIM. As professionals, members are expected to continually update their knowledge base and skills through CE and lifelong learning. HIM professionals and managers are expected to promote high standards of HIM practice, education, and research. Additionally, they are expected to promote and protect the confidentiality and security of health records and health information.

AHIMA Membership

To accommodate the diversity in AHIMA membership, the organization has established five membership categories.

Active membership is open to all individuals who are interested in AHIMA's purpose and willing to abide by the code of ethics. Active members in good standing are entitled to all membership privileges including the right to vote and to serve in the House of Delegates (discussed later in this chapter). Active membership provides HIM professionals the opportunity to participate in the organization and to offer input to the current and future practices of the profession.

Student membership includes any student who does not have an AHIMA credential, has not previously been an active member of AHIMA, and who is formally enrolled in a Professional Certificate Approval Program or Approved Committee for Certificate Programs, or in a CAHIIM-accredited HIM program. The student membership category gives entry-level professionals an opportunity to participate on a national level in promoting sound HIM practices. Student members can serve on committees and subcommittees in designated student positions with a voice, but they do not have a vote.

New graduate membership is for student members who are recent graduates of accredited associate, bachelor's and master's degree programs as well as AHIMA-approved coding programs. This membership level allows the students to continue their membership at a reduced rate for one year. This membership level has all membership rights including voting.

Emeritus membership allows AHIMA members who are 65 years or older to be a member at a reduced rate. This membership level has all membership rights including the right to vote.

Group membership allows multiple individuals from an organization to join at one time. Student and business groups are eligible for this membership type (AHIMA 2015b).

AHIMA Structure and Operation

Every organization needs a management structure to operate effectively and efficiently. AHIMA is made up of two components—a volunteer component and a staff component. The volunteer structure establishes the organization's mission and goals, develops policy, and provides oversight for the organization's operations. Figure 1.3 shows AHIMA's volunteer structure. The staff component of the organization carries out the operational tasks necessary to support the organization's mission and goals. The staff works within the policies established by the volunteer component.

Association Leadership

As a nonprofit membership association, AHIMA depends on the participation and direction of volunteer leaders from the HIM community. AHIMA's members elect the delegates who serve in the governing bodies of the organization.

AHIMA's **board of directors** leads the volunteer structure. The board of directors is responsible for managing the association and determining its direction. The board of directors is also responsible for ensuring that the organization is fiscally sound. This body is charged with tremendous responsibility. Its members include the president/chair, the president/chair-elect, the past president/chair, speaker of the House of Delegates, nine elected directors, the chief executive officer of the organization, and the advisor to the board. Except for the chief executive officer, who is selected by the board of directors, all members of the board of directors are elected by the membership and serve three-year terms of office; members must be active members of the association.

In addition to the board of directors, CCHIIM is elected by the membership. CCHIIM is responsible for overseeing AHIMA's certification process and for setting policies and procedures.

Engage

Engage is a virtual network of AHIMA members who communicate via a web-based program managed by AHIMA. Engage is open only to AHIMA members and provides the following benefits:

- Provides opportunities for members to contact other members for quick problem solving, support, advice, shared best practices, and career-building tips and opportunities

Figure 1.3 AHIMA volunteer organizational structure

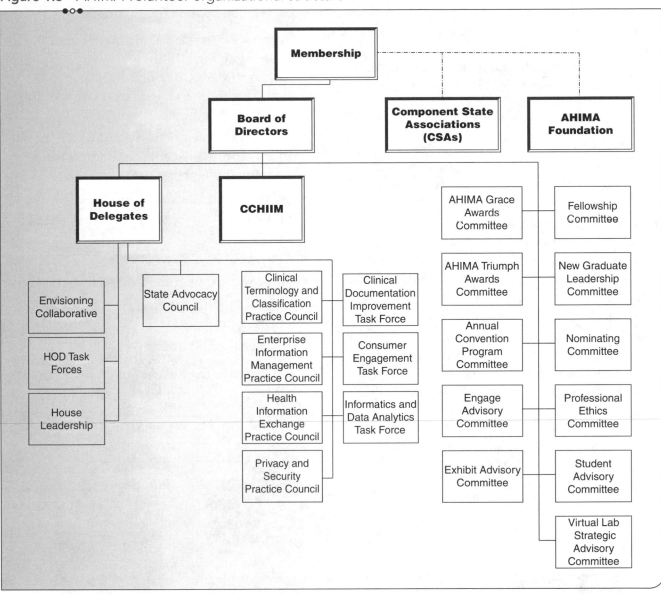

Source: AHIMA 2015c.

- Makes it possible for members to search for other members with similar interests and backgrounds
- Provides links to other sites that have specialized HIM information
- Includes a professional library of HIM standards, guidelines, practice briefs, and other resources

National Committees

AHIMA's president appoints the members of the association's national committees, practice councils, and workgroups. These groups support the mission of the organization and work on specific projects as designated by the president and the board of directors. Examples of the national committees include the Annual Convention Program Committee, the Professional Ethics Committee, and the Fellowship Review Committee. Practice councils are established for ad hoc projects. Once the project is completed, the practice council is disbanded. Examples of practice councils include councils in clinical classification and terminology, health information exchange, and privacy and security practice, which all advise and provide AHIMA with expertise related to best practice in their specific areas of HIM. Practice councils and committees can last for years. In addition, AHIMA also utilizes workgroups to address challenges. These workgroups do the same thing as a practice council, but they are established for short-term projects and then disbanded. An example of a workgroup is the EHR-HIE Interoperability Workgroup.

House of Delegates

The **House of Delegates** is an extremely important component of the volunteer structure because it governs the profession (AHIMA 2014). The annual face-to-face business meeting of the House of Delegates is held in conjunction with AHIMA's national convention, however, the House of Delegates work virtually year round. The House of Delegates will create ad hoc task forces as necessary to address the business of the profession.

Each component state association, defined later in this chapter, elects representatives to the House of Delegates to serve for a specified term of office. For that reason, the House of Delegates is similar

to the legislative branch of the US government. Its specific powers include the following:

- Approving the standards that govern the profession, including:
  o AHIMA's Code of Ethics
  o The guide to the interpretation of the code of ethics
- Electing the members of AHIMA's nominating committee, except the chairman and appointed members
- Advising the board of directors in the development and modification of the association's plans
- Levying special assessments
- Approving amendments to AHIMA's bylaws
- Approving the standing rules of the House of Delegates
- Approving resolutions

Figure 1.4 shows the formal governance structure of AHIMA.

Figure 1.4 Governance structure of AHIMA

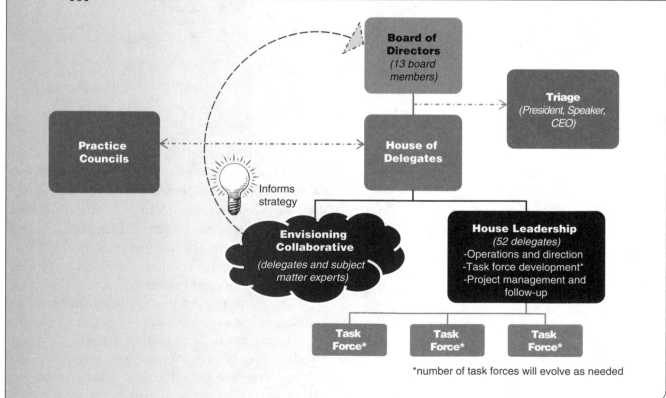

Source: AHIMA 2015d.

State and Local Associations

In addition to its national volunteer organization, AHIMA supports a system of component organizations in every state, plus Washington, DC, and Puerto Rico. Component state associations (CSAs) provide their members with local access to professional education, networking, and representation. CSAs also serve as an important forum for communicating information relevant to national issues and keeping members informed of regional affairs that affect HIM.

Many states also have local or regional organizations. For newly credentialed professionals, the state and local organizations are ideal avenues for becoming involved with volunteer work within the professional organization. Most HIM professionals who serve in the House of Delegates or serve on AHIMA's Board of Directors got their start in volunteer services with local, regional, and state associations.

Staff Structure

AHIMA's headquarters are located in Chicago, Illinois. The chief executive officer (CEO) is the individual responsible for overseeing day-to-day operations. A team of executives, managers, and staff support the CEO. Examples of the staff departments include, among others, member services, professional practice services, AHIMA Press, marketing, and policy and government relations.

Accreditation of Educational Programs

AHIMA has a long tradition of commitment to HIM education. As discussed previously, the first prescribed educational curriculum for the training of health record professionals was proposed in 1929. The first educational programs were accredited in 1934. Since that time, the association has developed and maintained a rigorous accreditation process for academic programs, continuously developed up-to-date curriculum models, and supported educational programs in a variety of ways.

In 2004, AHIMA's House of Delegates voted to establish an independent accreditation commission (CAHIIM) with sole and independent authority in all matters pertaining to accreditation of educational programs in health informatics and information management. CAHIIM serves the public interest by establishing quality standards for the educational preparation of future HIM professionals. When a program is accredited by CAHIIM, it means that it has voluntarily undergone a rigorous review process and has been determined to meet or exceed the standards established by CAHIIM. CAHIIM accreditation is a way to recognize and publicize best practices for HIM education programs.

CAHIIM reviews formal applications from college programs that apply for candidacy status, which is a preliminary approval process. After a successful review of the application documentation, a program may be deemed a candidate for accreditation for up to two years. Students enrolled in programs that are placed in candidacy status are eligible to join AHIMA as student members. The steps of the accreditation process are:

- The college program prepares a self-assessment document
- Accreditation site visitors visit the campus to review documents and interview faculty, students, and others
- A report of the site visit is reviewed by the CAHIIM Board of Commissioners
- A final determination is made as to the ability of the college program to meet the accreditation standards for curriculum, facility, resources, and other requirements.

The accreditation of educational programs is important because only those individuals who graduate from an approved program may sit for the national credentialing examinations for the RHIT and RHIA.

Certification and Registration Program

As the field of HIM became more complex, the association recognized the need to control its credentialing program. In 2008, CCHIIM was established. CCHIIM is dedicated to assuring the competency of professionals practicing HIM. CCHIIM serves the public by establishing, implementing, and enforcing standards and procedures for certification and recertification of HIM professionals. CCHIIM provides strategic oversight of all AHIMA certification programs. This standing commission of AHIMA is empowered with the sole and independent authority in all matters pertaining to both the initial certification and ongoing recertification (certification maintenance) of HIM professionals.

Today, AHIMA's certification program encompasses several credentials, including:

- Registered Health Information Technician (RHIT)
- Registered Health Information Administrator (RHIA)
- Certified Coding Associate (CCA)
- Certified Coding Specialist (CCS)
- Certified Coding Specialist—Physician-based (CCS-P)
- Certified in Healthcare Privacy and Security (CHPS)
- Certified Health Data Analyst (CHDA)
- Clinical Documentation Improvement Practitioner (CDIP)
- Certified Healthcare Technology Specialist (CHTS)

Each of these credentials has specific eligibility requirements and a certification examination. To achieve certification from CCHIIM, individuals must meet the eligibility requirements for certification and successfully complete the certification examination.

Because the HIM profession is constantly changing, certified individuals must demonstrate that they are continuing to maintain their knowledge and skill base. Therefore, to maintain their certification, individuals who hold any of AHIMA's credentials must complete a designated set of continuing education units (CEU). Activities that qualify for CEUs include attending workshops and seminars, taking college courses, participating in independent study activities, and engaging in self-assessment activities. The CCHIIM website provides information on the most recent requirements for maintenance of certification.

Fellowship Program

AHIMA's fellowship program is a program of earned recognition for AHIMA members who have made significant and sustained contributions to the HIM profession through meritorious service, excellence in professional practice, education, and advancement of the profession through innovation and knowledge sharing. Individuals who earn fellowship use the designation Fellow of the American Health Information Management Association (FAHIMA).

Fellowship is open to any individual who is an active or senior member of AHIMA and who meets the eligibility requirements. Fellows must have a minimum of 10 years full-time professional experience in HIM or a related field, a minimum of 10 years continuous AHIMA membership at the time of application (excluding years as a student member), hold a minimum of a master's degree, and provide evidence of sustained and substantial professional achievement that demonstrates professional growth and use of innovative and creative solutions. Once conferred, the fellowship is a lifetime recognition as long as the individual remains an AHIMA member and complies with AHIMA's Code of Ethics. At the time of this writing, only 179 members have been awarded fellowship status.

AHIMA Foundation

AHIMA Foundation actively promotes education and research in the HIM field. It also works to advance the HIM profession. Founded in 1962, AHIMA Foundation is a separately incorporated philanthropic and charitable arm of AHIMA.

The HIM profession is based on the belief that high-quality healthcare requires high-quality information. The Foundation provides leadership in research, workforce development, and education for the HIM profession. Its role is to envision the future direction and needs of the field and to respond with strategies, information, planning, and programs that will keep the HIM profession on the cutting edge.

One of the ways that AHIMA supports education is the Council for Excellence in Education (CEE). The council brings together representatives of the HIM education stakeholders, including industry representatives, to address issues related to the future of the profession and HIM education. The CEE has a number of workgroups to conduct the work of the commission. These workgroups include faculty development, curricula, educational programming, professional practice experience, research and workforce (AHIMA Foundation 2015). These workgroups set the future of HIM education, identifying the future needs of the profession and then setting the college curriculum required to ensure the future HIM professionals have those skills.

They also assist educators by helping the educator to keep skills current and by assisting with establishing standards for professional practice experiences.

Some of the initiatives that have been spearheaded by the Foundation include the *Perspectives in Health Information Management* publication, establishing education competencies and providing resources to educators. In addition, the Foundation administers a number of programs, including the scholarship and the professional certificate approval program.

Health Information Management Specialty Professional Organizations

HIM professionals frequently specialize in an area of the HIM profession. Examples of these specialties include clinical documentation improvement, coding, tumor registry, medical transcription, information governance, privacy and security, standards, and information systems. A number of specialty organizations support these areas.

Healthcare Information and Management Systems Society

Healthcare Information and Management Systems Society (HIMSS) is a not-for-profit organization who is "focused on better health through information technology (IT). HIMSS leads efforts to optimize health engagements and care outcomes using information technology" (HIMSS 2015). In other words, HIMSS strive to improve the quality of care by using technology. HIMSS sponsors exams for health information and information systems professionals—the certified professional in Healthcare Information and Management Systems (CPHIMS) certification and Certified Associate Professional in Healthcare Information and Management Systems (CAHIMS). The CPHIMS exam covers topics such as healthcare environment, technology environment, system analysis, system design, system selection and implementation, privacy and security, and administration. The CAHIMS certification covers administration,

healthcare information and systems management, organization environment, and technology environment (HIMSS 2015).

Association for Healthcare Documentation Integrity

The **Association for Healthcare Documentation Integrity (AHDI)** is a professional organization dedicated to the capture of health data and documentation. It was formerly known as the American Association for Medical Transcription but changed its name to fit their broadened scope. AHDI sponsors the Registered Healthcare Documentation Specialist (RHDI) and Certified Healthcare Documentation Specialist (CHDS) credentials. The RHDS is designed to determine if the candidate has the skills to be a medical transcriptionist. It covers clinical medicine, health information technology, and transcription standards and style. The CHDS determines if the candidate is qualified to be a transcriptionist in a multidisciplinary environment. It covers clinical medicine and health information technology (AHDI 2015).

American Academy of Professional Coders

The **American Academy of Professional Coders (AAPC)** educates and certifies medical coders.

They sponsor certifications in coding, medical compliance, and medical auditing. The certifications include:

- Certified Professional Coder (CPC)
- Certified Professional Coder—Payer (CPC-P)
- Certified Professional Medical Auditor (CPMA)
- Certified Professional Compliance Officer (CPCO)
- Certified Inpatient Coder (CIC)
- Certified Outpatient coder (COC)
- Certified Risk Adjustment Coder (CRC)

They also offer many specialty coding certifications (AAPC 2015).

National Cancer Registrars Association

The **National Cancer Registrars Association (NCRA)** represents cancer registrar professionals. Their mission is to "serve as the premier education, credentialing, and advocacy resource for cancer data professionals" (NCRA 2015). The NCRA sponsors the Certified Tumor Registrar (CTR) certification. This exam includes information on registry organization and operations, abstracting, coding, follow-up, data analysis, and interpretation as well as coding and staging.

Check Your Understanding 1.2

Instructions: **Answer the following questions.**

1. Our college has applied to become accredited by CAHIIM. Which of the following is the name of the interim stage of accreditation?
   A. Certification
   B. Candidacy
   C. Fellowship
   D. Credentialing

2. Which of the following is the virtual network used by AHIMA members?
   A. Engage
   B. Fellowship
   C. House of Delegates
   D. Communities of Practice

3. Which of the following functions governs the HIM profession?
   A. Board of Directors
   B. House of Delegates
   C. CCHIIM
   D. CAHIIM

4. The primary focus of AHIMA is to:
   A. Ensure that health records are complete
   B. Implement an electronic record in hospitals
   C. Foster professional development of its members
   D. Set and implement standards

5. Which of the following certifications is administered by CCHIIM?
   A. Registered Healthcare Documentation Specialist
   B. Registered Health Information Technician
   C. Certified Professional in Healthcare information and Management Systems
   D. Certified Professional Coder

Real-World Case 1.1

The EHR is causing many changes in both the HIM profession and the structure of the HIM department itself. Because of the EHR, many functions of the HIM department can be performed remotely. Some HIM staff such as coders and transcriptionists are now working from home. The file areas where the paper records are housed are disappearing as more and more of the health records are electronic. These changes enable the healthcare facility to use the space previously occupied by the HIM staff and the file areas to be used for other purposes. Some healthcare organizations with multiple locations have centralized their HIM functions enabling them to standardize the HIM functions and to share staff between the facilities. The staff at the central location is able to perform most of the functions of the HIM department. There may be some staff at the healthcare facility to attend committee meetings, take authorization for release of information from patients, and perform other functions that require staff on site. Even though the employees work from home or a centralized location, the privacy and security of the patient information must be ensured at all of the locations and their productivity must meet the standards established by the organization.

Real-World Case 1.2

One of the strengths of the HIM profession is the ability for a career path to evolve over time. Kathryn has an RHIT credential. She began working in utilization review, and then she worked in HIM department management. After 15 years of working in hospitals she was ready for a change, so she left the hospital and worked first in a consulting firm and then for an information system vendor. In both of these roles she traveled around the country. Quickly tiring of the travel, Kathryn decided to change the focus of her career path once again. Now she is an HIM educator. While Kathryn has earned both a master's degree and a doctorate degree, it was her HIM degree and skills that allowed her to move from one career path to another.

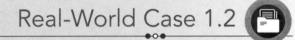

References

AHIMA Foundation. 2015. Council for Excellence in Education (CEE). http://www.ahimafoundation.org/education/cee.aspx.

AHIMA Foundation. 2012 (September 26). Reality 2016: The Council for Excellence in Education's Recommendation for HIM Education. http://www.ecu.edu/cs-dhs/hsim/upload/Reality_2016_Presentation-9_26_12_NC.pdf.

American Academy of Professional Coders. 2015. Medical Certification Overview. http://www.aapc.com/certification.

American Health Information Management Association. 2015a. Mission Vision and Values. http://www.ahima.org/about/aboutahima?tabid=mission.

American Health Information Management Association. 2015b. Membership Types and Payment Options. http://www.ahima.org/membership/types.

American Health Information Management Association. 2015c. 2015 Volunteer Organization Chart. http://www.ahima.org/~/media/AHIMA/Files/Volunteers/Volunteer%20Org%20Chart.ashx.

American Health Information Management Association. 2015d. Governance. http://www.ahima.org/about/governance#.

American Health Information Management Association. 2014. Bylaws of the American Health Information Management Association. http://bok.ahima.org/doc?oid=107453.

Association for Healthcare Documentation Integrity. 2015. http://www.ahdionline.org/?page=typescredentials.

The Caviart Group. 2015. A Workforce Study of the Future Direction and Skill Set for HIM Professionals. http://bok.ahima.org/PdfView?oid=300801.

Healthcare Information Management Systems Society. 2015. http://www.himss.org/aboutHIMSS/.

Huffman, E.K. 1985. *Medical Record Management,* 8th ed. Berwyn, IL: Physicians' Record Company.

Huffman, E.K. 1941. Requirements and advantages of registration for health record librarians. *Bulletin of the American Association of Medical Record Librarians.*

Johns, M.L. 1991. Information management: A shifting paradigm for medical record professionals? *Journal of the American Medical Record Association.* 62(8):55–63.

National Cancer Registrars Association. 2015. About Us. http://www.ncra-usa.org/i4a/pages/index.cfm?pageid=3862.

2

Healthcare Delivery Systems

Donald W. Kellogg, PhD, CPEHR, RHIA, FAHIMA

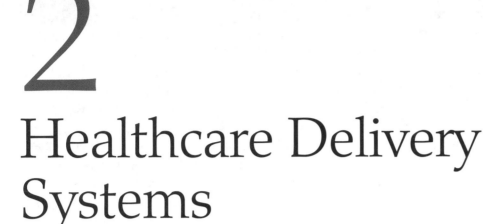

Learning Objectives

- Understand the basic organization of the various types of hospitals and healthcare organizations
- Describe how internal and external forces have shaped the healthcare industry
- Differentiate the roles of various stakeholders throughout the healthcare delivery system

- Describe the influence of federal legislation on healthcare delivery
- Identify the various functional components of an integrated delivery system
- Recognize the role of government in healthcare services

Key Terms

Accountable care organizations (ACOs)
Allied health professional
American Recovery and Reinvestment Act (ARRA)
Average length of stay (ALOS)
Case management
Centers for Disease Control and Prevention (CDC)
Chief executive officer (CEO)
Chief financial officer (CFO)
Chief information officer (CIO)
Chief nursing officer (CNO)

Chief operating officer (COO)
Clinical privileges
Continuum of care
Critical access hospital
Extended care facility
Health Information Technology for Economic and Clinical Health (HITECH) Act
Home healthcare
Hospice
Hospital
Integrated delivery network (IDN)
Integrated delivery system (IDS)

Managed care organization (MCO)
Medicaid
Medical staff bylaws
Medical staff classification
Medicare
Peer review organization (PRO)
Public health service
Quality improvement organization (QIO)
Skilled nursing facility (SNF)
Subacute care
Utilization review
Utilization Review Act

A broad array of healthcare services are available in the United States today, from simple preventive measures such as vaccinations to complex life-saving procedures such as heart transplants. An individual's contact with the healthcare delivery system often begins before he or she is born, with family planning and prenatal care, and continues through the end of life, with long-term or hospice care.

Physicians, nurses, and other clinical providers deliver healthcare services in a variety of healthcare settings. Those care settings include ambulatory, acute care, rehabilitative, psychiatric, long-term care, hospice, home care, assisted living centers, industrial medical clinics, and public health department clinics. In other words, wherever people need access to the healthcare system, there are healthcare professionals providing that care.

Integrated delivery systems (IDSs) are healthcare systems that combine the financial and clinical aspects of healthcare and use a group of healthcare providers, selected on the basis of quality and cost management criteria, to furnish comprehensive health services across the continuum of care. The IDS ensure patients get the right care at the right time from the right provider. The continuum of care places an emphasis on treating individual patients at the level of care required by their course of treatment and extends from their primary care providers to specialists and ancillary providers. The goal of IDS is to deliver high-quality, cost-effective care in the most appropriate setting.

While most hospitals are integrated into their communities through ties with area physicians and other healthcare providers, clinics and outpatient facilities, and other practitioners, almost half the nation's hospitals also are tied to larger organizational entities such as multihospital and integrated healthcare systems (IHCSs), integrated delivery networks (IDNs), and alliances. An IDN comprises a group of hospitals, physicians, other providers, insurers, or community agencies that work together to deliver health services. In 2015, 55 percent of all hospitals in the United States belonged to an IDN (AHA 2015).

This chapter discusses healthcare delivery in the United States and how political, societal, and other factors have influenced its development. Well-known legislation affecting healthcare and healthcare information systems in the United States is examined. Different types of healthcare delivery facilities and the services they provide are explained.

Standardization of Medical Care

In the 1990s, US hospitals faced growing pressure to contain costs, improve quality, and demonstrate their contributions to the health of the communities they serve. They adapted to these pressures in various ways. Some merged with, or bought out, other hospitals and healthcare organizations. Others created IDSs to provide a full range of healthcare services along the continuum of care, from ambulatory care to inpatient care to long-term care. Still others concentrated on improving the care they provided by focusing on patients as customers. Many hospitals responded to local competition by quickly entering into affiliations and other risk-sharing agreements with acute and nonacute-care providers, physicians' groups, and managed care organizations (MCOs)—a type of healthcare organization that delivers medical care and manages all aspects of patient care or the payment for care by limiting providers of care, discounting payments to providers of care, or limiting access to care.

By the end of 2010, healthcare organizations faced the challenges of a stressed economy. With higher unemployment rates and more uninsured individuals throughout the nation, hospital reimbursement payments continued to shrink and hospitals reached out for opportunities to control costs, streamline operations, implement efficient information technologies, engage in quality initiatives, and pursue joint ventures and consolidation. In 2014, healthcare expenditures in the United States were approximately $3.0 trillion, which represented 17.5 percent of the total American economy (CMS 2015). In response to increasing costs and shrinking access to care, the government initiated steps for reforming healthcare by instituting temporary measures to make healthcare coverage more affordable, providing incentives for computerizing health records, and investing in wellness and disease prevention.

Medical Practice

There are many providers included under the term *medical practice*, all of which are referred to as "doctor." It should be noted that *doctor* is an educational degree, not a profession. Some of the most common healthcare practitioners are:

- Chiropractor (DC—Doctor of Chiropractic) focuses on the diagnosis, treatment, and prevention of disorders of the neuromusculoskeletal system.
- Dentist (DDS or DMD—Doctor of Dental Surgery or Doctor of Medicine in Dentistry) focuses on the diagnosis, prevention, and treatment of diseases and condition of the oral cavity.
- Medical (MD—Doctor of Medicine) focuses on the diagnosis, treatment, and education of any human disease or condition.
- Optometry (OD—Doctor of Optometry) focuses on vision, visual systems, and are trained to prescribe and fit lenses to improve vision.
- Osteopath (DO—Doctor of Osteopathic Medicine) not only focuses on manipulation of muscles and bones but also incorporates the diagnosis and treatment of diseases.
- Podiatrist (DPM—Doctor of Podiatric Medicine) focuses on the treatment of disorders of the foot, ankle, and lower extremity.

The most prevalent medical practitioner in the United States is the MD (Doctor of Medicine). Two types of practitioners can hold this degree: physicians and surgeons. MDs (also known as allopathic physicians) diagnose and treat diseases and act

as a pathway for prescription drugs and medical procedures in private offices, clinics, or hospitals. MDs generally have three to four years of undergraduate work, four years of medical school, and then additional training through a residency that varies depending on the specialty in which they want to practice. Physicians can be divided into two groups—generalists (those who are the first point of contact between a patient and access to healthcare services, such as family medicine) and specialists (those who focus their practice on a very specific body system, such as cardiology). Ideally a ratio of 60:40 of specialists to generalist is recommended as it is the generalist who initially diagnoses the patient's condition and then sends a referral for the patient to see the specialist (Sultz and Young 2014). Generalists include family medicine, internal medicine, pediatrics, and obstetrics and gynecology. Listed as follows are a few of the medical specialties for physicians:

- Internal medicine: Provides care to diagnosis and treatment to adults
- Pediatrics: Provides care to infants, children, and adolescents, birth to 18 years of age
- Family practice: Provides comprehensive care to all ages
- Cardiology: Focuses on disorders of the heart
- Psychiatry: Focuses on diagnosis and treatment of mental disorders
- Neurology: Focuses on the diagnosis and treatment of the nervous system
- Oncology: Focuses on diagnosis and treatment of tumors, both malignant and benign
- Radiology: Uses imaging techniques to diagnose and treat disease
- Urology: Focuses on diagnosis and treatment of urinary tract system and male reproductive organs

The most common surgical specialties include:
- Anesthesiology: Focuses on relief of pain during surgery
- Cardiovascular surgery: Surgery on the heart and great vessels

- Gynecology and obstetrics: Surgery for cesarean sections or other female health-related surgeries
- Orthopedics: Surgery on the musculoskeletal system
- Ophthalmology: Surgery on the eye
- Otorhinolaryngology: Surgery on the ear, nose, and throat
- Plastic and reconstructive surgery: Surgery to restore the form of the body
- Neurosurgery: Surgery on the brain, spinal cord, and peripheral nerves

Some physicians and healthcare organizations employ physician assistants (PAs) or surgeon assistants (SAs) to help them carry out their clinical responsibilities. Such assistants may perform routine clinical assessments, provide patient education and counseling, and perform simple therapeutic procedures. Most PAs work in primary care settings and most SAs work in hospitals and ambulatory surgery clinics. PAs and SAs always work under the supervision of licensed physicians and surgeons.

Nursing Practice

Most registered nurses (RN) have either a two-year associate's degree or a four-year bachelor's degree from a state-approved nursing school, though some schools offer a master's degree that allows the graduate to sit for the licensure examination. Nurse practitioners, researchers, educators, and administrators generally have a four-year degree in nursing and additional postgraduate education in nursing. The postgraduate degree may be a master's of science or a doctorate in nursing. Nurses who graduate from nonacademic training programs are called licensed practical nurses (LPNs) or licensed vocational nurses (LVNs). Non-degreed nursing personnel work under the direct supervision of registered nurses. Nurses in all 50 states must pass an exam to obtain a license to practice.

Today's registered nurses (RN) are highly trained clinical professionals. Many specialize in specific areas of practice such as surgery, psychiatry, and intensive care. Nurse-midwives complete advanced training and are certified by the American College of Nurse-Midwives. Similarly, nurse-anesthetists are certified by the Council on Certification/Council on Recertification of Nurse Anesthetists. Nurse practitioners also receive advanced training at the master's level that qualifies them to provide primary care services to patients. They are certified by several organizations (for example, the National Board of Pediatric Nurse Practitioners) to practice in the area of their specialty.

The need for registered nurses is expected to rise over the next decade. Hospitals in the United States report continued vacancies for registered nurses. The Bureau of Labor Statistics estimates that between the years 2012 and 2022 approximately 526,800 more registered nurses will be needed over the projected supply (BLS 2015).

Professionalization of the Allied Health Professions

After World War I, many roles previously assumed by nurses and nonclinical personnel began to change. With the advent of modern diagnostic and therapeutic technology in the mid-20th century, the complex skills needed by ancillary medical personnel fostered the growth of specialized training programs and professional accreditation and licensure.

According to the American Medical Association (AMA), allied health incorporates the healthcare-related professions that function to assist, facilitate, or complement the work of physicians and other clinical specialists. The Health Professions Education Extension Amendment of 1992, which amended the Public Health Service Act, describes **allied health professionals** as health professionals (other than registered nurses, physicians, and physician assistants) who have received a certificate, an associate's degree, a bachelor's degree, a master's degree, a doctorate, or postdoctoral training in a healthcare-related science. Such individuals share responsibility for the delivery of healthcare services with clinicians (physicians, nurses, and physician assistants).

Allied health occupations are among the fastest growing in healthcare. Unlike the case in medicine, women dominate most of the allied health professions, representing between 75 and 95 percent in most of the occupations. All 50 states require licensure for some allied health professions (physical therapy, for example). Practitioners in other allied health professions (respiratory therapy, for example) may be licensed in some states but not in others. Significant shortages of personnel in many of the allied health disciplines are projected to reach 1.6 to 2.5 million by 2020 (US Census Bureau 2011).

The following list briefly describes some of the major occupations usually considered to be allied health professions:

- *Audiology:* Audiology is the branch of science that studies hearing, balance, and related disorders. Audiologists treat those with hearing loss and proactively prevent related damage. According to the American Speech-Language-Hearing Association, audiologists provide comprehensive diagnostic and treatment or rehabilitative services for auditory and related impairments. These services are provided to all individuals regardless of age, socioeconomic, ethnicity, or cultural backgrounds (ASHA 2016).

- *Clinical laboratory science:* Originally referred to as medical laboratory technology, this field is now known as clinical laboratory science. Clinical laboratory technicians perform a wide array of tests on body fluids, tissues, and cells to assist in the detection, diagnosis, and treatment of diseases and illnesses. The clinical laboratory is divided into two sections—anatomic pathology and clinical pathology. Anatomic pathology deals with human tissues and provides surgical pathology, autopsy, and cytology services. Clinical pathology deals mainly with the analysis of body fluids—principally blood, but also urine, gastric contents, and cerebrospinal fluid. Physicians who specialize in performing and interpreting the results of pathology tests are called pathologists. Laboratory technicians are allied health professionals trained to operate laboratory equipment and perform laboratory tests under the supervision of a pathologist.

- *Diagnostic medical sonography or imaging technology:* Originally referred to as x-ray technology and then radiologic technology, this field is now referred to as diagnostic imaging. The field continues to expand to include nuclear medicine, radiation therapy, and echocardiography. These services are provided by physician specialists (radiologists) and technologists including radiation therapists, cardiosonographers (ultrasound technologists), and magnetic resonance technologists. Nuclear medicine involves the use of ionizing radiation and small amounts of short-lived radioactive tracers to treat disease, specifically neoplastic disease (that is, nonmalignant tumors and malignant cancers). Radiation therapy uses high-energy x-rays, cobalt, electrons, and other sources of radiation to treat human disease. In current practice, radiation therapy is used alone or in combination with surgery or chemotherapy (drugs) to treat many types of cancer. In addition to external beam therapy, radioactive implants (as well as therapy performed with heat—hyperthermia) are available.

- *Dietetics and nutrition:* Dietitians (also clinical nutritionists) are trained in nutrition. They are responsible for providing nutritional care to individuals and for overseeing nutrition and food services in a variety of settings, ranging from hospitals to schools.

- *Emergency medical technology:* Emergency medical technicians (EMTs) and paramedics provide a wide range of services on an emergency basis for cases of traumatic injury and other emergency situations and in the transport of emergency patients to a medical facility.

- *Health information management:* Health information management (HIM) professionals (formerly called medical record administration) oversee health record systems and manage health-related information to ensure that it meets relevant medical, administrative, and legal requirements. Health records are the responsibility of Registered Health Information Administrators (RHIAs) and Registered Health Information Technicians (RHITs).

- *Occupational therapy:* Occupational therapists (OTs) use work and play activities to improve patients' independent functioning, enhance their development, and prevent or decrease their level of disability. Occupational therapy activities may involve the adaptation of tasks or the environment to achieve maximum independence and to enhance the patient's quality of life and improve his or her activities of daily living (ADL). An occupational therapist may treat developmental deficits, birth defects, learning disabilities, traumatic injuries, burns, neurological conditions, orthopedic conditions, mental deficiencies, and psychiatric disorders. Working under the direction of physicians, occupational therapy is made available in acute-care hospitals, clinics, and rehabilitation centers.

- *Optometry:* Optometry is a health profession that is focused on the eyes and related structures, as well as vision, visual systems, and vision information processing in humans. Optometrists provide treatments such as contact lenses and corrective and low-vision devices, and are authorized to use diagnostic and therapeutic pharmaceutical agents to treat anterior segment disease, glaucoma, and ocular hypertension. As primary eye care practitioners, optometrists often are the first ones to detect such potentially serious conditions as diabetes, hypertension, and arteriosclerosis.

- *Pharmacy:* The scope of pharmacy practice includes traditional roles such as compounding and dispensing medications, as well as modern services including reviewing medications for safety and efficacy, and providing drug information to physicians and patients. Pharmacists are the experts on drug therapy and are the primary health professionals who optimize medication use to provide patients with positive health outcomes.

- *Physical therapy:* Physical therapists (PTs), who work under the direction of a physician, evaluate and treat patients to improve functional mobility, reduce pain, maintain cardiopulmonary function, and limit disability. PTs treat movement dysfunction resulting from accidents, trauma, stroke, fractures, multiple sclerosis, cerebral palsy, arthritis, and heart and respiratory illness. Treatment modalities include therapeutic exercise, therapeutic massage, biofeedback, and applications of heat, low-energy lasers, cold, water, electricity, and ultrasound.

- *Respiratory therapy:* Respiratory therapists (RTs) evaluate, treat, and care for patients with acute or chronic lung disorders. They work under the direction of qualified physicians and provide services such as emergency care for stroke, heart failure, and shock. In addition, they treat patients with emphysema and asthma. Respiratory treatments include the administration of oxygen and inhalants such as bronchodilators, and setting up and monitoring ventilator equipment.

- *Speech-language pathology and audiology:* Speech-language pathologists and audiologists identify, assess, and provide treatment for individuals with speech, language, or hearing problems.

- *Surgical technologist:* Surgical technologists provide surgical care to patients in a variety of settings; the majority are hospital operating rooms. Surgical technologists work under medical supervision to facilitate the safe and effective conduct of invasive surgical procedures (Kickman and Kovner 2015).

Check Your Understanding 2.1

Instructions: **Answer the following questions.**

1. The acronym IDS refers to:
   A. Integrated Disease Syndrome
   B. Independent Delivery Systems
   C. Independent Dietitian Service
   D. Integrated Delivery Systems

2. Which healthcare professional assists physicians in clinical assessments and patient education?
   A. Diagnostic medical sonographer
   B. Health information manager
   C. Clinical laboratory technician
   D. Physician assistant

3. Which of the following medical practitioner is not considered a generalist?
   A. Internal medicine
   B. Cardiology
   C. Pediatrics
   D. Obstetrics and gynecology

4. Which healthcare provider utilizes ultrasound, computed tomography, or MRIs?
   A. Nuclear medicine technologist
   B. Orthoticists
   C. Podiatrist
   D. Radiologic technologist

5. Which of the following is a surgical specialty?
   A. Internal medicine
   B. Oncology
   C. Neurology
   D. Orthopedics

6. Which of the following statements is true about registered nurses (RNs)?
   A. RNs only provide clinical services within a healthcare entity.
   B. RNs are required to have a license in the state in which they practice.
   C. RNs are graduates of nonacademic training programs.
   D. RNs must have a bachelor's degree from an approved nursing school.

7. Which of the following perform a wide array of tests on body fluids, tissues, and cells to assist in the detection, diagnosis, and treatment of diseases and illnesses?
   A. Clinical laboratory scientists
   B. Sonographers
   C. Licensed practical nurses
   D. Surgical technologists

8. True or false: Respiratory therapists treat patients with limited mobility.

9. True or false: Audiologists provide comprehensive diagnostic and treatment/rehabilitative services for auditory, vestibular, and related impairments.

10. True or false: Physical therapy assistants carry out the treatment plans created by the physical therapists.

Modern Healthcare Delivery in the United States

Until World War II, most healthcare was provided in the home. Quality in healthcare services was considered a product of appropriate medical practice and oversight by physicians and surgeons. Even the minimum standards used to evaluate the performance of hospitals were based on factors directly related to the composition and skills of the hospital medical staff.

The 20th century was a period of tremendous change in American society. Advances in medical science promised better outcomes and increased the demand for healthcare services. But medical care has never been free. Even in the best economic times, many Americans have been unable to take full advantage of what medicine has to offer because they cannot afford it.

Concern over access to healthcare was especially evident during the Great Depression of the 1930s. During the Depression, America's leaders were forced to consider how the poor and disadvantaged could receive the care they needed. Before the Depression, medical care for the poor and elderly had been handled as a function of social welfare agencies. During the 1930s, however, few people were able to pay for medical care. The problem of how to pay for the healthcare needs of millions of Americans became a public and governmental concern. Working Americans turned to prepaid health plans to help them pay for healthcare, but the unemployed and the unemployable needed help from a different source.

During the 20th century, Congress passed many pieces of legislation that had a significant impact on the delivery of healthcare services in the United States.

Social Security Act of 1935

The Great Depression revived the dormant social reform movement in the United States as well as more radical currents in American politics. The Depression also brought to power the Democratic administration of Franklin D. Roosevelt, which was more willing than any previous administration to involve the federal government in the management of economic and social welfare.

Although old-age pension and unemployment insurance bills were introduced into Congress soon after his election, Roosevelt refused to give them his strong support. Instead, he created a program of his own and appointed a Committee on Economic Security to study the issue comprehensively and report to Congress in January 1935.

Sentiment in favor of health insurance was strong among members of the Committee on Economic Security. However, many members of the committee were convinced that adding a health insurance amendment would spell defeat for the entire Social Security legislation. Ultimately, the Social Security bill included only one reference to health insurance as a subject that the new Social Security Board might study. The Social Security Act was passed in 1935.

Public Law 89–97 of 1965

In 1965, passage of a number of amendments to the Social Security Act brought Medicare and Medicaid into existence. The two programs have greatly changed how healthcare organizations are reimbursed. Recent attempts to curtail Medicare and Medicaid spending continue to affect healthcare organizations.

Medicare (Title XVIII of the Social Security Act) is a federal program that provides healthcare benefits for people age 65 and older who are covered by Social Security. The program was inaugurated on July 1, 1966. Over the years, amendments have extended coverage to individuals who are not covered by Social Security but are willing to pay a premium for coverage, to the disabled, and to those suffering from end-stage renal disease (ESRD).

The companion program, **Medicaid** (Title XIX of the Social Security Act), was established at the same time to support medical and hospital care for persons classified as medically indigent. Originally targeting recipients of public assistance (primarily single-parent families and the aged, blind, and disabled), Medicaid has expanded to additional groups so that it now targets poor children, the disabled, pregnant women, and very poor adults (including those age 65 and older).

Today, Medicaid is a federally mandated program that provides healthcare benefits to low-income people and their children. Medicaid programs are administered and partially paid for by individual states. Medicaid is an umbrella for 50 different state programs designed specifically to serve the poor. Beginning in January 1967, Medicaid provided federal funds to states on a cost-sharing basis to ensure welfare recipients would be guaranteed medical services. Coverage of four types of care was required: inpatient and outpatient services, other laboratory and x-ray services, physician services, and nursing facility care for persons over 21 years of age.

Many enhancements have been made in the years since Medicaid was enacted. Services now include family planning and 31 other optional services such as prescription drugs and dental services. With few exceptions, recipients of cash assistance are automatically eligible for Medicaid. Medicaid also pays the Medicare premium, deductible, and coinsurance costs for some low-income Medicare beneficiaries. More information on Medicaid can be found in chapter 15.

Since the implementation of the Affordable Care Act, the number of people covered under Medicaid has increased 13.8 percent between the years 2014 and 2015. Medicaid spending has also increased over that time period with a 13.9 percent increase. The increase in spending is attributed to the growth in enrollment, increased provider rates, increased in prescription costs, and other costs spread out over the healthcare system. Not every state is required to provide expansion of Medicaid services, and as of the end of fiscal year 2015, 29 states had increased their Medicaid coverage (Kaiser Family Foundation 2015).

Public Law 92–603 of 1972

In an effort to curtail Medicare and Medicaid spending, additional amendments to the Social Security Act were instituted in 1972. Public Law 92–603 required concurrent review for Medicare and Medicaid patients. It also established the professional standards review organization (PSRO) program to implement concurrent review. PSROs performed professional review and evaluated patient care services for necessity, quality, and cost-effectiveness.

Utilization review (UR) is the process of determining whether the medical care provided to a specific patient is necessary according to pre-established objective screening criteria at time frames specified in the organization's utilization management plan. UR was a mandatory component of the original Medicare legislation. Medicare required hospitals and **extended care facilities,** which are facilities licensed by applicable state or local law to offer room and board, skilled nursing by a full-time registered nurse, intermediate care, or a combination of levels on a 24-hour basis over a long period of time. Extended care facilities are required to establish a plan for UR as well as a permanent utilization review committee. The goal of the UR process is to ensure the services provided to Medicare beneficiaries are medically necessary.

Utilization Review Act of 1977

In 1977, the **Utilization Review Act** made it a requirement for hospitals to conduct continued-stay reviews for Medicare and Medicaid patients. Continued-stay reviews determine whether it is medically necessary for a patient to remain hospitalized. This legislation also included fraud and abuse regulations. More information on fraud and abuse can be found in chapter 16.

Peer Review Improvement Act of 1982

In 1982, the Peer Review Improvement Act redesigned the PSRO program and renamed the agencies **peer review organizations (PROs)**. At that time, hospitals began to review the medical necessity and appropriateness of certain admissions even before patients were admitted. PROs were given a new name in 2002 and now are called **quality improvement organizations (QIOs)**. They currently emphasize quality improvement processes. Each state and territory, as well as the District of

Columbia, now has its own QIO. The mission of the QIOs is to ensure the quality, efficiency, and cost-effectiveness of the healthcare services provided to Medicare beneficiaries in its locale.

Tax Equity and Fiscal Responsibility Act of 1982

In 1982, Congress passed the Tax Equity and Fiscal Responsibility Act (TEFRA). TEFRA required extensive changes in the Medicare program. Its purpose was to control the rising cost of providing healthcare services to Medicare beneficiaries. Before this legislation was passed, healthcare services provided to Medicare beneficiaries were reimbursed on a retrospective, or fee-based, payment system. TEFRA required the gradual implementation of a prospective payment system (PPS) for Medicare reimbursement.

In a retrospective payment system, a service is provided, a claim for payment for the service is made, and the healthcare provider is reimbursed for the cost of delivering the service. In a PPS, a predetermined level of reimbursement is established before the service is provided. More information on PPSs can be found in chapter 15.

Public Law 98–21 of 1983

The PPS for acute hospital care (inpatient) services was implemented on October 1, 1983, according to Public Law 98–21. Under the inpatient PPS, reimbursement for hospital care provided to Medicare patients is based on diagnosis-related groups (DRGs). Each case is assigned to a DRG based on the patient's diagnosis at the time of discharge. For example, under inpatient PPS, all cases of viral pneumonia would be reimbursed at the same predetermined level of reimbursement no matter how long the patients stayed in the hospital or how many services they received. PPSs for other healthcare services provided to Medicare beneficiaries have been gradually implemented since 1983.

Health Insurance Portability and Accountability Act of 1996

The Health Insurance Portability and Accountability Act of 1996 (HIPAA) addresses issues related to the portability of health insurance after leaving employment, establishment of national standards for electronic healthcare transactions, and national identifiers for providers, health plans, and employers. A portion of HIPAA addressed the security and privacy of health information by establishing privacy standards to protect health information and security standards for electronic healthcare information. HIPAA privacy and security standards are covered in chapters 9 and 10. Another provision of HIPAA was the creation of the Healthcare Integrity and Protection Data Bank (HIPDB) to combat fraud and abuse in health insurance and healthcare delivery. A purpose of the HIPDB is to inform federal and state agencies about potential quality problems with clinicians, suppliers, and providers of healthcare services. The American Recovery and Reinvestment Act (ARRA) includes important changes in HIPAA privacy and security standards that are discussed in chapters 9 and 10.

American Recovery and Reinvestment Act of 2009

The **American Recovery and Reinvestment Act of 2009 (ARRA)**, is considered one of the major health information technology laws that provided stimulus funds to the US economy in the midst of a major economic downturn. A substantial portion of the bill, Title XIII of the Act entitled the **Health Information Technology for Economic and Clinical Health (HITECH) Act**, allocated funds for implementation of a nationwide health information exchange and implementation of electronic health records. The bill provides for investment of billions of dollars in health information technology and incentives to encourage doctors and hospitals to use information technology; $19.2 billion was dedicated to implementing and supporting health information technology. ARRA requires the government to take a leadership role in developing standards for exchange of health information nationwide, strengthens federal privacy and security standards, and established the Office of the National Coordinator for Health Information Technology (ONC) as a permanent office (Rode 2009). Four major components of the bill include: meaningful use (that providers are using certified EHRs to improve patient outcomes); EHR standards and certifications; regional extension centers (used to assist providers with selection and implementation of EHRs); and breach notification guidance. Though challenged in court, the US Supreme Court up held the law in a 6–3 decision. Meaningful use is discussed in chapter 16.

Patient Protection and Affordable Care Act of 2010

This federal statute was signed into law on March 23, 2010, and is the most significant healthcare reform legislation of the first decade of the 21st century. The Congressional Budget Office (CBO) projected savings of $143 billion over the first decade and a second decade deficit reduction of $1.2 trillion. Its major provisions include:

- Health insurance market reforms including:
  - Subsidized premiums for people with pre-existing conditions
  - Eliminating lifetime limits on benefits
  - The option of covering children on parents' insurance until the age of 26
- Development of state-based and state-administered health insurance exchanges
- Consumer Operated and Oriented Plan program
- Expansion of Medicaid to individuals under age 65 with incomes up to 133 percent of federal poverty level
- Individual mandate to have minimum acceptable coverage or pay a tax penalty
- Employers with 50 or more employees must provide healthcare coverage
- Premium subsidies to individuals
- Small employer tax credits (CRS 2010)

Check Your Understanding 2.2

Instructions: **Answer the following questions.**

1. Which of the following laws created the HITECH Act?
   A. Health Insurance Portability and Accountability Act
   B. American Recovery and Reinvestment Act
   C. Consolidated Omnibus Budget Reconciliation Act
   D. Healthcare Quality Improvement Act

2. Until the World War II, where was most healthcare provided?
   A. Government clinic
   B. Physician's office
   C. Home
   D. Hospital

3. An HIM student has asked you why Medicare reimburses healthcare providers through prospective payment systems. Which of the following pieces of legislation would you use as your explanation?
   A. Peer Review Improvement Act of 1982
   B. Consolidated Budget Reconciliation Act of 1986
   C. Tax Equity and Fiscal Responsibility Act of 1982
   D. Omnibus Budget Reconciliation Act of 1986

4. Which of the following legislation authorized the creation of the Office of National Coordinator for Health Information Technology?
   A. PPACA
   B. HIPAA
   C. ARRA
   D. TEFRA

5. Which of the following best describes Medicaid?
   A. Federal program targeted principally for those age 65 and older
   B. Federally mandated healthcare program for low-income people
   C. Healthcare program limited to those under age 65
   D. Healthcare program for low-income persons regardless of age that is totally financed and operated by the states

Match the descriptions with the appropriate legislation.

6. _____ Tax Equity and Fiscal Responsibility Act of 1982

7. _____ Social Security Act of 1935

8. _____ Public Law 92–603 of 1972

9. _____ Patient Protection and Affordable Care Act of 2010

10. _____ Utilization Review Act of 1977

   A. Required that hospitals conduct continued-stay reviews for Medicare and Medicaid patients
   B. Required concurrent review of Medicare and Medicaid patients
   C. Provided an individual mandate to have minimum acceptable coverage or pay a tax penalty
   D. Gave the states funds on a matching basis for maternal and infant care, rehabilitation of crippled children, general public health work, and aid for dependent children under age 16.
   E. Required the gradual implementation of a prospective payment system (PPS) for Medicare reimbursement.

Organization and Operation of Modern Hospitals

The term **hospital** can be applied to any healthcare facility that:

- Has an organized medical staff
- Provides permanent inpatient beds
- Offers around-the-clock nursing services
- Provides diagnostic and therapeutic services

Most hospitals provide acute-care services to inpatients. Acute care is the short-term care provided to diagnose or treat an illness or injury. The individuals who receive acute-care services in hospitals are considered inpatients. Inpatients receive room-and-board services in addition to continuous nursing services. Generally, patients who spend more than 24 hours in a hospital are considered inpatients.

The **average length of stay (ALOS)** in an acute-care hospital is 25 days or less. Hospitals that have ALOSs longer than 25 days are considered long-term acute-care facilities. Long-term care is discussed in detail later in this chapter. With recent advances in surgical technology, anesthesia, and pharmacology, the ALOS in an acute-care hospital is much shorter today than it was only a few years ago. In addition, many diagnostic and therapeutic procedures that once required inpatient care now can be performed on an outpatient basis.

For example, before the development of laparoscopic surgical techniques, a patient might be hospitalized for 10 days after a routine appendectomy (surgical removal of the appendix). Today, a patient undergoing a laparoscopic appendectomy might spend only a few hours in the hospital's outpatient surgery department and go home the same day. The influence of managed care and the emphasis on cost control in the Medicare or Medicaid programs also have resulted in shorter hospital stays.

In large acute-care hospitals, hundreds of clinicians, administrators, managers, and support staff must work closely together to provide effective and efficient diagnostic and therapeutic services. Most hospitals provide services to both inpatients and outpatients. A hospital outpatient is a patient who receives hospital services without being admitted for inpatient (overnight) clinical care. Outpatient care is considered a kind of ambulatory care. (Ambulatory care is discussed later in this chapter.)

Modern hospitals are extremely complex organizations. Much of the clinical training for physicians, nurses, and allied health professionals is conducted in hospitals. Medical research is another activity carried out in hospitals.

Types of Hospitals

There are many different types of hospitals providing care within the United States healthcare system. The five major ways they are classified are:

- Number of beds
- Types of services provided
- Types of patients served
- For-profit or not-for-profit status
- Type of ownership

Number of Beds A hospital's number of beds refers to the number of beds that are equipped and staffed for patient care. The term *bed capacity* sometimes is used to reflect the maximum number of inpatients for which the hospital can care. *Licensed beds* are the number of beds that the state has authorized the hospital to have available for patients and *staffed beds* refers to the number of beds for which the hospital actually has nursing staffing covered. Hospitals with fewer than 100 beds are usually considered small. Most US hospitals fall into this category. Some large, urban hospitals may have more than 500 beds. The number of beds is usually broken down by adult beds and pediatric beds. The number of maternity beds and other special categories may be listed separately. Hospitals also can be categorized according to the number of outpatient visits per year.

Types of Services Provided Some hospitals specialize in certain types of service and treat specific illnesses. For example:

- *Rehabilitation hospitals* generally provide long-term care services to patients recuperating from debilitating or chronic illnesses and injuries such as strokes, head and spine injuries, and gunshot wounds. Patients often stay in rehabilitation hospitals for several months.

- *Psychiatric hospitals* provide inpatient care for patients with mental and developmental disorders. In the past, the ALOS for psychiatric inpatients was longer than it is today. Rather than months or years, most patients now spend only a few days or weeks per stay. However, many patients require repeated hospitalization for chronic psychiatric illnesses.

- *General hospitals* provide a wide range of medical and surgical services to diagnose and treat most illnesses and injuries.

- *Specialty hospitals* provide diagnostic and therapeutic services for a limited range of conditions such as burns, cancer, tuberculosis, obstetrics, or gynecology.

Types of Patients Served Some hospitals specialize in serving specific types of patients. For example, children's hospitals provide specialized pediatric services in a number of medical specialties and rehabilitation hospitals provide postacute-care for patients recovering from an injury, illness, or disease.

For-Profit or Not-for-Profit Status Hospitals also can be classified based on their ownership and profitability status. Not-for-profit healthcare organizations use excess funds to improve their services and to finance educational programs and community services. For-profit healthcare organizations are privately owned. Excess funds are paid back to the managers, owners, and investors in the form of bonuses and dividends.

Type of Ownership The most common ownership types for hospitals and other kinds of healthcare organizations in the United States include:

- *Government-owned hospitals* are operated by a specific branch of federal, state, or local government as not-for-profit organizations. (Government-owned hospitals sometimes are called public hospitals.) They are supported, at least in part, by tax dollars. Examples of federally owned and operated hospitals include those operated by the Department of Veterans Affairs (VA) to serve retired military personnel. The Department of Defense operates facilities for active military personnel and their dependents. Many states own and operate psychiatric hospitals. County and city governments often operate public (municipal) hospitals to serve the healthcare needs of their communities, especially those residents who are unable to pay for their care.

- *Proprietary hospitals* may be owned by private foundations, partnerships, or investor-owned corporations. Large corporations may own a number of for-profit hospitals, and the stock of several large US hospital chains is publicly traded.

- *Voluntary hospitals* are not-for-profit hospitals owned by universities, churches, charities, religious orders, unions, and other not-for-profit entities. They often provide free care to patients who otherwise would not have access to healthcare services.

Critical Access Hospitals

As part of the Balanced Budget Act of 1997, the Centers for Medicare and Medicaid Services (CMS) was authorized to allow to give certain healthcare facilities the designation of critical access hospital (CAH). By meeting certain requirements these hospitals were allowed a separate payment system that allows reimbursement for Medicare patients of 101 percent of reasonable costs and are not subject to the inpatient prospective payment system (IPPS) or the hospital outpatient prospective payment system (OPPS). The criteria to qualify as a CAH are as follows:

- Be located in a state that accepted a grant under the Medicare Rural Hospital Flexibility Program, which helps states to strengthen their rural healthcare infrastructure.

- Be located in a rural area

- Furnish 24-hour emergency care services 7 days a week

- Maintain no more than 25 inpatient beds that may also be used as swing beds

- Have an annual length of stay 96 hours or less per patient for acute-care services

- Be located more than a 35-mile distance from any other hospital

- Be certified as a CAH prior to January 1, 2006 (CMS 2014)

Organization of Hospital Services

The organizational structure of every hospital is designed to meet its specific needs. For example, most acute-care hospitals are comprised of a professional medical staff and hospital administrative services, which includes an executive administrative staff, medical and surgical services, patient care (nursing) services, diagnostic and laboratory services, and support services (for example, nutritional services, environmental safety, and HIM services). Both are overseen by a board of directors.

Board of Directors The board of directors has primary responsibility for setting the overall direction of the hospital. (In some hospitals, the board of directors is called the governing board or board of trustees.) The board works with the chief executive officer (CEO) and the leaders of the organization's medical staff to develop the hospital's strategic direction as well as its mission (statement of the organization's purpose and the customers it serves), vision (description of the organization's ideal future), and values (descriptive list of the organization's fundamental principles or beliefs).

Other specific responsibilities of the board of directors include:

- Establishing bylaws in accordance with the organization's legal and licensing requirements

- Selecting qualified administrators

- Approving the organization and makeup of the clinical staff

- Monitoring the quality of care

The board's members are elected or appointed for specific terms of service (for example, five years). Most boards also elect officers, commonly a chairman, vice-chairman, president, secretary, and treasurer. The size of the board varies considerably. Individual board members are called directors, board members, or trustees. Individuals serve on one or more standing committees such as the executive committee, joint conference committee, finance committee, strategic planning committee, and building committee.

The makeup of the board depends on the type of hospital and the form of ownership. For example, the board of a community hospital is likely to include local business leaders, representatives of community organizations, and other people interested in the welfare of the community. The board of a teaching hospital, on the other hand, is likely to include medical school alumni and university administrators, among others.

Increased competition among healthcare providers and limits on managed care and Medicare or Medicaid reimbursement have made the governing of hospitals especially difficult in the past two decades. In the future, boards of directors will continue to face strict accountability in terms of cost containment, performance management, and integration of services to maintain fiscal stability and to ensure the delivery of high-quality patient care.

Medical Staff The medical staff consists of physicians who have received extensive training in various medical disciplines (internal medicine, pediatrics, cardiology, gynecology and obstetrics, orthopedics, surgery, and so on). The medical staff's primary objective is to provide high-quality patient care to the patients who come to the hospital. The physicians on the hospital's medical staff diagnose illnesses and develop patient-centered treatment regimens. Moreover, they may serve on the hospital's governing board, where they provide critical insight relevant to strategic and operational planning and policy making.

The medical staff is the aggregate of physicians who have been granted permission to provide clinical services in the hospital. This permission is called clinical privileges. An individual physician's privileges are limited to a specific scope of practice. For example, an internal medicine physician would be permitted to diagnose and treat a patient with pneumonia, but not to perform a surgical procedure. Traditionally most members of the medical staff have not been employees of the hospital, although this is changing as many hospitals are purchasing physician practices.

Medical staff classification refers to the organization of physicians according to clinical assignment. Depending on the size of the hospital and on the credentials and clinical privileges of its physicians, the medical staff may be separated into departments such as medicine, surgery, obstetrics, pediatrics, and other specialty services. Typical medical staff classifications include active, provisional, honorary, consulting, courtesy, and medical resident assignments.

Officers of the medical staff usually include a president or chief of staff, a vice president or chief of staff elect, and a secretary. These offices are authorized by a vote of the entire active medical staff. The president presides over all regular meetings of the medical staff and is an ex officio member of all medical staff committees. The secretary ensures that accurate and complete minutes of the meetings are kept and that correspondence is handled appropriately.

The medical staff operates according to a predetermined set of policies called the medical staff bylaws. The bylaws spell out the specific qualifications that physicians must demonstrate before they can practice medicine in the hospital. They are considered legally binding. Any changes to the bylaws must be approved by a vote of the medical staff and the hospital's governing body.

Administrative Staff The leader of the administrative staff is the CEO or chief administrator. The CEO is responsible for implementing the policies and strategic direction set by the hospital's board of directors. He or she also is responsible for building an effective executive management team and coordinating the hospital's services. Today's healthcare organizations commonly designate a chief financial officer (CFO), a chief operating officer (COO), and a chief information officer (CIO) as members of the executive management team.

The executive management team is responsible for managing the hospital's finances and ensuring that the hospital complies with the federal, state, and local rules, standards, and laws that govern the delivery of healthcare services. Depending on the size of the hospital, the CEO's staff may include healthcare administrators with job titles such as vice president, associate administrator, department director or manager, or administrative assistant. Department-level administrators manage and coordinate the activities of the highly specialized and multidisciplinary units that perform clinical, administrative, and support services in the hospital.

Healthcare administrators may hold advanced degrees in healthcare administration, nursing, public health, or business management. A growing number of hospitals are hiring physician executives to lead their executive management teams.

Patient Care Services   Most direct patient care delivered in hospitals is provided by professional nurses. Modern nursing requires a diverse skill set, advanced clinical competencies, and postgraduate education. In almost every hospital, patient care services constitutes the largest clinical department in terms of staffing, budget, specialized services offered, and clinical expertise required.

Nurses are responsible for providing continuous, around-the-clock treatment and support for hospital inpatients. The quantity and quality of nursing care available to patients are influenced by a number of factors, including the nursing staff's educational preparation and specialization, experience, and skill level. The level of patient care staffing also is a critical component of quality.

Traditionally, physicians alone determined the type of treatment each patient would receive. However, today's nurses are playing a wider role in treatment planning and **case management**. They identify timely and effective interventions in response to a wide range of problems related to the patients' treatment, comfort, and safety. Their responsibilities include performing patient assessments, creating care plans, evaluating the appropriateness of treatment, and evaluating the effectiveness of care. At the same time that they provide technical care, effective nursing professionals also offer personal care that recognizes the concerns and emotional needs of patients and their families.

A registered nurse qualified by advanced education and clinical and management experience usually administers patient care services. Although the title may vary, this role is usually referred to as the **chief nursing officer (CNO)** or vice president of nursing or patient care. The CNO is a member of the hospital's executive management team and usually reports directly to the CEO.

Diagnostic Services   The services provided to patients in hospitals go beyond the clinical services provided directly by the medical and nursing staff. Many diagnostic and therapeutic services involve the work of allied health professionals. Allied health professionals receive specialized education and training, and their qualifications are registered or certified by a number of specialty organizations.

Diagnostic and therapeutic services are critical to the success of every patient care delivery system. Diagnostic services include clinical laboratory, radiology, and nuclear medicine. Therapeutic services include the clinical laboratory services, radiology, and radiation therapy.

Rehabilitation Services   Rehabilitation services are dedicated to eliminate the patients' disability or alleviate it as fully as possible. The goal is to improve the cognitive, social, and physical abilities of patients impaired by chronic disease or injury. Rehabilitation services can be provided within the acute-care setting or in specialty hospitals dedicated to providing many forms of rehabilitation to patients needing extra work to either return to work or home. The rehabilitation team may include physicians, nurses, occupational therapists, physical therapists, respiratory therapist, speech therapists, social workers, and other healthcare personnel.

Ancillary Support Services   The ancillary units of the hospital provide vital clinical and administrative support services to patients, medical staff, visitors, and employees.

The clinical support units provide the following services:

- Pharmaceutical services (provided by registered pharmacists and pharmacy technologists)
- Food and nutrition services (managed by registered dietitians who develop general and special-diet menus and nutritional plans for individual patients)
- HIM services (managed by RHIAs and RHITs)
- Social work and social services (provided by licensed social workers and licensed clinical social workers)
- Patient advocacy services (provided by several types of healthcare professionals, most commonly registered nurses and licensed social workers)

- Environmental (housekeeping) services
- Purchasing, central supply, and materials management services
- Engineering and plant operations

In addition to clinical support services, hospitals need administrative support services to operate effectively. Administrative support services provide business management and clerical services in several key areas, including:

- Admissions and central registration
- Claims and billing (business office)
- Accounting
- Information services
- Human resources
- Public relations
- Fund development
- Marketing

Check Your Understanding 2.3

Instructions: **Answer the following questions.**

1. Which of the following is NOT an example of an administrative support services?
   A. Admissions
   B. Marketing
   C. Billing
   D. HIM

2. Who has the primary responsibility to guide the direction of the hospital?
   A. Board of directors
   B. Chief executive officer
   C. Medical staff
   D. Chief operating officer

3. Which of the following is an example of a federally run hospital?
   A. VA
   B. Psychiatric
   C. Not-for-profit
   D. Community

4. Which service diagnoses and treats patients who have acute and/or chronic lung disorders?
   A. Occupational therapy
   B. Physical therapy
   C. Respiratory therapy
   D. Clinical laboratory services

5. Dr. Smith has been granted permission by Community hospital to perform cardiac catheterizations. This permission is called:
   A. Clinical privileges
   B. Clinical assignment
   C. Clinical classification
   D. Case management

6. True or false: Acute-care hospitals provide short-term care to diagnose or treat an illness.

7. True or false: A registered nurse performs patient assessments, creates care plans, and evaluates the appropriateness of treatment and effectiveness of care.

8. True or false: Pharmaceutical services are considered part of the clinical support services.

9. True or false: The average length of stay for an acute-care hospital is 21 days or less.

10. True or false: Physical therapists are only one member of the rehabilitation service team.

Other Types of Healthcare Services

Healthcare delivery is more than hospital-related care. It can be viewed as a continuum of services that cuts across care settings, including ambulatory, acute, subacute, long-term, and residential care, among others. The American Health Information Management Association (AHIMA) has also defined the continuum of care as the range of healthcare services provided to patients, from routine ambulatory care to intensive acute care; the emphasis is on treating individual patients at the level of care required by their course of treatment with the assurance of communication between caregivers.

Ambulatory Care

Ambulatory care may be defined as the preventive or corrective healthcare provided in a practitioner's office, a clinic, or a hospital on a nonresident (outpatient) basis. The term usually implies that patients go to locations outside their homes to obtain healthcare services and return the same day.

Ambulatory care encompasses all the health services provided to individual patients who are not residents in a healthcare facility. Such services include the educational services provided by community health clinics and public health departments.

Primary care, emergency care, and ambulatory specialty care (which includes ambulatory surgery) all may be considered ambulatory care. Ambulatory care services are provided in a variety of settings, including urgent care centers, school-based clinics, public health clinics, and neighborhood and community health centers.

Current medical practice emphasizes performing healthcare services in the least costly setting possible. This change in thinking has led to decreased utilization of emergency services, increased utilization of nonemergency ambulatory facilities, decreased hospital admissions, and shorter hospital stays. The need to reduce the cost of healthcare also has led primary care physicians to treat conditions they once would have referred to specialists.

Physicians who provide ambulatory care services fall into two major categories—physicians working in private practice and physicians working for ambulatory care organizations. Physicians in private practice are self-employed. They work in solo, partnership, and group practices set up as for-profit organizations.

Alternatively, physicians who work for ambulatory care organizations are employees of those organizations. Ambulatory care organizations include health maintenance organizations (HMOs), hospital-based ambulatory clinics, walk-in and emergency clinics, hospital-owned group practices and health promotion centers, freestanding surgery centers, freestanding urgent care centers, freestanding emergency care centers, health department clinics, neighborhood clinics, home care agencies, community mental health centers, school and workplace health services, and prison health services.

Ambulatory care organizations also employ other healthcare providers, including nurses, laboratory technicians, podiatrists, chiropractors, physical therapists, radiology technicians, psychologists, and social workers.

Private Medical Practice

Private medical practices are physician-owned entities that provide primary care or medical or surgical specialty care services in a freestanding office setting. The physicians have medical privileges at local hospitals and surgical centers but are not employees of the other healthcare entities.

Hospital-Based Ambulatory Care Services

In addition to providing inpatient services, many acute-care hospitals provide various ambulatory care services such as the ones discussed as follows.

Emergency Services and Trauma Care More than 90 percent of community hospitals in the United States provide emergency services. Hospital-based emergency departments provide specialized care for victims of traumatic accidents and life-threatening illnesses. In urban areas, many also provide walk-in services for patients with minor illnesses and injuries who do not have access to regular primary care physicians.

Many physicians on the hospital staff also use the emergency care department as a setting to assess patients with problems that may either lead to an inpatient admission or require equipment or diagnostic imaging facilities not available in a private office or nursing home. Emergency services function as a major source of unscheduled admissions to the hospital.

Outpatient Surgical Services Generally, the term *ambulatory surgery* refers to any surgical procedure that does not require an overnight stay in a hospital. It can be performed in the outpatient surgery department of a hospital and in a freestanding ambulatory surgery center.

Outpatient Diagnostic and Therapeutic Services Outpatient diagnostic and therapeutic services are provided in a hospital or one of its satellite facilities. Diagnostic services are those services performed by a physician to identify the disease or condition from which the patient is suffering. Therapeutic services are those services performed by a physician to treat the disease or condition that has been identified.

Hospital outpatients fall into different classifications according to the type of service they receive and the location of the service. For example, emergency outpatients are treated in the hospital's emergency or trauma care department for conditions that require immediate care. Clinic outpatients are treated in one of the hospital's clinical departments on an ambulatory basis. Referral outpatients receive special diagnostic or therapeutic services in the hospital on an ambulatory basis, but responsibility for their care remains with the referring physician.

Community-Based Ambulatory Care Services

Community-based ambulatory care services are those services provided in freestanding facilities that are not owned by or affiliated with a hospital. Such facilities can range in size from a small medical practice with a single physician to a large clinic with an organized medical staff.

Among the organizations that provide ambulatory care services are specialized treatment facilities. Examples of these facilities include birthing centers, cancer treatment centers, renal dialysis centers, and rehabilitation centers.

Freestanding Ambulatory Care Centers Freestanding ambulatory care centers provide emergency services and urgent care for walk-in patients. Urgent care centers provide diagnostic and therapeutic care for patients with minor illnesses and injuries. They do not serve seriously ill patients, and most do not accept ambulance cases.

Two groups of patients find these centers attractive. The first group consists of patients seeking the convenience and access of emergency services without the delays and high costs associated with using hospital services for non-urgent problems. The second group consists of patients whose insurance treats urgent care centers preferentially compared with physicians' offices.

As they have increased in number and become familiar to more patients, many freestanding ambulatory care centers now offer a combination of walk-in and appointment services.

Freestanding Ambulatory Surgery Centers   Freestanding ambulatory surgery centers generally provide surgical procedures that take anywhere from 5 to 90 minutes to perform and require less than a four-hour recovery period. Patients must schedule their surgeries in advance and be prepared to return home on the same day. Patients who experience surgical complications are sent to an inpatient facility for care.

Most ambulatory surgery centers are for-profit entities. Individual physicians, MCOs, or entrepreneurs may own them. Generally, ambulatory care centers can provide surgical services at lower cost than hospitals can because their overhead expenses are lower.

Public Health Services

The states have constitutional authority to implement public health measures, and many of them are assisted by a wide variety of federal programs and laws. The Department of Health and Human Services (HHS) is the principal federal agency that ensures health and provides essential human services. All HHS agencies have some responsibility for prevention. Through its 10 regional offices, HHS coordinates closely with state and local government agencies and many HHS-funded services are provided by these agencies as well as by private-sector and nonprofit organizations.

Two units in the Office of the Secretary of HHS are important to public health—the Office of the Surgeon General of the United States and the Office of Disease Prevention and Health Promotion (ODPHP). The surgeon general is appointed by the president of the United States and provides leadership and authoritative, science-based recommendations about the public's health. He or she has responsibility for the **public health service (PHS)** workforce and the ODPHP provides an analysis and leadership role for health promotion and disease prevention.

Home Care Services

Home healthcare is the fastest-growing sector to offer services for Medicare recipients. The primary reason for this is increased economic pressure from third-party payers who want patients released from the hospital more quickly than they were in the past. Moreover, patients generally prefer to be cared for in their own homes. In fact, most patients prefer home care, no matter how complex their medical problems.

In 1989, Medicare rules for home care services were clarified to make it easier for Medicare beneficiaries to receive them. Patients are eligible to receive home health services from a qualified Medicare provider when they are homebound, when they are under the care of a specified physician who will establish a home health plan, and when they need physical or occupational therapy, speech therapy, or intermittent skilled nursing care.

Skilled nursing care is defined as both technical procedures, such as tube feedings and catheter care, and skilled nursing observations. *Intermittent* is defined as up to 28 hours per week for nursing care and 35 hours per week for home health aide care. Many hospitals have formed their own home healthcare agencies to increase revenues and at the same time to enable them to discharge patients from the hospital earlier.

Voluntary Agencies

Voluntary agencies provide healthcare and healthcare planning services, usually at the local level and to low-income patients. Their services range from giving free immunizations to offering family planning counseling. Funds to operate such agencies come from a variety of sources, including local or state health departments, private grants, and funds from different federal bureaus.

One common example of a voluntary agency is the community health center. Sometimes called neighborhood health centers, community health centers offer comprehensive, primary healthcare services to patients who otherwise would not have access to them. Often patients pay for these services on a sliding scale based on income or according to a flat rate, discounted fee schedule supplemented by public funding.

Some voluntary agencies offer specialized services such as counseling for battered and abused women. Typically, these are set up within local communities. An example of a voluntary agency that offers services on a much larger scale is the Red Cross.

Subacute Care

Patients needing ongoing rehabilitative care or treatments using advanced technology sometimes are eligible to receive subacute care. **Subacute care** offers patients access to constant nursing care while recovering at home. In the past, patients could receive comprehensive rehabilitative care only while in the hospital. Today, however, the availability of subacute-care services allows patients to optimize their functional gain in a familiar and more comfortable environment. In essence, subacute care in most IDNs emphasizes patient independence. The patient is given an individualized care plan developed by a highly trained team of healthcare professionals. Patients considered appropriate for subacute care are those recovering from stroke, cardiac surgery, serious injury, amputation, joint replacement, or chronic wounds.

Long-Term Care

Generally speaking, long-term care is the healthcare rendered in a nonacute-care facility to patients who require inpatient nursing and related services for more than 30 consecutive days. SNFs, nursing homes, and rehabilitation hospitals are the principal facilities that provide long-term care. Rehabilitation hospitals provide recuperative services for patients who have suffered strokes and traumatic injuries as well as other serious illnesses. Specialized long-term

care facilities serve patients with chronic respiratory disease, permanent cognitive impairment, and other incapacitating conditions.

Long-term care encompasses a range of health, personal care, social, and housing services provided to people of all ages with health conditions that limit their ability to carry out normal daily activities without assistance. People who need long-term care have many different types of physical and mental disabilities. Moreover, their need for the mix and intensity of long-term care services can change over time.

Long-term care is mainly rehabilitative and supportive rather than curative. Moreover, healthcare workers other than physicians can provide long-term care in the home or in residential or institutional settings. For the most part, long-term care requires little or no technology.

Long-Term Care in the Continuum of Care

The availability of long-term care is one of the most important health issues in the United States today. There are two principal reasons for this. First, people are living longer today than they did in the past as a result of advances in medicine and healthcare practices. The number of people who survive previously fatal conditions has been growing, and more and more people with chronic medical problems are able to live reasonably normal lives. Second, there was an explosion in birth rate after World War II. Children born during that period (1946 to 1964), the so-called baby-boomer generation, are today in their 50s and 60s. These factors combined mean that the need for long-term care will only increase in the years to come.

As discussed earlier, healthcare is now viewed as a continuum of care. In the case of long-term care, the patient's continuum of care may have begun with a primary provider in a hospital and then continued with home care and eventually care in skilled nursing facility. The patient's care is coordinated from one care setting to the next.

Moreover, the roles of the different care providers along the patient's continuum of care are continuing to evolve. Health information managers play a key part in providing consultation services to long-term care facilities with regard to developing systems to manage information from a diverse number of healthcare providers.

Delivery of Long-Term Care Services

Long-term care services are delivered in a variety of settings, including skilled nursing facilities or nursing homes, residential care facilities, hospice programs, and adult day-care programs.

Skilled Nursing Facilities and Nursing Homes

The most important providers of formal, long-term care services are nursing homes, which provide medical, nursing, or rehabilitative care, in some cases, around the clock. Most skilled nursing facilities (SNFs) have residents that are over age 65 and often are classified as the frail elderly.

Many nursing homes are owned by for-profit organizations. However, SNFs also may be owned by not-for-profit groups as well as local, state, and federal governments. In recent years, there has been a decline in the total number of nursing homes in the United States, but an increase in the number of nursing home beds.

Nursing homes are no longer the only option for patients needing long-term care. Various factors play a role in determining which type of long-term care facility is best for a particular patient, including cost, access to services, and individual needs.

Residential Care Facilities

New living environments that are more homelike and less institutional are the focus of much attention in the current long-term care market. Residential care facilities now play a growing role in the continuum of long-term care services. Having affordable and appropriate housing available for elderly and disabled people can reduce the level of need for institutional long-term care services in the community. Institutionalization can be postponed or prevented when the elderly and disabled live in safe, accessible settings where assistance with daily activities is available.

Hospice Programs

Hospice care is provided mainly in the home to patients who are diagnosed with a terminal illness with a limited life expectancy of six months or less and to their families. Hospice is based on a philosophy of palliative care imported from England and Canada that holds that during the course of terminal illness, the patient should be able to live life as fully and as comfortably as possible, but without artificial or mechanical efforts to prolong life.

In the hospice approach, the family is the unit of treatment. An interdisciplinary team provides medical, nursing, psychological, therapeutic, pharmacological, and spiritual support during the final stages of illness, at the time of death, and during bereavement. The main goals are to control pain, maintain independence, and minimize the stress and trauma of death.

Hospice services have gained acceptance as an alternative to hospital care for the terminally ill. The number of hospices is likely to continue to grow because this philosophy of care for people at the end of life has become a model for the nation.

Adult Day-Care Programs

Adult day-care programs offer a wide range of health and social services to elderly persons during the daytime hours. Adult day-care services are usually targeted to elderly members of families in which the regular caregivers work during the day. Many elderly people who live alone also benefit from leaving their homes every day to participate in programs designed to keep them active. The goals of adult day-care programs are to delay the need for institutionalization and to provide respite for caregivers.

Data on adult day-care programs are still limited, but there were about 5,000 programs in 2015 providing services to 260,000 participants in a variety of programs (NADSA 2015). Most adult day-care programs offer social services, crafts, current events discussions, family counseling, reminiscence therapy, nursing assessment, physical exercise, activities of daily living, rehabilitation, psychiatric assessment, and medical care.

Behavioral Health Services

From the mid-19th century to the mid-20th century, psychiatric services in the United States were based primarily in long-stay institutions supported by state governments and patterns of practice were relatively stable. During the past 50 years, however, remarkable changes have occurred. These changes include a reversal of the balance between institutional and community care, inpatient and outpatient services, and individual and group practice.

Today, the number of long-stay residents in state mental hospitals is estimated to be well below 50,000. In 1955, it was more than 500,000 (NASMHPD 2015). The shift to community-based settings began in the public sector and community settings remain dominant. The private sector's bed capacity increased in the 1970s and 1980s, including psychiatric units in nonfederal general hospitals, private psychiatric hospitals, and residential treatment centers for children. Substance abuse centers and child and adolescent inpatient psychiatric units grew particularly quickly in the 1980s, as investors recognized their profitability. In the 1990s, the growth of inpatient private mental health facilities leveled off and the number of outpatient and partial treatment settings increased sharply.

Some patients with treatment-resistant schizophrenia, severe mood disorders, or chronic cognitive impairment may be dangerous to themselves or others. State and county hospitals may be returning to their traditional role by providing asylum to disabled patients who are unable to function in their communities.

Residential treatment centers for emotionally or behaviorally disturbed children provide inpatient services to children under 18 years of age. The programs and physical facilities of residential treatment centers are designed to meet patients' daily living, schooling, recreational, socialization, and routine medical care needs.

Day-hospital or day-treatment programs occupy one niche in the spectrum of behavioral healthcare settings. Although some provide services seven days a week, many programs provide services only during business hours, Monday through Friday. Day-treatment patients spend most of the day at the treatment facility in a program of structured therapeutic activities and then return to their homes until the next day. Day-treatment services include psychotherapy, pharmacology, occupational therapy, and other types of rehabilitation services. These programs provide alternatives to inpatient care or serve as transitions from inpatient to outpatient care or discharge. They also may provide respite for family caregivers and a place for rehabilitating or maintaining chronically ill patients. The number of day-treatment programs has increased in response to pressures to decrease the length of hospital stays.

Insurance coverage for behavioral healthcare has always lagged behind coverage for other medical care. Although treatments and treatment settings have changed, rising healthcare costs, the absence of strong consumer demand for behavioral health coverage, and insurers' continuing fear of the potential cost of this coverage have maintained the differences between medical and behavioral healthcare benefits (non-parity).

Although most individuals covered by health insurance have some outpatient psychiatric coverage, the coverage is often quite restricted. Typical restrictions include limits on the number of outpatient visits, higher copayment charges, and higher deductibles.

Behavioral healthcare has grown and diversified, particularly during the past 40 years, as psychopharmacologic treatment has made possible the shift away from long-term custodial treatment. Psychosocial treatments continue the process of care and rehabilitation in community settings. Large state hospitals have been supplemented—and in many cases replaced—by psychiatric units in general hospitals, new outpatient clinics, community mental health centers, day-treatment centers, and halfway houses. Treatment has become more effective and specific, based on our growing understanding of the brain and behavior.

Managed Care Organizations

Managed care is a generic term for a healthcare reimbursement system that manages cost, quality, and access to services. Most managed care plans do not provide healthcare directly. Instead, they enter into service contracts with the physicians, hospitals, and other healthcare providers who provide medical services to enrollees in the plans.

Managed care systems control costs primarily by presetting payment amounts and restricting patient access to healthcare services through precertification and utilization review processes. (Managed care is discussed in more detail in chapter 15.) Managed care delivery systems also attempt to manage cost and quality by:

- Implementing various forms of financial incentives for providers
- Promoting healthy lifestyles
- Identifying risk factors and illnesses early in the disease process
- Providing patient education

There are three basic types of managed care plans:

- Health maintenance organizations (HMO) where healthcare is provided within a closed network
- Preferred provider organizations (PPO) that provides reduced costs if the plan member stays within the network but will contribute if the member goes outside the network, but a reduced cost
- Point of service (POS) that allows the patient to choose between an HMO or PPO each time you have a medical encounter (NIH 2015).

Accountable Care Organizations

The Patient Protection and Affordable Care Act of 2010 has had a significant impact on physicians and hospitals, namely in the establishment of **Accountable Care Organizations (ACOs)**. The law allows CMS to create ACOs by developing voluntary partnerships between hospitals and physicians to coordinate and deliver quality care to Medicare patients and allow the participating organizations to share the savings that would result from improvement of care for those Medicare populations. CMS has established three primary ACO programs whereby participating ACOs would assume the accountability for improving quality care while reducing costs for a defined Medicare patient population. The beneficiaries will be assigned to the ACO based on utilization of primary care services provided by primary care physicians. The three ACO models are:

- Medicare Shared Savings program that gives Medicare fee-for-service providers an opportunity to become an ACO
- Advance Payment ACO model designed as a supplementary incentive program for selected participants
- Pioneer ACO model created for early adopters of coordinate care, though CMS is no longer accepting applications for this model

CMS has outlined a series of 33 quality measures in four categories (patient or caregiver experience; care coordination or patient safety; preventative health; and at-risk population) to assess the quality of care furnished by the ACO (RTI International 2015). As of the first quarter of 2015, 744 organizations have received status as an ACO serving 23.5 million patients (Leavitt Partners 2015).

Biomedical and Technological Advances in Medicine

Rapid progress in medical science and technology during the late 19th and 20th centuries revolutionized the way healthcare was provided. The most important scientific advancement was the discovery of bacteria as the cause of infectious disease. The most important technological development was the use of anesthesia for surgical procedures. These 19th-century advances laid the basis for the development of antibiotics and other pharmaceuticals and the application of sophisticated surgical procedures in the 20th century.

To further medical advances in the 21st century, National Institutes of Health (NIH) sought the input of more than 300 recognized leaders in academia, industry, government, and the public to create a Roadmap program to accelerate biomedical advances, create effective prevention strategies and new treatments, and bridge knowledge gaps. The program, which involves a plethora of NIH institutes and centers, has three main strategic initiatives:

1. New Pathways to Discovery, which includes a comprehensive understanding of building blocks of the body's cells and tissues; how

complex biological systems operate; structural biology; molecular libraries and imaging; nanotechnology; bioinformatics; and computational biology

2. Research Teams of the Future, including interdisciplinary research and public–private partnerships

3. Re-engineering the Clinical Research Enterprise

Through these efforts, NIH will boost the resources and technologies needed for 21st-century biomedical science (NIH 2008).

Surgical procedures were performed before the development of anesthesia requiring surgeons to work quickly on conscious patients to minimize the risk and pain. The availability of anesthesia made it possible for surgeons to develop more advanced surgical techniques. Ether, nitrous oxide, and chloroform were used as anesthetics by the middle of the 19th century. By the 1860s, the physicians who treated the casualties of the American Civil War on both sides had access to anesthetic and pain-killing drugs.

During the latter 1800s, significant improvements in healthcare were being made. In 1885, Louis Pasteur developed a vaccine that prevented rabies. Joseph Lister was the first to apply Pasteur's research to the treatment of infected wounds. His discovery was called the antiseptic principle, which helped reduce the mortality rate in Lister's own hospital. Wilhelm Roentgen made observations that led to the development of x-ray technology.

Diagnostic radiology and radiation therapy have undergone huge advances in the past 50 years. In 1971 an imaging modality called computed tomography (CT) was first invented. The first CT scanners were used to create images of the skull. Whole-body scanners were introduced in 1974. In the 1980s, another powerful diagnostic tool was added—magnetic resonance imaging (MRI). MRI is a noninvasive technique that uses magnetic and radio-frequency fields to record images of soft tissues.

Surgical advances have been remarkable as well. Cardiac bypass surgery and joint replacement surgery was developed in the 1970s. Organs are now successfully transplanted, and artificial organs are being tested. New surgical techniques have included the use of lasers in ophthalmology, gynecology, and urology. Microsurgery is now a common tool in the reconstruction of damaged nerves and blood vessels. The use of robotics, such as da Vinci, in surgery holds great promise for the future. In the future surgeons will use 3-D printers to make patient models for patient education as well as in the training of surgeons (Lasalandra 2013).

Today, it is human genetics and progress toward sequencing the human genome that promise to change the healthcare paradigm. New research on cellular and molecular changes underlying disease processes will necessitate new approaches to diagnosis and treatment.

The current paradigm for treating disease is to meet with the patient, diagnose the patient's symptoms, and prescribe therapy to treat them. The hope is that genetic medicine will enable the provider to identify gene patterns that underlie the process of cellular dysfunction that leads to injury before even meeting with the patient. Thus, diseases will be diagnosed much earlier, enabling physicians to provide treatment to stop or slow the disease process.

The study of cell-based technologies is controversial. Cell-based technologies include:

- Tissue engineering, which involves the use of biomaterials to develop new tissue and even whole organs with or without transplanting cells
- Human embryonic stem cells or adult stem cells used for transplantation and in regenerative medicine
- Gene therapy or cell transplantation

The year 2003 saw completion of the Human Genome Project (HGP), a 13-year-long international effort with three principal goals: (1) to determine the sequence of the three billion DNA subunits, (2) to identify all human genes, and (3) to enable genes to be used in further biological study. The Human Genome Project also sought to develop new tools for researching the genome as well as to ensure that all information was made widely available (NIH 2016).

Check Your Understanding 2.4

Instructions: **Answer the following questions.**

1. Which of the following statements is true about behavioral health?
   A. It provides only day-hospital and day-treatment programs.
   B. The quality of the treatment provided has not changed in the past 20 years.
   C. Psychiatric care is restricted to ambulatory care settings.
   D. Insurance coverage generally places restrictions on the psychiatric care such as a limit on the number of outpatient visits.

2. My daughter fell and cut herself tonight. Though it is not an emergency, I believe she needs stitches and she should see someone tonight for treatment. What type of setting would I most likely access?
   A. Hospital emergency department
   B. Community-based ambulatory care services
   C. Private medical practice
   D. Freestanding ambulatory care center

3. Most patients in long-term care facilities require inpatient nursing and related services for more than how many consecutive days?
   A. 14
   B. 30
   C. 60
   D. 100

4. What type of facility offers palliative care for end-of-life care so that the patient may live life as fully and as comfortably as possible?
   A. Hospice
   B. Adult day-care
   C. Skilled nursing facilities
   D. Nursing home

5. Which of the following settings provides ambulatory care to low-income patients and receives funding from many sources?
   A. Voluntary agency
   B. Subacute-care service
   C. Private medical practice
   D. Skilled nursing facility

Match the descriptions provided with the terms to which they apply.

6. _____ Managed care

7. _____ Freestanding ambulatory care centers

8. _____ Human Genome Project

9. _____ Subacute care

10. _____ Continuum of care
   A. A 13-year-long international effort with three principal goals—(1) to determine the sequence of the three billion DNA subunits, (2) to identify all human genes, and (3) to enable genes to be used in further biological study
   B. Provides emergency services and urgent care for walk-in patients
   C. Care that offers patients access to constant nursing care while recovering at home
   D. Care provided by different caregivers at several different levels of the healthcare system
   E. Manages cost, quality, and access to services

Policy Making and Healthcare Delivery

The American healthcare system is a patchwork of independent and governmental entities that provide healthcare services to those in need. Institutions ranging from not-for-profits, profits, and governmental agencies provide not only services but also policy on how Americans are to receive and pay for their healthcare.

The government's role in healthcare services is extensive from the federal level down to the county and local levels. By setting policies on how healthcare is provided, delivered, and reimbursed, government agencies have a significant impact on our healthcare delivery system.

The following sections list five ways that healthcare policies affect the American people. All are dedicated to providing the best services in a system that is constrained by increasing costs generally at the expense of access and quality.

Healthy People 2020

Launched in December 2010 by the Office of Disease Prevention and Heath Promotion of the Department of Health and Human Services, Healthy People 2020 sets out a plan to improve the nation's health with a vision of "a society in which all people live long, healthy lives" (HealthyPeople.gov 2015). This is the third Healthy People initiative (starting with Healthy People 2000) since its inception 30 years ago. The overall goals of Healthy People 2020 are to:

- Attain high-quality, longer lives free of preventable disease, disability, injury, and premature death
- Achieve health equity, eliminate disparities, and improve the health of all groups
- Create social and physical environments that promote good health for all
- Promote quality of life, healthy development, and healthy behaviors across all life stages (HealthyPeople.gov 2015)

Healthy People 2020 is the outcome of extensive stakeholder feedback that resulted in 13 topic areas:

- Adolescent health
- Blood disorders and blood safety
- Dementias, including Alzheimer's disease
- Early and middle childhood
- Genomics
- Global health
- Health-related quality of life and well-being
- Healthcare-associated infections
- Lesbian, gay, bisexual and transgender health
- Older adults
- Preparedness
- Sleep health
- Social determinants of health

Healthy People 2020 also recognizes the important role that health information technology and health communication are an integral part of the implementation process of the initiative. The goal is to develop a feasible, public health information technology (IT) infrastructure in conjunction with the national health information network.

National Academy of Medicine Reports

The National Academy of Medicine (NAM), formerly known as the Institute of Medicine, was established in 1970 as a nongovernmental agency to provide unbiased advice to decision makers and the public. The National Academy of Medicine has written over 1,000 reports since 1970. Six quintessential publications dealing with the public's health are listed as follows:

- *To Error is Human* (1999) reported that as many as 98,000 people die each year from preventable medical errors (IOM 1999).
- *Crossing the Quality Chasm* (2001) identified gaps in the delivery of patient care services resulting from a complex medical system as well as the rapid advancement in medical knowledge (IOM 2001).

- *Envisioning a National Health Care Quality Report* (2001) addressed the collection, measurement, and analysis of quality data (Hurtado et al. 2001).

- *Leadership by Example* (2002) addressed the duplication and contrasting approaches to performance measures by the six major governmental healthcare programs that serve nearly 100 million Americans (IOM 2002).

- *Priority Areas for National Action* (2003), which recognized priorities from earlier reports and suggested a framework for action (IOM 2003).

- *Health IT and Patient Safety* (2012) stated that the improvement in safety of health IT is essential and can help improve healthcare providers' performance, better communication between patients and providers, and enhance patient safety (IOM 2012).

Center for Disease Control and Prevention

Founded in 1946, the **Centers for Disease Control and Prevention (CDC)** is the leading federal agency charged with protecting the public health and safety through the control and prevention of disease, injury, and disability. The CDC leads the nation in:

- Detecting and responding to diseases and conditions (attention deficit hyperactivity disorder, sexually transmitted diseases, cancer, heart disease, diabetes, flu)

- Promoting healthy living (adolescents and school health, food safety, tobacco and alcohol use, overweight and obesity, vaccines and immunizations)

- Providing information for travelers' health (destinations, travel notices, find a clinic)

- Educating for emergency preparedness (natural disasters and severe weather, recent outbreaks and incidents, bioterrorism, chemical emergencies, radiation emergencies, mass casualties)

With over 9,000 employees, the CDC—organized into 15 distinct centers, institutes, and offices (CIOs)—collects, analyzes, and creates national statistical databases and publishes papers on important health issues (CDC 2015).

Local, State, and Federal Policies

All levels of government create policies affecting the nation's healthcare. At the local and community level, leaders decide where public funds will finance community health centers and municipal hospitals, which provide care to those without regard of the patient's ability to pay.

At the state level, decisions on access, eligibility, and level of treatments for Medicaid recipients, where state and federal dollars will be spent on items like tobacco cessation and gambling addiction centers (for those states with casinos), and how to provide services to people with special needs, as well as funding for mental health facilities are a large component of most state budgets.

At the federal level, six agencies provide healthcare to over 100 million Americans (Medicare, Medicaid, State Children's Health Insurance Program [SCHIP], Veterans Health Administration [VHA], TRICARE, Indian Health Service [IHS]). All three branches of government have input on the cost, access, and quality of care provided to Americans through these federal agencies as well as the various policy-making institutions that provide carefully considered input to the decision makers.

Unfortunately, the American healthcare system is not developed from a master plan but is instead a patchwork quilt of measures passed not from thought as to how it would affect the whole, but rather based on ideology. Much attention today is focused on the cost of healthcare often at the expense of patient access and the quality of care provided.

Patient-Centered Outcomes Research Institute

The Patient-Centered Outcomes Research Institute (PCORI) was created in 2010 from the passage of the Patient Protection and Affordable Care Act (PPACA) as a nonprofit, nongovernmental organization mandated to improve the quality and applicability of evidence available to help all stakeholders (patients, caregivers, clinicians, employers, insurers, and policy makers) to make knowledgeable healthcare choices. While PCORI is not the first organization focusing on patient-centered care, it is the largest single research funder that has comparative effectiveness research (CER) as its main focus, and incorporates patients and other stakeholders throughout the process more consistently and intensively than others have before. PCORI has established five national priorities:

- Assessment of prevention, diagnosis, and treatment options
- Improving healthcare systems
- Communication and dissemination research
- Addressing disparities
- Accelerating patient-centered outcomes research and methodological research (PCORI 2015)

Check Your Understanding 2.5

Instructions: **Answer the following questions.**

1. The publication *To Error Is Human* stated that as many as how many patients die each year from preventable medical mistakes?
   A. 10,000
   B. 46,000
   C. 72,000
   D. 98,000

2. To "create social and physical environments that promote good health for all" is a goal of which of the following organizations?
   A. CDC
   B. Healthy People 2020
   C. PCORI
   D. VHA

3. Which of the following is a nonprofit, nongovernmental organization?
   A. SCHIP
   B. CDC
   C. National Academy of Medicine
   D. Healthy People 2020

4. Which federal agency monitors healthy precautions for international travelers?
   A. CDC
   B. VHA
   C. IHS
   D. PCORI

5. Which of the following documents from the National Academy of Medicine addressed the duplication and contrasting approaches to performance measures by the six major governmental healthcare programs that serve nearly 100 million Americans?
   A. *To Error is Human*
   B. *Leadership by Example*
   C. *Envisioning a National Health Care Quality Report*
   D. *Priority Areas for National Action*

6. True or false: There are six federal agencies that provide healthcare to over 100 million people.

7. True or false: Healthcare policy is only formulated at the federal level.

8. True or false: The delivery of healthcare in the United States is based on a well-researched master plan designed to contain costs, increase patient access to providers, and ensure excellent quality of care.

9. True or false: Healthy People 2020 is the third iteration of this document.

10. True or false: Comparative effectiveness research is a major focus of the Patient-Centered Outcomes Research Institute.

 # Real-World Case 2.1

The American healthcare system is a patchwork of not-for-profit and for-profit entities that provide comprehensive diagnostics and treatment services. Marsha, the supervising coder at her local hospital, became a veteran of this system after she noticed neuropathy in her right arm. She first noticed a tingling in her right shoulder and elbow in February and by July the discomfort had increased so that the tingling had become painful throughout the entire length of the arm to such a degree that the arm was almost unusable and she had to take time off from work. She set up an appointment with her family practitioner and was seen seven days later. He ordered x-rays of the arm as well as a cervical MRI. While the x-rays did not show any involvement in the affected joints, the MRI indicated cervical stenosis at the C4–C6 levels. Her physician prescribed pain medication and recommended that she see a neurologist. Her physician ordered a neurological consult, which took place three weeks later. The neurologist performed an assessment, looked over the MRI results, and referred her to a neurosurgeon at another hospital in a major city to the east to have her neck evaluated and fused. Four weeks later she was seen by a neurosurgeon who wanted her to have a cervical CT scan with contrast. The CT confirmed the cervical stenosis. Surgery was set for November 1. The surgery was successful and after six weeks of convalescence she was able to go back to work. Marsha was convinced that she had the best possible care, though the cost was extremely expensive. During the process she was involved with six medical doctors (her family physician, the neurologist, a radiologist to read the MRI scans, the neurosurgeon, another radiologist to evaluate the CT scans, and an anesthesiologist who was present during surgery) and five different facilities (her family physician office, the hospital where the x-rays and MRI were done, the neurologist's office, the neurosurgeon's office, and the hospital where the CT scans and the surgery on her cervical spine were conducted). Throughout the entire process Marsha was required to carry her medical record from one facility to another as the family physician and neurologist were not part of the EHR with the local hospital where she worked, nor was her hospital able to electronically share her information with the hospital where the neurosurgeon practiced. She also made sure to check her patient portal at each hospital to verify appointments and to ensure that the correct information was being entered for each of her visits.

Real-World Case 2.2

A municipal medical center in a city of 100,000 residents decided that they needed to diversify if they were going to survive the ups and downs of the economy. The board of directors met with the chief of the medical staff to determine the best course of action. They mutually decided to emphasize a cradle-to-grave approach by acquitting a few selected physician practices and a local nursing home, starting a home health agency, and creating a hospice unit within the medical center. The board then decided to link all of their new acquisitions to the medical center's existing EHR but ran into a problem with patient identification for medical record purposes. The issue was that the same patient may have been or were going to be in multiple facilities within the new enterprise. However, at each of the present facilities (physician office, medical center, and nursing home) the same patient would have different medical record numbers. A plan for an enterprise medical record number was needed. The medical center administration decided to bring in the HIM director of the medical center to provide expertise and experience in resolving the problem.

References

American Hospital Association. 2015. Fast Facts on US Hospitals. http://www.aha.org/aha/resource-center/Statistics-and-Studies/fast-facts.html.

American Speech-Language-Hearing Association. 2016. http://www.asha.org/public/hearing.

Bureau of Labor Statistics. 2015. Occupational Outlook Handbook. http://www.bls.gov/ooh/healthcare/registered-nurses.htm.

Centers for Disease Control and Prevention. 2015. Fast Facts about CDC. http://www.cdc.gov/about/facts/cdcfastfacts/cdcfacts.html.

Centers for Medicare and Medicaid Services. 2015. National Health Expenditures 2014 Highlights. https://www.cms.gov/research-statistics-data-and-systems/statistics-trends-and-reports/nationalhealthexpenddata/downloads/highlights.pdf.

Centers for Medicare and Medicaid Services. 2014. Critical Access Hospitals. http://www.cms.gov/Outreach-and-Education/Medicare-Learning-Network-MLN/MLNProducts/downloads/CritAccessHospfctsht.pdf.

Congressional Research Service. 2010. Private Health Insurance Provisions in the Patient Protection and Affordable Care Act (PPAA). http://www.ncsl.org/documents/health/privhlthins2.pdf.

HealthyPeople.gov. 2015. http://www.healthypeople.gov/2020/About-Healthy-People.

Hurtado, M.P., E.K. Swift, and J.M. Corrigan. 2001. *Envisioning the National Health Care Quality Report.* Washington, DC: National Academies Press.

Institute of Medicine. 2012. Health IT and Patient Safety: Building Safer Systems for Better Care. http://iom.nationalacademies.org/Reports/2011/Health-IT-and-Patient-Safety-Building-Safer-Systems-for-Better-Care.aspx.

Institute of Medicine. 2003. Priority Areas for National Action: Transforming Health Care Quality. http://iom.nationalacademies.org/reports/2003/priority-areas-for-national-action-transforming-health-care-quality.aspx.

Institute of Medicine. 2002. Leadership by Example: Coordinating Government Roles in Improving Health Care Quality. http://iom.nationalacademies.org/reports/2002/leadership-by-example-coordinating-government-roles-in-improving-health-care-quality.aspx.

Institute of Medicine, Committee on Quality of Health Care in America. 2001. *Crossing the Quality Chasm: A New Health System for the 21st Century.* Washington, DC: National Academies Press.

Institute of Medicine. 1999. To Error is Human: Building a Safer Health System. http://iom.nationalacademies.org/~/media/Files/Report%20Files/1999/To-Err-is-Human/To%20Err%20is%20Human%201999%20%20report%20brief.pdf.

Kaiser Family Foundation. 2015. Medicaid Enrollment and Spending Growth: FY 2015 and 2016. http://kff.org/medicaid/issue-brief/medicaid-enrollment-spending-growth-fy-2015-2016.

Kickman, J.R. and A.R. Kovner. 2015. *Jonas and Kovner's Healthcare Delivery in the United States*, 11th ed. New York: Springer.

Lasalandra, M. 2013. Surgery of the Future: Surgeons Using Printers to make 3-D Patient Models. Beth Israel Deaconess Medical Center. http://www.bidmc.org/YourHealth/Health-Notes/SurgicalInnovations/Advances/SurgeryOfTheFuture.aspx.

Leavitt Partners. 2015. Projected Growth of Accountable Care Organizations. http://leavittpartners.com/category/white-papers/.

National Adult Day Services Association. 2015. http://www.nadsa.org.

National Association of State Mental Health Program Directors. 2015. http://www.nasmhpd.org/.

National Institutes of Health. 2016. What Were the Goals of the Human Genome Project? http://ghr.nlm.nih.gov/handbook/hgp/goals.

National Institutes of Health. 2015. Managed Care. Medline Plus. https://www.nlm.nih.gov/medlineplus/managedcare.html#summary.

National Institutes of Health. 2008. Roadmap for Medical Research. http://pubs.niaaa.nih.gov/publications/arh311/12-13.pdf.

Patient-Centered Outcomes Research Institute. 2015. About Us. http://www.pcori.org/about-us.

Rode, D. 2009. Recovery and privacy: Why a law about the economy is the biggest thing since HIPAA. *Journal of AHIMA* 80(5):42–44.

RTI International. 2015. Accountable Care Organization 2015: Program Analysis Quality Performance Standards Narrative Measure Specification. Prepared for CMS. https://www.cms.gov/medicare/medicare-fee-for-service-payment/sharedsavingsprogram/downloads/ry2015-narrative-specifications.pdf.

Sultz, H.A. and K.M. Young. 2014. *Healthcare USA—Understanding Its Organization and Delivery*, 8th ed. Sudbury, MA: Jones and Bartlett.

US Census Bureau. 2011. Income, Poverty, and Health Insurance Coverage in the United States: 2010. http://www.census.gov/newsroom/releases/archives/income_wealth/cb11-157.html.

3

Health Information Functions, Purpose, and Users

Nanette B. Sayles, EdD, RHIA, CCS, CHDA, CHPS, CPHIMS, FAHIMA

Learning Objectives

- Define the term health record
- Understand the purposes of the health record
- Identify the different users of the health record and how they use it
- Identify processes in paper-based and electronic health records

- Manage the master patient index
- Identify quality controls that can be put into place to manage health information management functions
- Explain the health record processes
- Explain the health information management information systems

Key Terms

Abstracting
Addendum
Aggregate data
Alphabetic filing system
Alphanumeric filing system
Amendment
Analysis
Assembly
Audit trail
Centralized unit filing system
Clinical coding
Clinical decision support
Computer-assisted coding
Concurrent review
Correction
Data

Data mining
Deficiency slip
Delinquent record
Demographics
Deterministic algorithm
Document management system
Duplicate health record
Electronic health record
Encoder
Enterprise master patient index
Free-text data
Grouper
Guidelines
Health record
Hybrid health record
Index

Information
Loose material
Master patient index
Meaningful Use
Natural language processing
Numeric filing system
Outguide
Overlap
Overlay
Paper health record
Patient account number
Probabilistic algorithm
Qualitative analysis
Quantitative analysis
Record reconciliation
Registry

Release of information
Requisition
Retrospective review
Rules-based algorithm

Serial numbering system
Serial-unit numbering system
Standard
Straight numeric filing system

Terminal-digit filing system
Turnaround time
Unit numbering system
Voice recognition technology

The **health record** contains information relating to the physical or mental health or condition of an individual, as made by or on behalf of a health professional in connection with the care ascribed that individual The health record contains the who, what, where, why and how of patient care and is used for different reasons by many people.

When discussing these usages and users, it is important to understand the difference between two terms—*data* and *information*. The terms *data* and *information* are often used interchangeably but they are distinctly different. **Data** are raw facts and figures and **information** is data that has been turned into something meaningful.

Purposes of the Health Record

The health record has many primary and secondary purposes. The primary purposes are those for which it is developed and used—patient care. The secondary purposes are those where the health record is used for healthcare purposes not directly related to patient care.

Primary Purposes

The primary purposes of the health record are related to providing care to the patient. Patient care includes the direct care provided and the day to day business of the organization. These usages can be categorized in the following ways:

- *Patient care:* One of the most important uses of the health record for patient care is the documentation of the care provided by physicians, nurses, and allied health professionals. This documentation serves as a communication tool between these professionals (refer to chapter 2) and may contain treatments and the patient's response to the treatment. For more information on health record documentation, see chapter 4.

- *Management of patient care:* The health record is an important part of managing patient care services performed at the healthcare facility. It includes the development of

patient care standards; conducting research at the local, state, and national levels; and evaluating the quality of care provided. For more on quality, see chapter 18.

- *Administrative purposes:* The health record is used for administrative purposes including billing for services provided, making decisions about the future of the healthcare facility, monitoring the fiscal health of the organization, and scheduling staffing. Many administrative purposes are discussed in detail in chapters 13, 14, 15, and 18.

Secondary Purposes

Healthcare is a sophisticated industry and information from the health record is used for many purposes not related specifically to patient care. These secondary purposes include:

- *Education of healthcare professionals:* Health records are used by medical, nursing, and other allied health professionals including health information management (HIM) to teach present and future healthcare providers how to document care provided, and how to manage the healthcare information. See chapter 20 for more on training.

- *Legal, accreditation, and policy development:* The health record is used to protect the healthcare facility from medical malpractice and other lawsuits, to monitor compliance with laws and regulations, and to adhere to accreditation standards. Information from the health record is also used at the national level to determine where funding will be allocated, as well as the direction the healthcare industry should take. For additional information on how the record is used for legal purposes, see chapters 8, 9, and 10. For additional information public health and research usage, see chapter 14.
- *Public health and research:* Data in the health record is aggregated and turned into information that is used at the national level to establish best practices of patient care, conduct research on new medications and technologies, and to study patient outcomes. New diseases are continuously identified while current ones evolve, making them resistant to traditional treatment. The information from the health record is used to determine treatment for these new diseases and conditions to determine what traditional and nontraditional treatments are effective. Local health departments use health information to identify outbreaks in diseases early so the source of the disease can be managed and epidemics can be managed or prevented.

Formats of the Health Record

To understand how the health record is used, it is important to understand the three types of health records: paper, electronic, and hybrid. The paper health record is completely available in paper media. Some portions of it may have been created electronically, like lab results, but they are printed and filed in the paper record. The electronic health record (EHR) is a digital record of an individual's health-related information that conforms to nationally recognized interoperability standards and that can be created, managed, and consulted by authorized clinicians and staff across more than one healthcare organization. The hybrid health record is a combination of the paper record and the EHR. In the hybrid health record, the laboratory results, radiology results, and other components of the record are stored in the EHR while the progress notes, nurse's notes, and other documents are in the paper record. The electronic documents may or may not be printed and stored in the paper health record.

Users of the Health Record

Healthcare providers are the primary users of the health record, however, others use the health record to manage the healthcare facility and the healthcare industry. Some use the health record directly while others use data or information that has been aggregated from multiple health records. Aggregate data is data that has been extracted from individual health records and combined to form deidentified information about groups of patients that can be compared and analyzed. For example, aggregate data can be used to determine survival rates for various kinds of cancer or to determine if a new drug is safe. Deidentification is the removal of all data elements that can identify the patient.

Individual Users

Individual users are those who depend on the health record in order to complete their job.

The way the record is used varies by individual user. For example, nurses use physician orders with the intention of knowing how to care for the patient. A description of these individual users follows.

- *Patient care providers:* Patient care providers include physicians, nurses, and other allied health professionals who rely on information from the health record in order to make decisions about the care provided to the patient and for documentation of care. Allied health professionals include respiratory therapists, nutritionists, physical therapists, and many more. See chapter 4 for more information on allied health professionals.

- *Patient care managers and support staff:* Patient care managers evaluate the services provided by their employees. As care is documented in the health record, it becomes a key resource in their evaluation of the quality of care provided. The managers look for patterns and trends to recommend changes to the process to improve outcomes and efficiency of the care provided. Support staff gathers information for the patient care managers to use.

- *Coding and billing staff:* Documentation in the health record is the basis for reimbursement or payment for the care provided. The coding staff at the healthcare facility must read the entire health record and assign the appropriate diagnoses and procedure codes for treatment received during the encounter. The billing staff obtains the codes from the coders and submits the bill to the insurance company. See chapter 15 for more information on reimbursement.

- *Patients:* Patients are informed consumers of their healthcare. As informed consumers, patients may obtain access to and be informed about their health record through copies of records or via a personal health record. Personal health records are discussed later in this chapter. See chapter 9 to learn more about patient rights in regard to their health record.

- *Employers:* Employers may use health records when processing health insurance claims and in managing wellness programs. Another use

of the health record by employers in determining when employees are well enough to return to work, although this is generally limited to a note from the physician giving his or her approval. When an employee claims disability due to a work-related incident it is the information found in the health record that supports or refutes the claim.

- *Lawyers:* Lawyers may need access to support a client (the patient) for life insurance claims and lawsuits such as those related to automobile accidents, disability, and such. In order to protect themselves from medical malpractice and other lawsuits, healthcare facilities may grant lawyers access to patient records. See chapter 9 for more on access to the health record.

- *Law enforcement officials:* Law enforcement officials need access to health record documentation to investigate gunshot wounds and other injuries resulting from a crime. They also may access documentation for information that will help protect the security of the country.

- *Healthcare researchers and clinical investigators:* Healthcare researchers use health records to study the safety and efficacy of drugs or the value of care provided. The researcher's aggregate data and information based on these findings are used to approve new treatments and to stop unsafe treatments. Chapter 14 includes more information about how the health record is used in research.

- *Government policy makers:* The health record may be used to develop and evaluate current and future laws, regulations, and standards related to healthcare. The data collected can help determine best practices, gaps in current legislation, and other issues that need to be addressed to improve care and prevent fraud.

Institutional Users

Institutional users are organizations that need access to health records in order to accomplish their mission. These institutional users include healthcare delivery organization, third party payers, medical review organizations, research organizations, educational organizations, accreditation organizations, government licensing agencies, and policy-making bodies.

- *Healthcare delivery organizations:* Healthcare delivery organizations—including hospitals, physician offices, home health agencies, and others—use the health record to provide care, submit claims for reimbursement, and evaluate the quality of care provided.
- *Third-party payers:* Third party payers are organizations responsible for the reimbursement of healthcare services through an insurance program. These insurance programs include commercial insurance, managed care organizations, government insurance programs, accountable care organizations, as well as self-insured employers. The health record is used to justify the care provided and therefore the reimbursement. For additional information, refer to chapter 16.
- *Medical review organizations:* Medical review organizations evaluate the quality and appropriateness of the care provided to the patient. Medicare hires organizations known as quality improvement organizations to determine if the care provided to the patient was medically necessary. See chapter 18 for more information on quality improvement organizations.
- *Research organizations:* Research organizations conduct medical research and include state

disease registries such as the cancer registry, research centers, and others who explore diseases and their treatment.

- *Educational organizations:* Colleges and universities train healthcare professionals in their medical schools as well as nursing and allied health programs. The students in these programs use the health records as case studies as a part of the educational program.
- *Accreditation organizations:* In order to be granted and maintain accreditation, a healthcare organization must show compliance with the accrediting body standards. This frequently requires review of the health record to determine compliance with documentation and patient care standards. To learn more about accreditation, see chapter 8.
- *Government licensing agencies:* Government agencies at the local, state, and federal level review the health record in order to ensure compliance with state licensing requirements and in verifying compliance with standards that enable the healthcare facility to receive federal funding. To learn more about licensing, see chapter 8.
- *Policy-making bodies:* The data submitted for healthcare claims to governmental databases and other sources is analyzed and utilized for decision making related to healthcare programs. For example, the Centers for Medicare and Medicaid Services (CMS) utilize a wide range of data to make revisions to reimbursement systems each year.

Check Your Understanding 3.1

Instructions: **Answer the following questions.**

1. Which of the following is an example of a primary purpose of the health record?
   A. Education
   B. Policy making
   C. Research
   D. Patient care

2. I work for an organization that utilizes health record data to prove or disprove the efficacy of a healthcare treatment. What type of organization do I work for?
   A. Education
   B. Policy making
   C. Research
   D. Third-party payer

3. Which of the following is an example of an institutional user of the health record?
   A. Third-party payer
   B. Patient
   C. Physician
   D. Employer

4. Which of the following is an example of an individual user?
   A. Policy-making body
   B. Government licensing agency
   C. Patient
   D. Accreditation organization

5. Health departments use the health record to monitor outbreaks of diseases. Which type of use is this?
   A. Education
   B. Public health and research
   C. Accreditation
   D. Patient care

HIM Functions

The HIM department performs many functions to support patient care and the healthcare organization. The functions focus on ensuring the quality, security, and availability of the health record. While every HIM department is different, the functions of the department typically include:

- Record processing
- Monitoring of record completion
- Transcription
- Release of patient information
- Clinical coding, abstracting, and clinical data analysis

Other functions that may be found in the department include:

- Research and statistics
- Registries, including, cancer, trauma, birth defects, and organ transplant
- Birth and death certificate completion

The HIM department does not operate in isolation but in conjunction with other departments to support and enhance their services including patient care, information governance, quality management, billing, and patient registration.

Master Patient Index

The master patient index (MPI) is the permanent record of all patients treated at a healthcare facility. It is used by the HIM department to look up patient demographics, dates of care, the patient's health record number, and other information. Demographics are basic information about the patient such as their name, address, date of birth, and insurance information. The MPI is an important element of a numeric filing system (discussed later in this chapter) as it allows the user to look up the patient health record number so the record can be located. When a healthcare enterprise has more than one facility and the patient is seen at two or more places, the **enterprise master patient index (EMPI)** links the patient's information at the different facilities. The recommended core data elements for the EMPI are:

- Internal patient identification
- Person name
- Date of birth
- Gender
- Race
- Ethnicity
- Address
- Telephone number
- Alias, previous, or maiden names
- Social Security number

- Facility identification
- Universal patient identifier
- Account or visit number
- Admission or visit number
- Admission, encounter, or visit data
- Discharge or departure date
- Encounter service type
- Encounter primary physician
- Patient disposition (AHIMA 2010)

Before computerization, the MPI was maintained on index cards; now the MPI is generally electronic, which allows for alphabetic and phonetic search capabilities, as well as the ability to search numerous data elements such as patient name, health record number, and billing number. Figure 3.1 provides an example of an input screen for an electronic MPI system.

The health record number is created by the MPI and the numbers are issued in sequential numeric order.

Figure 3.1   Input screen for an electronic MPI system

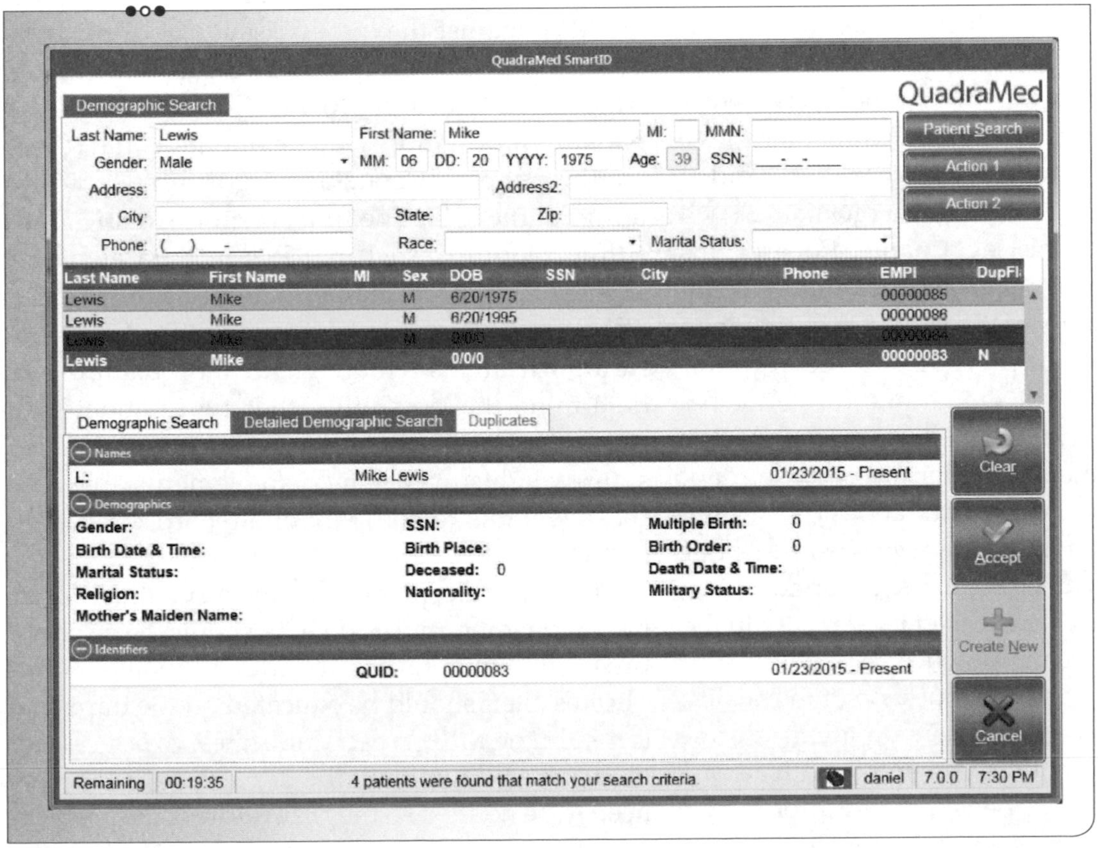

Source: AHIMA Virtual Lab QuadraMed MPI.

For example, Ms. Smith is admitted to the healthcare facility at 4:00 p.m. and is issued the health record number of 156876. When Ms. Jones, the next new patient, is admitted at 4:06 p.m., she is issued the health record number of 156877.

Unfortunately, there are data quality issues that result from improper issuance of the health record, as described in the next section.

Quality Issues in MPI Systems

Typographical errors, outdated demographic information, and other data quality issues are always present in the MPI. For example, patients change their name, identify themselves by their nickname, move, or change phone numbers. The erroneous information is then shared with other information systems, exacerbating the problem. It takes a lot of time to identify and correct the erroneous information. Some of the more common problems include duplicates, overlays, and overlaps.

Duplicate, Overlay, and Overlap Health Record Numbers

When the patient is registered in the admission department, previous MPI information may not be retrieved. The clerk may not conduct a thorough search for the patient or the patient may give a different name. For example, the patient may give her new married name rather than her maiden name. The patient may also give a nickname, such as Bob, rather than his legal name, Robert. This results in a duplicate health record number being issued. A duplicate health record results when the patient has two or more health record numbers issued. The patient's medical information becomes fragmented with some information under the first number and the remainder under the second. When this happens, duplicate laboratory testing may occur, causing unnecessary expenses, poor decisions such as misdiagnoses or unnecessary tests, and the facility's increased legal risk with the potential for medical malpractice.

Another problem with the question of the quality of the MPI is an overlay, where a patient is erroneously assigned another person's health record number. When this happens, patient information from both patients becomes commingled and care

providers may make medical decisions based on erroneous information, increasing the legal risks to the healthcare organization and quality of care risks to the patient as well. For example, a patient with the name Jeffery Johnson, date of birth January 1, 1962, may be mistaken for Jeffery Johnson, date of birth January 1, 1957. One of the more common reasons for this is an error in selecting the correct patient by the hospital staff.

A third issue is an overlap, or when a patient has more than one health record number at different locations in an enterprise. This frequently becomes an issue when organizations merge or create an EMPI.

MPI Quality Control

A healthcare facility must work to protect the integrity of the data in the MPI. Most errors are human, such as transposition of numbers and typographical errors, the user may use poor search strategies and the patient is not found in the system, or the patient may give inaccurate information.

All healthcare facilities and organizations must have processes in place to maintain and correct the MPI against the quality issues of duplicates, overlays, and overlaps on a continuous basis. Algorithms are used to match patients so the patient information can be merged and there are three types of matching algorithms typically found in the MPI. The first, a deterministic algorithm, requires exact matches in data elements such as the patient name, date of birth, and Social Security number. The second, a probabilistic algorithm, uses mathematical probabilities to determine the possibility that two patients are the same. The third, a rules-based algorithm, assigns weights to specific data elements and uses those weights to compare one record to another (AHIMA 2010).

This clean-up process is not a one-time effort but an ongoing process. There should be a formal process to help prevent and identify potential duplicates. Staff should be educated on the impact of errors in the MPI. When duplicates, overlays, and overlaps are identified, the department managers need to be notified so they can address the problem with the staff making the errors.

Identification Systems

Identification systems link the patient to the health record. The health record number is a key data element in the MPI as it is a unique identifier for the patient. It is important in numeric filing system as the MPI is used to look up the patient's health record number. The health record number is typically assigned during the patients initial registration encounter at the facility. The Social Security number should not be used for the health record due to confidentiality concerns.

Identification Systems for Paper-Based Health Records

There are several ways to identify records in a paper-based health record system. These include numeric, alphabetic, and alphanumeric systems. For the numeric systems to work, the health record number has to be accessed in the MPI before the health record can be retrieved. The identification systems are serial numbering systems, unit numbering systems, serial-unit numbering systems, and alphabetic filing systems.

Serial Numbering System

In the **serial numbering system**, a patient is issued a unique numerical identifier for every encounter at the healthcare facility. If a patient is admitted to the healthcare facility five times he or she will have five different health record numbers. The documentation for each of the encounters is filed in the health record for that encounter so the information is filed separately and all health records must be retrieved in order to view the complete health information. The serial numbering system is inefficient and more costly because of the extra costs to manage the folders as well as to purchase the folders.

Unit Numbering System

The **unit numbering system** is commonly used in large healthcare facilities as it does not have many of the inefficiencies of the serial numbering systems. The patient is issued a health record number at the first encounter and that number is used for all subsequent encounters. This system consolidates all of the information on the patient in one location and is therefore more efficient than the serial numbering system.

Serial-Unit Numbering System

The **serial-unit numbering system** is a combination of the serial and unit numbering systems. The patient is issued a new health record number with each encounter but all of the documentation is moved from the last number to the new number.

Alphabetic Filing System

The **alphabetic filing system** is typically used by small clinics and physician offices. The folders are filed alphabetically by the patient's last name. If there is more than one person with the same last name, then the first and middle initial are used. The disadvantage of this system is that more than one person may have the same or similar name.

Identification Systems Used for Electronic Health Records

The unit numbering system is the most common system used in the EHR. The advantage of the EHR is that identifiers other than the health record number—such as the patient name and patient account number—can be used to retrieve the information. The **patient account number** is "a number assigned by a healthcare facility for billing purposes that is unique to a particular episode of care; a new account number is assigned each time the patient receives care or services at the facility" (AHIMA 2014, 111). It is easy to select the wrong person in the EHR so it is important to double check to make sure that the correct person is retrieved.

HIM Functions in a Paper-Based Environment

While the EHR is becoming more prevalent, the existing paper records have not disappeared. While HIM professionals operate in the EHR environment, the paper records must still be managed.

The following sections address the HIM processes for the creation, storage, and maintenance of paper-based records.

Record Storage and Retrieval Functions

The HIM department is responsible for the storage and retrieval of the paper-based record. Policies and procedures should be in place to ensure access to the health records for authorized users but to prevent access for unauthorized access. In a paper-based record, the documentation is typically stored alphabetically or numerically in a special file folder. Healthcare facilities may also file their paper-based records off-site, on microfilm, or digitally as a scanned document.

Filing Systems for Paper-Based Health Records

In a paper-based record filing system, the folder containing the health records are stored in shelving units or in filing cabinets based on the health record number or patient name.

Alphabetic Filing System   In the alphabetic filing system, records are filed in alphabetical order. This system works well with a small volume of records such as in a physician practice. Employees are comfortable with it and the system is easy

to create and use. A disadvantage is that there is no unique identifier as patients can have the same name. Another problem is the alphabetic filing system does not expand evenly. Statistically almost half of the files fall under the letters B, C, H, M, S and W. Figure 3.2 contains rules for alphabetic filing.

Numeric Filing Systems   In a numeric filing system, the health records are filed by the health record number. The MPI is consulted to identify the health record number and then the number is used to locate the health record. This may seem like more work than the alphabetic system but there are many advantages for the numeric filing system. The most common types of numeric filing systems are as follows.

- The **straight numeric filing system** files the records in straight numeric order based on the health record number. This filing system is easy to teach to new employees however the most active area in the files is the higher numbers, which are the most current files, making it difficult to manage. Management problems include the higher number of department staff in the area and the space required by the health records may exceed the amount available.

Figure 3.2   Rules for alphabetic filing

1. File each record alphabetically by the last name, followed by the first name and middle initial. For example:

   Brown, Michelle L.
   Brown, Michelle S.
   Brown, Robert A.

   When the patient has identical last and first names and middle initial, order the records by date of birth, filing the record with the earliest birthdate first.

2. Last names beginning with a prefix or containing an apostrophe are filed in strict alphabetical order, ignoring any apostrophes or spaces. For example, the names D'Angelo would be filed as Dangelo.

3. Names beginning with the abbreviation St. such as St. Clair, are filed as S-a-i-n-t.

4. In hyphenated names such as Burchfield-Sayles, the hyphenation is ignored and the record is filed as Burchfieldsayles

5. In the event that a name is given as an initial, the rule is "file nothing before something." For example, Smith, J would be filed before Smith, Jane.

6. Mac and Mc can be filed either way but there should be a policy stating whether Mac or Mc will be used.

Source: Huffman 1994.

Figure 3.3 Terminal-digit filing system example

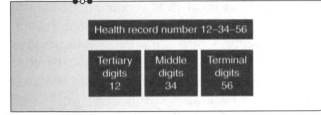

- Microfilm
- Off-site storage
- Image-based storage

The storage choice for health records depends on the needs and storage capacity of the facility.

- The **terminal-digit filing system** may sound backward, but it is typically considered the most efficient of the numeric filing systems in part because it distributes charts evenly throughout the filing units. It is also effective for facilities with a heavy record volume. The health records are filed by the last two digits, called the terminal digits, then the middle two digits, known as the secondary unit. The health records are then filed by the first two or three numbers, known as the tertiary units. See figure 3.3 for an example.

Alphanumeric Filing System As the name alphanumeric filing system indicates, both alphabetic and numeric characters are used to sort health records in this system. The first two letters of the patient's last name are followed by a unique numeric identifier such as SA2567. This system is appropriate for small organizations. Like numeric systems, alphanumeric filing systems require an MPI.

Centralized Unit Filing Systems In a centralized unit filing system, all of the patient's encounters are filed together in a single location. For example, a patient may be seen in radiology for a mammogram and in the laboratory for a urinalysis. These test results will be filed together. This type of filing system is usually associated with the unit numbering system; the unique identifiers can be alphabetic, alphanumeric or numeric depending on the needs of the facility.

Storage Systems for Paper-Based Records Several different options are available for storing paper records including:

- Filing cabinets
- Shelving units

Filing Cabinets or Shelving Units Vertical and lateral filing cabinets, open-shelves, or compressible filing units can all be used for storage of records. The vertical and lateral filing cabinets are seen in most office settings and usually contain two or four drawers. These small filing cabinets are only appropriate for low-volume storage as the drawers are challenging to quickly access health records.

Typically, an HIM department uses open shelving—units that resemble bookcases and can store large volumes of files that are easy to view and access. Multiple shelves separated by aisles large enough for a person to walk through to access the files can be used. A common variation is compressible filing units, where there is not an aisle between each shelving unit but instead one or two aisles while the rest of the units are collapsed together. These shelving units move and the aisles open and close as needed. The units are on tracks, which allow the units to be moved to open up the aisle.

Files of patients who have not been at the facility for a specified period, such as two years, may be purged or removed from the active filing area. The time period and frequency of purging depends on the space available, patient readmission rate, and the need for access to the health record. For more information on retention and destruction, see chapter 9.

An important role of the HIM professional is to determine the space requirements needed to store the paper health record by evaluating the volume indicators such as number of discharges, size of records, and the capacity of the storage units. For example, the space needed can be estimated with the following information:

Shelving unit shelf width = 36 inches
Number of shelves per unit = 8 shelves
Average record thickness = ½ inch
Average annual inpatient discharges = 10,200

The following demonstrates how these statistics are used to estimate the number of shelving units to store one year of health records.

1. Determine the linear inch capacity of each shelving unit.

   36 inches per shelf x 8 shelves per unit = 288 inches per shelving unit

2. Determine the linear filing inches needed for the volume of records.

   10,200 average annual inpatient discharges x ½ inch average record thickness = 5,100 inches required to store one year of inpatient discharge records

3. Determine the number of shelving units required by dividing the required filing space by the shelving unit linear inch capacity.

   5,100/288 = 17.7 = 18 shelving units

Since it is impossible to purchase a part of a shelving unit, the number of shelving units required should always be rounded up to a whole number. This example only included inpatient discharges for simplicity; however outpatient health records would also have to be considered.

File Folders   File folders are used to hold paper health records. File folders used for health records are usually purchased in one of two standard weights or thicknesses—11 points and 14 points—although to the weight may be as much as 20 points. The higher the points, the more durable the file folder. The amount of filing and retrieval activity will impact the decision. Typically side tabs are used for health records but top tabs may be used in lateral shelving units. Two-pronged record fasteners should be placed at the top or sides of the file folder in order to hold the health record forms in place.

File folders should be color coded for easy filling and retrieval. For example, the tab on the file folder has a label that displays a single digit of the health record number in a specific color. This makes it easy to identify misfiled records. For example, a yellow label would stand out in a row of green and red. Typically the file folders are purchased with the color coding already applied but labels can be applied manually.

Microfilm-Based Storage Systems   Paper health records require a great deal of space. One way to reduce the amount of space required is to microfilm the health record, which is a photographic process that reduces an original paper document into a small static image on film. Microfilm has been used for decades by healthcare facilities and works well for inactive or infrequently used health records. A picture of each page of the health record is taken and stored as a small negative. A microfilm viewer is required in order to be able to read the image. There are a number of formats:

- *Roll microfilm*: The microfilm images are stored on a long roll of film. Each roll can store thousands of images for hundreds of patients. The major problem with this format is that patient encounters can be stored on multiple rolls making retrieval difficult.

- *Jacket microfilm:* A roll of microfilm is cut and inserted into four-by-six inch jackets with sleeves. Multiple jackets containing all episodes of care that have been microfilmed can be filed together to maintain the unit-record. The same type of filing systems that apply to paper records can be used.

- *Microfiche:* This format is a copy of the jacket microfilm. Microfiche is the same size as the microfilm jacket. Some facilities use microfiche rather than allow the original jacket microfilm outside of the HIM department (for example, microfiche would be sent to the nursing unit for patient care).

Off-site Storage Systems   Inactive records can be stored off-site and copied on microfilm. The off-site location may be under the control of the healthcare facility or a commercial company that stores and retrieves the facility's health records for a fee. The healthcare facility must meet privacy and security regulations in terms of storage of health record. The vendor must be able to protect the health records from fire, pests, burglary, and other hazards. The commercial vendor must be able to return the records to the healthcare facility within a predetermined time. The records can be faxed, scanned and e-mailed, or hand-delivered to the healthcare facility.

Image-Based Storage Systems Document imaging is scanning the document and storing it digitally on hard drives, CD, or other storage media. The file formats also vary but are typically picture file formats such as .tif or .jpg. The advantage of image-based storage over microfilm is that each document can be indexed or identified by patient or document type. The image itself cannot be searched but the indexed information is used to retrieve patient information. Retrieval of the images with a few keystrokes is a much quicker method than microfilm retrieval.

Retrieval and Tracking Systems for Paper-Based Records Health records must be accessible to authorized users. A common way of tracking the location of a health record is the outguide. The **outguide** identifies where the health record is located and when it was removed. It is generally made of colored vinyl with two plastic pockets and it is placed in the shelving unit where the health record should be. The outguide is approximately the size of the health record. The larger plastic pocket can hold documentation that needs to be filed in the health record, known as **loose material,** which includes dictated reports, reports not filed on the nursing unit, and such. The small pocket can be used to hold a slip of paper that tells where the record has been moved to and when it was checked out.

Traditionally when a record is needed by a patient care area or other department in the healthcare facility, they submit a **requisition** or request for the health record. The requisition tells the HIM department the name, health record number, date or request, name of requester, and where the record needs to be delivered. The requisition can be handwritten or be generated by a computer system.

Today automated systems frequently create the requisition and replace the outguide. In an automated chart tracking system, the computer keeps up with the location of the health record by "checking out" the chart to the nursing unit or other location. Because of this, an outguide is not needed to record the location of the chart but may still be used to hold the documents to be filed.

Record Processing of Paper-Based Records Record processing ensures that health records are organized and meet standards. These functions help ensure the accessibility and completeness of the health record. When the quality of the health record is not maintained, patient care suffers due to missing, inaccurate, or incomplete information and it also impacts billing, research, and other purposes.

Admission and Discharge Record Reconciliation for Paper-Based Records When a patient is admitted to the healthcare facility, a search of the MPI is performed to identify if the patient has been at the facility before. If so, then the paper health records from the previous encounters will be made available for patient care. Once the patient is discharged from the health facility, the health record is taken to the HIM department for processing. The first task is to ensure that all health records have been received. This process is known as **record reconciliation.**

Record Assembly Function for Paper-Based Records **Assembly** is the process of ensuring that each page in the health record is organized in a standardized format, which varies by facility. During the assembly process each page should be reviewed to ensure that all pages belong to the same patient and same encounter.

Analysis for Paper-Based Records Analysis, or review, of the health record is performed by HIM department personnel to determine the completeness of the health record. There are two types of analysis that should be performed—qualitative and quantitative.

Qualitative analysis is monitoring the quality of the documentation. This is a collaborative effort among the HIM department, risk management, healthcare providers, and others. While the physicians must review the quality of physician documentation, nurses review nurse documentation, and so forth, HIM professionals can review legibility, timeliness of documentation, use of approved abbreviations, and other documentation standards.

Quantitative analysis is a review of the health record to determine if there are any missing reports, forms, or signatures. This analysis can be performed by concurrent review—in an ongoing manner while the patient is still in the healthcare facility. It can also be reviewed after discharge from the healthcare facility, known as retrospective review. The review involves the following:

- All forms and reports contain correct patient identification (name, health record number, encounter number, and date of service).
- All forms and reports are present.
- Reports requiring signatures are signed.

When a document or signature is missing, a deficiency slip is created. The deficiency slip identifies the pertinent document and what needs to be done (dictated, completed, and signed). and is often created by a computer system. An example of the deficiency slip is shown in figure 3.4.

When a deficiency is identified in the health record, it must be corrected. This may require locating a missing document or asking the physician or other healthcare provider to either sign or complete a document. The specific analysis performed depends on the medical staff bylaws, rules, and regulations, as well as state licensing and accreditation requirements.

Monitoring Completion of Paper-Based Records Physicians and other practitioners are notified when they have incomplete health records requiring their attention. They usually come to the HIM department to complete the necessary documentation in the chart. The records are then reanalyzed to make sure everything has been completed. If no deficiencies are identified, the deficiency slip is removed and the health record can be filed away in the permanent file. If a health record remains incomplete for a specified number of days

Figure 3.4 Sample deficiency slip

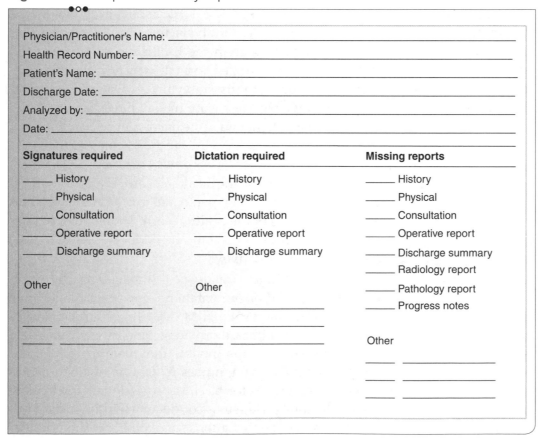

Source: Cerrato and Roberts 2012.

as defined in the medical staff rules and regulations, the record is considered to be a **delinquent record**. The specific number of days varies by facility, but is generally 15 to 30 days.

Handling Corrections, Errors, and Addendums in Paper-Based Records Occasionally health records must be corrected, amended, or deleted. Information may be written in the wrong patient's chart, information may have been omitted, or an error may have been made in documentation. Policies must be in place to ensure the integrity of the health record.

Corrections to the health record should be made by drawing a single line through the erroneous information and writing the word "error" above the mistake. The practitioner should sign, date, and time the correction. An **addendum** is additional information provided in the health record. The addendum should be dated the day it was written—not the date it is referencing. It should be signed and the time of entry should be recorded. An **amendment** is a clarification made to healthcare documentation after the original document has been signed. It should be dated, timed, and signed.

Forms Design, Development, and Control for Paper-Based Records Forms should be designed using appropriate form design principles that will enhance the documentation on the form. The form must meet the needs of the end user, which means it should be easy to use and include all necessary data.

The purpose should be identified before developing the form so that all necessary and appropriate data are included; and the form should not duplicate one that is already in use. The users should be involved in the development form to ensure their needs are met. Effective form design principles include the following.

- All forms should contain a unique identifying number for positive identification and easy inventory control.
- Each form should include original and revised dates for the tracking and purging of obsolete forms.

- Each form should have a concise title that clearly identifies the form's purpose.
- The facility's name and logo should appear on each page of the form, preferably in the same location on each.
- For clinical forms, patient identification information (name, health record number, billing number, physician name and number, date of birth, admission date, and room number) should appear on every page.
- For clinical forms, a signature line should appear at the bottom and there should be no question about what has been authenticated. If initials are used, space also should be provided for the full name and title so that each set of initials is identified.
- Data-entry methodology should be considered when the information is to be keyed into a computer. The order of the form should mirror the data-entry order to ensure that information is entered consistently.
- Optical character reader codes and barcodes should be printed in the upper left-hand corner of the form when imaging the health record is a possibility.
- A standard of 8.5 by 11 inches is the best size for a document.
- Form colors should be black ink on white paper. If color coding is desired, a strip of color along one margin is the best option.
- Documents that contain punched holes should have a margin of at least 3/4 inch. All other margins should be at least 3/8-inch wide.
- Vertical and horizontal lines assist the user in completing and reviewing the form. Bold lines should be used to draw the reader's eye to an important field.
- Sufficient space should be provided to complete the entry (for example, 1/16 inch for typed letters and 1/3-inch high for handwritten entries).

- Titles for boxes and fields should be located in the top left-hand corner of the box or field.

- Paper ranging from 20 to 24 pounds in weight is recommended for use in copiers, scanners, and fax machines.

- Type size should be no smaller than 9 points for lowercase letters and 10 points for upper-case letters (AHIMA 1997).

When a document imaging system is used, form design is critical as the color in both the paper and the ink can negatively impact the quality of the image and should be eliminated or reduced. Forms that will be scanned should have a barcode imprinted on them allowing the automatic indexing into the chart.

Every healthcare facility should have a clinical forms committee to establish standards for design and to approve new and revised forms. The committee should also have oversight of computer screens and other data capture tools. The committee should be comprised of users of health information and include representatives from the following areas:

- HIM
- Medical staff
- Nursing staff
- Purchasing
- Information services
- Performance improvement
- Support or ancillary departments
- Forms vendor representatives

Representatives from the area that will use the form should attend the committee meeting to explain the form and the need for it.

Without oversight the number of forms can become overwhelming to manage and there can be duplication. A forms control program includes the following.

- *Establishing standards*: Written standards and guidelines ensure that effective forms design as previously discussed are used. These standards should be recorded in a forms manual. **Standards** are fixed rules that must

be followed. A guideline provides general direction about the design of the form.

- *Establishing a number and tracking system*: A unique number should be assigned to each form. There should be a master form index and a copy of all forms should be maintained. The master form index should include the title, number, origination date, revision dates, purpose, and legal requirements.

- *Establishing a testing and evaluation plan*: New and revised forms should be tested prior to their implementation to ensure that data elements are not missing and that there is enough space to write.

- *Checking the quality of new forms*: A process should be in place to guarantee that the printed forms were printed correctly.

- *Systematizing storage, inventory, and distribution*: There must be a process to store and distribute the forms where and when they are needed.

- *Establishing a forms database*: An electronic database should be used to store and facility updating forms.

Quality Control Functions in Paper-Based Systems There must be processes in place to safeguard the quality of analysis and forms design. Each function should have its own acceptable level of performance and monitoring should be performed to confirm the standards are met. If not, corrective actions should be taken. See chapter 18 for more on quality improvement.

There are several components of storage and retrieval that are monitored. Managers monitor misfiles, timeliness of storage and retrieval to calculate filing accuracy, and timeliness rates. Examples of standards include:

- An average of 50 health records will be filed in an hour

- Records for the emergency department will be retrieved within 10 minutes of the request

- Loose materials will be filed in either the health record or the outguide pocket within 24 hours of receipt in the HIM department

To complete health records in a paper media, the physician must come to the HIM department to dictate, sign, or otherwise complete the record. If records are unavailable to the physician when they try to complete the record, the completion record is delayed. The manager monitors the number of charts not available to physician, usually weekly.

Check Your Understanding 3.2

Instructions: **Answer the following questions.**

1. What microfilm format is inefficient when patients have multiple admissions on microfilm?
   A. Roll
   B. Jacket
   C. Microfiche
   D. Both roll and jacket

2. What type of paper-based storage system conserves floor space by eliminating all but one or two aisles?
   A. Open-shelf units
   B. Carousel systems
   C. Mobile filing units
   D. Filing cabinets

3. What feature of the filing folder helps locate misfiles within the paper-based filing system?
   A. Fasteners
   B. Folder weight
   C. Color coding
   D. Barcodes

4. Which of the following is a tool used to track paper-based health records?
   A. Compliance documentation
   B. Outguide
   C. Requisition
   D. MPI

5. What should be done when the HIM department's error or accuracy rate is too high based on policy?
   A. Corrective action should be taken.
   B. The problem should be treated as an isolated incident.
   C. The formula for determining the rate may need to be adjusted.
   D. Re-audit the problem area.

6. The forms design committee:
   A. Provides oversight for the development, review, and control of forms and computer screens
   B. Is responsible for the EHR implementation and maintenance
   C. Is always a subcommittee of the quality improvement committee
   D. Is an optional function for the HIM department

7. In a paper-based system, individual health records are organized in a standardized order in which of the following processes?
   A. Retrieval
   B. Assembly
   C. Analysis
   D. Reordering

8. Reviewing a health record for missing signatures and missing medical reports is called:
   A. Assembly
   B. Indexing
   C. Analysis
   D. Coding

9. Two patient's records were filed together by mistake. This is an example of:
   A. Overlap
   B. Overlay
   C. Duplicate
   D. Purge

10. Which of the following describes incomplete records that are not completed by the physician within the time frame specified in the healthcare facility's policies?
    A. Suspended records
    B. Delinquent records
    C. Loose records
    D. Default records

HIM Functions in an Electronic Environment

The functions of the HIM department have changed dramatically with the introduction of the EHR. The EHR is an electronic record of health-related information on an individual that conforms to nationally recognized interoperability standards and that can be created, managed, and consulted by authorized clinicians and staff across more than one healthcare organization.

Record Filing and Tracking of EHRs

Filing of health records is significantly reduced or even completely eliminated in the EHR environment. As more data is captured directly into the EHR, there is no need for paper nor the storage of paper-based records. The EHR is able to track who has access to a record through the audit trail. An **audit trail** is a chronological set of computerized records that provides evidence of information system activity (logins and logouts, file accesses) used to determine security violations For more information on audit logs, please see chapter 10.

Record Processing of EHRs

In the EHR, the assembly process is eliminated; however, even if the facility does not use paper documents, they may receive papers from the patient or other sources. These loose reports are scanned and indexed for inclusion in the EHR. **Indexing** is the linking of patient name, health record number, document type, and other identifying information to the scanned document.

Record completion in the EHR is performed via computer so healthcare professionals can complete them from any accessible location. An electronic work queue, or workflow, allows the record to be routed to all healthcare professionals who have deficiencies so that they can access, complete, and authenticate the health record. The work queue is also used to route the health record to HIM for processing. With a document management system, one function does not have to be completed before the next one so the chart is available for all functions. For example, the chart does not have to be analyzed before it is coded. Also, if coding cannot be performed for some reason, workflow will reroute the health record to coding once the problem has been resolved.

Version Control of EHRs

The health record may have multiple versions of the same document; for example, a signed and unsigned copy of a document. Additional versions are also created when addendums, corrections, or amendments are made to original documents. To address the issues that result from having multiple versions of the same document, policies and procedures addressing version control must be developed. Version control identifies which version(s) of the documents is available to the user. All versions must be maintained but access to all except the current version should be controlled so that there is no confusion about which version is correct.

Management of Free Text in EHRs

Free-text data is the unstructured narrative data that is the result of a person typing data into an information system. It is undefined, unlimited, and unstructured, meaning that the typist can type anything into the field or document. The amount of free-text in the EHR should be limited as the ability to manipulate data is diminished. For example, with structured data, the term used would be consistent where in free text synonyms would be used making it more difficult to retrieve. The preferred data type is structured text where you point and click or otherwise select the data. For example, you would have two choices with the data element gender: male and female. The user simply points and clicks the appropriate choice rather than typing it in.

In the EHR, the user is able to copy and paste free text from one patient or patient encounter to another. This practice is dangerous as inaccurate information can easily be copied. Specific risks to documentation integrity of using copy functionality include:

- Inaccurate or outdated information
- Redundant information, which makes it difficult to identify the current information
- Inability to identify the author or intent of documentation
- Inability to identify when the documentation was first created

- Propagation of false information
- Internally inconsistent progress notes
- Unnecessarily lengthy progress notes (AHIMA 2014, 4)

Policies and procedures need to be in place in order to reduce some of the risks.

Management and Integration of Digital Dictation, Transcription, and Voice Recognition

A common method to capture dictation in the EHR is digital dictation. The physician or other healthcare provider dictates a medical report and the transcriptionist types what is said into an electronic, or digital, format. These reports are electronically transmitted into the EHR where the physician is able to sign the document.

With voice recognition technology a computer captures the dictation and converts what is said directly into text and no transcriptionist is needed. The transcriptionist becomes an editor and therefore focuses on data quality. More specifically, natural language processing is a technology that converts human language (structured or unstructured) into data that can be translated then manipulated by computer systems. It is the software used for speech recognition.

Reconciliation Processes for EHRs

As in the paper-record environment, the HIM professional must verify that there is a complete health record for every episode of care including both inpatient and outpatient patients. HIM professionals also need to verify that documents sent to the EHR from the transcription system and others arrive in the system as expected.

Managing Other Electronic Documentation

In an electronic record environment, many documentation sources can be included in the health record that were not previously stored in the paper-health record. Examples of these documentation sources include e-mail, voice mail, audio, monitoring strips, images (radiology, pathology), video (heart catheterization), and monitoring (fetal, electrocardiogram).

E-mail is being used in healthcare to share patient information. Policies and procedures need to be in place to address privacy and security as well as the creation, storage, and maintenance of the messages. The e-mail management system should allow e-mails that contain patient information to be stored in the EHR.

Voice mail that contains patient information can also be included in the EHR. The message should include the provider and patient identification, date and time of message, and the date of time of entry into the EHR.

Handling Materials from Other Facilities

When materials are received from other facilities such as paper-health records or diagnostic images, they should be handled per policy; these typically are added to the health records. Some states have laws that address these external health records. If state law does not address health records from other facilities, then the facility attorney should be consulted regarding whether or not to include them in the health record (AHIMA 2011).

Search, Retrieval, and Manipulation Functions of EHRs

One of the advantages of the EHR is the ability to search, retrieve, and manipulate health data quickly and easily. This information can be used for patient care, research, and monitoring patient care. In the paper-health record, each patient record had to be reviewed individually and data abstracted into a database or other data collection tool. In the EHR, data mining can be performed. Data mining is the process of extracting and analyzing large volumes of data from a database for the purpose of identifying hidden and sometimes subtle relationships or patterns and using those relationships to predict behaviors. Data mining could be used to determine why one physician's outcomes are better or which medication is the most effective.

Handling Amendments and Corrections in EHRs

Policies and procedures need to be in place to address amendments and corrections in the EHR. Once a document is authenticated, the document should be locked in order to prevent changes. In the event that an amendment, addendum, or deletion needs to be made, the document would need to be unlocked. Not everyone should have the ability to unlock the documents; the policies should state who has the rights to unlock the document (Brown et al. 2012). The EHR should retain the previous version of the document and identify who made the change along with the date and time that the change was made. If the change impacts data that is sent to other information systems, then the change must be made in the other systems as well.

Quality Control Functions for EHRs

Data is collected in a number of ways: scanning, data entry, barcodes, and transfer of data from other systems. The information system should have measures in place to control the data entered into the EHR. For example, when entering fields such as the Social Security number (SSN), an input mask should be used. An input mask shows the format that the data will be displayed. Entering the SSN the user should be able to input the number 123456789 and it will appear in the system as 123-45-6789. This prevents one user from entering the SSN as 123456789 and the other as 123-45-6789. A drop-down box that is pre-populated with acceptable entries is another way of controlling what is entered. For example, a drop-down box can be used for states as there are a finite number of states as choices. A checkbox can be used for yes or no type entries. Radio buttons allow the user to select from a small number of choices such as male and female in the gender field.

Best practices for designing or evaluating the entry screens are as follows. All of these features help ensure the quality of documentation and therefore the quality of patient care.

General guidelines

- Clear navigational buttons that direct the user to the next step in the documentation process and buttons to move from one screen to another
- Clear labeling of buttons and data fields
- Limiting the use of abbreviations on buttons and data fields
- Consistent location on the screen of navigation buttons
- Built-in alerts to notify the user of possible errors
- Availability of references at the appropriate data field
- Prompt for more information where appropriate
- Checks for warning signs or errors

Navigation design

- All controls should be clear and placed in an intuitive location on the screen
- Use neutral colors and limit highlighting, flashing, and so forth to reduce eye fatigue
- Limit choices and label commands
- Provide undo buttons to make mistakes easy to override
- Use consistent grammar and terminology
- Provide a confirmation message for any critical function (such as deleting a file)
- Required fields identified

Input design

- Simplify data collection
- Sequence data input to follow workflow

- Provide a title for each screen
- Minimize keystrokes by using pop-up menus
- Use text-specific boxes to enter text
- Use number-specific boxes to enter numbers
- Use a selection box to allow the user to select a value from a predefined list:
    - Check boxes (used for multiple selections)
    - Radio buttons (used for single selections)
    - On-screen list boxes
        - Drop-down list boxes
        - Combo boxes

Data validation

- Perform a completeness check to ensure that all required data have been entered
- Perform a format check to ensure that data are the right type (numeric, alphabetic, and so on)
- Perform a range check to ensure that numeric data are in the correct range such as appropriate range for temperature
- Perform a consistency check to ensure that combinations of data are correct
- Perform a database check to compare data against a database or file to ensure data are correct as entered

Output design

- Minimize the number of clicks needed to reach data or a specific screen
- Combine data into a single, organized menu to eliminate layers of screens (Williams 2006)

Hybrid Record

A healthcare organization cannot move from a paper-based record to an electronic record overnight. The transition can take years and often involves a hybrid record—part of the health record on paper and part of it electronic. During this time, some functions will be handled as described in the paper-based record environment while others may be handled electronically.

As the percentage of the record is digitized increases, more of the functions will be as described in the electronic record environment.

A common system that is used during this transition period is the document management system (DMS). The DMS scans the paper record and stores it digitally. The user has the benefits of immediate access but unfortunately the user is not able to manipulate the data as the document is stored as a picture not data. One of the advantages of a DMS is the ability to control the workflow electronically. This workflow is not limited to the HIM department but can be automatically routed to other users throughout the healthcare facility.

During the period of transition to an EHR, it is difficult to identify the legal health record as some of it is paper, some electronic (and may be a multitude of information systems), and some documents are created electronically but may be printed and stored in the paper health record. (See chapter 4 for more information on the legal health record.) This period is also challenging as the HIM department must manage both the paper and the electronic documents.

 ## Check Your Understanding 3.3

Instructions: **Answer the following questions.**

1. One of the advantages of a DMS is that it can:
   A. Control workflow
   B. Decrease the time records should be retained
   C. Improve communications with physicians
   D. Eliminate all of the problems encountered with the paper record

2. How are amendments handled in the EHR?
   A. Automatically appended to the original note. No additional signature is required.
   B. Amendments must be entered by the same person as the original note.
   C. Amendments cannot be entered after 24 hours of the event.
   D. The amendment must have a separate signature, date, and time.

3. Version control of documents in the EHR requires:
   A. The deletion of old versions and the retention of the most recent
   B. Policies and procedures to control which version(s) is displayed
   C. Signed and unsigned documents not to be considered two versions
   D. Previous versions to be accessible to administration only

4. Which of the following is a risk of copying and pasting?
   A. Reduction in the time required to document
   B. System may not save data
   C. Copying the note in the wrong patient's record
   D. System thinking that the information belongs to the patient from whom the content is being copied

5. When I key in 10101963, the computer displays it as 10/10/1963. What enables this?
   A. Toolkit
   B. Input mask
   C. Check box
   D. Radio button

Medical Transcription

Medical transcription, the process of deciphering and typing medical dictation, may be a part of the HIM department or it may be a separate centralized department where all transcription services are performed. Transcription services may also be outsourced to another company. In that case, there should be a liaison between the HIM department and the transcription company. This liaison would work with physicians, monitor turnaround time, monitor the quality of the work, and more. Commonly transcribed reports include history and physical, discharge summary, pathology reports, and radiology reports. See chapter 4 for a description of these reports.

The transcription manager is responsible for monitoring the quality of the documents and services performed. The transcription supervisor should review a sample of the documents typed to ensure that proper formatting was used, there were no typographical or other errors and it was transcribed in a timely manner. The date dictated and the date transcribed should be recorded on the document. The expected turnaround time is determined by the facility and may vary by document. For example, a radiology report may be transcribed within 24 hours and a discharge summary within three days of dictation.

Today healthcare facilities may use speech recognition to go directly from dictation to a typed document. There are two strategies to be considered. Front-end speech recognition occurs when physicians review and edit the document directly upon dictation and then are able to sign it immediately. The document is available quickly with this strategy. The other strategy is back-end speech recognition. In this strategy, the transcriptionists become editors, making corrections to the document rather than typing it. Because they review and edit the document after dictation, the physician cannot sign the document until a later time. The advantage is that the physician is able to focus on patient care rather than correcting any issues in the document.

Release of Information

One of the responsibilities of the HIM department is release of information. Release of information (ROI) is the process of disclosing patient-identifiable information from the health record to another party. The HIM department receives a request for access to patient information, ensures that the request is appropriate for release and then submits the information for use in patient care, insurance claims, or legal claims. For more information on release of information and privacy requirements, see chapter 9.

Quality Control

The ROI supervisor is responsible for ensuring policies and procedures are followed, the requests are processed in a timely manner, and the staff meets their productivity requirements. Quality control for the ROI function includes ensuring the records are available first and foremost for patient care. It also includes ensuring the requested documents and only the requested documents are submitted.

ROI Turnaround Time Monitoring

The supervisor is responsible for ensuring turnaround times are met. Turnaround time is the time between receipt of request and when the request is sent to requester. The ROI system discussed later in this chapter can report this statistic.

Tracking and Reporting of Disclosures

The ROI staff is responsible for documenting to whom they released information, when it was released, and specifically what was released. This includes specific document(s) and the dates of service. A copy of the formal request for copies of patient information must be retained by the HIM department.

Clinical Coding

Clinical coding, or assigning codes to represent diagnoses and procedures, is a key responsibility of the HIM department. A number of coding systems can be used. During the coding process, data is abstracted into the information system. **Abstracting** can be either the process of extracting information from a document to create a brief summary of a patient's illness, treatment, and outcome, or the process of extracting elements of data from a source document or database and entering them into an automated system. The amount of data varies by facility but includes data such as date of surgery, surgeon, and disposition of patient upon discharge (went home, transferred to another hospital, and so forth). The codes are included on the bill and are used to determine reimbursement that the healthcare facility will receive. The coding supervisor must ensure the quality of code assignment and the timeliness of the coding process. If the coding process gets behind, the encounters cannot be billed, thus ensuring that reimbursement for patient care is delayed.

HIM Interdepartmental Relationships

Managing information cannot be performed by the HIM department in isolation. The HIM department must work with a number of departments, including the following, to ensure that they have the information that they need to perform their jobs.

- *Patient registration:* The health record typically begins in patient registration with the capture of patient demographic information. This information is entered into the MPI as discussed earlier. The health record is assigned to new patients during the patient registration process. The HIM department works with patient registration to ensure the quality of the data collected and to correct duplicate and other issues with the MPI.

- *Billing department:* The billing department uses the codes assigned and data abstracted by the coders as part of the billing process. Because of this, the billing department cannot perform their responsibilities until the HIM department completes theirs. The two departments must work together to ensure that all of the information required for billing is available.

- *Patient care departments:* The HIM department works closely with nursing units, emergency department, and other patient care areas to ensure they have access to the patient's health records from previous encounters. In a paper-based environment, the records are delivered by the HIM staff or picked up by the patient care areas and then the records are returned once they are no longer needed. The departments may send loose reports found to the HIM department for filing if the health record has already been returned.

- *Information systems:* The interaction between the HIM department and the information systems department will continue to increase as the EHR becomes more and more important to the organization. The HIM staff works with the information systems staff to plan, implement, and maintain information systems that impact the health record and other systems related to HIM. The information system also assists the HIM department with technical issues related to computers, printers, and other hardware. For more information, see chapter 11.

- *Quality management:* The quality management department depends on the health record to complete their functions. They need health records for committee meetings, audits, and outcome monitoring. HIM staff may collect some of the data needed, provide the records, generate statistics, write reports, mine data, or assist in other ways.

- *Virtual HIM:* Much of the work of the HIM department can be performed remotely due to the implementation of the EHR. Some healthcare corporations have centralized their HIM services into a single location while others have staff that work at home. Common functions that can be performed from home include coding and transcription, but others can be performed remotely as well. The manager must ensure that the employees are able to work independently so that productivity standards can still be met. Refer to chapter 1 to learn more about the future of the HIM profession.

HIM Software

The HIM department cannot perform the functions of the department efficiently without the use of software. Some of these systems are becoming more and more important with the implementation of the EHR and others may be phased out completely as the EHR makes it obsolete.

Release of Information

The ROI system tracks requests for information. HIM staff enters basic information from the request such as the patient name, health record number, and who is requesting the health record. Once the information is released, the staff records what is released and the date. The system is able to bill requesters for the copies of records, when appropriate. It can monitor productivity and turnaround time.

Chart Tracking

This system currently tracks the location of the health record but will eventually become obsolete when paper records are eliminated. It records who checked it out, where it went, and how long it has been checked out. It also records when the health record returns to the HIM department.

Coding

Coders use two specialty information systems—encoders and groupers. An **encoder** assigns the diagnosis and procedure codes. The encoder can query the coder to determine if related codes should be assigned. The **grouper** uses the codes assigned to determine the diagnostic-related group or other grouping. (See chapter 15 for specifics on diagnostic related groups.) Some healthcare facilities are now using **computer-assisted coding**, which uses EHR data to assign the codes. The HIM professional monitors the quality of the codes assigned by the computer system.

Registries

A **registry** is a database on specific diseases and procedures; for example, cancer and transplant registries are common ones. Information of the condition is captured and can be used for research, patient care, and quality monitoring. For more details on registries, see chapter 7.

Billing

The HIM department may or may not directly use the billing system. The encoder and grouper may submit the codes and other data directly to the billing system or it may be entered manually by the coder. The HIM department does not create the bill but rather provide information that is included on the bill.

Quality Improvement

Quality improvement systems go by many different names and perform a number of functions but characteristically they are a repository of data that is used to monitor trends, generate statistics, monitor outcomes, and improve the quality of the documentation in the EHR.

Electronic Health Records

The electronic health record (EHR) utilizes a number of information systems to capture patient information. These source systems supply the EHR with demographic information, test results, dictated reports, and more. The EHR also has **clinical decision support (CDS)**, which assists physicians and other users when making decisions regarding medications, diagnoses, and such based on the information entered into the EHR. The EHR contains alerts and reminders to notify the user of medication allergies, tests that should be performed, immunizations due, and so forth. Benefits of the EHR include reduction in administrative costs and improvement in quality of care. The organization becomes more efficient with the improved accessibility to health information.

One of the programs managed by the Centers for Medicare and Medicaid Services is Meaningful Use. **Meaningful Use** is "using certified electronic health record (EHR) technology to:

- Improve quality, safety, efficiency, and reduce health disparities
- Engage patients and family
- Improve care coordination, and population and public health
- Maintain privacy and security of patient health information

Ultimately, it is hoped that the Meaningful Use compliance will result in:

- Better clinical outcomes
- Improved population health outcomes
- Increased transparency and efficiency

- Empowered individuals
- More robust research data on health systems" (HealthIT 2015)

Certified electronic health record technology is an EHR that has been verified by organizations approved by CMS to ensure that the EHRs meet minimum standards. In order to receive incentive payments for implementing the EHR, the healthcare organizations must choose one of the certified EHR technologies. For more on Meaningful Use, see chapter 16.

Personal Health Records

Personal health records are "an electronic or paper health record maintained and updated by an individual for himself or herself; a tool that individuals can use to collect, track, and share past and current information about their health or the health of someone in their care" (myPHR 2015). The PHR provides a way for patient's involvement in his or her healthcare. It is not the same as an EHR, but rather is a subset of the information that is available to and controlled by the patient. The patient can add information to the PHR, such as over the counter medications and self-administered blood glucose test results. The PHR is especially useful for patients with complex, chronic conditions. The PHR may be provided by the healthcare provider, the insurance company, or the patient may purchase or subscribe to it from a commercial vendor.

 Check Your Understanding 3.4

Instructions: **Answer the following questions.**

1. Which of the following is controlled by patients?
   A. Electronic health record
   B. Health record in any format
   C. Personal health record
   D. Certified health record

2. Where will you find clinical decision support?
   A. Electronic health record
   B. Health record in any format
   C. Personal health record
   D. Natural language processing

3. Which of the following systems is used to track whether or not a request for information has been processed?
   A. Chart tracking
   B. Release of information
   C. Encoder
   D. Registry

4. With which department does the HIM department interact to perform audits and monitor outcomes?
   A. Billing
   B. Quality improvement
   C. Patient care departments
   D. Virtual HIM

5. What type of speech recognition is used when the physician edits the document?
   A. Front-end
   B. Back-end
   C. Provider
   D. Enhanced

Real-World Case 3.1

General Hospital knew they had a problem with duplicate health records and needed to clean up the MPI before the implementation date for the EHR in order to get the best results. A consulting firm was hired and a review of the data confirmed this problem when they 3,000 potential duplicate health records issued over the past five years were identified. The hospital started the MPI clean-up process by educating their patient registration staff on proper search strategies, questions to ask the patient, the importance of a unit health record, and other related topics. This education was an important first step so that additional duplicate health records would not be assigned while the clean-up process was going on. Once the training was complete, the consulting firm began cleaning up the MPI. The consultants reviewed the potential duplicate health records and merged the records where appropriate. They also ensured the health records were merged in other information systems used throughout the healthcare facility. They provided documentation to General Hospital showing which health records were and were not duplicates based on their review.

Real-World Case 3.2

The University of Wisconsin Hospital and Clinics (UWHC) received AHIMA's first Grace Award. This award is given to a healthcare organization that is innovative in the use of health information. UWHC collects all documentation electronically either through direct entry, scanning, or from a variety of information systems throughout the organization. Information from other facilities can be directly faxed into the EHR and be available for access within two hours. Patients are able to access information to schedule appointments and access test results. Physicians are reminded that the patient is due for tests or other services (Dooling and Wiedemann 2012).

References

American Health Information Management Association. 2014. Appropriate Use of the Copy and Paste Functionality in Electronic Health Records. http://bok.ahima.org/PdfView?oid=300306.

American Health Information Management Association. 2011. Fundamentals of the legal health record and designated record set. *Journal of AHIMA.* 82(2):44–49.

American Health Information Management Association. 2010. Fundamentals for building a master patient index/enterprise master patient index (updated). *Journal of AHIMA.* http://bok.ahima.org/doc?oid=10622.

American Health Information Management Association. 1997. Practice brief: Developing information capture tools. *Journal of AHIMA.* 68(3):Supplement.

Brown, L., P. Komara, D. Warner, L.A. Wiedemann. 2012. Amendments in the Electronic Health Record Toolkit. http://bok.ahima.org/PdfView?oid=105672.

Cerrato, L.A. and J. Roberts. 2012. Health Information Functions. Chapter 7 in *Health Information Management Technology: An Applied Approach*, 4th ed. Chicago: AHIMA.

Dooling, J. and L.A. Wiedemann. 2012 (November). AHIMA issues first Grace Award: University of Wisconsin Hospital and Clinics receives HIM excellence award. *Journal of AHIMA.* 83(11):26–27.

HealthIT. 2015. Meaningful Use and Objectives. http://www.healthit.gov/providers-professionals/meaningful-use-definition-objectives.

Huffman, E.K. 1994. *Health Information Management.* Berwyn, IL: Physician Record Co.

myPHR. 2015. What Is a Personal Health Record (PHR)? https://www.myphr.com/StartaPHR/what_is_a_phr.aspx.

Williams, A. 2006. Design for better data: How software and users interact on screen matters to data quality. *Journal of AHIMA.* 77(2):56–60.

Part II
Data Content Structures and Standards

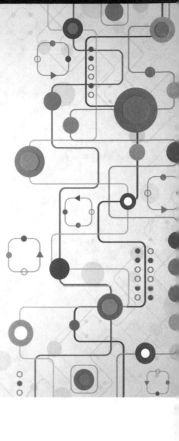

4

Health Record Content and Documentation

Megan R Brickner, MSA, RHIA

Learning Objectives

- Define documentation standards and describe how medical staff bylaws, accreditation entities, and state and federal regulations influence the documentation practice standards of healthcare provider organizations
- Articulate how documentation standards drive patient safety and quality within the healthcare industry
- Describe how the definition of a legal health record has changed as healthcare providers have more

widely adopted electronic health record (EHR) technologies
- Identify and describe the documentation content of health records within different healthcare settings
- Compare different health record media and evaluate the potential advantages and disadvantages of each
- Describe the differences among consents, authorizations, and acknowledgments
- Describe the roles that various healthcare professionals play in health record documentation

Key Terms

Accreditation
Accreditation organizations
Acknowledgments
Administrative data
Ambulatory
Ambulatory surgery center/
   ambulatory surgical center
   (ASC)
American Association for
   Accreditation of Ambulatory
   Surgery Facilities (AAAASF)
Ancillary services

Anesthesia report
Authentication
Authorization
Auto-authentication
Autopsy report
Care area assessments (CAAs)
Care plan
Centers for Medicare and Medicaid
   Services (CMS)
Certification
Clinical data
Clinical observations

Commission for the Accreditation
   of Birth Centers
Commission on Accreditation
   of Rehabilitation Facilities
   (CARF)
Conditions for Coverage
Conditions of Participation
Consent to treatment
Consultation report
Deemed status
Discharge summary
Documentation

Documentation standards
Documents imaging
Emergency Medical Treatment and
    Active Labor Act (EMTALA)
Expressed consent
History and physical (H&P)
Hybrid record
Implied consent
Informed consent
Integrated health record
Joint Commission
Legal health record
Licensure

Medical history
Medical staff
Medical staff bylaws
Medical staff privileges
Minimum Data Set (MDS) for
    Long-Term Care
Operative report
Pathology report
Patient assessment instrument
    (PAI)
Physical examination
Physician orders
Problem list

Problem-oriented health record
Progress notes
Recovery room report
Resident assessment instrument
    (RAI)
Source-oriented health record
Subjective, objective, assessment,
    plan (SOAP)
Standard
Standing orders
Statute
Transfer record
Universal chart order

Documentation is the recording of pertinent healthcare findings, interventions, and responses to treatment as a business record and form of communication among caregivers. The health record, specifically, centralizes a patient's healthcare visit and treatment history in an official, permanent, and recorded format. For thousands of years, individuals have found documentation essential for the retelling of stories or the recording of actual events occurring at the present time, codifying such stories and events in written form, in order to be shared and re-shared with future generations. Healthcare documentation is no exception. The health record, specifically the documentation maintained within it, has historically allowed and presently enables the patient's healthcare providers to make well-informed concurrent treatment decisions for the patient and establishes a healthcare history for the patient for future reference.

Documentation Standards

A **standard** is a set of principles, codes, beliefs, guidelines, and regulations that have been vetted and agreed upon by an individual or a group of individuals who are regarded as an authority on a particular subject matter. Standards are evaluated conformance with a generally accepted rule. Within the context of healthcare, **documentation standards** describe those principles, codes, beliefs, guidelines, and regulations that guide health record documentation. Documentation standards dictate how healthcare providers should document the treatment and services (rendered to the patient) within the health record. The basis for healthcare-related documentation standards is to promote healthcare quality and safety, as well as provide for optimized continuity of care for the patient. As the health record and the health record documentation has become more computer-based, documentation standards have become even more important, not only from a clinical documentation standpoint but also from a organizational standpoint. How health record documentation is used within the electronic health record (EHR) has become a focus of many health information management (HIM) professionals.

When the EHR first began replacing traditional paper-based health records, a common belief was the standards addressing the documentation contained within the EHR (covered in chapter 11) were somehow different from those standards addressing the documentation in a paper-based chart; however, this is not the case. In general, the standards that traditionally applied to paper-based documentation hold true for documentation generated and maintained within the EHR. As healthcare provider organizations have come to realize the great benefits of EHR technologies as they relate to documentation quality and overall patient safety, those same technologies have also presented a number of challenges. One example is the use of a template. A template is a pattern used in EHRs to capture data in a structured manner and specify the information to be collected. For example, a birthrecord template would require data such as date of birth, time of birth, APGAR scores, length, weight, and so forth. It helps the care provider ensure key information is not forgotten. It also certifies the data is captured in a specific order and format. Whether the patient's health record is electronic or paper-based, accurate and appropriate documentation is key to meeting compliance standards—namely, those for medical necessity and the justification for treating the patient.

Standards

Over the years, documentation standards have become more detailed and focus on patient care quality, appropriate reimbursement, and the prevention of fraud and abuse from a regulatory perspective now more than ever. Centers for Medicare and Medicaid Services (CMS) defines *fraud* as the intentional deception or misrepresentation that an individual knows, or should know, to be false or does not believe to be true, knowing the deception could result in some unauthorized benefit to himself or some other person(s) and *abuse* describes practices that either directly or indirectly result in unnecessary costs to the Medicare Program (CMS 2015). Abuse includes any practice that is not consistent with the goals of providing patients with services that are medically necessary, meet professionally recognized standards, and priced fairly. (See chapter 16 for additional information on fraud and abuse.) The application of the standards varies depending upon the content of health record; whether the record is an inpatient, ambulatory, behavioral health, or physician office record; and from where the standards originate. Sources for standards include insurance companies and payers, government regulatory agencies, licensing boards, accrediting bodies, facility policies and procedures, and healthcare provider organization medical staff bylaws.

With the focus on patient care quality, appropriate reimbursement, and the prevention of fraud and abuse, the goal of documentation standards is to ensure what is documented in the health record is complete and accurately reflects the treatment provided to the patient. This provides an inherent level of acceptable quality so other healthcare providers have a clear and accurate understanding of the patient's condition and how the patient is responding to treatment. In addition, documentation standards drive appropriate reimbursement through accurate code capture during the revenue cycle process, reducing the chances that inaccurate or fraudulent claims are processed and sent to commercial or governmental payers for reimbursement.

Medical Staff Bylaws

A healthcare provider organization's **medical staff bylaws**—the standards governing the practice of medical staff members typically voted upon by the organized medical staff and the medical staff executive committee and approved by the facility's board of directors—play an important role in documentation standards mandates and development. Accreditation organizations measure the compliance of the healthcare organization with the standards developed by the accreditation organization. **Licensure** organizations are the legal authority or formal permission from the authorities to carry on certain activities that require such permission and federal and state regulatory agencies mandate the content, specifically the breadth and depth of these bylaws as well as the application of the bylaws. In addition, although there are many content requirements related to medical staff bylaws they will vary slightly from one organization to another. Before addressing the medical staff bylaws themselves, it is important to understand the function and responsibility of an organization's medical staff.

A healthcare organization's **medical staff** is a group of physicians and nonphysicians such as nurse practitioners and physician assistants who have **medical staff privileges**, specific services and procedures that the medical staff member is deemed qualified to perform, to practice medicine at a particular healthcare provider organization (ACEP 2015). The medical staff are governed by medical staff bylaws. These bylaws govern the business conduct, rights, and responsibilities of the medical staff; medical staff members must abide by these bylaws in order to continue to practice in the healthcare facility. It is through the medical staff and enforcement of the medical staff bylaws that the overall quality of care and treatment provided to patients by the physicians credentialed and privileged at a healthcare organization is governed (Adelman 2012, 3). Credentialing is the process of reviewing and validating the qualifications (degrees, licenses, and other credentials) of physicians and other licensed independent practitioners for granting medical staff privileges to provide patient care services.

A number of accrediting, licensing, and regulatory entities drive the configuration of the medical staff and the content and application of the medical staff bylaws of an organization. The **Centers for Medicare and Medicaid Services (CMS)** is the federal agency within the US Department of Health and Human Services (HHS). (CMS and its roles and responsibilities are discussed in chapter 15.) CMS is known for its operational oversight of the Medicare program and in collaboration with state governments. CMS also plays an important regulatory role in an organization's medical staff makeup and the content of the medical staff bylaws. CMS and the Joint Commission both mandate the content of the bylaws. Additional information on The Joint Commission can be found in chapter 4. The required content includes a healthcare provider organization's processes for self-governance and general oversight obligations, due process rights as they relate to potential disciplinary action, peer review policies and procedures, medical staff appointment, privileging, and credentialing (CMS 2015). CMS mandates the medical staff bylaws must:

- Be approved by the governing body of the medical staff;

- Address the duties and privileges of each medical staff category (active, courtesy, and such);

- Describe the organization of the medical staff;

- Describe the qualifications that must be met by any individual wishing to seek appointment to the medical staff (42 CFR 482.22(c)).

In addition, through its **Conditions of Participation (CoPs)**—the administrative (policy and procedure requirements) and operational guidelines (how the policies and procedures are carried out) under which facilities are allowed to take part in the Medicare and Medicaid programs—CMS dictates medical staff bylaws must address certain documentation requirements that include the requirement that a medical **history and physical (H&P)** be documented for every patient no more than 30 days before or 24 hours after admission to the hospital. The H&P contains pertinent information about the patient including chief complaint, past and present illnesses, family history, social history, and review of body systems and must be documented and in the chart prior to any surgery or procedure requiring the patient to receive anesthesia. If, however, the physical exam is completed within the 30 days of a surgery or procedure, an updated exam must be documented within 24 hours of admission and prior to the surgery or procedure. This updated exam must include any changes in the patient's condition since the time of the first exam. Autopsies are also addressed in the CoPs as a component of the medical staff bylaws (42 CFR 482.22(c)).

Accreditation

Accreditation is a voluntary process of institutional or organizational review in which a quasi-independent body created for this purpose periodically evaluates the quality of the entity's work against pre-established written criteria. CMS CoPs and **Conditions for Coverage (CFCs)** ensure patient care quality, safety, and improvement of clinical outcomes. CFCs are standards applied to facilities that choose to participate in federal government reimbursement programs such as Medicare and Medicaid (CMS 2015). In order for a healthcare organization to participate in federal government reimbursement programs, healthcare provider organizations must demonstrate they at least meet, if not exceed, the CoPs and CFCs.

Auditing and monitoring are the main ways the government, whether state or federal, measure a healthcare provider organization's compliance with the CoPs and CFCs standards and criteria. (For additional information on auditing and monitoring, see chapter 17.) The government allows healthcare provider organizations that are accredited by an approved accreditation organization to be exempt from direct government auditing and monitoring. The accreditation organization—a professional organization that establishes the standards against which healthcare organizations are measured for compliance with the CoPs and CFCs standards and criteria—must go through its own CMS review in order to receive deemed status, an official designation indicating that a healthcare facility is in compliance with the Medicare Conditions of Participation (CMS 2015). It is through this obtained deemed status that the accreditation organization is permitted to evaluate other healthcare provider organizations for CoP and CFC compliance through its accreditation process.

Many healthcare provider organizations seek accreditation because it gives the organization an opportunity to measure its own compliance as well as see what operational improvements it can make based upon the findings of the accreditation organization. Patients also want to see that the healthcare provider they are entrusting their care to is in compliance with quality and clinical outcome measures. Accreditation enhances reputation among healthcare organizations that take part in the process. In most cases the accreditation process is voluntary, but for specific programs and services

the healthcare organization must be accredited by an accreditation organization in order to participate in the Medicare and Medicaid programs. There are currently nine national accreditation organizations that have obtained deemed status by CMS and are responsible for surveying healthcare provider organizations who are currently participating in the Medicare and Medicaid programs (see table 4.1).

Although there are many high quality accreditation organizations in existence today, all with the common goals of patient safety and the delivery of high quality healthcare to patients, the Joint Commission has been an industry leader in the area of healthcare provider organization accreditation. The Joint Commission has performed better in the area of its own continuous improvement in terms of its survey processes and the updating of its criteria and standards to better reflect industry changes in clinical and operational practices and understanding (Pollack 2013). The Joint Commission also provides its member organizations with education and compliance outreach services.

Over the years, the Joint Commission has expanded its accreditation program offerings and currently provides accreditation for ambulatory healthcare, behavioral health, critical access hospitals, homecare, hospital, laboratory, nursing care centers, physician offices, and office-based surgery centers. In addition to the different types of healthcare provider organizations that can seek and obtain Joint Commission accreditation, specific programs addressing specific disease processes can also obtain

Table 4.1 CMS-approved accrediting organizations

Accreditation organization	Program
Accreditation Association for Ambulatory Health Care (AAAHC)	Ambulatory surgery centers
Accreditation Commission for Health Care (ACHC)	Home health, hospice
American Association for Accreditation of Ambulatory Surgery Facilities (AAAASF)	Ambulatory surgery centers, occupational therapy, rural health clinics
American Osteopathic Association/Healthcare Facilities Accreditation Program (HFAP)	Ambulatory surgery centers, critical access hospitals, hospital
Center for Improvement in Healthcare Quality (CIHQ)	Hospital
Community Health Accreditation Program (CHAP)	Home health, hospice
DNV GL Healthcare	Critical access hospitals, hospital
The Compliance Team	Rural health clinics
Joint Commission	Ambulatory surgery centers, critical access hospitals, hospital, home health, hospice, psychiatric hospital

Source: CMS 2015.

accreditation through the Joint Commission certification process (Joint Commission 2016a).

Certification is the process by which a duly authorized body evaluates and recognizes an individual, institution, or educational program as meeting predetermined requirements. The more commonly known programs that often obtain certification address asthma, diabetes, and heart failure (Joint Commission 2016b–d).

Compliance, quality, and patient safety have become the focal points of the healthcare industry's clinical and operational practices. The Joint Commission responded to this shift in focus by moving from announced reviews that occurred once every three years to unannounced reviews, coupled with changes to the review process itself. Much like many other accreditation organizations. The Joint Commission provides organizations that choose to obtain or maintain their accreditation with an accreditation manual. The manual is comprised of chapters addressing various areas of clinical and operational practice, including but not limited to:

- Environment of Care
- Leadership
- Provision of Care, Treatment, and Services
- Life Safety
- Information Management (Joint Commission 2016e)

The chapters contain specific standards and elements that describe in detail the continuous compliance expectations for the healthcare organization. Each standard and element has a corresponding explanation and scoring procedure associated with it.

The Joint Commission places emphasis on appropriate and standardized health record documentation. Those standards and elements address health record content, legibility and completeness, dating and timing of entries, order sets, abbreviations, history and physical component requirements, and informed consent, among many other standards and elements. With the proliferation of electronic health record technologies, accreditation manuals now address documentation issues in relation to health record documentation standards within the electronic realm.

State Statutes

A **statute** is a piece of legislation written and approved by a state or federal legislature and then signed into law by the state's governor, or President of the United States. State statutes, as they relate to health record documentation, vary by state in terms of what components of health record documentation are regulated and to what degree it is regulated by law. In many instances, state statutes address the documentation requirements according to the type of health record. For example, Ohio law addresses the specific documentation requirements for inpatient psychiatric service providers. The Ohio Administrative Code describes how involved a patient should be in his or her care plan and how the care plan should be documented.

Legal Health Record

In the past, the term *health record* and *legal health record* were used interchangeably, and the subtle nuances of these two terms provided little impact to the operations of a healthcare provider (for more information about the health record, refer to chapter 3). The **legal health record**, by definition was simple when health records were primarily paper-based and included the contents of the paper health record in addition to diagnostic radiographic films or x-rays; the health record and the legal health record were one and the same. This changed when electronic health record technology was adopted and healthcare provider organizations moved from strictly paper-based to a more **hybrid record** model, and then to a fully electronic format.

The current definition of what is considered a legal health record is complicated. Each healthcare organization must define what its legal health record contains. The role of the legal health record includes documentation to support decisions made in the course of treating a patient, support documentation for the revenue pursued by payers, as well as documentation used for legal testimony related to the patient's disease process, injury, treatment, decisions related to the treatment, and the patient's response to the treatment (AHIMA 2011, 2). One issue raised by healthcare organizations who have an EHR is what to do with records from a different healthcare provider organization when those records in one way or another make their way into the patient's health record. Do those other provider's records become part of the legal health record of another organization? At one time, there was no doubt that not only incorporating another provider's health record into the legal health record but also the releasing of that documentation was part of an organization's legal health record. The healthcare organization should consult with their attorney in order to assist with making a decision about whether or not to include these records in the legal health record. Some state laws dictate what can and cannot be included in the healthcare organization's legal medical record and, in many cases, the hospital's attorney is in the best position to decide to include or exclude the records from other providers. In order for the EHR to be a legal health record and meet the requirements as such there are several concepts that need to be considered, including how documentation is actually created and signed off on by the healthcare providers; how the documentation is managed and preserved; how the documentation impacts and interacts with the revenue cycle functions of billing and claims submission; and how the documentation is displayed both electronically to the user as well as in hard copy form, should the data be printed (HIMSS 2011). Once an organization defines its legal health record, necessary policies and procedures should be developed in order to formalize the organization's approach to defining such a record. See chapter 8 for more information about the legal health record.

Check Your Understanding 4.1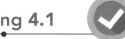

Instructions: **Answer the following questions.**

1. The overall goal of documentation standards is:
   A. To ensure physicians have access to the health record information they need to care for the patient
   B. To ensure that the healthcare provider organization is reimbursed appropriately by payers
   C. To ensure that CMS does not find reason to fine the healthcare provider organization
   D. To ensure what is documented in the health record is complete and accurately reflects the treatment provided to the patient

2. A hospital that participates in the Medicare and Medicaid programs must follow:
   A. The medical bylaws of the healthcare provider organization
   B. The Conditions of Participation
   C. The accreditation organization
   D. The plan

3. When defining its legal health record, a healthcare provider organization must do which of the following?
   A. Assess the legal environment
   B. Determine what other healthcare provider organizations are doing
   C. Decide if a legal health record is needed
   D. Include only the paper components of the health record

4. Which of the following is the health record component that addresses the patient's current complaints and symptoms and lists the patient's past medical, personal, and family history?
   A. Problem list
   B. Medical history
   C. Physical examination
   D. Clinical observation

General Documentation Guidelines

General documentation guidelines apply to all categories of healthcare records. These guidelines address the uniformity, accuracy, completeness, legibility, authenticity, timeliness, frequency, and format of health record entries. The American Health Information Management Association (AHIMA) developed the following general documentation guidelines:

- Every healthcare organization should have policies that ensure the uniformity of both the content and the format of the health record. The policies should be based on all applicable accreditation standards, federal and state regulations, payer requirements, and professional practice standards.

- The health record should be organized systematically in order to facilitate data retrieval and compilation.

- Only individuals authorized by the organization's policies should be allowed to enter documentation in the health record.

- Organizational policy and medical staff rules and regulations should specify who may receive and transcribe verbal physician's orders.

- Health record entries should be documented at the time the services described are rendered.

- The authors of all entries should be clearly identified in the record.

- Only abbreviations and symbols approved by the organization and medical staff rules and regulations should be used in the health record.

- All entries in the health record should be permanent.

- Errors in paper-based records should be corrected according to the following process: Draw a single line in ink through the incorrect entry. Then print the word "error" at the top of the entry along with a legal signature or initials, the date, time, and reason for change, and the title and discipline of the individual making the correction. The correct information is then added to the entry. Errors must never be obliterated. The original entry should remain legible, and the corrections should be entered in chronological order. Any late entries should be labeled as such.

- Any corrections or information added to the record by the patient should be inserted as an addendum (a separate note). No changes should be made in the original entries in the record. Any information added to the health record by the patient should be clearly identified as a patient addendum (Smith 2001, 56).

- When errors in the EHR are corrected, the erroneous information should not be displayed; however, there should be a method to view the previous version of the document with the original data (Wiedemann 2010).

From a governmental regulatory perspective, CMS and federal regulations also address what would be considered general documentation guidelines and further explains what this guidance means.

- All health record entries must be legible. Orders, progress notes, nursing notes, or other entries in the health record that are not legible may be misread or misinterpreted and may lead to medical errors or other adverse patient events.

- All entries in the health record must be complete. A health record is considered complete if it contains sufficient information to identify the patient; support the diagnosis or condition; justify the care, treatment, and services; document the course and results of care, treatment, and services; and promote continuity of care among healthcare providers.

- The time and date of each entry (orders, reports, notes) must be accurately documented. Timing establishes when an order was given, when an activity happened, or when an activity is to occur. Timing and dating entries is necessary for patient safety and quality of care. Timing and dating of entries establishes a baseline for future actions or assessments and establishes a timeline of events.

- There must be a method to establish the identity of the author of each entry.
- There must be a method to require that each author takes a specific action to verify that the entry being authenticated is his or her entry or that he or she is responsible for the entry and the entry is accurate (42 CFR 482.24(c)(1)).

Authentication is the process of identifying the source of health record entries by attaching a hand-written signature, the author's initials, or an electronic signature. CMS defines what authentication methods are to be used for health record entries such as written signatures, initials, computer key, or other code; the requirements healthcare provider organizations need to have in place; and controls to

prevent any changes from being made to the health record after and the entries have been authenticated (42 CFR 482.24(c)(1)).

Auto-authentication is a procedure that allows dictated reports to be considered automatically signed unless the HIM department is notified of needed revisions within a certain time limit or a process by which the failure of an author to review and affirmatively approve or disapprove an entry within a specified time period results in authentication. For example, a physician dictated an operation, the operative report is transcribed, but the physician never accesses the report to review for accuracy and completeness. The EHR system is set up to show the physician signed the operative report even though he or she never reviewed the document. Auto-authentication does not meet standards for appropriate timing, dating, and signing-off of documentation by healthcare providers and therefore should not be used.

Check Your Understanding 4.2

Instructions: **Answer the following questions.**

1. General documentation guidelines apply to:
   A. Only electronic health records
   B. All categories of healthcare records
   C. Only emergency health records
   D. Clinical observations

2. True or false: Health record entries should be documented at the time the services they describe are rendered.

3. True or false: Only individuals authorized by the organization's policies should be allowed to enter documentation in the health record.

4. True or false: Auto-authentication is the preferred method of authentication.

5. True or false: When an error is made, the erroneous information can be obliterated.

Documentation by Setting

Despite the different settings in which healthcare can be provided—hospitals, ambulatory surgery centers, physician offices, long-term care facilities—health records contain two distinct types

of information: *clinical* and *administrative*. A significant portion of administrative data is demographic data. Healthcare provider organizations provide each patient his or her own health record whether in paper-based, electronic, or hybrid format. The HIM industry is beginning to use a comprehensive and centralized health record for the patient within the health provider organization. This comprehensive and centralized health record allows hospitals to see the documentation of the patient's outpatient providers and these outpatient providers can also see the patient's hospital-based (inpatient) documentation. Both the inpatient and outpatient health record documentation is maintained in one health record rather than separate and distinct records. Whether the health record is paper-based, electronic, or hybrid, there are distinct differences among the health record documentation an HIM professional will encounter within the health record itself. It is important to understand these differences so the HIM professional can navigate the health record more efficiently despite the setting or format. Inpatient, emergency department, ambulatory, ambulatory surgery, ancillary, physician office, long term care, rehabilitation, and behavioral health settings are discussed below in more detail.

Inpatient Health Record

The inpatient health record is generated when a patient is provided with room, board, and continuous general nursing care in an area of an acute-care facility, such as a hospital, where the patient generally stays overnight at that facility. The documents that one may typically find in an inpatient health record includes, but is not limited to, history and physical (H&P), consultation reports, physician's orders and progress notes, nursing assessments and progress notes, as well as a discharge summary. Over the years, there has been a dramatic shift in the delivery of healthcare treatment and services. Many services such as surgery, infusions, and other diagnostic procedures that once required a patient to stay overnight in the hospital can be performed on an outpatient basis. Only the most severely ill patients and the most invasive procedures require an overnight stay and therefore the inpatient health record is the most complex.

Within the inpatient care services continuum, there are three major health records categories that will be addressed—medical and surgical, obstetric, and newborn.

Medical and Surgical

The medical and surgical health record is found in a variety of settings including inpatient care units, long-term care facilities, home health, surgical centers, and ambulatory care units. Medical and surgical health record documentation pertains to adult patients with various acute and active disease processes or injuries. The medical and surgical health record contains documentation originating from physicians, nurses, diagnostic procedures, as well as from the dietary, pharmacy, and social services departments. The medical and surgical record is a common type of health record that HIM professionals will encounter. The categories of information found in the medical and surgical record include clinical data, administrative data, and consents, authorizations, and acknowledgments.

Clinical Data   Clinical data is the information that reflects the treatment and services provided to the patient as well as how the patient responded to such treatment and services; it is also the basis for the reimbursement of the treatment and service rendered to the patient. The clinical data portion of the acute-care record constitutes the largest portion of the health record and consists of nine separate and distinct parts.

Medical History   The medical history portion of clinical data addresses the patient's current complaints and symptoms and lists his or her past medical, personal, and family history. In inpatient care, the medical history is the responsibility of the attending physician. Medical histories obtained by specialists such as gynecologists and cardiologists concentrate on the organ systems involved in the patient's current illness. Table 4.2 shows the information that is usually included in a medical history.

It is important to note that the *chief complaint* is a component of the medical history that is told to the healthcare provider by the patient and in the patient's own words. Examples of a chief complaint include vomiting, headache, and abdominal pain.

Table 4.2 Information included in a complete medical history

Components of the history	Complaints and symptoms
Chief complaint	Nature and duration of the symptoms that caused the patient to seek medical attention as stated in his or her own words
Present illness	Detailed chronological description of the development of the patient's illness, from the appearance of the first symptom to the present situation
Past medical history	Summary of childhood and adult illnesses and conditions, such as infectious diseases, pregnancies, allergies and drug sensitivities, accidents, operations, hospitalizations, and current medications
Social and personal history	Marital status; dietary, sleep, and exercise patterns; use of coffee, tobacco, alcohol, and other drugs; occupation; home environment; daily routine
Family medical history	Diseases among relatives in which heredity or contact might play a role such as allergies, cancer, and infectious, psychiatric, metabolic, endocrine, cardiovascular, and renal diseases; health status or cause of and age at death for immediate relatives
Review of systems	Systemic inventory designed to uncover current or past subjective symptoms that includes the following types of data: • *General:* Usual weight, recent weight changes, fever, weakness, fatigue • *Skin:* Rashes, eruptions, dryness, cyanosis, jaundice; changes in skin, hair, or nails • *Head:* Headache (duration, severity, character, location) • *Eyes:* Glasses or contact lenses, last eye examination, glaucoma, cataracts, eyestrain, pain, diplopia, redness, lacrimation, inflammation, blurring • *Ears:* Hearing, discharge, tinnitus, dizziness, pain • *Nose:* Head colds, epistaxis, discharges, obstruction, postnasal drip, sinus pain • *Mouth and throat:* Condition of teeth and gums, last dental examination, soreness, redness, hoarseness, difficulty in swallowing • *Respiratory system:* Chest pain, wheezing, cough, dyspnea, sputum (color and quantity), hemoptysis, asthma, bronchitis, emphysema, pneumonia, tuberculosis, pleurisy, last chest x-ray • *Neurological system:* Fainting, blackouts, seizures, paralysis, tingling, tremors, memory loss • *Musculoskeletal system:* Joint pain or stiffness, arthritis, gout, backache, muscle pain, cramps, swelling, redness, limitation in motor activity • *Cardiovascular system:* Chest pain, rheumatic fever, tachycardia, palpitation, high blood pressure, edema, vertigo, faintness, varicose veins, thrombophlebitis • *Gastrointestinal system:* Appetite, thirst, nausea, vomiting, hematemesis, rectal bleeding, change in bowel habits, diarrhea, constipation, indigestion, food intolerance, flatus, hemorrhoids, jaundice • *Urinary system:* Frequent or painful urination, nocturia, pyuria, hematuria, incontinence, urinary infections • *Genitoreproductive system:* Male—venereal disease, sores, discharge from penis, hernias, testicular pain, or masses; female—age at menarche, frequency and duration of menstruation, dysmenorrhea, menorrhagia, symptoms of menopause, contraception, pregnancies, deliveries, abortions, last Pap smear • *Endocrine system:* Thyroid disease; heat or cold intolerance; excessive sweating, thirst, hunger, or urination • *Hematologic system:* Anemia, easy bruising or bleeding, past transfusions • *Psychiatric disorders:* Insomnia, headache, nightmares, personality disorders, anxiety disorders, mood disorders

Source: Petterson 2013, 79.

Physical Examination The **physical examination** represents the physician's assessment of the patient's current health status after evaluating the patient's physical condition. The physician performs the physical examination so appropriate treatment and services may be ordered for the patient. Table 4.3 lists the components that are included in the physical examination documentation.

CMS guidance and regulations, Joint Commission standards, and healthcare provider organizational policies and procedures will dictate when the medical history and physical exam must be completed by the physician. There are also

Table 4.3   Information documented in the report of a physical examination

Report components	Content
General condition	Apparent state of health, signs of distress, posture, weight, height, skin color, dress and personal hygiene, facial expression, manner, mood, state of awareness, speech
Vital signs	Pulse, respiration, blood pressure, temperature
Skin	Color, vascularity, lesions, edema, moisture, temperature, texture, thickness, mobility and turgor, nails
Head	Hair, scalp, skull, face
Eyes	Visual acuity and fields; position and alignment of the eyes, eyebrows, eyelids; lacrimal apparatus; conjunctivae; sclerae; corneas; irises; size, shape, equality, reaction to light, and accommodation of pupils; extraocular movements; ophthalmoscopic exam
Ears	Auricles, canals, tympanic membranes, hearing, discharge
Nose and sinuses	Airways, mucosa, septum, sinus tenderness, discharge, bleeding, smell
Mouth	Breath, lips, teeth, gums, tongue, salivary ducts
Throat	Tonsils, pharynx, palate, uvula, postnasal drip
Neck	Stiffness, thyroid, trachea, vessels, lymph nodes, salivary glands
Thorax, anterior and posterior	Shape, symmetry, respiration
Breasts	Masses, tenderness, discharge from nipples
Lungs	Fremitus, breath sounds, adventitious sounds, friction, spoken voice, whispered voice
Heart	Location and quality of apical impulse, trill, pulsation, rhythm, sounds, murmurs, friction rub, jugular venous pressure and pulse, carotid artery pulse
Abdomen	Contour, peristalsis, scars, rigidity, tenderness, spasm, masses, fluid, hernia, bowel sounds and bruits, palpable organs
Male genitourinary organs	Scars, lesions, discharge, penis, scrotum, epididymis, varicocele, hydrocele
Female reproductive organs	External genitalia, Skene's glands and Bartholin's glands, vagina, cervix, uterus, adnexa
Rectum	Fissure, fistula, hemorrhoids, sphincter tone, masses, prostate, seminal vesicles, feces
Musculoskeletal system	Spine and extremities, deformities, swelling, redness, tenderness, range of motion
Lymphatics	Palpable cervical, axillary, inguinal nodes; location, size, consistency; mobility and tenderness
Blood vessels	Pulses, color, temperature, vessel walls, veins
Neurological system	Cranial nerves, coordination, reflexes, biceps, triceps, patellar, Achilles, abdominal, cremasteric, Babinski, Romberg, gait, sensory, vibratory
Diagnosis(es)	

Source: Petterson 2013, 80.

documentation standards that address when a previously completed H&P can be utilized when a patient is admitted to the hospital (discussed later in this chapter).

Diagnostic and Therapeutic Procedure Orders   There are a number of diagnostic and therapeutic order types. Diagnostic orders include orders for x-rays, CT, MRI, and lab tests for the purpose of diagnosing a patient's symptoms of illness. Therapeutic orders are orders for treatment that either prevent or address illness by way of medication administration, surgery, or counseling. **Physician orders** are the instructions the physician gives to other healthcare professionals who actually perform diagnostic tests and treatments, administer medications, and provide specific services to a particular patient. Admission and discharge orders should be found for every patient unless the patient leaves the facility against medical advice (AMA), but other orders will vary from patient to patient. All orders must be legible and include the date and the physician's signature. In electronic systems, signatures are attached via an authentication process.

Standing orders are orders the medical staff or an individual physician established as routine care for a specific diagnosis or procedure. Standing orders authorize other healthcare providers (such as nurses) to begin treating the patient before the physician actually examines the patient. Standing orders are commonly used for disease processes and injuries requiring prompt attention. Like other physician's orders, they must be signed, verified, and dated.

Physicians may communicate orders verbally or via telephone when the hospital's medical staff rules allow. State law and medical staff rules specify which practitioners (for example, only registered nurses) are allowed to accept and execute verbal and telephone orders. How the orders are to be signed as well as the time period allowed for authentication also may be specified. Currently, there is technology that allows orders to be sent via mobile devices, such as smart phones and tablets and healthcare organizations are beginning to explore the possibility of using this technology.

Clinical Observations In acute-care hospitals, the documentation of **clinical observations** is usually provided in a **progress note**. Clinical observations are the comments of physicians, nurses, and other caregivers in order to create a chronological report of the patient's condition and response to treatment during his or her hospital stay. Progress notes serve to justify further acute-care treatment in the facility. In addition, they document the appropriateness and coordination of the services provided. The patient's condition determines the frequency of the notes.

The rules and regulations of the hospital's medical staff specify which healthcare providers are allowed to enter progress notes in the health record. Typically, the patient's attending physician, consulting physicians who have medical staff privileges, house medical staff, nurses, nutritionists, social workers, and clinical therapists are authorized to enter progress notes. Depending on the record format used by the hospital, each discipline may maintain a separate section of the health record or the observations of all the providers may be combined in the same chronological

or **integrated health record**. Guidelines for the frequency of notations may also be found in the medical staff rules and regulations.

Special types of notes are frequently found in a record. For example, prior to the administration of anything other than local anesthesia, the anesthesiologist visits the patient and documents important factors about the patient's condition that may have an impact on the anesthesia chosen or its administration. Allergies and drug reactions would be noted. A postanesthesia note also should be found describing the patient's recovery from the anesthetic. Similarly, the surgeon responsible for a major procedure must document both pre- and post-surgical patient evaluations.

In the case of a death, the attending physician should add a summary statement to the patient's health record to document the circumstances surrounding the patient's death. The statement can take the form of a final progress note or a separate report. The statement should indicate the reason for the patient's admission, his or her diagnosis and course in the hospital, and a description of the events that led to his or her death.

Just as physician documentation begins with the H&P, nurses and allied health professionals may begin their care with assessments focused on understanding the patient's condition from the perspective of their specialized body of knowledge. Often a **care plan**— a summary of the patient's problems from the nurse or other professional's perspective with a detailed plan for interventions—may follow the assessment. In addition, nurses are responsible for specific patient admission and discharge notes and for documenting the patient's condition at regular intervals throughout the patient's stay. If a patient should die while hospitalized, nursing notes regarding the circumstances leading to and of death are important for quality and patient health outcomes improvement, risk management activities, and, in some cases, payer reimbursement considerations.

In certain situations when the patient has died, an autopsy may be requested or required and a subsequent **autopsy report**, a description of the examination of a patient's body after he or she has died, is completed. Also called necropsies, autopsies are usually conducted when there is some question about the cause of death or when information is needed for educational or legal purposes. The purpose of the autopsy is to determine or confirm the cause of death or to provide more information about the course of the patient's disease.

The autopsy report is completed by a pathologist and becomes part of the patient's permanent health record. Autopsy report content and the format of the content is standardized and governed by the National Association of Medical Examiners. Every autopsy report will contain the diagnosis, toxicology, opinion, circumstances of death, identification of the decedent, general description of clothing and personal effects, evidence of medical intervention, external examination, external evidence of injury, internal examination, and samples obtained. Because reports from tissue examination or laboratory testing can take weeks or even months, a preliminary report including preliminary diagnoses is often documented until findings are received and the final report is completed. The authorization for the autopsy, signed by the patient's next of kin or by law enforcement authorities, must be obtained prior to the autopsy and also should become part of the record.

Nursing professionals also maintain chronological records of the patient's vital signs (blood pressure, heart rate, respiration rate, and temperature) and documentation of medications ordered and administered. Other chronological monitors such as measures of a patient's fluid input and output may be ordered and recorded depending on the patient's diagnosis. Sometimes these records are referred to as flow records because they show trends over time, or the data may be represented in graphic form for ease of communication. Special interventions such as the use of restraints also require documentation. For example, restraint information must include the type of restraint used, time frame used, and regular vital signs monitors and descriptions of the patient's physical condition while restrained.

After an initial assessment, documentation by other allied health professionals varies by specialty. Each facility will define appropriate content and frequency of recording using specific regulations and standards in addition to the profession's practice guidelines. For example, respiratory therapy treatments may be documented via samples and social work interventions may appear as dictated reports.

Diagnostic and Therapeutic Procedure Reports   The results of all diagnostic and therapeutic procedures become part of the patient's health record. Diagnostic procedures include the following:

- Laboratory tests performed on blood, urine, and other samples from the patient
- Pathological examinations of tissue samples and tissues or organs removed during surgical procedures
- Imaging procedures of the patient's body and specific organs (radiology, scans, ultrasounds, MRIs, PETs)
- Monitors and tracings of body functions

The results of most laboratory procedures are generated electronically by automated testing equipment. In contrast, the results of monitors, imaging, and pathology procedures require interpretation by specially trained physicians such as cardiologists, radiologists, and pathologists. These physicians document their findings in reports that then become part of the patient's permanent record, along with copies or samples of the tracing, images, and scans (figure 4.1).

Surgical Procedure Documentation   Any surgical procedure requires special documentation. Preoperative notes are made by the anesthesiologist and surgeon prior to the procedure, and nurses report preoperative patient preparations. The entire procedure itself is then recorded, along with an anesthesia record, an operative report, and a postanesthesia or **recovery room report**. When tissue is removed for evaluation, a pathology report also must be present.

The **anesthesia report** notes any preoperative medication and response to it, the anesthesia administered with dose and method of administration, the duration of administration, the patient's vital signs while under anesthesia, and any additional products given to the patient during

Figure 4.1 Electronic lab report

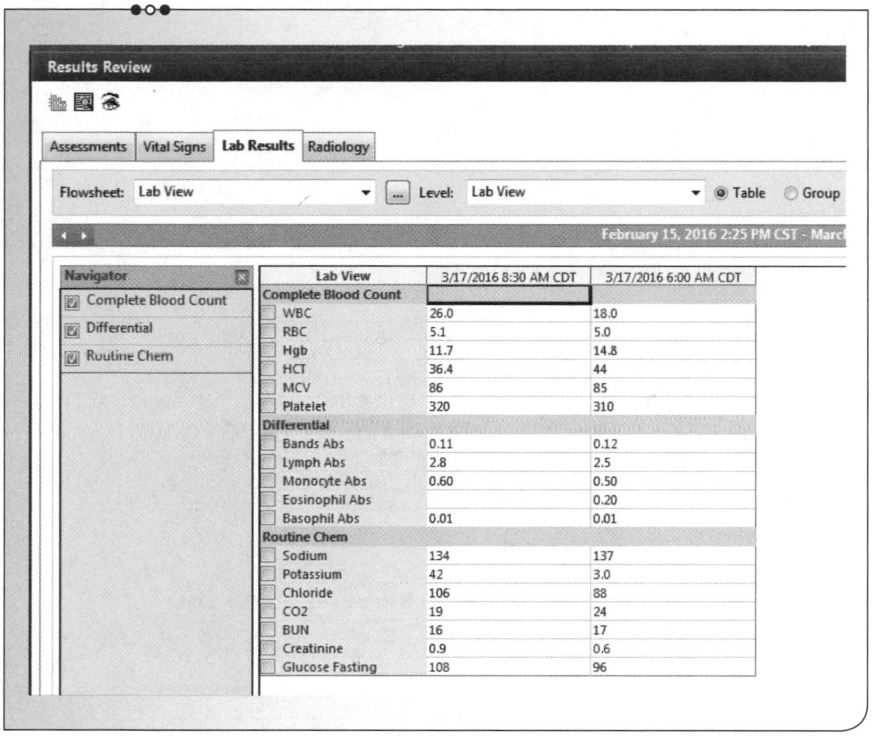

Lab View	3/17/2016 8:30 AM CDT	3/17/2016 6:00 AM CDT
Complete Blood Count		
WBC	26.0	18.0
RBC	5.1	5.0
Hgb	11.7	14.8
HCT	36.4	44
MCV	86	85
Platelet	320	310
Differential		
Bands Abs	0.11	0.12
Lymph Abs	2.8	2.5
Monocyte Abs	0.60	0.50
Eosinophil Abs		0.20
Basophil Abs	0.01	0.01
Routine Chem		
Sodium	134	137
Potassium	42	3.0
Chloride	106	88
CO2	19	24
BUN	16	17
Creatinine	0.9	0.6
Glucose Fasting	108	96

the procedure. The anesthesiologist or nurse anesthetist is responsible for this documentation.

The **operative report** describes the surgical procedures performed on the patient. Each report usually includes the following information:

- Patient's preoperative and postoperative diagnosis
- Descriptions of the procedures performed
- Descriptions of all normal and abnormal findings
- Description of the patient's medical condition before, during, and after the operation
- Estimated blood loss
- Descriptions of any specimens removed
- Descriptions of any unique or unusual events during the course of the surgery
- Names of the surgeons and their assistants
- Date and duration of the surgery

Figure 4.2 shows an operative report in electronic format. The operative report should be written or dictated by the surgeon immediately after surgery and become part of the health record as soon as possible. When there is a delay in dictation or transcription, a progress note describing the surgery should be entered into the patient's record. Reports of other procedures or treatments may or may not be associated with surgery. For example, administration of blood transfusions may occur prior to, during, or after surgery, but chemotherapy documentation is usually separate from that of other procedures.

Immediately after the procedure, the patient is evaluated for a period of time in a special unit called a recovery room. Monitoring is important to make sure the patient sufficiently recovers from the anesthesia and is stable enough to be moved to another location. The **recovery room report** includes the postanesthesia note (if not found elsewhere), nurses' notes regarding the patient's condition and surgical site, vital signs, intravenous fluids, and other medical monitoring.

A **pathology report** is dictated by a pathologist after examination of tissue received for evaluation. This report usually includes descriptions of the tissue from a gross or macroscopic (with the eye) level and representative cells at the microscopic

Figure 4.2 Electronic operative report

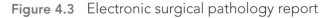

SURGEON: CHANDLER BLOCK, DO

PRE-OPERATIVE DIAGNOSIS:
  Painful swallowing

POST-OPERATIVE DIAGNOSIS:
  Significant Barrett's esophagus, acute GE junction inflammation secondary to reflux. Moderate gastritis.

OPERATION: Gastroscopy, biopsy, and Clo test.

According to his wife, this male is being seen at the request of Dr. Swenson, after developing painful swallowing. The patient and his wife were told the reasons for the procedure and the possible esophageal dilation including other risks.

PROCEDURE: Following local anesthesia with Cetacaine, 25 mg of Demerol and 1 mg Versed IV, the GIF. 100 was with some difficulty passed into the esophagus where starting at about 26 cm to the GE junction, scattered area of what looked like typical Barrett's esophagus. It was a little more prominent distally at the GE junction where there was no stricturing process. The scope was easily passed into the small hiatus hernia into the stomach where the gastric mucosa and the body and the antrum were significantly inflamed and, therefore, Clo test was taken of pyloric ring and duodenum which was negative. The scope was the withdrawn back up into the esophagus where random biopsy from the inflamed area was taken.

IMPRESSION: I wonder if the patient has had a greater degree of reflux during hospitalization when he has had more bed rest.

PLAN: Anti-reflux program. Prev acid.

level along with interpretive findings. Sometimes an initial tissue evaluation occurs while the surgery is in progress to give the surgeon information important to the remainder of the operation. A full written report would follow (see figure 4.3).

Consultation Reports The **consultation report** documents the clinical opinion of a physician other than the primary or attending physician. The consultation is usually requested by the primary or attending physician, but occasionally may be the request of the patient or the patient's family. The report is based on the consulting physician's examination of the patient and a review of his or her health record.

Some organizations allow consultation requests by telephone and provide the consultant with selected information from the patient's record. The consultant then dictates his or her findings and returns them to the requesting physician.

Figure 4.3 Electronic surgical pathology report

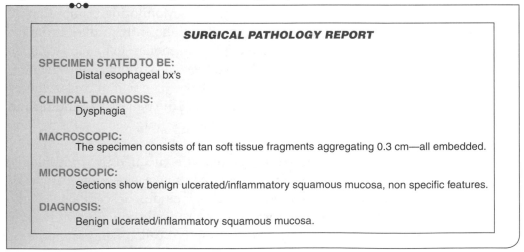

SURGICAL PATHOLOGY REPORT

SPECIMEN STATED TO BE:
  Distal esophageal bx's

CLINICAL DIAGNOSIS:
  Dysphagia

MACROSCOPIC:
  The specimen consists of tan soft tissue fragments aggregating 0.3 cm—all embedded.

MICROSCOPIC:
  Sections show benign ulcerated/inflammatory squamous mucosa, non specific features.

DIAGNOSIS:
  Benign ulcerated/inflammatory squamous mucosa.

Discharge Summary The **discharge summary** is a concise account of the patient's illness, course of treatment, response to treatment, and condition at the time of patient discharge (official release) from the hospital. The summary also includes instructions for follow-up care to be given to the patient or his or her caregiver at the time of discharge. Because it provides an overview of the entire medical encounter, it is used for a variety of purposes:

- Ensures the continuity of future care by providing information to the patient's attending physician, referring physician, and any consulting physicians
- Provides information to support the activities of the medical staff review committee
- Provides concise information that can be used to answer information requests from authorized individuals or entities

The discharge summary is the responsibility of and must be signed by the attending physician. If the patient's stay is not complicated and lasts less than 48 hours or involves an uncomplicated delivery or normal newborn, a discharge note in place of a full summary is often acceptable.

Patient Instructions and Transfer Records It is vital that the patient be given clear, concise instructions upon discharge so the recovery progress begun in the hospital continues. Ideally, patient instructions are communicated both verbally and in writing. The healthcare professional who delivers the instructions to the patient or caregiver should sign the record to indicate that he or she has issued them. In addition, the person receiving the instructions should sign to verify that he or she has received and understands them. A copy of these instructions should be filed in the health record.

When someone other than the patient assumes responsibility for the patient's aftercare, the record should indicate the instructions were given to the responsible party. Documentation of patient education may be accomplished by using formats that prompt the person providing instruction to cover important information.

When a patient is being transferred from the acute setting to another healthcare organization, a **transfer record** may be initiated. This record is also called a referral form. A brief review of the patient's acute stay along with current status, discharge and transfer orders, and any additional instructions will be noted. Social service and nursing personnel often complete portions of the transfer record.

Administrative Data **Administrative data** is coded information contained in secondary records (such as billing records) describing patient identification, diagnosis, procedures, and insurance. Patient registration information would be considered administrative data as would patient account information.

Patient Registration Information Patient registration information includes those data elements obtained during the patient registration process. The majority of the patient registration process usually takes place before the physician examines or begins treating the patient. During the registration process, demographic information (a type of administrative data) is collected. Registration information simply identifies the patient and uniquely identifies the patient with the EHR system. Registration information that is obtained or generated includes:

- Patient's full name (in addition to any aliases that may be used for example, Bob instead of Robert)
- Establishing a medical record number if the patient was not seen at a particular facility before as well as establishing an account number for this particular visit
- Patient address
- Patient contact phone number
- Date of birth
- Patient gender
- Patient marital status
- Patient's religious affiliation (if patient has one and choses to disclose it)
- Race (often this is optional)

- Next of kin information
- Healthcare power of attorney or advanced directives (if the patient has these documents)
- If the patient wants to be a private or confidential patient under HIPAA, where the patient opts-out of the healthcare facility's directory

Historically speaking, it was common to ask for a patient's social security number (SSN); some insurance policy numbers were the patient's or the policy holder's actual SSN. In recent years, due to the increase in healthcare related identity theft, more and more healthcare provider organizations are moving away from requesting patient disclosure of his or her SSN. The healthcare industry in general is moving now toward biometric identifiers for patient identification and patient identity verification, such as finger or palm prints.

Patient Account Information   Patient account information is the financial information associated with a particular patient. Patient account information usually includes:

- Insurance payer information (this would include a patient who was considered to be self-pay or no insurance)
- Insurance policy holder information
- Patient's relationship to the insurance policy holder
- Insurance policy number

Patient registration and account information can also generate tertiary administrative data that is often used for statistical analysis.

Consents, Authorizations, and Acknowledgments   From the moment a patient walks through the doors of the healthcare facility, he or she must provide the healthcare provider organization or physician permission to treat, perform procedures, and use and disclose his or her protected health information. The healthcare provider must also provide the patient notice as to how treatment will proceed and how the patient's information will be safeguarded. There are three separate categories of permissions and notices that will be addressed in this section—consents, authorizations, and acknowledgments.

Consents   Within the healthcare setting, general **consent to treatment** means the patient gives the physician or other healthcare provider permission to touch them. Often a general consent document is signed by the patient or his or her authorized personal representative at nonemergent visits during the registration process. This consent to treat document normally contains a general statement regarding treatment, as well as an agreement for payment. In some cases, the patient can limit the extent of the consent within the general consent document. The general consent document will also address picture-taking for treatment (for reasons such as wound evaluation and treatment) as well as medical education purposes; and in some states a statement regarding HIV testing with patient blood should a healthcare provider sustain a significant exposure is also included.

General consent can either be expressed or implied and more often than not the general consent to treat takes the form of **expressed consent**, or consent given by the patient by either his or her words or in writing. **Implied consent** is consent that is inferred by the patient's action or inaction and most commonly asserted by the patient when he or she presents to the emergency department. For example, the patient sticks out his or her arm in order for the nurse to take a blood pressure. It is imperative that treatment, when there is an emergent situation, is started right away; thus inferred consent allows the healthcare provider to start the treatment without the patient directly expressing his or her wishes. In the case of invasive treatment or procedures that carry significant risk, general consent is not always adequate in terms of communicating with the patient about the treatment or procedure and providing the patient the opportunity to make an informed healthcare decision. In these cases, informed consent must be obtained. **Informed consent** is the process by which the healthcare provider informs or makes the patient knowledgeable about the risks and benefits of the proposed treatment or procedure. The physician will speak with the patient in detail about the treatment or procedure, risks, and alternatives allowing the patient to make an intelligent decision regarding the performance or nonperformance of the treatment or procedure.

Authorizations An **authorization** is a document that is required under the Privacy Rule of the Health Insurance Portability and Accountability Act (HIPAA) for the use and disclosure of protected health information (PHI). An authorization is a document that provides healthcare providers the authority to use or disclose PHI for a specific purpose. For more details on authorizations, see chapter 9.

Acknowledgments Acknowledgments are documents that the patient or the patient's authorized personal representative sign, confirming the receipt of important and applicable information. The following are the three most common acknowledgments that patients receive.

- *Notice of privacy practices (NPP):* Under the Privacy Rule of HIPAA, healthcare providers must provide patients notice that tells them how the healthcare provider will use or disclose their PHI, as well as how the healthcare provider will safeguard the PHI in its possession and what HIPAA rights the patient can exercise.
- *Patient rights*: CMS requires that healthcare providers inform their patients about general patient rights afforded to them. These rights include the patient's right to know who is treating him or her, the right to be informed about the treatment that will be received, and the patient's right to be an active participant in the decision making of that treatment. The patient has the right to refuse treatment and be safe from abuse. The patient is required to sign an acknowledgment that demonstrates that the patient has been informed of his or her rights as described and that he or she understands those rights.

- *Property and valuables list-* Normally healthcare providers ask that the patient leave any valuables at home and not to wear any jewelry. If a patient brings valuables or wears jewelry into the facility, the facility will very often have the patient sign an acknowledgment demonstrating that the facility is not responsible for any loss of or damage to the patient's belongings.

Obstetric

Some health records have unique requirements because of the specialized services provided. Specifically, the following kinds of information should be maintained for both obstetric and gynecologic patients in addition to other ambulatory care documents.

- Medical history to include history of abuse or neglect and sexual practices
- Periodic laboratory testing, including Pap tests and mammography, cholesterol levels, and fecal blood tests
- Additional laboratory testing needed for high-risk groups such as tuberculosis skin testing and testing for sexually transmitted diseases

As an additional resource, the American College of Obstetricians and Gynecologists (ACOG) provides guidelines to members for perinatal and women's healthcare that impact health record content. Another group whose voluntary accreditation process includes perinatal documentation standards is the **Commission for the Accreditation of Birth Centers**.

Prenatal Prenatal health record documentation captures the treatment and services a pregnant patient receives before giving birth. During the initial prenatal visit, the healthcare provider establishes a treatment relationship with the patient and obtains patient information that will drive the healthcare provider's clinical decision making for the patient. The healthcare provider evaluates the patient for any obstetrical risks that will affect the patient or the baby. During subsequent prenatal patient visits, the healthcare provider continuously evaluates the health status of both patient and baby through a variety of evaluation methods, including but not limited to physician exams, laboratory tests, and other diagnostic testing.

As health records move from paper-based to electronic formats, prenatal record content has begun to reflect a standardization, both in the actual information found within prenatal documentation as well as the organization of that documentation. Typically, within the prenatal visit documentation you will find data on the patient's menstrual history, obstetric history, medical and surgical history, physical exams, nutritional evaluation, behavioral evaluation, and laboratory test results. In addition, the healthcare provider, will determine if the patient is high risk or not based upon various criteria. Throughout the duration of the patient's prenatal visits, documentation reflecting provider-given obstetrical education based on patient need is also found within the prenatal health record. Finally, after a thorough evaluation, the healthcare provider will document a plan of care based upon the health issues found or not found during patient examination.

Labor and Delivery Labor and delivery health record documentation reflects the events that occur during the time the pregnant patient goes into labor through the actual birth of the baby. Labor and delivery documentation includes fetal monitoring strips, a record of medications given and stopped, as well as nursing progress notes. The events that occur during the actual birth of the baby are documented by the patient's healthcare providers, including the time of the actual birth and the type of delivery.

Newborn

Within the hospital and acute-care setting, a newborn's health record documentation is handled separately from the mother's health record information. With that said, the newborn's health record will contain documentation and other information from the mother's chart. The newborn's health record will contain an examination

performed upon birth and an examination performed prior to discharge. Immediately after birth, the baby's physical condition is evaluated in order to determine if the baby is in distress and needs additional care or treatment. The evaluation determines the baby's APGAR score. APGAR stands for **a**ppearance and skin color, **p**ulse and heart rate, **g**rimace response and reflexes, **a**ctivity and muscle tone, and **r**espiratory and breathing rate. Each evaluation element is a score from 0 to 10, 10 being the best possible score. The newborn health record also will contain physician's orders, nursing notes, and progress notes, the same as what is found within an adult health record.

Emergency Department Record

The emergency department record is a health record that is generated when a patient visits an emergency department (ED) seeking treatment. Any patient who presents to an ED must be examined in compliance with the **Emergency Medical Treatment and Active Labor Act (EMTALA)** to determine if an emergency condition exists. If an emergency condition exists, the patient must be stabilized before discharge or transfer. EMTALA prohibits healthcare providers from refusing to treat patients or delaying treatment due to the patient not having insurance or not having the ability to pay. The emergency department record must reflect certain elements in compliance with regulations governing emergency treatment. The emergency department record itself is sometimes incorporated within the inpatient health record and at other times, is kept separately.

The emergency department record should include:

- Patient demographic information
- Arrival time
- Means of arrival (ambulance, car, private car)
- Name of the person bringing the patient to the ED
- Pertinent history of illness
- Physical findings
- Diagnostic tests
- Treatment provided

- Disposition of patient (whether the patient was admitted, transferred, or admitted)
- Condition of patient upon discharge
- Patient discharge instructions
- Signatures of patient

If the patient leaves before treatment is complete or AMA, documentation must reflect that the patient has been apprised of the risks of doing so. Healthcare provider organizations normally have the patient sign an AMA form for documentation and liability purposes.

Ambulatory Record

Ambulatory means that treatment is provided on an outpatient basis. Patients receiving ambulatory care do not require admission to the hospital. The ambulatory record is very similar to an inpatient hospital-based health record. In general, documentation in ambulatory care patient records typically includes the following materials:

- Registration forms including patient identification data
- Problem lists
- Medication lists
- Patient history questionnaires
- History and physicals
- Progress notes
- Results of consultations
- Diagnostic test results
- Miscellaneous flow sheets (for example, pediatric growth charts and immunization records and specialty-specific flow sheets)
- Copies of records of previous hospitalizations or treatment by other healthcare practitioners
- Correspondence
- Consents to disclose information
- Advance directives

Ambulatory care records also include several elements unique to the ambulatory setting. For example, ambulatory records usually contain a problem list whose function is to facilitate ongoing patient care management. The **problem list** describes any significant current and past illnesses and conditions as well as the procedures the patient has undergone. Sometimes problems are separated into acute (short term, such as otitis media) and chronic (such as diabetes mellitus) categories. The problem list also may include information on the patient's previous surgeries, allergies, and drug sensitivities.

Ambulatory Surgery Record

Ambulatory facilities that perform surgery are called **ambulatory surgery centers (ASC)**. Patients who have surgery in an ASC still must have a history and physical prior to surgery present within the health record. The patient must also have signed the appropriate consent documentation prior to the procedure. Much like an inpatient health record containing a surgery component, an ambulatory surgery record must contain operative reports and notes, diagnostic and therapeutic documentation, consultations, and discharge notes at the conclusion of the treatment.

Ambulatory surgery centers also perform discharge follow-up phone calls, where a nurse will call the patient within 24 to 48 hours post discharge to check on the patient, assessing pain levels, and addressing any immediate or future needs the patient has or will have related to the treatment. This conversation must be documented in the health record. The Joint Commission and the **American Association for Accreditation of Ambulatory Surgery Facilities (AAAASF)** have requirements applicable to the ambulatory surgery center setting. CMS's Conditions of Coverage for ambulatory surgical centers govern those that seek Medicare reimbursement.

Ancillary Departments

Ancillary departments are considered the departments that provide treatment and services that support the patient's overall care plan. Ancillary departments perform **ancillary services**—tests and procedures sometimes ordered by a physician—and these services assist the physician with diagnosing and treating the patient. Ancillary departments also consist of departments that play an indirect patient care role, but are absolutely necessary for the overall management of the patient care. These departments include pharmacy, nutrition, HIM, social services, and patient advocacy and patient relations. Many ancillary departmental services must be documented within the patient health record according to the governing standards and regulations within a specific department.

Physician Office Record

Routine healthcare treatment commonly occurs within the physician office setting. Routine services include preventative services such as yearly physicals and blood tests, in addition to diagnosis and treatment of minor illnesses and injuries. In many instances, hospital-based health records can feed into the physician office record if the hospital and physician office records are electronic and information can be exchanged from one health record system to another. Much like a paper-based physician office record, the physician office record that is EHR-based, is often in an integrated health record format.

The physician office record content consists of:

- Medical history
- Family history
- Social history
- Vital signs
- Chief complaint
- Progress notes
- Allergies
- Medication list
- History of present illness
- Review of systems
- Assessment and diagnosis
- Plan of treatment

Long-Term Care

Long-term care is provided in a variety of facilities, including: skilled nursing facilities (SNFs) or units; subacute-care facilities; nursing facilities (NFs) (nursing homes, long-term care facilities); and assisted-living facilities.

The regulations that govern long-term care facilities vary among these settings. Most SNFs and NFs are governed by both federal and state regulations, including the Medicare CoP. Assisted-living facilities are usually governed only by state regulations. Most long-term care providers do not participate in voluntary accreditation programs, although the Joint Commission does have long-term care facility standards.

Because the stay for a patient or resident in long-term settings can be lengthy, health records are based on ongoing assessments and reassessments of the patient's (or resident's) needs. An interdisciplinary team develops a plan of care for each patient upon admission to the facility, and the plan is updated regularly over the patient's stay. The team includes the patient's physician and representatives from nursing services, nutritional services, social services, and other specialty areas (such as physical therapy), as appropriate.

In SNFs, the care plan is based on a format required by federal regulations. The care plan format is called the **resident assessment instrument (RAI)**. The RAI is based on the **Minimum Data Set (MDS) for Long-Term Care**. The overall RAI framework includes the MDS, triggers, utilization guidelines, and **care area assessments (CAAs)**. The patient is assessed and reassessed at defined intervals and whenever there is a significant change in his or her condition.

The RAI is a critical component of the health record. In addition to development of the care plan, Medicare uses the form to determine reimbursement. Many states also use it to determine Medicaid payments, and accreditation surveyors use information from it during the survey process.

The RAI is submitted electronically to each state health department and then to CMS. CMS compiles demographic and quality indicator information and is provided as feedback to each facility.

The physician's role in a long-term care facility is not as visible as it is in other care settings. The physician develops a plan of treatment, which includes the medications and treatments to be given to the resident. The physician visits the resident in the facility on a 30- or 60-day schedule unless the resident's condition requires more frequent visits. At each visit, the physician reviews the plan of care and physician's orders and makes changes as necessary. Between visits, the physician is contacted when nursing personnel identify changes in the resident's condition.

The following list identifies the most common components of long-term care records:

- Registration forms including resident identification data
- Personal property list, including furniture and electronics
- History and physical and hospital records
- Advance directives, bill of rights, and other legal records
- Clinical assessments
- RAI and care plan
- Physician's orders
- Physician's progress notes and consultations
- Nursing notes
- Rehabilitation therapy notes (physical, occupational, and speech therapy)
- Social services, nutritional services, and activities documentation
- Medication and records of monitors, including administration of restraints
- Laboratory, radiology, and special reports
- Discharge or transfer documentation

If paper-based records are found in a long-term setting, a process called record thinning may occur at intervals during the patient's stay. Records of patients whose stay extends to months or years become cumbersome to handle. Selected material may be removed and filed elsewhere according to facility guidelines. Any material removed must remain accessible when needed for patient care and service evaluation.

Rehabilitation

The focus of services in physical medicine and rehabilitation settings is increasing a patient's ability to function independently within the parameters of the individual's illness or disability. The documentation requirements for rehabilitation facilities vary because facilities range from comprehensive inpatient care to outpatient services or special programs.

Inpatient rehabilitation hospitals and units within hospitals are reimbursed by Medicare under a prospective payment system. A **patient assessment instrument (PAI)** is completed shortly after admission and upon discharge. Based on the patient's condition, services, diagnosis, and medical condition, a payment level is determined for the inpatient rehabilitation stay. Comprehensive outpatient rehabilitation facilities have separate Medicare guidelines.

Many rehabilitation facilities are accredited through the **Commission on Accreditation of Rehabilitation Facilities (CARF)**, although the Joint Commission or American Osteopathic Association (AOA) also can be chosen. CARF requires a facility to maintain a single case record for any patient it admits. The documentation standard for the health record includes the following requirements:

- Patient identification data
- Pertinent history, including functional history
- Diagnosis of disability and functional diagnosis
- Rehabilitation problems, goals, and prognosis
- Reports of assessments and program plans
- Reports from referring sources and service referrals
- Reports from outside consultations and laboratory, radiology, orthotic, and prosthetic services
- Designation of a manager for the patient's program
- Evidence of the patient's or family's participation in decision making
- Evaluation reports from each service
- Reports of staff conferences
- Progress reports
- Correspondence related to the patient
- Release forms
- Discharge summary
- Follow-up reports (CARF 2016)

Behavioral Health

Behavioral health records are more commonly referred to as mental health records and contain much of the same content as a non-behavioral health record such as discharge summary, H&P, or physician's orders. Behavioral health records contain a treatment plan that often includes family and caregiver input and information as well as assessments geared toward the transition to outpatient, nonacute treatment. CMS requires that the social workers assigned to a patient assess and document the family or home environment and community services that are compatible with the patient's needs. The behavioral health record also contains a psychiatric evaluation that is performed by a healthcare provider appropriately trained to do such an evaluation and that evaluation consists of a patient history, current mental status, and cognitive function.

✓ Check Your Understanding 4.3

Instructions: **Answer the following questions.**

1. A patient's gender, phone number, address, next of kin, and insurance policy holder information would be considered what kind of data?
   A. Clinical data
   B. Authorization data
   C. Administrative data
   D. Consent data

2. Patient history questionnaires, problem lists, diagnostic tests results, and immunization records are commonly found in which type of record?
   A. Ambulatory record
   B. Emergency department record
   C. Long-term care record
   D. Rehabilitative care record

3. What type of health records may contain family and caregiver input?
   A. Behavioral health records
   B. Ambulatory surgery health records
   C. Emergency department health records
   D. Obstetric health record

4. The ambulatory surgery record contains information most similar to which of the following?
   A. Physician's office records
   B. Emergency care records
   C. Hospital operative records
   D. Hospital obstetric records

5. Which group focuses solely on accreditation of rehabilitation programs and services?
   A. CARF
   B. AOA
   C. AAAHC
   D. Joint Commission

6. Which type of health record contains information about the means by which the patient arrived at the healthcare setting and documentation of care provided to stabilize the patient?
   A. Ambulatory care
   B. Emergency care
   C. Long-term care
   D. Rehabilitative care

7. A patient's registration forms, personal property list, RAI, care plan, and discharge or transfer documentation would be found most frequently in which type of health record?
   A. Rehabilitative care
   B. Ambulatory care
   C. Behavioral health
   D. Long-term care

8. Which of the following would not be found in a physical exam?
   A. Chief complaint
   B. Vital signs
   C. General condition
   D. Present illness

9. An attending physician requests the advice of a second physician who then reviews the health record and examines the patient. The second physician records his or her evaluation in what type of report?
   A. Consultation
   B. Progress note
   C. Operative report
   D. Discharge summary

10. Written or spoken permission to proceed with care is classified as:
    A. Expressed consent
    B. Acknowledgment
    C. Advance directive
    D. Implied consent

11. Which specialized type of progress note provides healthcare professionals impressions of patient problems with detailed treatment action steps?
    A. Flow record
    B. Vital signs record
    C. Care plan
    D. Surgical note

12. Which of the following reports provides information on tissue removed during a procedure?
    A. Operative report
    B. Laboratory report
    C. Pathology report
    D. Anesthesia report

13. A growth and development record may be found in what type of record?
    A. Rehabilitative care
    B. Pediatric
    C. Behavioral health
    D. Obstetric

14. True or false: Many services such as surgery, infusions, and other diagnostic procedures that once required an overnight hospital stay for the patient, no longer requires that level of care.

15. True or false: CMS requires that healthcare providers inform their patients about general patient rights afforded to them.

16. True or false: Healthcare provider organizations normally have patients sign an acknowledgment acknowledging that the healthcare provider organization is not responsible for the loss of or damage to the patient's valuables.

Health Information Media

Over the years, healthcare documentation media has transformed from a basic paper-based chart that sat on a shelf in an HIM department shelf to a fully interoperable EHR that can be shared. Many of the same rules, standards, and quality measures that held true for the paper-based chart hold true now for the EHR. Healthcare documentation integrity is paramount regardless of its form. Integrity of healthcare documentation includes information governance, patient identification, authorship validation, and record corrections, in addition to ensuring that the health record documentation appropriately supports the claims submitted to payers for reimbursement (AHIMA 2013, 58).

Paper Health Record Documentation

Paper-based health records are what most individuals working within the healthcare industry are accustomed to. The health record can take the source-orientated health record format in which the documentation contained within the record is organized by source or originating department. For instance, all nursing notes are together and all of the physician progress notes are grouped together. With each source, the health record documentation is placed in reverse chronological order, where the most current or recent documentation is first. This reverse chronological order is kept while the patient is being treated. Many times post patient discharge, the health record is kept in its source orientation, but within each source section the documentation is then rearranged and placed in chronological order. Other times, the health record post patient discharge is kept in reverse chronological order; this is called universal chart order.

Documentation within an integrated health record is placed in chronological order regardless of source. Lab results, nursing notes, physician's orders, and physician progress notes will all be placed in the order in which they occurred. The order of the health record is determined by when the documentation was entered into the health record, when the service or treatment was rendered, or when a test result was processed.

The subjective, objective, assessment, plan (SOAP) is a method used to construct physician progress notes and the acronym is a technique physicians use to remember what elements of documentation must be included within a progress note. The SOAP methodology came from the problem-oriented health record developed by Lawrence Reed in the 1970s which defines and documents clinical problems individually (AAPC 2015). The problem-oriented health record consists of a problem list, the history and physical examination and initial lab findings (the database), the initial plan (test, procedures), and progress notes. The HIM professional must be able to read and understand the documentation structure in order to locate information needed for coding, audits, and other usages.

As EHR technologies have advanced, the paper-based health record is considered antiquated by many. There are numerous shortcomings to the paper-based health record, notably the inability to share needed health information with multiple healthcare providers at one time (access and availability), as well as the lack of controls that can be placed in and around the paper-based medical record in terms of data security. Refer to chapter 10 for more on security.

Electronic Health Record Documentation

Computer-based health record documentation via EHRs has been in existence for 50 years. Over time, as EHR systems became more sophisticated, the manner in which healthcare providers document the treatment and services that they render to the patient also dramatically changed. Before EHR adoption, healthcare providers would carry paper-based health records into the patient's room to reference as the healthcare provider discussed and rendered treatment to the patient. It was not until the healthcare provider left the patient did he or she document what occurred while seeing the patient. With EHR systems used today, point-of-care documentation takes place—the healthcare provider can log into the EHR system in the same exam or treatment room as the patient and document within the patient's health record concurrently with the actual exam or treatment. This change in the way healthcare documentation is captured has impacted treatment workflow in some of the most

meaningful ways. For additional information on the EHR, refer to chapter 11.

Web-Based Document Imaging

Document imaging is the process by which paper-based documentation is captured, digitized, stored, and made available for retrieval by the end user (AIIM 2015). Although many healthcare provider organizations have an EHR, there still remains a good deal of paper-based documentation that must be integrated and included within the patient's EHR. Current EHR systems contain documentation-imaging and document management technologies that provide for the capture, digitization, integration, storage, and retrieval of paper-based health record documentation.

Check Your Understanding 4.4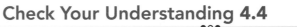

Instructions: **Answer the following questions.**

1. The subjective, objective, assessment, plan (SOAP) method came from the:
   A. Source-oriented health record
   B. Problem-oriented health record
   C. Hybrid health record
   D. Integrated

2. Which of the following electronic record technological capabilities would allow paper-based health records to be incorporated into a patient's EHR?
   A. Database management
   B. Documentation-imaging technology
   C. Text processing
   D. Vocabulary standards

3. The problem list is part of which of the following?
   A. SOAP note
   B. Problem-oriented health record
   C. Imaging
   D. Adoption of health record

4. The paper health record has been scanned and is now available digitally. What is this known as?
   A. It is still known as the paper record since it was originally paper
   B. It is known as imaging
   C. It is known as the EHR
   D. It is known as the problem-oriented health record

Role of Healthcare Professionals in Documentation

Authenticated, accurate, legible, complete, and timely documentation is paramount to patient safety, quality of care provided to those patients, and appropriate reimbursement. Healthcare providers have an obligation to document appropriately, reflecting a true picture of the treatment and services rendered to the patient. Not only does the health record documentation itself need to be of the highest quality, the health record also must be organized and available to the healthcare providers who need it to care for the patient. Physicians, nurses, allied health professionals, and HIM professionals all play vital roles in meeting the documentation standards from an organizational policy and procedural perspective and meeting regulatory requirements applicable to health record documentation.

Physicians

Patients place a significant level of trust in their physicians. Patients rely on their physicians to make sound medical decisions about them and document them accordingly. Payers and the government also trust physicians to document appropriately within the chart so quality care can be rendered and appropriate reimbursement issued by the payer. The information a physician documents within the health record impacts the patient first and foremost. All physicians caring for the patient and payers connected to the physicians need to coordinate their care and documentation. There are many regulatory laws that will be covered in chapter 16 that directly and indirectly govern physician documentation. Those laws fall into the general category of fraud and abuse laws, but namely the False Claims Act and Anti-Kickback Statute have significant documentation compliance jurisdiction for physicians.

Nurses

Nurses play an important role in the day-to-day caregiving of a patient and are an important member of the patient care team. Much like physicians, the manner in which a nurse documents within the health record will be based on the environment. Inpatient health record documentation will look slightly different from the documentation in the operating room, or in a long-term care facility. The elements or components that the nurse will capture in the documentation will also vary depending upon licensing and regulatory requirements, as well as internal policy and procedures of the health provider organization. However, the same rules apply to nursing documentation as they do to physician documentation. Legible, complete, and timely entries are required. In addition, though the documentation of a physician will be both subjective and objective, nursing documentation should only be objective in nature. At times when looking at the legal environment of nursing documentation versus physician documentation, nursing documentation standards tend to be more restrictive in nature due to the fact that it is the physicians who diagnose not the nurses.

Allied Health Professionals

Some allied health professionals work more independently than others when providing treatment and services to the patient. Many follow a treatment plan developed by the patient's physician. In this case, the allied health professional would document the treatment and the patient's response to the treatment.

The allied health professional usually falls into one of two categories of practice—technician (assistant) and therapist or technologist. In both categories of practice, allied health professionals may have certification and licensing requirements that must be met in addition to the standard documentation practices of an organization. Please refer to chapter 2 for additional information on allied heath professionals.

Health Information Management Professionals and Health Record Documentation

While HIM professionals do not document in the health record, the documentation in the record is important for them for coding, claim generation, data quality monitoring, release of information and such. Complete, accurate, and available health record information is essential for quality care and patient safety. Other healthcare providers, the government, and payers expect the health record documentation to accurately reflect the treatment and services provided to the patient so the patient receives the best quality healthcare available and the appropriate reimbursement is received for the treatment and services provided. Moreover, the governance of the health record documentation throughout its life cycle is of the utmost importance from not only a clinical perspective, but an operational perspective as well. HIM professionals are often in charge of ensuring physician documentation is complete and accurate and that the health record documentation is organized and readily accessible when needed for patient care. The American Health Information Management Association (AHIMA) defines information governance as "an organization-wide framework for managing information throughout its life cycle and supporting the organization's strategy, operations, regulatory, legal, risk, and environmental requirements" (AHIMA 2014). The governance or management of health record information is a fundamental component of the overall information governance model. Information governance applies to many categories of data, including health record information. HIM professionals play vital and different roles in the overall governance of health record information. For information on data governance, see chapter 6.

HIM professionals manage many aspects of the health record and its content. From scanning paper-based health record documentation into the EHR and organizing the overall content of the record, to analyzing the documentation for deficiencies like physician signatures, and coding the health record documentation for appropriate reimbursement, HIM professionals control the access and disclosure of the health record and its content across an organization. Within an EHR environment, HIM professionals are viewed as the experts to develop work flows and infrastructure around the EHR. As EHR technology proliferates, traditional HIM job roles continue to be more information technology (IT) focused. Continuing to learn and expand knowledge within the computer technology field and continuing to learn the many ways IT can be leveraged to improve the EHR infrastructure to support information governance is paramount. HIM professionals and the roles they play will continue to evolve—as they will be involved in clinical documentation improvement (CDI), forms design, screen design, data quality, and so much more.

Check Your Understanding 4.5

Instructions: **Answer the following questions.**

1. Nursing documentation within the health record will be:
   A. Subjective
   B. Objective
   C. Both subjective and objective
   D. Electronic

2. True or false: Payers and the government are not concerned with how a physician documents in a health record.

3. True or false: Only physicians document in the health record.

4. True or false: HIM professionals document in the health record.

5. True or false: Management of health record information is a fundamental component of information governance.

Real-World Case 4.1

When Anywhere Hospital began developing its EHR the EHR task force set out to develop an EHR that will serve as the organization's legal health record. The unofficial goal of the EHR task force was to compile all available health information into a single system and provide the means to deliver the needed administrative and clinical data instantaneously to end users when needed. Large volume of information, overcrowded computer screens, and lack of uniform structure soon proved overwhelming for the system's end users. Their feedback called for useful and needed health record information formatted in a usable structure.

In response to end-user frustration, the EHR task force took a hard look at the captured information and how that information was then presented to the end user. The task force considered the following questions:

- How is the health information captured, formatted, and structured into one system when pulling from many sources?
- How long is health information retained?
- What information is purged from the system and when is it purged?
- What health information is archived? Is there any information needed to be kept permanently?
- How much control should end users have over the information they are allowed to access?

Real-World Case 4.2

As an HIM professional within Anywhere Hospital's HIM department, you have been asked to review physician documentation within the hospital's new EHR system, implemented six months ago. Your goal of the review is to catch any documentation issues early and work with the appropriate hospital leadership to fix those issues.

As you review the documentation within your facility's EHR, you notice that physicians are utilizing the copy and paste functionality available within the EHR system, allowing physicians to select health record documentation from one source or from one section of the EHR and replicate it in another source or another section of the record. You notice in one particular instance that the health record identifies a patient as a 65-year-old male (as identified during the registration process) but in the progress notes is described as a 25-year-old female who has given birth. Clearly, the physician utilized the copy and paste functionality inappropriately and copied health record information from a health record of a patient who was a 25-year-old female and pasted that information accidentally into a health record of a 65-year-old male.

You find this concerning because this could have patient safety concerns, as well as billing and claims issues and the use of this functionality could open the facility up to potential claims of fraud and abuse by the payer. You take this concern to your leadership and a multidisciplined group of hospital employees including HIM professionals, nurses, physicians, and billing and revenue cycle employees to discuss and fix the problem. There are mixed opinions about the copy and paste functionality. Some individuals feel this feature is a time-saver and a productivity booster while others believe it only opens the hospital up to additional CMS scrutiny.

As the HIM professional, you present the following questions to the group for consideration:

- What, if any, are the regulatory requirements or prohibitions to using such a feature within an EHR?

- Does the design of the facility's EHR promote or detract from health record documentation quality and integrity?

- Are there any alternatives to this feature that will assist with documentation efficiency?

- How would the facility set forth organizational documentation standards related to this feature?

References

Adelman, T. 2012. Fundamentals of Health Law. *Fundamentals of Hospital Medical Staff Issues: Minimizing Risk and Maximizing Collaboration* (Session F). Chicago: AHLA.

American Academy of Professional Coders (AAPC). 2015. http://www.aapc.com.

American College of Emergency Physicians (ACEP). 2015. http://www.acep.org.

American Health Information Management Association. 2014. Information Governance Offers a Strategic Approach for Healthcare. *Journal of AHIMA*. 85(10):70–75.

American Health Information Management Association. 2013. Integrity of the healthcare record: Best practices for EHR documentation. *Journal of AHIMA*. 84(1):58–62.

American Health Information Management Association. 2011. Fundamentals of the legal health record and designated record set. *Journal of AHIMA*. 82(2):expanded online version. http://bok.ahima.org/doc?oid=104008#.Vw6KtvkrK9I.

Association for Information and Image Management (AIIM). 2015. http://www.aiim.org.

Centers for Medicare and Medicaid Services. 2015. http://www.cms.gov.

Commission on Accreditation of Rehabilitation Facilities. 2016. http://www.carf.org/Documentation_and_Time_Lines.

Health Information and Management Systems Society, HIMAA Practice Leadership Task Force and the HIMSS Knowledge Resources Task Force. 2011. *The Legal Electronic Health Record*. Chicago: HIMSS.

The Joint Commission. 2016a. About the Joint Commission. http://www.jointcommission.org/about_us/about_the_joint_commission_main.aspx.

The Joint Commission. 2016b. DSC Cardiovascular. http://www.jointcommission.org/certification/dsc_cardiovascular.aspx.

The Joint Commission. 2016c. DSC Endocrine. http://www.jointcommission.org/certification/dsc_endocrine.aspx.

The Joint Commission. 2016d. DSC Pulmonary. http://www.jointcommission.org/certification/dsc_pulmonary.aspx.

The Joint Commission. 2016e. Standards FAQs. http://www.jointcommission.org/standards_information/jcfaq.aspx.

Petterson, B. 2013. Content and Structure of the Health Record. Chapter 3 in *Health Information Management Technology: An Applied Approach*, 4th ed. Edited by Nanette B. Sayles. Chicago: AHIMA.

Pollack, R. 2013 (July 1). Letter to Marilyn Tavenner, CMS Administrator. http://www.aha.org/advocacy-issues/letter/2013/130701-cl-3255p-accred.pdf.

Smith, C.M. 2001. Documentation requirements for the acute care inpatient record (AHIMA Practice Brief). *Journal of AHIMA*. 72(3)2001:56A–G.

Wiedemann, L.A. 2010. Deleting errors in the EHR. *Journal of AHIMA*. 81(9):52–53.

42 CFR 482.22(c): Medical Staff Bylaws. 2015 (April 1).

42 CFR 482.24(c)(1): Interpretive Guidelines. 2009 (June 5).

5

Clinical Terminologies, Classifications, and Code Systems

Kathy Giannangelo, MA, RHIA, CCS, CPHIMS, FAHIMA

Learning Objectives

- Explain the importance of clinical terminologies, classifications, and code systems to healthcare
- Describe the content of SNOMED CT, Current Procedural Terminology, and terminologies used in nursing practice
- Examine the different classification systems and their purposes
- Identify code systems for laboratory and clinical

observations; professional services, procedures, and supplies; and drugs
- Define clinical terminologies, classifications, and code systems found in health data and information sets
- Recognize the need to have a database of clinical terminologies, classifications, and code systems

Key Terms

Classifications
Clinical terminologies
Code systems
Coding
Common Clinical Data Set
Concepts
Data set
Derived classification
Disability

Fully specified name (FSN)
Functioning
Granularity
Health information exchange
International Classification of Functioning, Disability, and Health (ICF)
Morbidity
Nomenclatures

Preferred term (PT)
Relationships
RxNorm concept unique identifier (RXCUI)
Semantic interoperability
SNOMED CT identifier
Unified Medical Language System (UMLS)

Health information management (HIM) professionals play a crucial role in coding clinical data. **Coding** is the process of assigning numeric or alphanumeric representations to clinical documentation. With the adoption of electronic health records (EHRs), the **nomenclatures** used to identify clinical data have increased in number and scope. Nomenclatures consist of a system of terms that follows pre-established naming conventions. They include clinical terminologies, classifications, and code systems. A **clinical terminology** is a set of terms representing the system of concepts for the medical field. **Classifications** are also a system where related entities are organized together. An accumulation of numeric or alphanumeric representations or codes for exchanging or storing information is a **code system**. Examples of each are SNOMED CT, International Classification of Diseases, Tenth Revision, Clinical Modification (ICD-10-CM), and Logical Observation Identifiers, Names, and Codes (LOINC) respectively.

This chapter discusses clinical terminologies, classifications, and code systems used in the healthcare industry to encode clinical data in a standardized manner. As this chapter will explain, certain nomenclatures are more appropriate for the collection of clinical data at a granular level such as SNOMED CT. Others are best utilized for the aggregation of clinical data for secondary data purposes, for example ICD-10-CM.

In addition, terminologies, classifications, and code systems are a key type of data managed by the data governance function. Understanding their purpose and use is necessary in order to succeed in managing the usability of the data employed by the healthcare organization or enterprise.

History and Importance of Clinical Terminologies, Classifications, and Code Systems

Clinical terminologies, classifications, and code systems exist to name and arrange medical content so it can be used for patient care, measuring patient outcomes, research, and administrative activities such as reimbursement. What started as a way to identify causes of death for statistical purposes, expanded to reporting diagnoses and procedures on claims for reimbursement. Today, the electronic health record (EHR) can capture the detail of diagnostic studies, history and physical examinations, visit notes, ancillary department information, nursing notes, vital signs, outcomes measures, and any other clinically relevant observations about the patient. Figure 5.1 illustrates a comparison of claims data and EHR data and the vast difference in clinical content.

Investigating the reasons for collecting data illustrates the importance of clinical terminologies, classifications, and code systems. If data **granularity,** or the detail is the goal, then clinical terminologies are the best option. On the other hand, if the objective is aggregate data, then classifications are the better choice. Aggregate data is data extracted from individual health records and combined to form deidentified information about groups of patients that can be compared and analyzed. With regards to code systems, some are for the collection of clinical data at a granular level while others are for aggregation. Table 5.1 lists examples of data uses and their data requirements. As the table shows, granular data is needed when the details are key to use whereas aggregate data suits when the combination of data provides information about related entities is sufficient.

Additionally, primary and secondary data uses are relevant to understanding clinical terminologies, classifications, and code systems. A nomenclature that allows for the collection of clinical data at a granular level is needed for primary data use such as for clinical decision support. Whereas, one that aggregates the data will work for secondary data use. An example of secondary data use is the identification of diagnoses and procedures

Figure 5.1 What lies beneath?

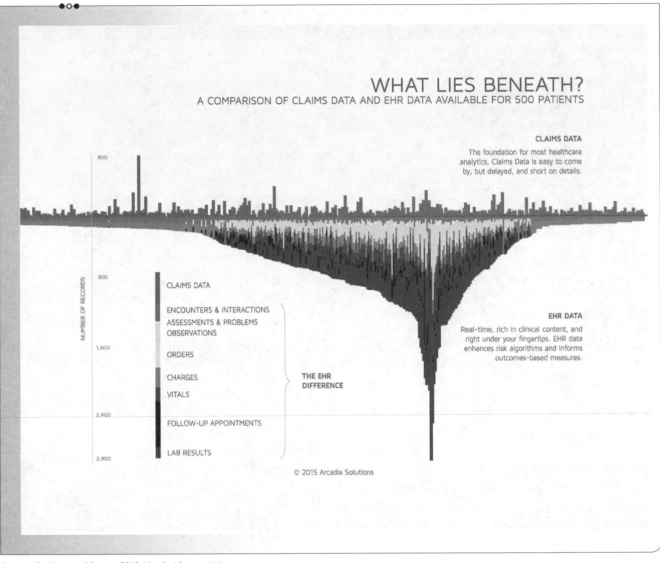

Source: Shulman and Stepro 2015. Used with permission.

for the purpose of billing and payment. For more information on primary and secondary data, refer to chapter 3.

The determination of which clinical terminologies, classifications, and code systems are used as the standard is primarily driven by regulation. Standards are critical for creating an interoperable health IT environment (ONC n.d.). An interoperable health IT environment is one in which seamless health information exchange is possible across diverse EHR systems and the information is understood and shared with those in need of it at the time it is needed. Clinical terminologies, classifications, and code system standards are one of the ONC's interoperability building blocks. They support system interoperability by providing the mutual understanding of the meaning of data exchanged between information systems.

Congress creates legislation authorizing the establishment of standards through regulatory agencies. For example, the Electronic Health Record Standards and Certification Criteria Rule defines the standards that must be used in order for EHR technology to be certified by the Office of the National Coordinator for Health Information Technology (ONC) Authorized Certification Bodies. Included in this rule are the content standards for representing electronic health information such as SNOMED CT for problems and RxNorm for clinical drugs, which will be discussed later in this chapter.

Table 5.1   Examples of data uses and their requirements

Data use	Requirement	Clinical terminologies, classifications, or code systems
To facilitate electronic data collection at the point of care with terms familiar to the user	Granular data	Clinical terminologies Code systems
To allow many different sites and different providers the ability to send and receive medical data in an understandable and usable manner, thereby speeding care delivery and reducing duplicate testing and duplicate prescribing	Granular data	Clinical terminologies Code systems
To allow the computer to manipulate standardized data and find information relevant to individual patients for the purpose of producing automatic reminders or alerts	Granular data	Clinical terminologies Code systems
To allow the computer to manipulate standardized data and find information relevant to individual patients for the purpose of producing automatic reminders or alerts	Granular data	Clinical terminologies Code systems
To allow collection and reporting of basic health statistics	Aggregate data	Classification systems Code systems
To provide data that are used in designing payment systems and determining the correct payment for healthcare services	Aggregate data	Classification systems Code systems
To provide data that are used in monitoring public health and risks	Aggregate data	Classification systems Code systems
To provide data to consumers on costs and outcomes of treatment options	Aggregate data	Classification systems Code systems

Source: Giannangelo 2015.

Clinical Terminologies

Clinical terminologies form the basis of coded data and provide the data structure required for semantic interoperability and health information exchange. Semantic interoperability is the mutual understanding of the meaning of data exchanged between information systems. Health information exchange is when health information is electronically traded between providers and others with the same level of interoperability. Clinical terminologies may also be reference terminologies. A reference terminology in the health information technology (HIT) domain is a set of concepts and relationships that provide a mutual understanding for clinical decision support and for exchanging data with meaning about the healthcare course (Giannangelo 2015, 5). Concepts are unique units of knowledge or thoughts created by a unique combination of characteristics whereas relationships are a type of connection between two concepts. Examples of clinical terminologies include SNOMED CT, Current Procedural Terminology, and various nursing terminologies.

SNOMED CT

The International Health Terminology Standards Development Organisation (IHTSDO) defines SNOMED CT as a "comprehensive clinical terminology that provides clinical content and expressivity for clinical documentation and reporting" (IHTSDO 2014a). According to IHTSDO, SNOMED CT is the most comprehensive, multilingual clinical terminology in the world.

There is no book of SNOMED CT codes and no coding professional assigns a SNOMED CT identifier. The terminology instead is implemented in software applications where healthcare providers record clinical information using identifiers that refer to concepts that are formally defined as part of the terminology during the process of care (IHTSDO 2014b). It allows for the collection of clinical data at a granular level. For example, at the point of care a physician using an EHR uses a drop-down list to view the clinical terms relevant to their practice and the patient's problem. While not seen by the physician, the clinical terms have SNOMED CT identifiers attached to them. By selecting the clinical term, the identifier is captured and thereby provides the primary source of information about the patient.

SNOMED CT Purpose and Use

SNOMED CT's overall purpose is to standardize clinical phrases, making it easier to produce accurate electronic health information. Doing so enables automatic interpretation and sharing of clinical information. Semantic interoperability is also possible.

With the consistent, reliable, and comprehensive capture of clinical phrases with SNOMED CT its uses and benefits are many:

> With the SNOMED CT encoded data sent securely during the transfer of care to other providers or to patients, the barriers to the electronic exchange are reduced resulting in improved quality of the information. Combining SNOMED CT coded data with other encoded data such as medication and lab results has a number of uses including clinical decision support, clinical quality measures, and registries. (Helwig 2013)

For additional information on registries, see chapter 7. Quality measures are covered in chapter 18.

SNOMED CT is also one of several standards chosen for the entry of structured data in certified electronic health record systems (ONC 2015). This includes patient problems, encounter diagnosis, procedures, family health history, and smoking status. The National Library of Medicine (NLM) produces the Clinical Observations Recording and Encoding (CORE) problem list subset of SNOMED CT. This subset includes SNOMED CT concepts commonly used for encoding clinical information at a summary level, such as the problem list.

SNOMED CT Content and Structure

SNOMED CT is made up of three main components—concepts, descriptions, and relationships. Concepts are a specific thought or abstract idea. Each concept is assigned a unique, numeric and machine-readable **SNOMED CT identifier.** The SNOMED CT identifier is a unique integer assigned to each SNOMED CT component. Examples of

clinical concepts are diagnoses (for example, coronary arteriosclerosis) and procedures (for example, coronary artery bypass grafting).

SNOMED CT contains 19 top-level hierarchies and each concept belongs to only one top-level hierarchy. For example, coronary arteriosclerosis belongs to the clinical finding hierarchy while coronary artery bypass grafting belongs to the procedure hierarchy. Figure 5.2 lists the 19 SNOMED CT hierarchies and shows how the concept arthritis of the knee belongs to only the clinical finding hierarchy.

Descriptions are human-readable representations of concepts. A SNOMED CT concept has at least two descriptions: a fully specified name and a preferred term. In SNOMED CT the **fully specified name (FSN)** is the unique text assigned to a concept that completely describes it and the **preferred term** is the description or name assigned to a concept that is used most commonly. In the example of transient cerebral ischemia, the fully specified name is transient ischemic attack (disorder). The term enclosed in parenthesis at the end is called the semantic tag and allows differentiation between concepts such as ulcer (disorder) from ulcer (morphologic abnormality). Synonyms are another type of description. Examples of synonyms for transient ischemic attack (TIA) (disorder) are transient cerebral ischemia, TIA, and temporary cerebral vascular dysfunction. Each concept has at least one synonym identified as a preferred term, which provides a common, agreed-upon way of referring to a concept. In the case of transient ischemic attack (disorder) the preferred term is *transient cerebral ischemia*. Concepts may have multiple synonyms.

Two main types of relationships link concepts to each other. Relationships define the meaning of a concept in a manner that allows a computer to process it (IHTSDO 2014b). The subtype relationship uses the "is a" relationship type to indicate the source concept is a subtype of the destination concept. These relationships form the poly-hierarchical structure of SNOMED CT. For example, figure 5.2 shows the "is a" relationship types indicating arthritis of knee is a subtype of arthropathy of knee joint, arthritis, knee joint inflamed, and inflammatory

Figure 5.2   SNOMED CT design and development

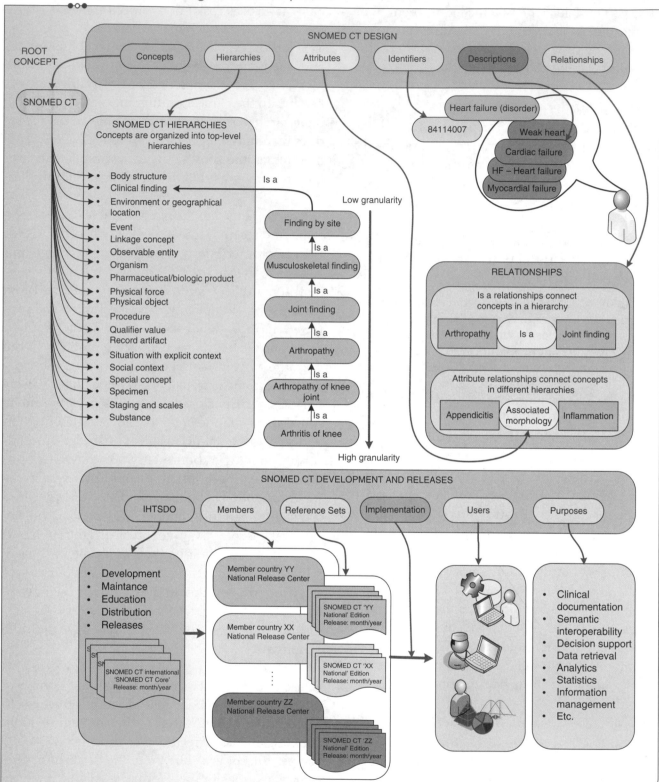

Source: IHTSDO 2014b. Used with permission.

disorder of extremity. Arthritis of knee, in turn, is a supertype of concepts such as rheumatoid arthritis of knee, synovitis of knee and monoarthritis of knee. The other main type of relationship is the attribute relationship, which is a factor in defining the source concept by associating it with the value of a defining characteristic (IHTSDO 2014b). For example, referring again to figure 5.2, the attribute relationships for arthritis of knee, associated morphology and finding site, are used to associate the source concept arthritis of knee to the target concepts of inflammation (associated morphology) and knee joint structure (finding site).

Current Procedural Terminology, Fourth Edition

The American Medical Association (AMA) owns and copyrights Current Procedural Terminology (CPT). According to the AMA, "CPT is the most widely accepted nomenclature for the reporting of physician procedures and services under government and private health insurance programs" (AMA 2015). The CPT Editorial Panel in consultation with medical specialty societies represented by the CPT Advisory Committee is responsible for maintaining the terminology.

CPT identifies the services rendered rather than the diagnosis on the claim. The International Classification of Diseases (ICD) identifies the diagnosis and is discussed later in this chapter. CPT and ICD form units of information about a patient visit in that the diagnosis represented by ICD supports the medical necessity of the service represented by CPT.

CPT is published annually as a print and e-book. It is also available in software applications such as physician practice management systems. Assignment of the CPT code is most often the responsibility of a professional coder based on the physician documentation of the medical services or procedures provided.

CPT Purpose and Use

The purpose of CPT is to provide a uniform language that allows for accurately descriptions of medical, surgical, and diagnostic services. It is designed to communicate consistent information about medical services and procedures among physicians, clinical staff, patients, accreditation organizations, and payers for administrative, financial, and analytical purposes.

Despite being copyrighted by the AMA, the Health Insurance Portability and Accountability Act (HIPAA) mandates the use of the CPT in healthcare data electronic transactions. HIPAA named CPT (including codes and modifiers) as the procedure code set for all but hospital inpatient procedures. CPT codes are the five-character identifiers that represent the service or procedure the individual receives from a healthcare provider and two-character modifiers indicate the service or procedure performed has been altered by some circumstance but not changed in its definition. Thus, physicians and hospitals must report medical and procedure services performed by physicians and other healthcare professionals to public as well as private insurers, using CPT.

CPT Content and Structure

CPT includes codes, descriptions, and guidelines and covers the breadth of health services physicians provide. Descriptions for evaluation and management services such as a new patient office visit, anesthetic services, surgical procedures, radiology services, pathology and laboratory tests, and medical care are all found in CPT. The Centers for Medicare and Medicaid Services (CMS) categorizes CPT as Level I of the Health Care Common Procedure Coding System (HCPCS) discussed later in this chapter.

CPT is divided into categories: Category I, Category II, and Category III. Category I is the major terminology. It contains a description along with a five-digit code for each service or procedure. Two-digit modifiers are available to qualify the service or procedure. For example, the modifier 50 is used to indicate a bilateral procedure. Criteria for inclusion in Category I include the US Food and Drug Administration has approved the service or procedure, many providers in different locations perform it, and it is clinically effective.

Category I CPT includes six main sections:

- Evaluation and Management (E/M)
- Anesthesia
- Surgery

- Radiology
- Pathology and Laboratory
- Medicine

The following are examples of Category I CPT services along with their identifiers:

33511 Coronary artery bypass, vein only: 2 coronary arteries

71020 Radiologic examination, chest 2 views, frontal and lateral

82951 Glucose; tolerance test (GTT), 3 specimens (includes glucose)

90839 Psychotherapy for crisis; first 60 minutes

Category II CPT is used for performance measurement. This category was created to support data collection about the quality of care rendered by coding certain services and test results that support nationally established performance measures and have an evidence base as contributing to quality patient care. They represent clinical findings or services where there is strong evidence of contribution to health outcomes and high quality care. The codes are alphanumeric consisting of four numbers followed by the letter F. The following is an example of a Category II CPT service along with its identifier:

1065F Ischemic stroke symptom onset of less than 3 hours prior to arrival

Category III CPT is for emerging technologies, services, and procedures. They are considered temporary and they may or may not eventually be moved to Category I. Category III codes are alphanumeric consisting of four numbers followed by the letter T. The following is an example of a Category III CPT procedure along with its identifier:

0345T Transcatheter mitral valve repair percutaneous approach via the coronary sinus

CPT also includes an introduction, an index, and appendices. The index is used to locate a code or code range and is organized by main and modifying terms. Appendices provide information to supplement the main portion of CPT. For example, Appendix A, Modifiers, describes all the modifiers available for use with a CPT code.

Nursing Terminologies

Just as the field of nursing covers a wide range of services, so do the terminologies available to identify those services. The choice of terminology depends on the nursing care documented. In addition, some are location specific. For example, the Nursing Outcomes Classification (NOC) may be used to represent the outcomes of nursing interventions in all settings and the Omaha System is used in the home health setting.

Nursing Terminologies Purpose and Use

Nursing terms provide an effective basis for use in contemporary data systems (Warren 2015, 218). Within the American Nursing Association (ANA) is a committee charged with reviewing and recognizing nursing terminologies that are considered useful in the support of the scope of nursing practice. Several organizations are responsible for nursing terminology development including universities and associations.

The purpose of nursing terminologies is to represent clinical information generated and used by nursing staff (Warren 2015, 207). They are designed to communicate consistent information about nursing services for a variety of reasons including directing patient care, measuring progress of treatment, as well as for administrative functions, education, and analytical purposes.

Although there is no mandate to use nursing terminologies, the ANA's board of directors published a position statement with regards to the inclusion of recognized terminologies within EHRs as well as other HIT applications. The ANA indicated support for the following recommendations:

- Plan implementation of terminologies
- Obtain consensus on which terminology to use
- Using the same terminologies facilitates data sharing
- Standards selected should be nationally recognized (ANA 2015)

Nursing Terminologies Content and Structure

Each nursing terminology covers content specific to its use. Table 5.2 lists the content coverage of some of the ANA-recognized nursing terminologies.

Table 5.2 Content coverage of ANA-recognized nursing terminologies

ANA-recognized nursing terminology	Content coverage
NANDA International	Thirteen domains: ● Health promotion ● Nutrition ● Elimination/exchange ● Activity/rest ● Perception/cognition ● Self-perception ● Role relationship ● Sexuality ● Coping/stress tolerance ● Life principles ● Safety/protection ● Comfort ● Growth/development
Nursing Interventions Classification (NIC)	Seven domains: ● Physiological: Basic ● Physiological: Complex ● Behavioral ● Safety ● Family ● Health system ● Community
Nursing Outcomes Classification (NOC)	Seven domains: ● Functional health ● Physiologic health ● Psychosocial health ● Health knowledge and behavior ● Perceived health ● Family health ● Community health
Clinical Care Classification (CCC)	Two taxonomies: ● CCC of nursing diagnoses and outcomes ● CCC of nursing interventions and actions
Omaha System	Three components: ● Assessment ● Intervention ● Outcomes
International Classification for Nursing Practice (ICNP)	Multiaxial representation with seven axes: ● Focus ● Judgment ● Means ● Action ● Time ● Location ● Client

Source: Warren 2015, 208–214.

The structure also varies among terminologies. For example, included with each nursing intervention in the Nursing Interventions Classification (NIC) is a label name, definition, unique number (code), set of activities to carry out the intervention, and background readings; whereas in the Nursing Outcomes Classification (NOC) each nursing outcome includes a definition, list of indicators for evaluating patient status in relation to outcome, a target outcome rating, a place to identify the source of the data, a scale to measure patient status, and a short list of references used in developing the outcome (Warren 2015, 209–210).

Check Your Understanding 5.1

Instructions: **Answer the following questions.**

1. True or false: If data granularity is the goal of collecting the data, clinical terminologies is the best choice.
2. True or false: The SNOMED CT preferred term includes the semantic tag.
3. True or false: The three main core components of SNOMED CT are the SNOMED CT identifier, concepts, and descriptions.
4. True or false: Category I CPT includes E/M, anesthesia, surgery, radiology, pathology and laboratory, and medicine.
5. True or false: Nursing terminologies are used for reimbursement of nursing care for Medicare patients.

Classifications

Classifications are key to secondary data use. They aggregate clinical data for healthcare statistics, design payment systems, and determine the correct payment for healthcare services. They also provide data that are used in monitoring public health and risks. Information can be obtained from data encoded with a classification to improve clinical, financial, and administrative performance. Some of these classification systems are discussed in the following sections.

International Classification of Diseases, Tenth Revision, Clinical Modification

The National Center for Health Statistics (NCHS) is the governmental body responsible for the development and maintenance of ICD-10-CM. It originates from the World Health Organization's International Statistical Classification of Diseases and Related Health Problems, Tenth Revision (ICD-10). However, ICD-10-CM greatly expands the classification resulting in greater specificity and clinical detail.

ICD-10-CM identifies the diagnosis established by the provider. For example, the ICD-10-CM code and the CPT code result in a package of information about a patient visit performed in the physician's office. This bundle is an example of aggregate data that can be used for a number of purposes.

ICD-10-CM can be updated twice a year by NCHS. The October update always occurs while the April update is available when necessary for improving the timeless of data collection. Twice a year the ICD-10 Coordination and Maintenance (C&M) Committee holds public meetings to review proposals for ICD-10-CM revisions. Representative from NCHS are members of this committee and, based on their advice, the director of NCHS makes the final decisions on ICD-10-CM revisions. Software vendors and publishers use NCHS available data files to produce coding resources such as online and print ICD-10-CM products.

Assignment of the ICD-10-CM code is most often the responsibility of a professional coder based on the physician documentation of the patient's diagnosis.

ICD-10-CM Purpose and Use

The purpose of ICD-10-CM is to provide a classification of diseases for **morbidity**. Morbidity is the state of being diseased including illness, injury, or deviation from normal health. It is intended to classify diagnoses established by physicians at the conclusion of a patient encounter.

ICD-10-CM has many uses. All of those identified previously for classifications apply to ICD-10-CM. One use is mandated by HIPAA, which specifies the use of national standards for electronic healthcare transactions. ICD-10-CM (including the official ICD-10-CM guidelines for coding and reporting) is named as the standard for diseases, injuries, impairments, other health related problems, their manifestations, and causes of injury, disease, impairment, or other health-related problems. Thus, healthcare providers must report diagnoses to public as well as private insurers using ICD-10-CM.

ICD-10-CM Content and Structure

ICD-10-CM contains three to seven character codes and descriptions for patient conditions. This includes symptoms, syndromes, diseases, and other reasons for patients requiring healthcare services. Instructions, referred to as conventions, are also a part of the classification. These are general rules to apply when using ICD-10-CM.

ICD-10-CM is divided into 21 chapters. Many are based on a body system; others are for certain types of conditions such as pregnancy. Within each chapter are blocks of conditions related in some manner, such as a single disease entity, categories, subcategories and, when appropriate, subclassifications. Figure 5.3 displays the blocks

for Chapter 4, Endocrine, Nutritional, and Metabolic Diseases, category E11, subcategory E11.2, and subclassification E11.21.

Another component of ICD-10-CM is the alphabetic index. There are two major sections to the alphabetic index—the Index to Diseases and Injuries and the Index to External Causes. Two tables—one for neoplasm and the other for drugs and chemicals—are also included the index. All content in the index is organized by main and modifying terms. Main terms represent the condition of the patient and modifying terms further explain the condition. For example, failure is the main term and congestive heart the modifying terms for the diagnosis of congestive heart failure.

ICD-10-Procedure Coding System

The Centers for Medicare and Medicaid Services (CMS) is the federal agency responsible for the ICD-10-Procedure Coding System (ICD-10-PCS). It was developed through a contract with 3M Health Information Systems and is being maintained by CMS.

Figure 5.3 Chapter 4, Endocrine, Nutritional, and Metabolic Diseases blocks, category, subcategory and subclassification

Blocks
E00-E07 Disorders of thyroid gland
E08-E13 Diabetes mellitus
E15-E16 Other disorders of glucose regulation and pancreatic internal secretion
E20-E35 Disorders of other endocrine glands
E36-E36 Intraoperative complications of endocrine system
E40-E46 Malnutrition
E50-E64 Other nutritional deficiencies
E65-E68 Overweight, obesity and other hyperalimentation
E70-E88 Metabolic disorders
E89-E89 Postprocedural endocrine and metabolic complications and disorders, not elsewhere classified

Category E11
E11 Type 2 diabetes mellitus

Subcategory E11.2
E11.2 Type 2 diabetes mellitus with kidney complications

Subclassification E11.21
E11.21 Type 2 diabetes mellitus with diabetic nephropathy

Source: NCHS 2015.

Just as CPT identifies the procedure performed by the provider so does ICD-10-PCS. However, it was created as the companion to ICD-10-CM and not as a replacement for CPT. A diagnosis coded in ICD-10-CM code combined with a procedure coded in ICD-10-PCS would be used by a hospital to explain the reason for a patient being admitted and discharged for care and the inpatient procedures performed during the stay. This aggregated data is used to determine hospital payment under the inpatient prospective payment system discussed in chapter 15.

Twice a year updates, on April 1 and October 1, are possible for ICD-10-PCS. The April update is available to address new technologies whereas the October 1st update is yearly. CMS representatives on the ICD-10 Coordination and Maintenance (C&M) Committee provide advice to the administrator of CMS who makes the final decisions on ICD-10-PCS revisions. CMS makes data files for software vendors and publishers to produce online and print ICD-10-PCS products available on their website.

Upon discharge of the patient from the hospital, a professional coder assigns the ICD-10-PCS code based on the physician documentation.

ICD-10-PCS Purpose and Use

The purpose of ICD-10-PCS is to provide a system for classifying procedures performed on hospital inpatients. It provides a unique code for all substantially different procedures, both currently known and those that may be identified at some future date in time.

Uses for ICD-10-PCS include those identified for classifications in general. Just as HIPAA mandates ICD-10-CM, there is also a requirement for ICD-10-PCS. ICD-10-PCS (including the official ICD-10-PCS guidelines for coding and reporting) is the standard for preventive, diagnostic, therapeutic or other management procedures or other actions taken for diseases, injuries, and impairments on hospital inpatients reported by hospitals. Hospitals are required to use ICD-10-PCS to report procedures to public as well as private insurers.

ICD-10-PCS Content and Structure

Although ICD-10-PCS replaces the volume of ICD-9-CM that classifies procedures, it is significantly different. ICD-10-PCS contains seven-character codes and descriptions for procedures. Most of ICD-10-PCS describes medical and surgical procedures. Divided into groups, the other sections are:

Medical and surgical-related sections

- Obstetrics
- Placement
- Administration
- Measurement and monitoring
- Extracorporeal assistance and monitoring
- Extracorporeal therapies
- Osteopathic
- Other procedures
- Chiropractic

Ancillary sections

- Imaging
- Nuclear medicine
- Radiation oncology
- Physical rehabilitation and diagnostic audiology
- Mental health
- Substance abuse treatment
- New technology

ICD-10-PCS is made up of number of parts including tables, an index, and definitions. The tables are arranged in alphanumeric order and are formatted as a grid that lays out the valid combinations of character values for a procedure code. There are two parts to the table. The upper portion lists the first three characters and their definition and the lower portion contains columns for the remaining four characters. Each column lists the possible options for completing the seven-character code. Figure 5.4 shows an ICD-10-PCS table.

ICD-10-PCS also has an alphabetic index organized by two types of main terms. One type is based common procedure names such as cholecystectomy and the other type on the value of the third character of the seven-character

Figure 5.4   Example of an ICD-10-PCS table

OFT

Section	**0**	Medical And Surgical
Body System	**F**	Hepatobiliary System and Pancreas
Operation	**T**	Resection: Cutting out or off, without replacement, all of a body part

Body Part	Approach	Device	Qualifier
0 Liver **1** Liver, Right Lobe **2** Liver, Left Lobe **4** Gallbladder **G** Pancreas	**0** Open **4** Percutaneous Endoscopic	**Z** No Device	**Z** No Qualifier
5 Hepatic Duct, Right **6** Hepatic Duct, Left **8** Cystic Duct **9** Common Bilc Duct **C** Ampulla of Vater **D** Pancreatic Duct **F** Pancreatic Duct, Accessory	**0** Open **4** Percutaneous Endoscopic **7** Via Natural or Artificial Opening **8** Via Natural or Artificial Opening Endoscopic	**Z** No Device	**Z** No Qualifier

Source: CMS 2015a.

ICD-10-PCS code. The meaning of the third character varies depending on the section. For example, the third character value for the medical and surgical procedure section is root operation or the objective of the procedure. Resection, as shown in table 5.3, is one of the root operations and is listed as a main term in the index.

Another part of ICD-10-PCS is the definitions. Arranged in section order, definitions are tied to values of characters 3 through 7 of the seven-character code. Explanations and examples may also be included with the definitions to aid in understanding how the character value is to be applied. To illustrate, the definitions and any associated explanation and examples for the third through fifth characters are shown as follows for T, 0, and 0 found in table 5.3.

International Classification of Functioning, Disability and Health

International Classification of Functioning, Disability, and Health (ICF) is one of the three reference classifications approved by the World Health Organization (WHO) Family of International Classification (WHO-FIC) Network. According to WHO, "ICF is the WHO framework for measuring health and disability at both individual and population levels" (WHO 2013).

Table 5.3   Example of ICD-10-PCS characters

Character 3 – Operation T Resection	
ICD-10-PCS Value	**Definition**
Resection	Definition: Cutting out or off, without replacement, all of a body part Includes/examples: Total nephrectomy, total lobectomy of lung
Character 4 – Body Part 0 Liver	
ICD-10-PCS Value	**Definition**
Liver	Includes: Quadrate lobe
Character 5 – Approach 0 Open	
ICD-10-PCS Value	**Definition**
Open	Definition: Cutting through the skin or mucous membrane and any other body layers necessary to expose the site of the procedure

ICD is also a WHO-FIC Network reference classification. ICD classifies heath conditions whereas ICF classifies states of functioning, disability and health. For example, a patient with a spinal cord injury with moderate impairment with control of voluntary movement would be represented with an ICD code for condition of the patient, spinal cord injury, and an ICF code for the level of functioning, moderate impairment with control of voluntary movement. ICF provides a standard language, terms and concepts and an organized data structure for health and disability information (WHO 2015).

ICF is updated once a year in October by WHO. While the application of the ICF concepts and framework in clinical practice is the responsibility of health professionals such as physical therapists, the individual or their advocate is an integral part of the assessment.

ICF Purpose and Use

WHO specifies four primary ICF purposes:

- To provide a scientific basis for understanding and studying health and health-related states, outcomes, and determinants
- To establish a common language for describing health and health-related states in order to improve communication between different users, such as healthcare workers, researchers, policy makers and the public, including people with disabilities
- To permit comparison of data across countries, healthcare disciplines, services and time
- To provide a systematic coding scheme for health information systems (WHO 2001)

ICF has a variety of uses including clinical practice, for population-based census or survey data, in educational systems, policy making, and advocacy. Although considered during clinical data content standards discussions, the United States has no federal mandate that requires ICF be used.

ICF Content and Structure

ICF is both a model and a classification. The ICF model is a nonlinear, systemic, biopsychosocial model consisting of multiple components including Health Condition, Body Functions and Structures, Activities and Participation, Contextual Factors (that is, Environmental and Personal Factors), and Umbrella Terms. **Functioning** is the umbrella term for Body Functions, Body Structures, Activities and Participation. It denotes the positive or neutral aspects of the interaction between the health condition and contextual factors. **Disability** is the umbrella term for impairments, activity limitations, and participation restrictions. It denotes the negative aspects of the interaction between an individual and that individual's contextual factors.

As a classification, ICF includes four code components—Body Structures, Body Functions, Activities and Participation, and Environmental Factors. The ICF model component health condition is described by ICD-10.

The first level of classification is the chapter and branches are the tiered levels of the classification (Porter 2015, 194). An example of this structure is shown as follows.

s Body Structures (code component)

s7 Chapter 7 Structures related to movement (chapter = first-level classification)

s730 Structure of the upper extremity (first branch = second-level classification)

s7301 Structure of the upper arm (second branch = third-level classification)

s 73010 Bones of forearm (third branch = fourth level of classification) (WHO 2001)

International Classification of Diseases for Oncology, Third Edition

International Classification of Diseases for Oncology, Third Edition (ICD-O-3) is a **derived classification** of the WHO Family of International Classifications and is based on ICD. A derived classification is one based on a reference classification such as ICD or ICF by adopting the reference classification structure and categories and providing additional detail or through rearrangement or aggregation of items from one or more reference classifications.

Tumor or cancer registries regard ICD-O-3 as their system for classifying the topography and morphology of neoplasms. Topography refers to the anatomical site of neoplasm's origin and morphology the structure and form. Specifically, morphology pertains to cell type or histology and the neoplasm's biological activity or behavior. The common source for the clinical content to be classified with ICD-O-3 is the pathology report.

ICD-O-3 was published in 2000 with corrections added in 2001 and 2003. WHO produced an additional update—ICD-O-3.1—in 2011. Both ICD-O-3 and ICD-O-3.1 are searchable online through WHO's International Agency for Research on Cancer webpage. The print product can be purchased from the WHO book store as well as online resellers.

ICD-O-3 Purpose and Use

The purpose of ICD-O-3 is to classify diseases for oncology, a branch of medicine that focuses on tumors. Data collected via ICD-O-3 is reported to state, national, and North American cancer registries.

The ICD-O-3 data have uses including:

- Planning and evaluating the patient's case management
- Administrative information for facility planners, cancer committees, and practitioners
- Developing and evaluating cancer control programs
- Cancer research (NCI n.d.)

ICD-O-3 Content and Structure

ICD-O-3 is a dual classification. It contains a set of codes for topography and morphology of tumors. The site of origin of the neoplasm is captured by the topography code. This code is the same four-character category as in the malignant neoplasm section of the second chapter of ICD-10. The exceptions are those categories that relate to secondary neoplasms and to specified morphological types of tumors. In addition, ICD-O-3 includes a topography for specific types of tumors.

With very few histological types available in ICD-10, ICD-O-3 provides greater detail of the

Figure 5.5 Example of the structure of a complete ICD-O-3 code

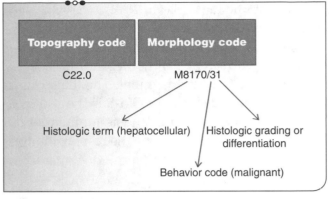

©AHIMA

histological classification. The morphology code describes the characteristics of the tumor itself, including cell type and biologic activity. For example, code M8170/3 is a hepatocellular carcinoma where the first four digits indicate the histological term (hepatocelluar), the fifth digit after the slash is the behavior code (malignant). A separate single digit indicates the histological grading or differentiation. Figure 5.5 shows the structure of a complete ICD-O-3 code.

There are five main sections of ICD-O-3: Instructions for Use; Topography-Numerical List; Morphology-Numerical List; Alphabetic Index; and Differences in Morphology Codes between the second and third editions. The Alphabetic Index is used for searching a noun or adjective in order to locate the code for topography identified with a leading C and morphology identified with a leading M.

Diagnostic and Statistical Manual of Mental Disorders, Fifth Edition

The American Psychiatric Association (APA) developed the Diagnostic and Statistical Manual of Mental Disorders (DSM). As the standard medical classification for mental disorders, the fifth edition provides a reliable source of clinical criteria for mental health and medical professionals when establishing a diagnosis. For example, contained within DSM-5 are diagnostic criteria for depressive, anxiety, feeding and eating, and personality disorders.

A clinician with the appropriate clinical training and experience uses DSM-5 to identify mental disorders. The codes incorporated into the classification are ICD-10-CM.

APA last updated DSM in 2013. Accessible via a link on the APA website, the DSM-5 Coding Supplement lists updates to reflect coding updates, changes or corrections, and other information relevant to mental health payment. The diagnosis of the mental disorder using DSM-5 is the responsibility of the clinician while the assignment of the ICD-10-CM code is most often the responsibility of a professional coder based on the documentation of the patient's diagnosis.

DSM-5 Purpose and Use

DSM-5 fills the need for "a clear and concise description of each mental disorder" (APA 2013, 5). It standardizes the clinician's diagnostic process for patients with mental disorders.

By including the ICD-10-CM codes, the clinician can report mental health disorders for administrative requirements such as requesting payment for psychiatric services or to report public health statistics.

DSM-5 may be used to conduct clinical assessments and to develop a comprehensive treatment plan. It is also used as a standard language for communicating between healthcare providers about mental disorders for a variety of purposes such as research. Although DSM-5 has forensic use, the APA warns there are risks and limitations to using it in this setting, as a clinical diagnosis of a DSM-5 mental disorder does not necessarily meet legal criteria for the presence of a mental disorder. It also does not determine a status such as competency or criminal responsibility.

DSM-5 Content and Structure

DSM-5 contains three sections, an Appendix, and an Index. The first section, DSM-5 Basics, provides an introduction along with instructions on how to use the manual. The APA's statement regarding forensic use is also a part of this section. Section II, Diagnostic Criteria and Codes, contains the diagnostic criteria, descriptive text, and ICD-10-CM codes.

Section III, Emerging Measures and Models, provides supplemental content that are not required for clinical use but could be helpful to the clinician. Included in this section are proposed mental disorders, which require further research.

 ## Check Your Understanding 5.2

Instructions: Answer the following questions by matching the classifications to what each classifies.

1. _____ ICD-10-CM

2. _____ ICD-10-PCS

3. _____ ICF

4. _____ ICD-O-3

5. _____ DSM-5

   A. Mental disorders
   B. Diseases for oncology
   C. Inpatient procedures
   D. States of functioning
   E. Diseases for morbidity

Code Systems

Code system is a very broad term. Given its definition at the beginning of this chapter, some of the terminologies and classifications previously covered could also be called code systems. Thus, a code system may have characteristics of a terminology or a classification. Depending on the system, it may be used at the point of care or for secondary data use. Common healthcare code systems are addressed in the following sections.

Logical Observation Identifiers, Names, and Codes

LOINC is "a universal code system for tests, measurements, and observations" (Regenstrief Institute n.d.). An observation is a measurement, test, or simple assertion and observation identifiers are the universal identifiers (names and codes) for the observation. LOINC provides names and codes for identifying laboratory and clinical test result or clinical observation. For example, the LOINC code 24356-8 and its long text name, Urinalysis complete panel—Urine, describes what was observed. Regenstrief Institute is the organization responsible for the development and maintenance of LOINC. The LOINC Committee, a group of experts organized by the Regenstrief Institute to study available standards, determined no code system available was granular enough for observation identifiers. Thus, LOINC was created to fill this gap.

Regenstrief Institute updates LOINC twice a year in June and December. No book of LOINC codes is produced. A number of file formats are released by Regenstrief Institute on their website for downloading. Regenstrief Institute also provides several tools for the industry. For example, they offer a web-based LOINC search application used to explore LOINC and a more extensive resource, Regenstrief LOINC Mapping Assistant (RELMA). The purpose of RELMA is to assist in the mapping of local terms to the universal LOINC codes.

LOINC Purpose and Use

The purpose of LOINC is to standardize names and codes for the identification of laboratory and clinical test results or observation. Those interested in LOINC include hospitals, clinical laboratories, doctors' offices, state health departments, governmental healthcare providers, third-party payers, and organizations responsible for quality assurance and utilization review (McDonald et al. 2015).

LOINC facilitates the exchange and aggregation of data between diverse electronic systems including the clinical laboratory information management and the EHR. This clinical data can then be used for clinical care and research. Another use is in outcomes management where the clinical data is examined in order to study the outcome and improve care.

LOINC is also one of several standards chosen for the entry of structured data in certified EHR systems (ONC 2015). This includes using LOINC for clinical lab test results and in the Common Clinical Data Set discussed later in this chapter. Having a structured format for laboratory test information in certified EHRs enables the exchange of data for use in clinical care and research.

LOINC Content and Structure

There are two major groups of LOINC content—laboratory and clinical. The laboratory piece includes just as the name suggests: laboratory tests such as chemistry, urinalysis, serology, toxicology. For the clinical piece LOINC, the scope is broad. Codes are available for observations like vital signs, obstetric ultrasound, radiology studies, clinical documents, and survey instruments to name a few.

The fully specified name of a test result or clinical observation is made up of five or six main parts:

- Name
- Property timing sample (urine, serum)
- Scale of measurement
- Method of measurement (McDonald et al. 2015)

In LOINC, each label is assigned a unique permanent code. The code identifies the test results in electronic reports in clinical laboratory information management and EHR systems thereby facilitating data exchange for use in clinical care, quality measurement, and research.

Healthcare Common Procedure Coding System Level II

HCPCS is made up of two code systems: Level I and Level II. Level I is made up of CPT, discussed previously. HCPCS Level II standardizes the reporting of professional services, procedures, products, and supplies. CMS publishes and maintains HCPCS Level II. One section within HCPCS Level II, the Dental Codes, or D codes, are a separate category and are published by the American Dental Association, not CMS.

CMS requires physicians to use HCPCS Level II to report services provided to Medicare and Medicaid patients. Hospitals must report ambulatory surgery services, radiology, and other diagnostic services using HCPCS Level II.

CMS updates HCPCS Level II quarterly on January 1, April 1, July 1, and October 1. A professional coder assigns the HCPCS Level II code based on the physician documentation.

HCPCS Purpose and Use

The primary purpose of HCPCS Level II is to meet the operational needs of Medicare and Medicaid reimbursement programs. Thus, as expected, HCPCS Level II is required for reimbursement of ambulatory services provided in healthcare settings. This includes physician and hospital outpatient reimbursement. Other uses of the code system include benchmarking, trending, planning, and measurement of quality of care.

HIPAA mandates HCPCS Level II as the standardized coding system for describing and identifying healthcare equipment and supplies in healtcare transactions that are not identified by the HCPCS Level I, CPT codes. Thus, healthcare providers must report these services to public as well as private insurers, using HCPCS Level II.

HCPCS Content and Structure

Level II of HCPCS contains products, supplies, and services. Included in HCPCS Level II are ambulance services, drugs, and durable medical equipment, prosthetics, orthotics, and supplies. Used with HCPCS Level II codes, modifiers are available to explain various circumstances of procedures and services. Modifiers also are used to enhance a code

narrative in order to describe the circumstances of each procedure or service and how it applies to an individual patient. In some situations, insurers instruct providers and suppliers to add a modifier in order to provide additional information regarding the service or item identified by the HCPCS Level II code.

HCPCS Level II is divided into chapters. They are:

- A Codes: Transportation Services including Ambulance, Medical and Surgical Supplies, Administration, Miscellaneous, and Investigation
- B Codes: External and Parental Therapy
- C Codes: Outpatient Prospective Payment System (Temporary)
- D Codes: Dental Procedures
- E Codes: Durable Medical Equipment
- G Codes: Procedures/Professional Services (Temporary)
- H Codes: Alcohol and Drug Abuse Treatment Services
- J Codes: Drugs Administered Other than by Oral Method
- K Codes: (Temporary Codes)
- L Codes: Orthotic and Prosthetic Procedures and Devices
- M Codes: Medical Services
- P Codes: Pathology and Laboratory Services
- Q Codes: (Temporary)
- R Codes: Diagnostic Radiology Services
- S Codes: Temporary National Codes (Non-Medicare)
- T Codes: Temporary National Codes
- V Codes: Vision and Hearing Services

The index for Level II codes lists terms alphabetically. Drugs are not included in the index but are found in their own table.

RxNorm

RxNorm is both a standardized nomenclature for clinical drugs and a semantic interoperability tool. The NLM, an institute of the National Institutes of Medicine, is responsible for the development and maintenance of RxNorm. The nomenclature is recognized as a standard for exchanging clinical drug information.

RxNorm normalizes names and unique identifiers for clinical drugs and links its names to the varying names of drugs present in many different vocabularies within the Unified Medical Language System (UMLS) Metathesaurus (NLM 2015a). A normalized name in RxNorm is the ingredient, strength, and dose form for a drug.

RxNorm is updated on an interim basis, weekly as well as a monthly full release cycle. The package includes the standardized nomenclature for clinical drugs and a tool for supporting semantic interoperation between drug terminologies and pharmacy knowledge base systems (Nelson 2015, 139). NLM also provides several tools for the industry including a web-based RxNorm browser application called RxNav.

RxNorm Purpose and Use

RxNorm's purpose is to allow computer systems to efficiently and unambiguously communicate drug-related information between hospitals, pharmacies, and other organizations (NLM 2015b). Its objective is to normalize names of generic and branded drugs and attach a unique identifier to that name.

Common RxNorm uses include:

- Cross-mapping among dissimilar drug vocabularies, which streamlines data exchange
- Facilitating medication-related clinical decision support by correctly identifying and categorizing medications
- Using RxNorm standard names and codes are commonly used to capture drug product information in an EHR (Nelson et al. 2011)

In addition, RxNorm was chosen as the standard for medications for the entry of structured data in certified EHR systems under the Meaningful Use program (ONC 2015).

RxNorm Content and Structure

The drug name and all of its synonyms represent a single concept, which is an **RxNorm concept unique identifier (RXCUI)**. Figure 5.6 shows the RxNorm graph for an amoxicillin 400 mg chewable tablet (brand name Amozil). This display shows a text string search using the form view. On the left is the ingredient (amoxicillin), ingredient plus strength (amoxicillin 400 mg), and ingredient plus strength plus dose form (amoxicillin 400 mg chewable tablet).

Figure 5.6 RxNorm graph for amoxicillin 400 mg chewable tablet

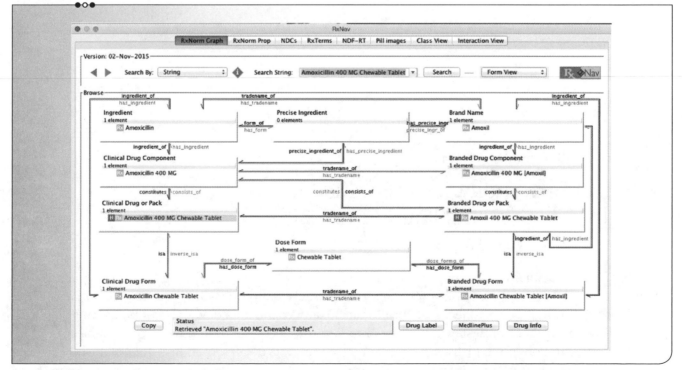

Source: NLM 2015c. Created from publicly available data from the U.S. National Library of Medicine (NLM), National Institutes of Health, Department of Health and Human Services.

The combination of ingredient plus strength plus dose form is known as a semantic clinical drug term type. Information about the branded name is found on the right. At the bottom are windows displaying the clinical drug form (bottom left), branded dose form (bottom right), and dose form (bottom middle).

Check Your Understanding 5.3

Instructions: **Answer the following questions.**

1   Which of the following is standard for drugs under the Meaningful Use program?
   A. RxNorm
   B. LOINC
   C. HCPCS
   D. ICD-10-PCS

2. Which of the following is standard for supplies under HIPAA?
   A. RxNorm
   B. LOINC
   C. HCPCS
   D. ICD-10-PCS

3. Which of the following is standard for clinical lab test results?
   A. RxNorm
   B. LOINC
   C. HCPCS
   D. CPT

4. Which type of HCPCS Level II code is not published by CMS?
   A. Dental Procedures
   B. Durable Medical Equipment
   C. Vision and Hearing Services
   D. Drugs Administered Other than by Oral Method

5. RxNorm names for clinical drugs contain information on which of the following?
   A. Manufactured drug
   B. Route
   C. Ingredients
   D. Packaged product

Clinical Terminologies, Classifications, and Code Systems Found in Health Data and Information Sets

There are many reasons for forming a **data set**, a list of recommended data elements with uniform definitions. One might be to collect statistical data for reporting to national and state registries. For additional information on registries, see chapter 7. Other purposes of data and information sets are to gather data for clinical decision support and for computation and reporting of clinical quality measures. Quality measures are covered in chapter 18. Many of the data elements contained in a data and information set are now captured electronically when data documentation is done at the time of care.

Data and information sets may come from federal data reporting requirements, such as

Meaningful Use, and others from public initiatives related to standardized performance measures. (Meaningful use is covered in chapter 16.) Data sets may be formed for such activities as research, clinical trials, quality and safety improvement, reimbursement, accreditation, and exchanging clinical information (Giannangelo 2007). Some of these data sets are listed as follows.

Outcomes and Assessment Information Set

The Outcomes and Assessment Information Set (OASIS) is standardized data set designed to provide the necessary data items to measure both outcomes and patient risk factors of Medicare beneficiaries who are receiving skilled services from a Medicare-certified home health agency. According to CMS, "OASIS data items address sociodemographic, environmental, support system, health status, functional status, and health service utilization characteristics of the patient" (CMS 2012).

OASIS has undergone several updates and refinements. OASIS-C1/ICD-10 version is the version of the OASIS data set that went into effect on October 1, 2015. It is the core data item set for collection on all adult home health patients whose skilled care is reimbursed by Medicare and Medicaid with the exception of patients receiving pre- or postnatal services only. Only a registered nurse (RN) or any of the therapies (physical therapy, speech-language pathology or speech therapy, occupational therapy) can conduct the comprehensive assessment and OASIS data collection (CMS 2015b).

A data collection instrument containing the data elements is used by those qualified to do so at various times such as the start of care or upon discharge from home care services. Submission of OASIS data is a CMS requirement if the agency participates in the Medicare program. The data are used in a variety of ways such as the assessment of the patient's ability to be discharged or transferred from home care services or the creation of patient case mix profile reports used by state survey staff in the certification process. The CMS Home Health Compare website's information on home health agency process and improvement outcome measures are based on OASIS data

submitted by home health agencies to state repositories. Medicare provides this information to anyone who may have an interest in comparing home health agency performance.

Healthcare Effectiveness Data and Information Set

The Healthcare Effectiveness Data and Information Set (HEDIS), sponsored by the National Committee for Quality Assurance (NCQA), is designed to collect administrative, claims, and health record review data. HEDIS contains more than 80 standard performance measures. Included are data related to patient outcomes and data about the treatment process.

Survey vendors certified by NCQA collect the data. HEDIS survey data and protocols standardize data about specific health-related conditions or issues in order to evaluate and compare the success of various treatment plans. These data form the basis of performance improvement (PI) efforts for health plans. HEDIS data also are important in the creation of physician profiles for use in positively shaping physician practice patterns by showing comparative clinical performance information to encourage quality improvement or utilization adjustments.

Clinics and hospitals collect the standardized HEDIS data elements from health records. Once gathered, this data are combined with enrollment and claims data and analyzed according to HEDIS specifications. Healthcare purchasers and consumers can use the information to compare the performance of managed healthcare plans to help decide which plan to contract with or enroll in.

Uniform Hospital Discharge Data Set

The Uniform Hospital Discharge Data Set (UHDDS) is required by Department of Health and Human Services (HHS). This core set of data elements is collected by acute care, short-term stay (usually less than 30 days) hospitals to report inpatient data elements in a standardized manner. Developed through the National Committee on Vital and Health Statistics (NCVHS).

Form CMS-1450, also known as the Uniform Bill UB-04, and the 837I, the institutional healthcare claim for electronic healthcare transactions, are the instruments for collecting UHDDS data elements. When diagnosis-related groups (DRGs) were implemented, UHDDS definitions were incorporated into the inpatient prospective payment system (PPS) regulations. For additional information on DRGs and the inpatient PPS, see chapter 15.

The UHDDS lists and defines a set of common data elements for the purpose of facilitating the collection of uniform and comparable health information from hospitals. Contained in the UHDDS's data dictionary are the definitions of the core data elements to be collected along with each data element's guidelines for use. For example, the UHDDS data element principal diagnosis is defined in the data dictionary as the condition, after study, to be chiefly responsible for occasioning the admission of the patient to the hospital for care. This element and its definition are used to determine a DRG.

Common Clinical Data Set

The Office of the National Coordinator for Health Information Technology (ONC) established a common set of data types and elements and associated standards for use across several certification criteria. The combination of these items is called the **Common Clinical Data Set**. Some but not all of the data types or elements have a standard attached to them. An example of a data element with specified standard is smoking status. It must be reported with one of the following SNOMED CT identifiers:

- Current every day smoker. 449868002
- Current some day smoker. 428041000124106
- Former smoker. 8517006
- Never smoker. 266919005

Table 5.4   Common Clinical Data Set 2015 edition health IT certification criteria

Data element
Patient name
Date of birth
Ethnicity
Smoking status
Medications
Laboratory test(s)
Vital signs (body height, body weight, diastolic blood pressure, systolic blood pressure, heart rate, respiratory rate, body temperature, pulse oximetry, and inhaled oxygen saturation, body mass index (ratio), and mean blood pressure)
Procedures
Immunizations
Assessment and plan of treatment
Health concerns
Sex
Race
Preferred language
Problems
Medication allergies
Laboratory value(s)/result(s)
Care plan field(s), including goals and instructions
Care team member(s)
Unique device identifier(s) for a patient's implantable device
Goals

Source: ONC 2015.

- Smoker, current status unknown. 77176002
- Unknown if ever smoked. 266927001
- Heavy tobacco smoker. 428071000124103
- Light tobacco smoker. 428061000124105

The Common Clinical Data Set is used across inpatient and ambulatory care settings. Table 5.4 lists the data elements in the data set.

Database of Clinical Terminologies, Classifications, and Code Systems

The number of clinical terminologies, classifications, and code systems in healthcare has grown substantially over the past few decades and some that have been around for several years have undergone revisions and updates expanding their size. Although consolidation in some instances may occur in the future, requirements for use are not limited to just one. With so many available and some of them being quite large, a centralized location is needed in order to maintain consistent terminology for implementation and use. One such centralized location of health and biomedical terminologies and standards is the **Unified Medical Language System (UMLS)**.

Having access to terminologies, classifications, and code systems from a single source is made possible through the efforts of the NLM via the UMLS. According to the NLM, "the UMLS integrates and distributes key terminology, classification and coding standards, and associated resources to promote creation of more effective and interoperable biomedical information systems and services, including electronic health records" (NLM 2015d).

The UMLS is a multipurpose resource. It contains the Metathesaurus, Semantic Network, and SPECIALIST Lexicon, which make up the UMLS Knowledge Resources. In addition, the UMLS has a number of software tools including the Lexical Tools and the UMLS Terminology Services (UTS). The Metathesaurus contains the codes and terms from over 150 terminology, classification,

and coding standards. Those found include terminologies designed for use in EHR systems (for example, SNOMED CT), disease and procedure classifications used for statistical reporting and billing (such as ICD-10-CM and CPT), and code systems such as LOINC. The UTS is set of web-based tools that serves as the gateway to the UMLS Knowledge Sources and the site to download the UMLS data files.

The following are UMLS uses:

- Linking health information, medical terms, drug names, and billing codes across different computer systems such as between the doctor, pharmacy, and insurance company; or for patient care coordination among different hospital departments
- Search engine retrieval
- Data mining
- Public health statistics reporting
- Interoperability support (NLM 2014)

Check Your Understanding 5.4

Instructions: **Answer the following questions.**

1. True or false: The Core Clinical Data Set definitions are incorporated into the inpatient prospective payment system.

2. True or false: Data elements specified in OASIS-C1 are collected on long-term care patients.

3. True or false: HEDIS collects standardized data from health records in clinics and hospitals.

4. True or false: The UMLS includes terminologies but excludes classifications.

5. True or false: The Common Clinical Data Set is used in home healthcare settings.

Real-World Case 5.1

Clinical quality measure developers create evidence-based standards used to assess the performance of providers in the provision of care. Developers include government agencies,

accreditation organizations, and physician specialty groups among others. They select terminologies, classifications, and code sets as a way to express healthcare performance data used in the measure. For example, the National Committee for Quality Assurance (NCQA) may want to author an electronic Clinical Quality Measure (eCQM) for breast cancer screening. Using the web-based Measure Authoring Tool (MAT), NCQA decides to include mammograms as a population criterion. Having identified mammogram as one of the criteria, NCQA determines LOINC and HCPCS are necessary for the measure. Mammogram codes from these two systems are then selected to create the content for the breast cancer screening eCQM.

 Real-World Case 5.2

The 2015 Edition EHR technology certification criteria states the following:

Smoking status: Enable a user to electronically record, change, and access the smoking status of a patient in accordance with the standard specified.

45 CFR 170.315(a)(11).Coded to one of the following SNOMED CT codes:

- Current every day smoker. 449868002
- Current some day smoker. 428041000124106
- Former smoker. 8517006
- Never smoker. 266919005
- Smoker, current status unknown. 77176002
- Unknown if ever smoked. 266927001
- Heavy tobacco smoker. 428071000124103
- Light tobacco smoker. 428061000124105

Objective: Record smoking status for patients 13 years or older.

Measure: More than 85 percent of all unique patients 13-years-old or older seen by the eligible professional or admitted to the eligible hospital's or critical care hospital's inpatient or emergency department during the EHR reporting period have smoking status records as structured data.

Included in the National Learning Consortium's resources is a quick reference guide from the American Academy of Family Physicians (AAFP) for meeting the smoking status Meaningful Use requirement. The AAFP supports the incorporation of tobacco cessation into EHR templates (AAFP n.d.). The quick reference provides guidance on what should be included in a tobacco cessation EHR template.

References

American Academy of Family Physicians (AAFP). n.d. Integrating Tobacco Cessation into Electronic Health Records. http://www.aafp.org/dam/AAFP/documents/patient_care/tobacco/ehr-tobacco-cessation.pdf.

American Medical Association. 2015. *Current Procedural Terminology*, 4th ed. Chicago: AMA.

American Nursing Association. 2015 (March 19). Inclusion of Recognized Terminologies within EHRs and Other Health Information Technology Solutions. http://www.nursingworld.org/

MainMenuCategories/Policy-Advocacy/Positions-and-Resolutions/ANAPositionStatements/Position-Statements-Alphabetically/Inclusion-of-Recognized-Terminologies-within-EHRs.html.

American Psychiatric Association. 2013. *Diagnostic and Statistical Manual of Mental Disorders*, 5th ed. Arlington, VA: APA.

Centers for Medicare and Medicaid Services. 2015a. ICD-10-PCS. http://www.cms.gov/Medicare/Coding/ICD10/2016-ICD-10-PCS-and-GEMs.html.

Centers for Medicare and Medicaid Services. 2015b. OASIS-C1/ICD-10 Guidance Manual. http://www.cms.gov/Medicare/Quality-Initiatives-Patient-Assessment-Instruments/HomeHealthQualityInits/HHQIOASISUserManual.html.

Centers for Medicare and Medicaid Services. 2012 (August 21). Outcomes and Assessment Information Set (OASIS): Data Set. http://www.cms.gov/Medicare/Quality-Initiatives-Patient-Assessment-Instruments/OASIS/DataSet.html.

Giannangelo, K., ed. 2015. Introduction. Chapter in *Healthcare Code Sets, Clinical Terminologies, and Classification Systems*, 3rd ed. Chicago: AHIMA.

Giannangelo, K. 2007. Unraveling the data set, an e-HIM essential. *Journal of AHIMA*. 78(2):60–61.

Helwig, A. 2013 (October 29). EHR Certification Criteria for SNOMED CT Will Help Doctors Transition to ICD-10. http://www.healthit.gov/buzz-blog/electronic-health-and-medical-records/ehr-certification-criteria-snomed-ct-doctors-transition-icd10/.

International Health Terminology Standards Development Organisation (IHTSDO). 2014a. Frequently Asked Questions. http://www.snomed.org/faq?t=faq_WhatIsSnomedCt.

International Health Terminology Standards Development Organisation (IHTSDO). 2014b. SNOMED CT Starter Guide. http://ihtsdo.org/fileadmin/user_upload/doc/download/doc_StarterGuide_Current-en-US_INT_20141202.pdf?ok.

McDonald, C.J., S. Huff, J. Deckard, K. Holck, S. Abhyankar, D. Vreeman, eds. 2015 (June). Logical Observation Identifiers Names and Codes (LOINC) Users' Guide. https://loinc.org/downloads/files/LOINCManual.pdf.

National Cancer Institute (NCI). n.d. SEER Training Modules: Data Standards. http://training.seer.cancer.gov/operations/standards/.

National Center for Health Statistics. 2015. ICD-10-CM. http://www.cdc.gov/nchs/icd/icd10cm.htm.

National Library of Medicine. 2015a. RxNorm Technical Documentation, Version 2015-1. http://www.nlm.nih.gov/research/umls/rxnorm/docs/2015/rxnorm_doco_full_2015-1.html.

National Library of Medicine. 2015b. RxNorm Overview. http://www.nlm.nih.gov/research/umls/rxnorm/overview.html.

National Library of Medicine. 2015c. RxNav, Version 02-Nov-2015. http://rxnav.nlm.nih.gov/.

National Library of Medicine. 2015d. Unified Medical Language System. http://www.nlm.nih.gov/research/umls/.

National Library of Medicine. 2014. UMLS Quick Start Guide. https://www.nlm.nih.gov/research/umls/quickstart.html.

Nelson, S.J. 2015. RxNorm. Chapter in *Healthcare Code Sets, Clinical Terminologies, and Classification Systems*, 3rd ed. Edited by K. Giannangelo. Chicago: AHIMA.

Nelson, S.J., K. Zeng, J. Kilbourns, T. Powell, and R. Moore. 2011 (July–August). Normalized names for clinical drugs: RxNorm at 6 years. *Journal American Medical Informatics Association*. 18(4):441–448.

Office of the National Coordinator for Health Information Technology (ONC). n.d. Interoperability Training Courses. http://www.healthit.gov/providers-professionals/interoperability-training-courses.

Office of the National Coordinator for Health Information Technology (ONC). 2015 (October 16). 2015 Edition Health Information Technology (Health IT) Certification Criteria, 2015 Edition Base Electronic Health Record (EHR) Definition, and ONC Health IT Certification Program Modifications. *Federal Register*. https://www.federalregister.gov/articles/2015/10/16/2015-25597/2015-edition-health-information-technology-health-it-certification-criteria-2015-edition-base.

Porter, H.R. 2015. International Classification of Functioning, Disability, and Health. Chapter in *Healthcare Code Sets, Clinical Terminologies, and Classification Systems*, 3rd ed. Edited by K. Giannangelo. Chicago: AHIMA.

Regenstrief Institute. n.d. LOINC from Regenstrief. https://loinc.org/.

Shulman, L. and N. Stepro. 2015 (June 3). What Lies Beneath. Arcadia Healthcare Solutions. http://arcadiasolutions.com/lies-beneath/.

Warren, J. 2015. Terminologies Used in Nursing Practice. Chapter in *Healthcare Code Sets, Clinical Terminologies, and Classification Systems*, 3rd ed. Edited by K. Giannangelo. Chicago: AHIMA.

World Health Organization (WHO). 2015. The International Classification of Functioning, Disability and Health (ICF). http://www.who.int/classifications/icf/en/.

World Health Organization. 2013. A Practical Manual for using the International Classification of Functioning, Disability and Health (ICF). http://www.who.int/classifications/drafticfpracticalmanual.pdf.

World Health Organization. 2001. *The International Classification of Functioning, Disability and Health (ICF)*. Geneva: WHO.

6

Data Management

Danika Brinda, PhD, RHIA, CHPS, HCISPP

Learning Objectives

- Identify the different sources where data are created, stored, or transmitted
- Distinguish among data elements, data sets, databases, indices, data mapping, and data warehousing
- Distinguish among data governance, information governance, data stewardship, data sharing, data integrity, and data interchange standards
- Explain the principles of information governance
- Illustrate the impact of data quality on the healthcare organization as it relates to patient care, reimbursement, and healthcare operations

- Apply the principles of AHIMA's data quality management model
- Examine the purpose of clinical documentation improvement and how it relates to data quality
- Identify the basics of clinical documentation improvement query processes
- Describe the reasons for establishing data quality and data management requirements in provider contracts, medical staff bylaws, and hospital bylaws

Key Terms

Bylaws
Clinical documentation
Critical thinking
Data
Database
Database life cycle
Data dictionary
Data element
Data governance
Data integrity
Data interchange standards
Data management

Data mapping
Data mining
Data sets
Data stewardship
Data warehouse
Data warehousing
Enterprise information
  management
Index
Information
Information assets
Information governance

Interoperability
Object-oriented database
Query
Relational database
Source data
Standards development
  organization
Structured data
System characterization
Target data
Unstructured data
Use case

With the advancement of technology within the US healthcare system, most healthcare organizations are inundated with data from multiple sources which are stored and maintained in a variety of locations. **Data** are a representation of basic facts and observations about people, processes, measurements, and conditions. Healthcare-specific data focuses on patients, which includes demographic, financial, and clinical data. **Data management** refers to the definition and structure of data elements and the creation, storage, and transmission of data elements (AHIMA 2015). Effective oversight and management of the data is an essential part of day-to-day operations of a healthcare organization. Knowing and understanding how data are produced, why certain types and formats of data are produced, how data are stored and managed, and maintaining data integrity become foundational steps to assure the data within organizations are properly managed.

Data Sources

A foundational step to the management of data within a healthcare facility is to understand the basic sources of data generated and stored by an organization. Data includes both clinical and administrative elements. The data elements stored in the electronic health record are an example of clinical data. Administrative data includes the data elements required for billing and quality improvement. Common data sources in healthcare are:

- Electronic health records (EHR) (see chapter 11)
- Practice management systems (see chapter 11)
- Lab information systems (see chapter 11)
- Radiology information systems (see chapter 11)
- Picture archival and communications (PACs) (see chapter 11)
- Other clinical documentation systems (home health, therapy, long-term care) (see chapter 11)
- Master patient index (see chapter 3 and 7)
- Other patient index (indices) (see chapter 7)
- Databases (see chapter 7)
- Registries (see chapter 7)

To manage the different aspects of data effectively, the facility should conduct system characterization. **System characterization** is the process of creating an inventory of all systems that contain data, including documenting where the data are stored, what type of data are created or stored, how they are managed, with what hardware and software they interact with, and providing basic security measures for the systems (Walsh 2013). This process helps identify all sources of data that exist within a healthcare organization.

Data Management

Managing the data that healthcare organizations create and produce is challenging. Data can exist in an information system, on a file on an employee's computer or file server, in an e-mail, and in many other formats and locations. Healthcare organizations are challenged with the proper management of the data in order to effectively use and preserve the data that exists.

The process of data collection has evolved over the years as healthcare organizations migrate from paper-based recordkeeping systems to electronic health records (EHR). For additional information on EHRs, refer to chapter 11. Additionally, healthcare organizations are collecting more patient data and using the data to support patient care and healthcare operations. The demand to properly collect, analyze, and utilize patient data is more important now than ever before. Not only are healthcare organizations using the data, but it is also being used by third-party payers, government agencies, accreditation organizations, and others within the healthcare industry to support and advance the healthcare delivery system and improve patient care. One of the challenges of healthcare systems managing data in an electronic environment is the vast differences in the collection of healthcare data throughout different electronic data systems such as EHRs, lab information systems, radiology information systems, and billing systems. There are many methods, formats, and processes used for the collection and storage of patient information such as direct entry into an electronic system, scanning of documentation, and uploading of transcribed documentation. Data management is further complicated because data is collected and stored in many locations in the healthcare organization. Given the various methodologies that exist for data collection, understanding data and data collection is important. Data management focuses on understanding data elements, data set, databases, indices, data mapping, and data warehousing.

Data Elements

The term *data* is actually the plural format of *datum*; however, it is more common to hear the term *data element* to describe one fact or measurement. A **data element** can be a single or individual fact that represents the smallest unique subset of a larger database sometimes referred to as the raw facts and figures. Examples of data elements include age, gender, blood pressure, temperature, test results, and date of birth. Data elements are entered into different formats through the EHR and other supporting patient systems. **Information** is different than data as it refers to data elements that have been combined and then manipulated into something meaningful regarding a patient or a group of patients. For example, a healthcare organization can create a report on the data element's most recent A1C test result and diagnosis of a heart attack analyze and determine if there is a relationship

between the A1C test score and a heart attack. By taking the specific data elements of the heart attack diagnoses and the most current A1C result, the healthcare organization can create best practices to enhance patient care based on the findings (Giannangelo 2013). For more on data and information, see chapter 3.

To help support and manage data elements within an electronic health record, the use of a data dictionary is implemented to support standardized input and understanding of all data elements. A **data dictionary** is a listing of all the data elements within a specific system that defines each individual data element, standard input of the data element, and specific data length. Common data elements within a data dictionary are:

- Data field (such as date of birth)
- Definition
- Data type (date, text, number, and so forth)
- Format (such as MM-DD-YYYY)
- Field size (such as 10 digit for phone number)
- Data values (such as M and F for gender)
- Data source (where data is collected)
- Data first entered (when the data element is first used)
- Why item is included (justification for collection of the data element) (AHIMA 2014a)

Defining a data dictionary can help with accuracy of patient data and create support for data comparison and data sharing (Clark et al. 2012). (Additional information on the sharing of data is found in chapter 12.) Table 6.1 provides a sample of a data dictionary defining the data elements in an EHR.

Defining a data dictionary is a fundamental step to understanding data elements, their meaning and usage. It also supports the creation of well-structured and defined data sets by creating standardized definitions of data elements to help ensure consistency of collection and use of the data. For example, the time of discharge could be the time the discharge order was written, the time the order was entered into the information system

Table 6.1   Sample data dictionary

DATA FIELD	NAME	DEFINITION	DATA TYPE	FORMAT	FIELD SIZE	VALUES	SOURCE SYSTEM	DATE FIRST ENTERED	WHY ITEM IS INCLUDED
Admission Date	ADMIT_DATE	The date the patient is admitted to facility as an inpatient	date	mmddyyyy	8	Admission date cannot precede birth date or 2007 No hyphens or slashes	Patient census	2/23/2008	Allows analysis of patients and service within a specific period that can be compared with other periods or trended
Census	CENSUS	The number of inpatients present in the facility at any given time	numeric	x to xx	3	Any whole number from 1 to 999	Patient census	2/23/2008	Provides analysis of budget variances, aids future budgetary decisions, and allows quicker response to negative trends
Ethnicity	PT_ETHNIC	Patient's ethnicity must be reported according to official office of management and budget categories	alphanumeric	Ex: letter must be uppercase	2	E1 - Hispanic or Latino ethnicity E2 - Non-Hispanic or Latino ethnicity	Patient census: Practice Management	2/23/2008	Patient demographics aid marketing and planning future budgets and services
Infant patient	INFANT_PT	A patient who has not reached 1 year of age at the time of discharge	alphanumeric	Age in months - xD to xxD OR xM to xxM	3	Must be > 0 AND < 1 year	Patient census: practice management	2/23/2008	Patient age affects types of services required and payer sources
Inpatient daily census	IP_DAY_CENSUS	The number of in-patients present at census-taking time each day, plus any inpatients who were both admitted and discharged after the previous day's census-taking time	numeric	x to xx	3	Any whole number from 0 to 999	Patient census	2/23/2008	Provides analysis of budget variances, aids future budgetary decisions, and allows quicker response to negative trends
Medical record number	MR_NUM	The unique number assigned to a patient's medical record The medical record is filed under this number	alphanumeric	xxxxxx: requires leading zeros	6	000001 to 999999	Patient census: practice management		Provides analysis of services, resource utilization, and patient outcomes at the physician level
Patient age	PT_AGE	Age of patient calculated by using most recent birthday attained before or on same day as discharge	numeric or alphanumeric	Age in days - xD to xxD OR Age in months - xM to xxM OR Age in years - x to xxx	3	Age must be > 0, and < OR - 124 years; children less than 1 year must be > 0 M AND < 1 year	Patient census: practice management	2/23/2008	Patient age impacts the services utilized and payer sources
Patient sex	PT_SEX	Patient sex	alphanumeric	Letter; must be uppercase	1	M - Male F - Female U - Unknown	Patient census: practice management	2/23/2008	Patient sex impacts the services and specialties utilized
Patient zip code	PT_ZIP_CODE	Zip code of patients residence	alphanumeric	xxxxx-xxxx	11	00000 to 99999; 00000 - Unknown 99999 - Foreign	Patient census: practice management	2/23/2008	Patient demographics aid marketing and planning future budgets/services

Source: AHIMA 2014a.

or the time the patient actually left the unit. These times could vary widely so it is important that the data dictionary defines which time should be used.

Data Sets

The concept of comparing data and the need for standardization became a common theme for healthcare organizations in the 1960s as a result of the work of the National Center for Health Statistics (NCHS) and National Committee on Vital and Health Statistics (NCVHS). It became evident that common structure and collection of data elements was needed to collect consistent data that allowed for comparison across all healthcare organizations. As a result, the concept of data sets was created. **Data sets** are a recommended list of data elements that have defined and uniform definitions that

are relevant for a particular use or are specific to a type of healthcare industry. One of the first defined and used data sets across the US healthcare industry was the Uniform Hospital Discharge Data Set (UHDDS), implemented in the mid-1970s. Created by NCHS, the National Center for Health Services Research and Development, and Johns Hopkins University, UHDDS collects uniform data elements from the health records of every hospital inpatient (Giannangelo 2013). The main data elements defined in the UHDDS data set are listed in figure 6.1.

Each of the data elements defined within the UHDDS has specific criteria for data collection. For example, the data of birth is defined as the month, day, and year of birth, with a recommendation to collect all four digits of the birth year. The four digits are important because a patient could be more than 100 years old. Another example is the definition of type of admission. There are two choices—unscheduled or scheduled admission. Each of the types of admissions is defined in the dataset for use of the UHDDS (Giannangelo 2013).

Shortly after the UHDDS was created and implemented, the need to expand uniform data sets across other healthcare settings became evident with the continuing movement from an inpatient, acute setting to outpatient care including surgical centers and emergency care settings.

Figure 6.1 UHDDS data elements

Data Element	Definition/Descriptor
01. Personal identification	The unique number assigned to each patient within a hospital that distinguishes the patient and his or her hospital record from all others in that institution.
02. Date of birth	Month, day, and year of birth. Capture of the full four-digit year of birth is recommended.
03. Sex	Male or female
04. Race and ethnicity	04a. Race American Indian/Eskimo/Aleut Asian or Pacific Islander Black White Other race Unknown
	04b. Ethnicity Spanish origin/Hispanic Non-Spanish origin/Non-Hispanic Unknown
05. Residence	Full address of usual residence Zip code (nine digits, if available) Code for foreign residence
06. Hospital identification	A unique institutional number across data collection systems. The Medicare provider number is the preferred hospital identifier.
07. Admission date	Month, day, and year of admission
08. Type of admission	Scheduled: Arranged with admissions office at least 24 hours prior to admission Unscheduled: All other admissions
09. Discharge date	Month, day, and year of discharge
10 & 11. Physician identification • Attending physician • Operating physician	The Medicare unique physician identification number (UPIN) is the preferred method of identifying the attending physician and operating physician(s) because it is uniform across all data systems.
12. Principal diagnosis	The condition established after study to be chiefly responsible for occasioning the admission of the patient to the hospital for care.
13. Other diagnoses	All conditions that coexist at the time of admission or that develop subsequently or that affect the treatment received and/or the length of stay. Diagnoses that relate to an earlier episode and have no bearing on the current hospital stay are to be excluded.

Figure 6.1 (*Continued*)

Data Element	Definition/Descriptor
14. Qualifier for other diagnoses	A qualifier is given for each diagnosis coded under "other diagnoses" to indicate whether the onset of the diagnosis preceded or followed admission to the hospital. The option "uncertain" is permitted.
15. External cause-of-injury code	The ICD-10-CM code for the external cause of an injury, poisoning, or adverse effect (commonly referred to as an E code). Hospitals should complete this item whenever there is a diagnosis of an injury, poisoning, or adverse effect.
16. Birth weight of neonate	The specific birth weight of a newborn, preferably recorded in grams
17. Procedures and dates	All significant procedures are to be reported. A significant procedure is one that is: • Surgical in nature, or • Carries a procedural risk, or • Carries an anesthetic risk, or • Requires specialized training. The date of each significant procedure must be reported. When more than one procedure is reported, the principal procedure must be designated. The principal procedure is one that is performed for definitive treatment rather than one performed for diagnostic or exploratory purposes or was necessary to take care of a complication. If there appear to be two procedures that are principal, then the one most closely related to the principal diagnosis should be selected as the principal procedure. The UPIN must be reported for the person performing the principal procedure.
18. Disposition of the patient	• Discharged to home (excludes those patients referred to home health service) • Discharged to acute care hospital • Discharged to nursing facility • Discharged home to be under the care of a home health service (including a hospice) • Discharged to other healthcare facility • Left against medical advice • Alive, other; or alive, not stated • Died
19. Patient's expected source of payment	Primary source Other sources All categories for primary and other sources are: • Blue Cross/Blue Shield • Other health insurance companies • Other liability insurance • Medicare • Medicaid • Worker's Compensation • Self-insured employer plan • Health maintenance organization (HMO) • CHAMPUS • CHAMPVA • Other government payers • Self-pay • No charge (free, charity, special research, teaching) • Other
20. Total charges	All charges billed by the hospital for this hospitalization. Professional charges for individual patient care by physicians are excluded.

Source: Giannangelo 2013.

Figure 6.2 UACDS data elements

Data Element	Definition/Descriptor
Provider identification, address, type of practice	Provider identification: Include the full name of the provider as well as the unique physician identification number (UPIN). Address: The complete address of the provider's office. In cases where the provider has multiple offices, the location of the usual or principal place of practice should be given. Profession: • Physician including specialty or field of practice • Other (specify)
Place of encounter	Specify the location of the encounter: • Private office • Clinic or health center • Hospital outpatient department • Hospital emergency department • Other (specify)
Reason for encounter	Includes, but is not limited to, the patient's complaints and symptoms reflecting his or her own perception of needs, provided verbally or in writing by the patient at the point of entry into the healthcare system, or the patient's own words recorded by an intermediary or provider at that time.
Diagnostic services	Includes all diagnostic services of any type.
Problem, diagnosis, or assessment	Describes the provider's level of understanding and the interpretation of the patient's reasons for the encounter and all conditions requiring treatment or management at the time of the encounter.
Therapeutic services	List by name all services done or ordered: • Medical (including drug therapy) • Surgical • Patient education
Preventive services	List by name all preventive services and procedures performed at the time of the encounter.

Disposition	The provider's statement of the next step(s) in the care of the patient. At a minimum, the following classification is suggested:
	1. No follow-up planned
	2. Follow-up planned
	  • Return when necessary
	  • Return to the current provider at a specified time
	  • Telephone follow-up
	  • Returned to referring provider
	  • Referred to other provider
	  • Admit to hospital
	  • Other

Source: Giannangelo 2013.

A standardized data set for the ambulatory setting was created known as the Uniform Ambulatory Care Data Set (UACDS). With less data elements than the UHDDS, the UACDS collects data specific to ambulatory care settings with an intent to improve data comparison across different settings of healthcare (see figure 6.2). After the success of the standardization of data elements with the UHDDS and UACDS, the standardization of data sets across healthcare settings commenced. Another key data set is Data Elements for Emergency Department Systems (DEEDS), which collects data for hospital-based emergency rooms. The following are other data sets that are defined within healthcare settings:

- Minimum Data Set (MDS)—Long-term care setting
- Outcomes and Assessment Information Set (OASIS)—Home healthcare setting
- Essential Medical Data Set (EMDS)—Emergency care setting

With the success of these data sets and the shift toward the ability to share data that is consistent across the entire healthcare spectrum, the need for additional standards to support standardized data sets continues to be a focus in the healthcare industry.

Databases

Databases are commonly used throughout the healthcare industry to support and store patient information entered into an EHR or maintained on a paper record. A **database** is a collection of data organized in such a way that its contents can be easily accessed, managed, reported, and updated. For proper management of data within an organization it is important to understand what databases exist, the purposes of the databases, the storage and backup of the databases, and who accesses and uses the databases. Common databases found in healthcare include Medicare Provider Analysis and Review File, National Practitioner Data Bank, and National Health Care Survey (Sharp 2013).

The database design and structure impacts how it can be used. A poorly designed database will result in redundant collection of data and data information errors. Understanding the **database life cycle (DBLC)** is an important step in the

proper execution, implementation, and management of databases within healthcare. There are six basis steps in the database life cycle:

1. Initial study (determining need for database)
2. Design (identify data fields, structure, and so forth)
3. Implementation (development of database)
4. Testing and evaluation (ensuring system works as expected)
5. Operation (use of database)
6. Database maintenance and evaluation (updating and backing up database and ensuring that it still meets needs)

Health information management (HIM) professionals should be involved in all stages of the database life cycle as they have the knowledge and skills needed to understand the essential steps of data collection privacy, security, and data integrity (Coronel and Morris 2015).

The two most common types of databases used in healthcare are relational database and object-oriented databases. A **relational database** stores data in tables that are predefined and contain both rows and columns of information. Typically a relational database is considered to be two-dimensional as it contains rows and columns. Relational databases are used frequently in the healthcare industry because they are easy to build, use, and query within the application. For example, a healthcare organization might choose to use a relational database to document the number of health record deficiencies a physician has at the time of evaluation for reporting to the organization's board (Sharp 2013). Table 6.2 provides a sample of a relational database for physician deficiency status.

Table 6.2   Relational database: physician deficiency status

Provider ID	Total # of deficiencies	History and physical deficiencies	Discharge summary deficiencies	Deficiencies greater than 30 days past due
1285	14	2	5	3
1965	2	1	1	0
8914	35	13	15	25
9462	6	3	2	2
3651	17	11	2	2

Table 6.3 Object-oriented database: fetal heart monitors (FHM)

Patient ID	FHM start date	FHM end date	FHM image
110011	6/30/15	7/1/15	Link to FHM image
123023	7/1/15	7/3/15	Link to FHM image
154623	7/2/15	7/2/15	Link to FHM image
948513	7/2/15	7/3/15	Link to FHM image

An **object-oriented database (OODB)** is designed to store different types of data including images, audio files, documents, videos, and data elements. OODBs are useful for storing fetal monitoring strips, electrocardiograms, PACs, and more. The OODB is dynamic because it provides the data as well as the object (image and document). Table 6.3 provides an example of an OODB. Using an OODB for the storage of fetal heart monitors allows an organization to query the database to retrieve an image for a specific person. Another potential use is to produce a report based on the date of the fetal heart monitor for retention and destruction of the images. When this type of database is used, the data is provided with the additional ability to retrieve the file when the link to the image is selected.

Indices

An **index** is a report or list from a database that provides guidance, indication, or other references to the data contained in the database. An index serves as a guide or indicator to locate something within a database or other systems storing data. For example, an index of a book will provide key terms and where to find the term within a book; the reader is able to find more information and detail regarding a specific topic. The indices used in healthcare identify where the desired information can be found, making it easier to aggregate and analyze data. There are many types of indices used within the healthcare industry. The following are the most common indices.

- *Master patient index:* A guide to locating specific demographic information about a patient such as the patient name, health record number, date of birth, gender, and dates of service. For more details, refer to chapter 3.

- *Disease index:* A listing of specific codes, such as International Classification of Disease, Tenth Revision, Clinical Modification (ICD-10-CM) codes that link a specific disease or diagnosis to a patient. (ICD-10-CM is explained later in this chapter.) Common data in a disease index would include diagnosis codes, health record number, gender, age, race, attending physician, hospital service, patient outcomes, and dates of encounter. A disease index can be used to query a specific diagnosis to determine other attributes of patients with the disease. For example, if an organization wanted to know the age range and gender of all patients diagnosed with a myocardial infarction, the disease index could be queried to get a listing of patients with that specific diagnosis code(s).

- *Operation or procedure index:* A listing of specific codes such as Current Procedure Terminology (CPT) for procedures or operations performed within the facility. (CPT is explained later in this chapter.) An operation or procedure code would include similar information as the disease index but would also include the specific code numbers as well as the operating physician. An operation or procedure index can be used to query specific information regarding procedures or operations done within the facility. For example, if an organization wanted to know the age range of the patients who had an appendectomy in the past year, the operation or procedure index could be queried to generate a listing of patients based on the procedure code.

- *Physician index:* A listing of all physicians within an organization with all the diagnosis and procedure codes linked to the provider within the index. The data collected in this index includes physician's identification (code or name), health record number, diagnosis, operations, dates of service, patient gender, patient age, and patient outcome from encounter. A provider index can be used to produce information regarding the work of the provider within an organization, which can be useful for certification and credentialing purposes. For example, an organization may need to produce a report for administration detailing the treatment of patients = and diagnoses and procedures performed in the past year by a specific provider (Sharp 2013). More information on indexes is found in chapter 7.

Indices support daily operations for healthcare organizations and are tools used to gather specific information quickly.

Data Mapping

Data mapping is a process that allows for connections between two systems. For example, mapping two different coding systems to show the equivalent codes allows for data initially captured for one purpose to be translated and used for another purpose. One system in a map is identified as the source while the other is the target. **Source data** is the location from which the data originates, such as a database or a data set; whereas **target data** is the location from which the data is mapped or to where it is sent. A data map creates a process to evaluate the disparity between two systems and links the data being collected together. The intent of conducting data mapping is to ensure the data exchange from one database to another is done in a meaningful way and maintains the integrity of the data (McBride et al. 2006).

During the process of data mapping, each data map should have a defined purpose that specifies why the data map is created and what purpose it serves. The purpose should describe why the data map is needed, what it represents, and how it will be used within the organization. For example, an organization may create a data map to show the relationship of the types of ambulatory services such as emergency room or ambulatory surgery, and map them directly to the ambulatory services.

Data mapping should be completed carefully to evaluate from where the data comes and the relationships of the source data to data in other systems. The process helps to ensure integrity of the data in all systems. When conducting data mapping

Table 6.4   Data map

ICD-10-CM code	ICD-10-CM name	Equivalence	SNOMED CT code	SNOMED CT name
A00.0	Cholera, unspecified	Equal	63650001	Cholera

Source: AHIMA 2013a, 2.

within an organization, evaluating the relationship of the data is fundamental to understanding the equivalence between the data. Equivalence of data is the relationship between the source data and target data in regards to how close or distant the data from the two systems are linked. The three common types of relationships are no match, approximate match, and exact match (AHIMA 2013a).

When creating data maps, organizations should create a common format for the output of the map to create consistency and ease the end user's ability to interpret the data map. Table 6.4 is an example of a data map that shows the relationship between ICD-10-CM codes and SNOMED CT codes, both explained later in this chapter.

Data mapping can be a long and tedious task for an organization; however, it is important from a data management perspective. To properly manage the data and ensure data integrity between systems, data maps serve as the tool to define the meaning and history of data elements within systems. Inaccurate data mapping can result in misinterpretation of data and inaccuracy of information stored and maintained in systems. For example, if the ICD-10-CM code was incorrectly mapped to the incorrect SNOMED CT code, data used and reported from the SNOMED system could show incorrect information regarding patients diagnosed with cholera, unspecified. Data map creators need to understand the data to be mapped between systems and the reasons for the data mapping. One way of doing this is to create a use case. A **use case** describes how the users will interact with the data map in a specific scenario. Some general data mapping steps are found in table 6.5.

Data Warehousing

Data warehousing is the process of collecting the data from different data sources within an organization and storing it in a single database that can be used for decision making. A **data warehouse** is

Table 6.5 AHIMA practice brief data mapping best practices: general data mapping steps

Develop a business case first. Questions to ask include:
- What is the reason for the project?
- What is the expected business benefit?
- What are the expected costs of the project?
- What are the expected risks?

Define a use case for how the content will be used within applications. Questions to ask include:
- Who will use the maps?
- Is the mapping between standard terminologies or between proprietary (local) terminologies?
- Are there delivery constraints or licensing issues?
- What systems will rely on the map as a data source?

Develop rules (heuristics) to be implemented within the project. Questions to ask when developing the rules include:
- What is the version of source and target schema to be used?
- What is included or excluded?
- How will the relationship between source and target be defined (such as are maps equivalent or related)?
- What mapping methodologies will be utilized?
- What procedures will be used for ensuring intercoder or interrater reliability (reproducibility) in the map development phase?
- What parameters will be used to ensure usefulness? (For example, a map from the SNOMED CT concept "procedure on head" could be mapped to hundreds of CPT codes, making the map virtually useless.)
- What tools will be used to develop and maintain the map?

Plan a pilot phase to test the rules. Maps must be tested and deemed "fit for purpose," meaning they are performing as desired. This may be done using random samples of statistically significant size. Additional pilot phases may be needed until variance from the expected result are resolved. Reproducibility is a fundamental best practice when mapping.

Develop full content with periodic testing throughout the process. Organizations should perform a final quality assurance test for the maps and review those data items unable to be mapped to complete the mapping phase. Any modifications from the review process should be retested to assure accuracy.
Organizations should release the map results to software configuration management where software and content are integrated. They should then perform quality assurance testing on the content within the software application (done in a development environment). They can then deploy the content to the production environment, or go-live.

Communicate with source and target system owners when issues are identified with the systems that require attention or additional documentation for clarity.

Source: AHIMA 2013b.

a single database that makes it possible to access data that exists in multiple databases through one single query and reporting interface.

Data warehouses allow healthcare organizations to obtain information needed to streamline processes and simplify access to the information that is stored among different databases within a healthcare system. If a user had to query each system, the amount of time needed to combine the data manually and then analyze the data would serve as a barrier to properly reporting and analyzing the data. With the use of a data warehouse, the data can be consolidated by pulling the data from multiple systems into a single database that allows for ease in reporting and analysis of the information.

Data mining is the processing of extracting from a database or data warehouse information stored in discrete, structured data format—that is, data that has a specific value. Examples of discrete data are a lab value or a diagnosis code. Advantages to the use of data warehouses are as follows.

- One consistent data storage area for reporting, forecasting, and analysis
- Easier and timely access to data
- Improved end-user productivity
- Improved information services productivity
- Reduced costs
- Scalability
- Flexibility
- Reliability (HIMSS 2009)

Since large amounts of data are being captured electronically within healthcare organizations, data warehousing will become a foundational aspect of healthcare operations due to its ability to gather data from multiple databases, incorporate the data, and then produce meaningful information.

Check Your Understanding 6.1

Instructions: **Answer the following questions.**

1. True or false: A data element is a single or individual fact that represents the smallest unique subset of larger data.

2. A data set is which of the following?
   A. A clearly defined data dictionary for the electronic health record
   B. A recommended list of data elements that support a specific healthcare industry
   C One element within an electronic health record
   D. A database where data is compiled from many sources into once central location

3. Which of the following is a purpose of the creation of a data dictionary?
   A. Identify the data elements that you want to college
   B. Create support for structured data collection
   C. Create use case
   D. Control security

4. Which of the following are the two most common types of databases found in healthcare?
   A. Relational and object-relational databases
   B. Object-relational and object-linking databases
   C. Relational and object-oriented databases
   D. Object-linking and object-oriented databases

5. True or false: An index creates a definition for terms that are within a database.

6. True or false: There is usually only one source of data within a healthcare organization.

Data Governance

Data governance is "enterprise authority that ensures control and accountability for enterprise data through the establishment of decision rights and data policies and standards that are implemented and monitored through a formal structure of assigned roles, responsibilities, and accountabilities" (Johns 2015, 81). Data governance focuses on how healthcare organizations create processes, policies, and procedures for keeping information that is relevant to patient care and healthcare operations. The goal of data governance is maintaining data accuracy and removing unnecessary data from the health record. Commonly, data governance is confused with the term *information governance*, even though there is a clear distinction between the two terms. Data governance focuses on managing the data as it is created within a system. **Information governance** focuses on principles and oversight to manage the information that is produced from the different systems within an organization (AHIMA 2013c). Simply stated, data governance manages the information put into the different systems used in healthcare and information governance manages the information output from those systems. The core processes of data governance within an organization are to establish policies and procedures on how data will be connected, who is responsible for the data, how the data will be stored, and how the data will be distributed within the organization.

AHIMA defined the following principles to support proper information governance across an organization.

- *Principle of accountability*: Create authority over the information governance process within an organization. A member of senior leadership should be assigned to oversee and implement a complete information governance program that aligns with the organization's goals and strategies.

- *Principle of transparency*: Create a clear and open documentation process for the information governance strategy and activities within an organization. Processes should be established to provide clear documentation and evidence that supports the organization's operations, decisions, activities, and performance as it relates to the creation, implementation, and maintenance of the information governance program.

- *Principle of integrity*: Create assurances that the data generated and maintained by an organization maintains authenticity and reliability. (This principle is discussed in detail later in this chapter.)

- *Principle of protection*: Create protections to safeguard data and information from improper use and disclosure to avoid data breaches. Regardless of the medium of the data, proper privacy and security safeguards need to be established to adequately protect the information from improper use and disclosure.

- *Principle of compliance*: Create a process for ensuring that all the information complies with appropriate laws, regulations, standards, and organizational policies. (Compliance is defined in more detail in chapters 9 and 16.)

- *Principle of availability*: Create processes and procedures to ensure that information is available when needed, and also accurate, timely, and can be retrieved with ease. Organizations need to build a program to guarantee that the right information is available at the right time.

- *Principle of retention*: Create a process for proper retention of information based on requirements from regulations, accrediting organizations, and company policy. (Chapter 8 contains more information regarding retention of information within an organization.)

- *Principle of disposition*: Create processes for secure and appropriate disposition of information that is no longer needed to be maintained by the organization based on

regulations and organizational policy (see chapter 8 for information regarding disposition of information) (AHIMA 2014b).

HIM professionals play a key role in the success of implementing information and data governance programs in organizations. Their training provides them with an understanding of healthcare's clinical, financial, regulatory, and technology environments, which allows them to lead the information governance within an organization and be the liaison between executive leadership and clinical leadership (AHIMA 2011; 2014b).

Data Stewardship

Data stewardship is an important component of the data governance process. **Data stewardship** creates responsibility for data through principles and practices to "ensure the knowledgeable and appropriate use of data derived from individuals' personal health information" (Kanaan and Carr 2009, 1). Data stewardship is important due to the increase in availability of health data, the use of the health data within the healthcare industry, the use of health information for population management, and the legal and financial risks associated with health data. Data stewardship is created to establish common and essential practices and principles for the management of health data. Benefits of data stewardship are:

- Improved access
- Alerts
- Reminders
- Rapid access
- Facilitates coordination of care
- Structured data collection
- Comprehensive data
- Supports research as well as disease prevention and control (Kallem 2009)

The National Committee on Vital and Health Statistics (NCVHS) recommends that the creation of principles for data stewardship fall into four categories: (1) individual's rights, (2) responsibilities of the data steward, (3) needed security safeguards and controls, and (4) accountability, enforcement, and remedies for data stewardship. Individual rights should be analyzed to assure:

- The individual has proper access to their protected health information
- The individual has a right to review and amend his or her own health information
- The individual is provided transparency of information allowing him or her to understand what information will exist and how it will be used
- Consent and authorization for use and disclosure of health information
- Provision of adequate information and education regarding the rights and responsibilities of health information (Kanaan and Carr 2009)

The data steward's responsibilities should be clearly defined to support adherence to the privacy and security of health information including requirements for uses and disclosures and guarantees gaining access to what is needed to perform job responsibilities. Data security safeguards and controls should be established to define what technical and nontechnical mechanisms are being used to protect the confidentiality, integrity, and accessibility of protected health information. Data stewardship should express accountability of appropriate use as well as sanctions in the event of noncompliance to the requirements (Kanaan and Carr 2009). The goal is to create and build trust and transparency through the entire organization as it pertains to the use of health data.

Data Integrity

Data integrity is the assurance that the data entered into an electronic system or maintained on paper are only accessed and amended by individuals with the authority to do so. Data integrity includes data governance, patient identification, authorship validation, amendments and record correction, and audit validation for reimbursement purposes. These functions ensure that the data is protected and altered by authorized individuals as per policy. Healthcare organizations need to implement proper safeguards to help

establish and manage data integrity in the health record. The Health Insurance Portability and Accountability Act (HIPAA) requires organizations implement policies and procedures to protect electronic protected health information from improper alteration or destruction and establish security measures to ensure that electronically transmitted electronic protected health information is not improperly modified. (For more detail, see chapter 10.) AHIMA recommends healthcare organizations institute policies and procedures for the management of data integrity. Some key components to include in data integrity policies are the documentation requirements, identification of who can document and the scope of that documentation, timeliness of documentation, and safeguards from changing and deleting documentation. Guidelines an organization establishes to reduce the likelihood of issues or damages to the patient data include:

- Committed to complying with laws and regulations, and in an ethical manner
- Requiring accurate data
- Holding individuals accountable for errors as per medical staff bylaws or rules and regulations.
- Identifying penalties for the falsification of information
- Requiring periodic training
- Defining management responsibility (AHIMA Workgroup 2013)

In addition to these policies and procedures, specific HIM department policies and procedures should be established to address the administrative documentation requirements, clinical documentation requirements, entering information into the EHR, correcting and amending the record, and timeframes for correcting the record (AHIMA 2013b). HIM professionals need to be a part of establishing proper integrity throughout the record as they are the custodian of the health record. It is common practice that the HIM department and HIM professionals ensure the health record is complete and accurate so it is available for the purposes of patient care and healthcare operations.

Data Sharing

Data sharing allows information to be exchanged via electronic formats to help support and deliver quality healthcare. Also known as health information exchange, data sharing is the electronic exchange of information between providers' electronic systems. The EHR Incentive Program, Meaningful Use, requires providers to successfully exchange information between organizations to support the quality of healthcare and reduce redundant testing. For example, if a CT scan was performed on a patient prior to referral to another healthcare organization, the results of the CT scan can be shared electronically to prevent the patient from having the same test replicated. Chapter 16 provides more information regarding the Meaningful Use program.

Data Interchange Standards

To help support and drive interoperability and data sharing between healthcare organizations, standards development organizations have created standards for the sharing of information in electronic formats. **Interoperability** is the capability of two or more information systems and software applications to communicate and exchange information. **Standards development organizations (SDOs)** are private or government agencies that are involved in the creation and implementation of healthcare standards. In this specific case, standards development organizations define standards to support the process of electronic exchange of data. **Data interchange standards** are developed in order to support and create structure with data exchanges to sustain interoperability. The goals of the data interchange standards are to facilitate consistent, accurate, and reproducible capture of clinical data. Data interchange standards help support data integrity and safeguard data quality when sharing between organizations. The goals of using data interchange standards for interoperability help to:

- Create a basis to enable the electronic exchange of data between two or more computer systems or application by creating consistent formats and sequence of data that are applied during data transmission

- Reflect the existing clinical and administrative data contained in both paper and electronic data systems to maintain patient data consistency in growing EHRs

- Transfer health data using appropriate business processes and necessary ethical and regulatory demands and guidance

- Foster electronic transmission as a business strategy to support patient care and better patient outcomes

- Promote efficient information sharing among individual computer systems and institutions (Murphy and Brandt 2001)

In the United States, SDOs are managed by the American National Standards Institute (ANSI). ANSI is the organization that oversees the creation of data standards from a variety of business sectors, including healthcare; some common SDOs are discussed as follows.

- *Health Level 7*: An ANSI-accredited SDO that was founded in 1987, established for the creation of standards to support the exchange of clinical information in multiple formats *Digital Imaging and Communication in Medicine:* The messaging standard for digital images; it is used by vendors, user organizations, government agencies, and trade associations to share radiology and other digital images such as cardiology

- *Institute of Electrical and Electronics Engineers (IEEE)*: A national organization that creates and develops different standards for hospital systems that need communication between bedside instruments and clinical information systems (for example, cardiac monitoring performed in the intensive care unit being integrated with the EHR); IEEE currently has standards that allow providers and hospitals to achieve interoperability between medical instrumentation and computer healthcare information system, and though used in multiple types of systems, it is most often used within acute-care settings

- *National Council for Prescription Drug Programs (NCPDP)*: A committee within the Designated and Standard Maintenance Organization focused on the development of standards regarding exchanging prescription information and payment information; NCPDP created multiple standards including a standardized data dictionary for pharmacy data, standards for transactions of file submissions between pharmacies and processors, standards for common billing unit language for submission of prescription claims, and standards to communicate formulary and benefit information to prescribers (AHIMA 2013d)

Information and Data Strategy Methods and Techniques

With the implementation of data governance and information governance, healthcare organizations must evaluate and implement different data strategy methods to promote the collection of quality healthcare data and proper use of the information. Data strategy should be a clear, concise method created to support proper collection and use of healthcare data within an organization that is approved by executive leadership. A data strategy will clearly define the organization's data policies and procedures, roles and responsibilities for data governance, business rules for data governance, process for controlling data redundancy, management of key master data, use of structured and unstructured data, storage for all healthcare data, and safeguards and protections of the data. The strategy must define the following:

- *Data standardization and integration*: This concept focuses on how the data is being entered into the system, where the data is going within the system, where the same data might exist in multiple areas, and how it is being integrated into other applications. The intent of data standardization is to document the location of data collection and ensure standardized formats and meaning of the data.
- *Data quality:* Data quality focuses on entering data into the system that is true, accurate, and relevant to patient care needs and business operations needs.

- *Metadata management*: This refers to managing and defining the metadata within the system. Metadata refers to the data that characterizes other data such as creation date of data, data sent, date received, last accessed date, and last modification date. It is important to clearly define what metadata will be collected and why it is being collected.
- *Data modeling:* This refers to the creation of documentation to justify business decisions made based on the different data collection and storage systems that are used within an organization. The creation of data models and defining the use of data in relation to business mission and vision allows for the support of data standardization across the organization.
- *Data ownership:* This refers to the creation of business owners over specific areas of the data. Based on the business need, the business owners are responsible to create business rules and definitions when collecting specific data to support patient care and their business operations.
- *Data stewardship:* Data stewardship is the evaluation of the data collection based on business need and strategy to ensure the data meets the requirements of patient care and organizational needs. Data stewardship and data ownership are closely connected (AHIMA 2011; Moss 2007).

A clearly defined data strategy approved by executive leadership supports management with one of the most important healthcare assets—patient data.

Enterprise Information Assets

Information assets are the reason for the addition of standards and safeguards to protect information and ensure data integrity is maintained. **Information assets** refer to the information collected during day-to-day operations of a healthcare organization that has value within an organization. For example, patient data collected to support patient care is an example of information assets for the organization. Without it, the organization would not be able to support the continuity of patient care or the billing of services provided to the patient. **Enterprise information management** is the set of functions created by an organization to plan, organize, and coordinate the people, processes, technology, and content needed to manage information for the purposes of data quality, patient safety, and ease of use (Johns 2015). As part of the creation of a data governance strategy, healthcare organizations should establish enterprise information management policies and procedures to address the collaboration and integrative efforts used across the system to protect the organization's enterprise information assets (Warner 2013). Discussions on the enterprise information assets of data visualization and presentation and critical thinking skills follow.

Data Visualization and Presentation

It is important that data is properly organized together and visualized when used for business purposes. Many tools exist to present data such as graphs, charts, and tables. It is easy to create different charts and graphs that provide information and detail regarding data, but it is important the data is presented in ways that are appropriate to the organization and the data being analyzed. For example, to present the frequency of a specific diagnosis by gender, a pie chart—meant to show the percentages of a total—would not be a good selection. A table could provide that information in a better format. Chapter 13 provides specific information regarding data visualization and presentation methods.

Another important aspect for the management and presentation of data is that the data and information needs to be meaningful and useful to the organization. Presenting data that does not support an initiative of the organization can be an unproductive use of company resources and time. Additionally, it may provide information and detail that elicits negative feedback. For example, if a healthcare organization is trying to determine if it wants to add an additional cardiac catheterization room, the healthcare organization may choose to evaluate and create data presentations for individuals within a specific geographic area who have been diagnosed with cardiac conditions. If graphs

that included detail regarding emergency room visits were also presented, it might not be pertinent and specific to the data needs to evaluate the expansion of a cardiac catheterization room. Understanding the data and properly managing it becomes an essential part of handling data assets appropriately.

Critical Thinking Skills

Another key aspect in the management of data assets in the organization is critical thinking skills. **Critical thinking** refers to the process of analyzing, assessing, and reconstructing a situation to provide enhanced solutions and outcomes to a problem (The Critical Thinking Community n.d.). As a healthcare organization produces more data that can be used to analyze and improve patient care and patient outcomes, it is important that individuals managing and overseeing data use within an organization are able to properly evaluate and understand the data.

The issues and challenges that face healthcare organizations and the healthcare industry continue to become more complex and require the effective evaluation of data to help support the change in the healthcare environment (Sharp et al. 2013). Many individuals can effectively analyze a situation and generate solutions to an issue; however, critical thinking skills enhance the process of analyzing the situations and producing a solution. During the critical thinking process it is common for data to be analyzed to effectively evaluate the current state and future solution in addition to generating a solution to the current issue. For example, a healthcare organization is currently evaluating a new line of service to add to an outpatient clinic being built in a small community where they currently only have family practice providers. Without critical thinking, an individual may only evaluate common types of care associated with family practice and add that new line of service to the outpatient clinic. From a critical thinking perspective, an organization may evaluate common referrals to other clinics for the patients seen and treated at the clinic. In addition, they may profile the community in which the clinic exists to understand the population and the care potentially needed. Based on this gathering and analysis of data, an enhanced decision on the nature of care can be made to support the community and its care needs.

With the implementation of EHRs, new roles are being established for the oversight and management of data collection within a healthcare organization as well as how information is used. While principles of information governance have been established by AHIMA and data governance is an essential component of daily operations, the ability to understand, evaluate, and apply the different principles becomes an essential part of a successful information and data governance program. Data management within a healthcare organization is complex and requires a deep knowledge and understanding of data management, data quality, data flow, and data protections. To be successful, critical thinking and processing of complex processes and practices is an essential skill.

✔ Check Your Understanding 6.2

Instructions: **Answer the following questions.**

1. True or false: Information governance and data governance are the same concept and can be used interchangeably.

2. Which of the following are components of AHIMA's principles of information governance?
   A. Accountability and accessibility
   B. Integrity and safeguards
   C. Safeguards and accessibility
   D. Accountability and integrity

3. True or false: Data stewardship is principles and practices established to ensure the knowledgeable and appropriate use of data derived from individuals' personal health information.

4. True or false: Data sharing is defined in multiple requirements under the meaningful use program.

5. Information assets are:
   A. Information considered to add value to an organization
   B. Data entered into a patient's health record by a provider
   C. Clearly defined elements required to be documented in the health record
   D. A list of all data elements added within a record

Data Quality

Clinical documentation is "any manual or electronic notation (or recording) made by a physician or other healthcare clinician related to a patient's medical condition or treatment" (Hess 2015). Clinical documentation is the foundation of every patient record in that it supports the care the patient received and the reimbursement that should be received for the care. Inaccurate information and poor documentation negatively impacts patient care and reimbursement, which can drive up the cost of healthcare (AHIMA 2015). Data quality has always been a focus for HIM professionals; with the implementation of the EHR, the need for more complete and accurate information is critical to support proper patient care and corresponding reimbursement.

Data quality serves as one of the most important elements of healthcare operations and patient care. Ensuring the data entered into the record are reliable and have integrity is a basic requirement for healthcare as it supports patient care and patient safety, provides evidence for reimbursement and accreditation, and affords documentation needed for quality initiatives and research (AHIMA 2015). Without complete and accurate data in a health record, a healthcare organization is at risk for patient safety issues. For example, if a provider does not document what medications were administered to a patient and the exact dosage, the patient may be prescribed another medication that could have adverse effects when combined with the first medication. In addition, there are risks such as having to return payment if the documentation does not support the organization's billing and reimbursement request. For example, if a physician billed that he performed a procedure but the documentation does not support the procedure, the physician may have to return the money and rebill the services.

Many accrediting organizations such as The Joint Commission require evidence of clinical care based on the data that is documented in the health record. If the accrediting organization has basic requirements for documentation in the health record, and the healthcare organization does not meet those requirements, it runs the risk of losing accreditation. Data quality is critical to both clinical care and administrative processes. AHIMA's Data Quality Model is important tool in ensuring the quality of the data collected.

AHIMA's Data Quality Management Model

AHIMA created a quality data management model to support the need for true and accurate data. Data quality management is "the business process that ensures integrity of an organization's data during collection, application, warehousing, and analysis" (AHIMA 2015, 62). Many areas such as patient care, patient outcomes, reimbursement, process improvement, and daily healthcare operations depend on detail quality of information. In order to get meaningful information from the data entered into the health record, core functions of enterprise information management must be established to create the ability to collect high-quality data.

The data quality management model defines four domains that link and support data quality.

The first domain is application, which is focused on understanding the purpose of the data collection. Since the amount of patient data collected through a patient encounter is immense, it is important to evaluate and understand why the data is being gathered and the purpose it serves for the organization. The second domain is collection, which concentrates on how the data elements are being collected throughout the encounter. Understanding where data is being entered and how it is being entered is an essential part of basic data quality management. This focus allows an organization to understand if duplicate or redundant information is being collected. The third domain is warehousing, which describes the processes as well as systems an organization uses to archive data; it also includes understanding where the data is being stored, and how it is being archived as well as managed. The last domain is analysis, which centers on how the data collected throughout the patient encounter is transformed into meaningful data for use throughout the entire spectrum of the healthcare setting (AHIMA 2015).

Ten characteristics of quality data defined within the AHIMA data quality model are accuracy, accessibility, comprehensiveness, consistency, currency, definition, granularity, precision, relevancy, and timeliness. Understanding and applying each of these characteristics to the data quality management domains is an essential part of effective oversight and management of data quality (AHIMA 2015).

Accuracy

Accuracy focuses on the data being free of errors. It is important that the data within the record is accurate across the entire record (that is, the data is valid with the appropriate test results and placed into the proper patient record). An example of monitoring the chart for data accuracy is the analysis of patient notes in the health record to ensure they support the diagnosis throughout the entire health record (AHIMA 2015). For instance, the information in an operative report should be compared to information in the discharge summary to confirm the operation performed and findings are accurate in both documents.

Accessibility

Proper safeguards must be established and employed to assure the data is available when needed while implementing proper precautions and safeguards to protect the information. An example of data accessibility is ensuring that the nurse has access to the health record of patients that he or she is treating (AHIMA 2015). (Refer to chapter 10 for additional information on access to health records.)

Comprehensiveness

Data comprehensiveness certifies all required data elements that should be collected throughout the health record are documented. Training and education should be conducted across the facility to ensure the staff collect all the required data elements are present in the health record (AHIMA 2015).

Consistency

Consistency means ensuring the patient data is reliable and the same across the entire patient encounter. In other words, patient data within the record should be the same and should not contradict other data also in the patient record; for example, a test result and diagnosis should be the same throughout the record (AHIMA 2015).

Currency

The data within the record needs to be current and up to date. EHRs present information across a broad spectrum of care, including data that may be outdated. Specific procedures should be established for updating data elements used for each patient encounter, including the discontinuation of collected data elements that are no longer current. An example of data currency is reviewing and updating patient medications at each patient encounter to remove medications are no longer being taken and adding any new medications (AHIMA 2015).

Definition

All data elements should be clearly defined to guarantee that all individuals using and collecting the data will understand the meaning of that data element. An example of data definition would be defining date of birth as the date the individual was born by month, day, and four digit year (AHIMA 2015).

Granularity

The data collected for patient care must be at the appropriate level of detail. An example of data granularity is documenting the results of a lab test with the appropriate number of decimal points (AHIMA 2015).

Precision

Data should be precise and collected in its exact form within the course of patient care; for example, documenting the exact measurement, such as the height or temperature of the patient. When information is entered precisely, there should be little to no variability of the data (AHIMA 2015).

Relevancy

Data relevancy is the extent to which the data elements being collected are useful for the purposes for which they are collected. If a healthcare organization collects data that is not relevant in supporting patient care and administration, it adds additional, unnecessary information to the record. For example, if a patient presents with pain during urination, data collection should be focused around the symptoms, testing, and treatment. Collecting additional data or data not relevant to support treatment, payment, and healthcare operations adds superfluous data to the record. An example of relevancy would be the creation of templates to collect the correct information during an emergency department visit for a patient, as this can help assemble accurate and relevant data to support the visit and help facilitate additional, nonrelevant information from being collected (AHIMA 2015).

Timeliness

Patient documentation should be entered promptly, ensuring up-to-date information is available within specified and required time frames.

Timeliness may vary throughout the patient record depending on for what the data is being used and how it is supporting patient care. An example of timeliness would be specifying when notes should be entered in the system such as discharge summaries or operative reports. Healthcare organizations frequently require specific forms such as orders or admitting evaluations to be entered within a defined period.

HIM professionals work in a variety of roles to support and manage the quality of data, especially as the implementation of the EHR continues. Some common HIM roles include clinical data manager, health data analysis, terminology asset manager, clinical documentation improvement specialist, data collection specialist, and EHR documentation specialist (AHIMA 2015). The HIM professional understands the need for quality data and can bring that knowledge and expertise into many different areas of the healthcare delivery system.

Data Collection Tools

The management of data quality depends on how the data are collected throughout the entire patient encounter. With data created, stored, and maintained on paper as well as in electronic format, it is important to assure that the data collection tools—such as forms and computer screens—used throughout an organization are effective and efficient. HIM professionals should be involved in the creation of data collection tools for both the electronic and paper-based tools.

In addition to data collection tools, standardization of the collection of patient data is essential to collect the proper information and reach data quality levels needed to support the enhancement of patient care and the healthcare industry. The two major ways to collect data elements are the use of forms within electronic systems or the use of paper-based data collection. It is important to remember that not all paper forms will convert to an electronic format easily so it is important to evaluate each of the different screens to assure data capture is correct. There are standards for both screen design and paper forms to facilitate data collection.

Screen Design

Most EHRs come with pre-built forms and templates for use within the system; the challenge is that these are noncustomized templates. For example, a template would contain all of the information required for inclusion in the discharge summary such as discharge diagnosis, discharge medications, and follow-up. Usually, prebuilt forms and templates do not match organization-specific paper forms and templates. One reason for this is that a screen typically holds approximately a third of what is contained on a form. In addition, the pre-built forms may not be constructed to collect the proper information needed to support the organization's patient care or payment processes. The Department of Health and Human Services Office of National Coordinator for Health Information Technology (ONC) discusses the need to evaluate workflow and customize patient data collection functions. They recommend the following for patient data collection functions:

- Create templates for common types of notes, visits, and procedures
- Configure patient data lists with multiple choices for diagnoses, medications, and orders
- Develop flow sheets for common vital signs and blood tests, allow for trending across a period of time
- Confirm that the EHR being used meets basic standards for interoperability and data sharing across systems (HHS 2015).

In addition, the EHR support staff within the organization should meet with each department that enters data into the health record to evaluate current data collection processes within the EHR and evaluate additional forms or tools necessary to support current workflow. Some key elements when evaluating forms design is deciding what should be in structured data format and what should be in unstructured data format. **Structured data** are data that are able to be read and interpreted by a computer. An example of structured data is a diagnosis code entered into the proper format within the system, such as an ICD-10-CM code format of XXX.XXXX. As long as the data element is in the proper format and in the proper location, the computer will read and perform analysis on that data. Other examples of structured data include check boxes, drop-down boxes, and radio buttons. Check boxes allow the user to select multiple values. For example, murmurs, gallops, and rubs can be chosen under the cardiac section of the physical exam. Drop-down boxes list all of the appropriate options, such as states, from which the user can choose. Radio buttons are used when there are few options, such as only male or female, from which the user should choose. Unstructured data, also known as free text, is data entered into the system with no format specified. An example of unstructured data would be a narrative discharge summary that does not follow a specific format or use a template. Unstructured data is unable to be interpreted by a computer and usually is not used in structured reports. When choosing how to collect data with an EHR, it is important to evaluate and make decisions based on how data is reported.

Since many organizations are unsure of what data they need, especially as they transition to the EHR, it is important to have a standardized committee or process evaluate data collection within electronic systems. This individual or group would be responsible for assuring quality data is entered into the system and proper data reporting is obtained from the system. The documentation should be used to support decisions for future evaluation.

Forms Design

Forms design is a major part of assuring data quality within an organization. With any new creation of a form, the following questions should be asked:

- What is the purpose of this form?
- Can the data be collected in electronic format versus paper format?
- When will this form be used during the patient encounter and in which type of patient encounters?
- Who will use this form within the organization?

- What will be done with the paper once it is created (scanned in system, stored in a paper health record)?

Answering these questions during the assessment of a new form will help the form be appropriate and direct whether it is needed to be created in paper or electronic format. The disadvantage of paper forms is that they will need to be entered into an EHR manually or by scanning the paper documents, which does not allow for reporting.

Recommended steps for control, tracking, and management of paper forms should include:

- Establishing data collection standards within the organization
- Establishing testing and evaluation process
- Evaluating the quality of new paper and electronic forms
- Systemizing storage, inventory, and distribution of forms
- Numbering, tracking, and using barcodes to manage paper forms Establishing a documentation system that supports decisions that are made by the forms committee

Proper and effective management of data collection requires quality data regardless of the media type. HIM professionals play a vital role with this process to certify the proper data is being collected in the best format as well as confirming the forms are designed properly to make processing the information the most efficient.

There is typically a clinical forms committee that manages both paper and electronic forms design. The clinical forms committee should be comprised of a multidisciplinary team across the healthcare organization and led by the HIM department. Some common recommended committee members are medical staff, nursing staff, purchasing, information services, performance improvement, support and ancillary departments, electronic health record support, and forms vendor liaison. In addition, anyone directly affected by the new form or computer view should be invited to attend the forms committee meeting. For example, when a form is being redesigned for use in the intensive care unit, nurses or physicians from that clinical area should be invited to give their input.

Forms control, tracking, and management are important issues. At a minimum, an effective forms control program includes the following activities:

- *Establishing standards:* Written standards and guidelines are essential to ensure that appropriate design and production practices are followed. A forms manual should be developed. **Standards** are fixed rules that must be followed for every form (for example, where the form title should be located). A guideline, on the other hand, provides general direction about the design of a form (for example, usual size of the font used).

- *Establishing a numbering and tracking system:* A unique numbering system should be developed to identify all organizational forms. A master form index should be established, and copies of all forms should be maintained for easy retrieval. At a minimum, information in the master form index should include form title, form number, origination date, revision dates, form purpose, and legal requirements. Ideally, the tracking system should be automated.

- *Establishing a testing and evaluation plan:* No new or revised form should be put into production or use without a field test and evaluation. Mechanisms should be in place to ensure appropriate testing of any new or revised form.

- *Checking the quality of new forms:* A mechanism should be in place to check all newly printed forms prior to distribution. This should be a quality check to confirm that the new form conforms to the original procurement order.

- *Systematizing storage, inventory, and distribution:* Processes should be in place to ensure that forms are stored appropriately. Paper forms should be stored in safe and environmentally appropriate environments. Inventory should be maintained at a cost-effective level, and distribution should be timely.

- *Establishing a forms database:* In an electronic system that supports document imaging, a forms database may be used to store and facilitate updating of forms. Such a database can provide information on utilization rates, obsolescence, and replacement of individual forms or documentation templates (Barnett 1996).

Check Your Understanding 6.3

Instructions: **Answer the following questions.**

1. True or false: Healthcare organizations do not need to evaluate the purpose of data collection for assuring data quality.

2. The four data quality management domains are:
   A. Accessibility, accuracy, consistency, and analysis
   B. Application, collection, warehousing, and relevancy
   C. Accessibility, collection, warehousing, and analysis
   D. Application, collection, warehousing, and analysis

3. Which of the following data quality characteristics means all data items are included within the information collected?
   A. Accuracy
   B. Consistency
   C. Comprehensiveness
   D. Relevancy

4. True or false: Data granularity is the detail level of the data where the attributes and values of the healthcare data are defined and documented.

5. Which of the following is not a recommended guideline for maintaining integrity in the health record?
   A. Specifying consequences for the falsification of information
   B. Requiring periodic training covering the falsification of information and information security
   C. Assuring documentation that is being changed is permanently deleted from the record
   D. Prohibiting the entry of false information into any of the organization's records

Clinical Documentation Improvement

Clinical documentation relates to the quality and integrity of patient data while supporting other functions such as timely coding and reimbursement. Historically, clinical documentation improvement (CDI) programs were created to support reimbursement; however, with the implementation of EHRs and the expanded uses of clinically coded data, CDI programs have shifted to facilitate an accurate representation of healthcare services through complete and accurate patient documentation within the record. Some basic goals of a CDI program are to:

- Obtain specific documentation that can be used to identify the patient's severity of illness
- Identify missing, conflicting, or unclear documentation
- Support code assignment and reimbursement
- Facilitate health record completion
- Support communication between care providers
- Facilitates education
- Improve quality of care (AHIMA 2014c)

CDI programs can help organizations enhance patient documentation, reduce errors within the health record, and improve the quality of the patient data entered in the system while supporting patient care and reimbursement for the organization.

A CDI program usually has dedicated staff that may include HIM professionals, physicians, nurses, and other healthcare professionals. CDI programs impact quality of care and finances within a healthcare organization along with other key stakeholders such as case management, utilization review, medical staff, physician leadership, executive leadership, patient financial services, revenue cycle management, quality and risk management, nursing, and compliance (AHIMA 2014c). The CDI program must have clear goals and strategies that align with the organization's requirement for clear and precise clinical documentation. There are a number of CDI tools that can be used to enhance the quality of the documentation. These tools are used by clinical documentation specialists.

CDI Tools

There are different ways to conduct the CDI review within an organization. Quality tools help manage and document the work of CDI professionals. Another tool that assists and helps with the CDI process is computer-assisted coding (CAC). CAC is software that has the ability to search and evaluate clinical documentation to produce information regarding potential areas for documentation improvement. Electronic documentation is passed through the CAC software application allowing the information to be analyzed. The CAC software will produce a report of procedure and diagnosis codes based on the electronic documentation evaluated. The codes are then manually evaluated for accuracy and completeness. The use of CAC software can speed up the coding process as it allows for evaluation of electronic assigned codes rather than having an individual analyze the entire electronic record and manually assign codes. While CAC is mainly used for the coding of the record for reimbursement purposes, it can be used to automate part of the CDI process as well as provide an electronic evaluation of documentation (AHIMA 2014c). When documentation is unclear or needs more information, a query or discussion with the healthcare provider to obtain the additional information is needed to properly code the chart. Other CDI tools include tip sheets, educational materials, and queries.

Queries The most common tool used for CDI is a query. A **query** is communication tool for CDI staff to communicate with providers to obtain clinical clarification, provide a documentation alert, clarify documentation, or ask additional questions regarding documentation. Traditionally, queries have been used to support coding and reimbursement; however, queries are expanding to the process of CDI outside the coding department. Queries may be used to help clarify a complex diagnosis within a record that does not have proper documentation or clarify procedures that may not be specific enough to support patient care or add a valid code. Queries are used to obtain appropriate reimbursement for the care and services provided to the patient, request more detail regarding the documentation that exists, or clarify contradictory documentation. Contradictory information exists when two parts of a patient's charts provide information that conflicts with one another. For example, if an operative report states that the patient had surgery on the right leg, but in the progress notes there is information regarding the surgical wound on the left leg, a query may be requested to confirm which leg was operated on. There are two formats of queries for CDI: electronic query and paper query. Both queries contain the same demographic information such as the patient name, admission date or date of service, health record number, account number, date query initiated, name and contact of the person who created the query, and a statement or issues trying to be resolved (AHIMA 2014c). For additional information on demographic information, refer to chapter 3.

An electronic query is conducted through an EHR and allows the healthcare provider to offer more clarification or specific information regarding the patient's treatment and diagnosis. The typical process for an electronic query is usually the same format as for a written query, however, the information will be sent electronically and will allow the provider to respond electronically or add an additional clarification note into the health record. A paper query uses a standardized physical document to request clarification or further specify a diagnosis. With the use of paper queries, the health record must be made available to the healthcare provider as he or she should review it and document the clarification in it. Additionally, the response of the query will be documented on paper and the coder or CDI professional will need access to the entire paper chart after the query is completed. The paper query is retained by the healthcare facility and can be stored within the paper health record or scanned into the EHR. Since the query will support patient care and reimbursement, the healthcare organization must create policies and procedures to manage how the query response will be incorporated into the record and if it will become part of the legal health record or designated record set (AHIMA 2014c).

Rules for Writing Queries When writing queries, regardless of medium, healthcare organizations must make sure they are not leading the physicians to document a particular response, but rather to request clarification or provide additional specification. Policies and procedures should delineate who to query, when to query, when not to query, the query format, and the management of the query response. In general, a query should be created when health record documentation meets one of the following criteria: "[it] is conflicting, imprecise, incomplete, illegible, ambiguous, or inconsistent; describes or is associated with clinical indicators without a definitive relationship to an underlying diagnosis; includes clinical indicators, diagnostic evaluation, or treatment not related to a specific condition or procedure; provides a diagnosis without underlying clinical validation; or is unclear for present on admission indicator assignment" (AHIMA 2013a).

There are multiple types of data queries: further specificity of a diagnosis, inconsistency in documentation, and missing clinical indicators. Figure 6.3 provides examples of inappropriate and appropriate queries.

The CDI process needs professional, objective communication. CDI specialists must have strong written and oral communication skills and have basic knowledge of clinical coding guidelines as well as clinical knowledge and knowledge of documentation requirements. All communication, verbal or written, between the CDI professional and the provider needs to be conducted in a professional manner. Most of the information and detail that will be discussed and concluded based on the findings from the CDI process or query process will need to be documented in the health record and may become part of the permanent health record. Both providers and CDI professionals must assure communication is professional and appropriate to support patient care and reimbursement (AHIMA 2013a).

Figure 6.3 Examples of appropriate and inappropriate queries

Example open-ended query

A patient is admitted with pneumonia. The admitting H&P examination reveals white blood count of 14,000; a respiratory rate of 24; a temperature of 102 degrees; heart rate of 120; hypotension; and altered mental status. The patient is administered an IV antibiotic and IV fluid resuscitation.

Leading: The patient has elevated white blood counts, tachycardia, and is given an IV antibiotic for Pseudomonas cultured from the blood. Are you treating for sepsis?

Nonleading: Based on your clinical judgment, can you provide a diagnosis that represents the below-listed clinical indicators?

In this patient admitted with pneumonia, the admitting H&P examination reveals the following:

- WBC 14,000
- Respiratory rate 24
- Temperature 102° F
- Heart rate 120
- Hypotension
- Altered mental status
- IV antibiotic administration
- IV fluid resuscitation

  Please document the condition and the causative organism (if known) in the health record.

Example multiple choice query

A patient is admitted for a right hip fracture. The H&P notes that the patient has a history of chronic congestive heart failure. A recent echocardiogram showed left ventricular ejection fraction (EF) of 25 percent. The patient's home medications include metoprolol XL, lisinopril, and furosemide.

Leading: Please document if you agree the patient has chronic diastolic heart failure.

Nonleading: It is noted in the impression of the H&P that the patient has chronic congestive heart failure and a recent echocardiogram noted under the cardiac review of systems reveals an EF of 25 percent. Can the chronic heart failure be further specified as:

- Chronic systolic heart failure_____
- Chronic diastolic heart failure_____
- Chronic systolic and diastolic heart failure_____
- Some other type of heart failure _____
- Undetermined _____

Source: AHIMA 2013a.

Role of Clinical Documentation Specialist

HIM professionals have always advocated for clear, accurate, and complete documentation in the health record. HIM professionals fit perfectly in the CDI role as they understand medical coding including guidelines, documentation requirements, the need for complete and accurate information, and billing and reimbursement requirements. The clinical documentation specialist is a new role established to improve work processes with documentation, communicating with providers, redesigning clinical documentation improvement, and ensuring accurate documentation to support the code assignment. The clinical documentation specialist must have a strong working relationship with the providers and feel comfortable requesting additional information via query processes.

Check Your Understanding 6.4

Instructions: **Answer the following questions.**

1. Which of the following are two types of queries?
   A. Manual and electronic
   B. Paper and electronic
   C. Manual and computer-assisted coding
   D. Electronic and computer-assisted coding

2. True or false: The response from a query will never go into the health record as it is just communication between the CDI professional and the provider.

3. Which of the following is a goal of a CDI program?
   A. Identify the providers who are not performing properly
   B. Ensure documentation is meeting minimum requirements of the medical staff bylaws
   C. Identify and clarify missing, conflicting, or nonspecific physician documentation related to diagnoses and procedures
   D. Analyze the records after the patient is discharged to document missing pieces of information

Data Management and Bylaws

To help with the facilitation of the collection and assurance of quality data within a healthcare organization, bylaws should be created. Bylaws are written documents that provide details and information regarding the rules and regulations established by a healthcare organization to help support healthcare operations. One of the concerns with healthcare operations is to assure the information documented in the health record supports patient care and healthcare operations such as quality improvement initiatives and accreditation activities. Data quality is a common area to analyze for the purposes of healthcare operations and creates a need for healthcare organizations to define minimum standards of clinical documentation. The most common location of minimum clinical documentation requirements are within the bylaws of the organization. Providers must abide by the bylaws when working in a healthcare facility. The establishment of data collection and data quality requirements in bylaws can help support and ensure proper documentation as required by the healthcare organization. Some other common formats of outlining expectations and ensuring compliance are the establishment of provider contracts, medical staff bylaws, and hospital staff bylaws.

Provider Contracts with Facilities

In the ambulatory care setting, healthcare providers will enter into a contract with a facility to provide patient care. The contracts delineate all expectations of the provider as they care for patients in a specific ambulatory care setting. When creating a provider contract, the need and requirements for data quality should be established. This includes documentation and timelines of documentation within the health record. For example, in a provider contract it will state all labs must be reviewed and signed within 24 hours of completion of the lab test. The contract will also include consequences if minimal requirements are not met, such as the cancellation of the contract in the event of a breach.

Medical Staff Bylaws

Medical staff bylaws describe the manner in which providers will practice medicine within an organization that aligns with the mission and values of the organization. In addition, medical staff bylaws have historically defined how records and documentation are assembled and authenticated. Bylaws should clearly state the contents of the health record, who can document within the

health record, the timelines of entries in the health record, and other clinical documentation expectations and requirements. Timelines and expectations of clinical documentation and data collection processes should be agreed upon and established between the hospitals and the medical staff practicing within the medical staff bylaws. This allows for expectations to be set and the ability to hold a provider accountable if the bylaws are not met adequately (AHIMA 2014b).

Hospital Bylaws

Outside of the medical staff bylaws, hospital bylaws are written documents that govern the staff members who create data within the record for additional support of patient care and reimbursement. Since providers are not the sole authors in the creation of clinical documentation, it is important for hospitals to define who can document within the record, the type of documentation that can occur, and the timeliness and completeness of that documentation. Common healthcare professionals who enter information are nurses, ancillary support, therapists, social work, health unit coordinators, and other support staff given rights to document within the record. As with the medical staff bylaws, clear and concise expectations of data entry and documentation should be established and training provided for all healthcare employees. The hospital bylaws create the foundation of supporting data governance and data quality across the entire spectrum of care.

 Check Your Understanding 6.5

Instructions: **Answer the following questions.**

1. True or false: When creating bylaws for the medical staff, expectations of data quality should be established and documented within the bylaws.

2. Documentation within medical staff bylaws defines how which of the following practitioners should document within the record?
   A. Nursing staff
   B. Therapy staff
   C. Providers
   D. Health unit coordinators

3. True or false: Without proper definition and requirements of data quality and data collection, healthcare organizations are challenged with the ability to hold providers and other patient care professionals accountable for documentation.

4. When creating requirements of documentation for the hospital bylaws, which of the following should be evaluated?
   A. The personal preferences of the healthcare practitioner
   B. The documentation needs based on accrediting bodies
   C. Information taught in the local nursing programs
   D. The wants of the department chairs in a hospital

5. True or false: When creating provider contracts, healthcare organizations should not define disciplinary actions in the event that the contract requirements are not met.

Real-World Case 6.1

A large urban healthcare system was experiencing the rapid implementation and use of the EHR as well as many mergers and partnerships to support clinics and create better business opportunity. In one year, the healthcare systems purchased three new clinics and became affiliates with two others. The affiliate structure allows for the clinics to use their EHR and have a clear referral process if a patient needed additional attention. While integrating the new clinics into the system, data and documents were being entered into the EHR with no common naming structure and with no common places to enter the information; the data was hard to find and inconsistent throughout the entire health record.

With the need to fix the issue as soon as possible, the eHIM manager was tasked with creating a process for the enterprise record management system. The objectives of the project were to define the organization's official health record, detail the record retention schedule for the organization, and create databases. A team consisting of members from across the organization strived to meet the goals of the project and help create information governance within the organization.

The project was a success and the organization now has processes, policies, procedures, and decisions documented to help manage and support health records throughout the entire organization. In addition, there will be efficient integration of records into the current enterprise record management process as new mergers occur. Better oversight of the records has not solved all the issues with the management of patient records, but it has created a foundation for success and a place to expand and build on information governance.

Source: Lundgren 2015

Real-World Case 6.2

A medium-sized hospital had been using an EHR for 12 months. They were having great success with getting the providers to document within a timely fashion; however, many of the notes did not provide enough information to code the record or key components to adequately code were missing. They had a process for physician query, as follows:

- Electronically flag the record for physician query
- Create a paper query form for the provider

- Send the electronic query to the HIM operations department to put in a physician completion folder
- HIM operations would add a deficiency to the patient chart to flag the provider that a coding query needed to be complete
- The provider would come in to the HIM department to complete the query
- The deficiency was removed, and the query was scanned into the chart
- HIM operations then notified the coder through an e-mail that the query was answered
- Chart is coded and sent to billing

While it was a strong process and the providers did answer the questions, it caused a spike in the time to get the charts coded and to billing, as providers usually came into the department once every 20 to 25 days. In some cases, providers would leave the coding queries unanswered for up to 60 days. The average turnaround time for a coding query was 28 days. The organization needed to change the process to help accelerate the query process and reduce the physicians' frustrations of having to come into the HIM department.

New functionality exists within the EHR to send an electronic query, which would automatically assign the deficiency and send a note to the provider's inbox within the EHR alerting him or her that a coding query exists. The new process had less steps and involved less people; however, the physicians were concerned about the new process. With careful training and education, the new process was implemented and reduced the steps, making the physician query process easier for coding, HIM operations, and the providers. The new processes steps were:

- Electronically flag the record for physician query
- Create the electronic physician query through predesigned templates and assign the correct physician (this would automatically assign the deficiency and send the coding query to the inbox)
- Physician electronically completes the coding query through the EHR
- The electronic deficiency is automatically removed and the coding query is electronically submitted to the physician and retained and the chart then automatically flagged to complete coding
- Chart is coded and sent to billing

With the change in the process, the HIM operations department has little involvement unless it is supporting the physician in completing the query. The turnaround time for completion of coding queries was reduced from 28 days to 15 days within the first 60 days of completion. The process was a success and the organization has significantly reduced the time it takes to code and bill all patient encounters.

References

American Health Information Management Association. 2015. Assessing and improving EHR data quality (updated). *Journal of AHIMA*. 84(2):48–53 [expanded online version]. http://library.ahima.org/PB/EHRDataQuality#.Vw55HfkrK9I.

American Health Information Management Association. 2014a. Health Data Analysis Toolkit. http://library.ahima.org/PdfView?oid=107504.

American Health Information Management Association. 2014b. Information Governance Principles for Healthcare. http://www.ahima.org/~/media/AHIMA/Files/HIM-Trends/IG_Principles.ashx.

American Health Information Management Association. 2014c. Clinical Documentation Improvement Toolkit. http://library.ahima.org/doc?oid=300359#.Vw576vkrK9I.

American Health Information Management Association. 2013a. Guidelines for achieving a compliant query practice. *Journal of AHIMA.* 84(2):50–53. http://library.ahima.org/doc?oid=106130#appxA.

American Health Information Management Association. 2013b. Data mapping best practices. *Journal of AHIMA.* 84(11). http://library.ahima.org/doc?oid=300264#.Vw58NvkrK9I.

American Health Information Management Association. 2013c. Breaking Down Information Governance Versus Data Governance. http://journal.ahima.org/2013/09/17/breaking-down-information-governance-versus-data-governance/.

American Health Information Management Association. 2013d. Data standards, data quality, and interoperability (updated). *Journal of AHIMA.* 84(11):64–69. http://library.ahima.org/doc?oid=107104#.Vw58evkrK9I.

American Health Information Management Association. 2011. HIM functions in healthcare quality and patient safety. Appendix B: HIM's role in data governance. *Journal of AHIMA.* 82(8). http://library.ahima.org/doc?oid=104977#.Vw581fkrK9I.

American Health Information Management Workgroup. 2013 (Update). Integrity of the Healthcare Record: Best Practices for EHR Documentation. *Journal of AHIMA.* 84(8):58–62.

Barnett, R. 1996. *Managing Business Forms.* Canberra, Australia: Robert Narnett and Associates.

Clark, J., B. Demster, and C.J. Solberg. 2012. Managing a data dictionary. *Journal of AHIMA.* 83(1):48–52. http://library.ahima.org/doc?oid=105176#.Vw586_krK9I.

Coronel, C. and S. Morris. 2015. *Database Systems: Design, Implementation, and, Management,* 11th ed. Stamford, CT: Cengage Learning.

Giannangelo, K. 2013. Healthcare Data Sets and Standards. Chapter 4 in *Health Information Management: An Applied Approach,* 4th ed. Edited by N. Sayles. Chicago: AHIMA.

Healthcare Information and Management Systems Society. 2009. Data Warehousing: A New Focus in Healthcare Data Management. http://s3.amazonaws.com/rdcms-himss/files/production/public/

HIMSSorg/Content/files/EHR/DataWarehousing.pdf.

Hess, P. 2015. *Clinical Documentation Improvement: Principles and Practices.* Chicago: AHIMA.

Johns, M. 2015. *Enterprise Health Information Management and Data Governance.* Chicago: AHIMA.

Kallem, C. 2009. Data stewardship: Global recommendations for local action. *Journal of AHIMA.* 79(9):58–59, 63. http://library.ahima.org/doc?oid=84417#.Vw59BfkrK9I.

Kanaan, S.B. and M.M. Carr. 2009. Health Data Stewardship: What, Why, Who, How. AN NCVHS Primer. http://library.ahima.org/PdfView?oid=94786.

Lundgren, K. 2015 (May 1). Minnesota Health Information Management Association Annual Meeting Presentation: Enterprise Record Management.

McBride, S., R. Gilder, R.T. Davis, and S. Fenton. 2006. Data mapping. *Journal of AHIMA.* 77(2):44–48. http://library.ahima.org/doc?oid=65895#.Vw59Q_krK9I.

Moss, L. 2007. Data Strategy. http://www.eiminstitute.org/library/eimi-archives/volume-1-issue-2-april-2007-edition/data-strategy.

Murphy, G. and M. Brandt. 2001. Health Informatics Standards and Information Transfer: Exploring the HIM Role (AHIMA Practice Brief). *Journal of AHIMA.* 72(1):68A–D. http://library.ahima.org/doc?oid=57544#.Vw59VfkrK9I.

Sharp, M. 2013. Secondary Data Sources. In *Health Information Management: An Applied Approach,* 4th ed. Edited by N. Sayles. Chicago: AHIMA.

Sharp, M., R. Reynolds, and K. Brooks. 2013. Critical thinking skills of allied health science students: A structured inquiry. *Educational Perspectives in Health Informatics and Information Management.* Summer 2013:1–13.

The Critical Thinking Community. n.d. Our Concept of Critical Thinking. http://www.criticalthinking.org/pages/our-concept-of-critical-thinking/411.

US Department of Health and Human Services Health Information Technology (HHS). 2015. How to Implement Your EHR System. http://www.hrsa.gov/healthit/toolbox/healthitimplementation/implementationtopics/implementsystem/implementsystem_4.html#Customize Patient Data Collection Functions.

Walsh, T. 2013. Security risk analysis and management: An overview (2013 update). *Journal of AHIMA*. 84(11). http://library.ahima.org/doc?oid=300266.

Warner, D. 2013 (December 11). IG 101: Enterprise Information Governance. http://journal.ahima.org/2013/12/11/ig-101-enterprise-information-governance/.

7

Secondary Data Sources

Marcia Sharp, EdD, RHIA

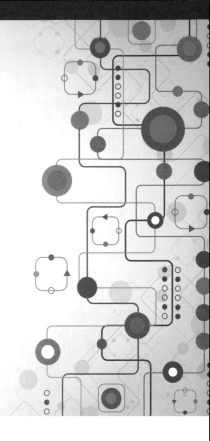

Physician index
Population-based registry
Primary data source
Protocol

Public health
Secondary data source
Stage of the neoplasm
Traumatic injury

Unified Medical Language
  System (UMLS)
Vital statistics

As a rich source of data about an individual patient, the health record's primary purpose is in patient care and reimbursement for individual encounters. (Refer to chapter 2 for details.) It is difficult to see trends in a population of patients by looking at individual records. For this purpose, data must be extracted from individual records and entered into databases. These data may be used in a facility-specific or population-based registry for research and improvement of patient care. In addition, the data may be reported to the state and become part of state- and federal-level databases used to set health policy and improve healthcare. With the electronic health record (EHR), it is possible for data to be collected once in the EHR and used many times (secondary records) for a variety of purposes as outlined in this chapter.

The health information management (HIM) professional can play a variety of roles in managing secondary records and databases. He or she plays a key role to help set up databases. This task includes determining the content of the database

and ensuring compliance with the laws, regulations, and accreditation standards that affect its content and use. All data elements included in the database or registry must be defined in a data dictionary. A data dictionary is a descriptive list of names, definitions, and attributes of data elements to be collected in an information system or database (AHIMA 2014a). The HIM professional may serve as a data steward to oversee the completeness and accuracy of the data abstracted for inclusion in the database or registry. Data stewardship is a responsibility guided by principles and practices to ensure the knowledgeable and appropriate use of data derived from individuals' personal health information (AHIMA 2008).

This chapter explains the difference between primary and secondary data and their users. It also offers an in-depth look at the types of secondary databases, including indexes and registries, and their functions. Finally, this chapter discusses how secondary databases are processed and maintained.

Differences between Primary and Secondary Data Sources

The health record is considered a primary data source because it contains information about a patient that has been documented by the professionals who provided care or services to that patient. Data derived from the primary patient record, such as an index or a database, are considered secondary data sources.

Data also are categorized as either patient-identifiable data, or aggregate data. With patient-identifiable data, the patient is identified within the data either by name or number. The health record consists entirely of patient-identified data. In other words, every fact in the record relates to

a particular patient identified by name. Secondary data also may be patient identified. In some instances, data are entered into a database along with information such as the patient's name maintained in an identified form. Registries are an example of patient-identified data in a secondary source.

Data are patient-identifiable if the identity of the patient is linked via address, age, or other identifier. For example, if an individual can be identified by using a combination of elements such as date of birth, zip code, gender, marital status, and phone number, this would be considered patient-identifiable data.

More often, however, secondary data are considered aggregate data. Aggregate data include data on groups of people or patients without identifying any particular patient individually. Examples of aggregate data are statistics on the average length of stay (ALOS) for patients discharged within a particular diagnosis-related group (DRG).

Purposes and Users of Secondary Data Sources

There are four major purposes for collecting secondary data. The first is for quality, performance, and patient safety. Healthcare facilities, for example, collect core measures information from the health record for the Centers for Medicare and Medicaid Services (CMS) to evaluate the quality of care within the facility.

The second area of secondary data use is research. Data taken from health records and entered into disease-oriented databases can help researchers determine the effectiveness of alternate treatment methods. They also can quickly demonstrate survival rates at different stages of diseases.

The third major use is for population health. For example, states require information be reported to them on certain diseases so the extent of the disease can be determined and steps taken to prevent its spread.

The final use of secondary data is for administration. For instance, in credentialing physicians, facilities are required to access a national database for information on previous malpractice or other adverse decisions against a physician (Mon 2007).

In healthcare, the record is a source for various types of data, and serves many purposes. There are also various users of healthcare data, addressed in the following sections.

Internal Users

Internal users of secondary data are individuals located within the healthcare facility. For example, internal users include medical staff and administrative and management staff. Secondary data enable these users to identify patterns and trends that are helpful in patient care, long-range planning, budgeting, and benchmarking with other facilities.

External Users

External users of patient data are individuals and institutions outside the facility. Examples of external users are state data banks and federal agencies. States have laws mandating cases of health of patients with diseases such as tuberculosis and AIDS be reported to the state department. Moreover, the federal government collects data from the states on vital events such as births and deaths.

The secondary data provided to external users are generally aggregate data and not patient-identifiable data. Thus, these data can be used as needed without risking breaches of confidentiality.

Check Your Understanding 7.1

Instructions: **Answer the following questions.**

1. Bob Smith is a 56-year-old white male. This is an example of what type of data?
   A. Patient-specific
   B. Primary
   C. Aggregate
   D. Secondary

2. Which of the following is an example of how an internal user utilizes secondary data?
   A. State infectious disease reporting
   B. Birth certificates
   C. Death certificates
   D. Benchmarking with other facilities

3. Secondary data is used for multiple reasons including:
   A. Assisting researchers in determining effectiveness of treatments
   B. Assisting physicians and other healthcare providers in providing patient care
   C. Billing for services provided to the patient
   D. Coding diagnoses and procedures treated

4. True or False: A registry is a secondary data source.

5. True or False: A patient health record contains aggregate data.

6. True or False: Administrative and management staff members are internal users of secondary data.

7. True or False: Medical staff members are external users of secondary data.

Types of Secondary Data Sources

Secondary data sources consist of facility-specific indexes; registries, either facility or population based; or other healthcare databases.

Facility-Specific Indexes

The most long-standing secondary data sources are those developed within facilities to meet their individual needs. These **indexes** enable health records to be located by diagnosis, procedure, or physician. Prior to extensive computerization in healthcare, these indexes were kept on cards. Today, most indexes are maintained as computerized reports based on data from databases routinely developed in the healthcare facility.

Disease and Operation Indexes

The **disease index** is a listing in diagnosis code number order of patients discharged from the facility during a particular time period. Each patient's diagnoses are converted from a verbal description to a numerical code, usually using the International Classification of Diseases (ICD). The patient's diagnosis codes are entered into the facility's health information system as part of the discharge processing of the patient's health record. The index always includes the patient's health record number as well as the diagnosis codes so records can be retrieved by diagnosis. Because each patient is listed with the health record number, which may be linked to the patient's name, the disease index is considered patient-identifiable data. The disease index also may include information such as the attending physician's name and the date of discharge.

The **operation index** is similar to the disease index except that it is arranged in numerical order by the patient's procedure code(s) using ICD or Current Procedural Terminology (CPT) codes. The other information listed in the operation index is generally the same as that listed in the disease index except that the surgeon may be listed in addition to, or instead of, the attending physician. For additional information on coding systems, please see chapter 5.

Physician Index

The **physician index** is a listing of cases in order by physician name or physician identification number. It also includes the patient's health record number and may include other information, such as date of discharge. The physician index enables users to retrieve information about a particular

Figure 7.1 Terminology associated with registries

Accession number: A number assigned to each case as it is entered in a cancer registry
Accession registry: A list of cases in a cancer registry in the order in which they were entered
Demographic information: Information used to identify an individual, such as name, address, gender, age, and other information linked to a specific person
Facility-based registries: A registry that includes only cases from a particular type of healthcare facility, such as a hospital or clinic
Incident: An occurrence in a medical facility that is inconsistent with accepted standards of care
Population-based registry: A type of registry that includes information from more than one facility in a specific geopolitical area, such as a state or region

©AHIMA

physician, including the number of cases seen during a specific time period.

Registries

Disease registries are collections of secondary data related to patients with a specific diagnosis, condition, or procedure. Registries are different from indexes in that they contain more extensive data. Index reports can usually be produced using data from the facility's existing databases. Registries often require more extensive entry of data from the patient record. Each registry must define the cases that are to be included; this process is called **case definition**. In a trauma registry, for example, the case definition might be all patients admitted with a diagnosis falling into the ICD trauma diagnosis codes.

After the cases to be included have been determined, the next step is usually **case finding**. Case finding is a method used to identify the patients who have been seen or treated in the facility for the particular disease or condition of interest to the registry. After cases have been identified, extensive information is abstracted from the patients' paper-based health records into the registry database or extracted from other databases and automatically entered into the registry database.

The sole purpose of some registries is to collect data from health records and make them available for users. Other registries take further steps to enter additional information in the registry database, such as routine follow-up of patients at specified intervals. Follow-up information might include rate and duration of survival and quality of life over time. General terminology associated with registries are defined in figure 7.1 and a list of major registries is displayed in table 7.1.

Cancer Registries

Cancer registries have a long history in healthcare. According to the National Cancer Registrars Association (NCRA), the first hospital cancer registry was founded in 1926 at Yale–New Haven Hospital (NCRA 2014a). It has long been recognized that information is needed to improve the diagnosis and treatment of cancer. Cancer registries were developed as an organized method to collect these data. The data may be facility based (for example, within a hospital or clinic) or population based (for example, from more than one facility within a state or region).

The data from facility-based registries are used to provide information for the improved understanding of cancer, including its causes and

Table 7.1 Major registries

Registry	Definition
Cancer registries	Tracks the incidence (new cases) of cancer
Trauma registries	Tracks patients with traumatic injuries from the initial trauma treatment to death
Birth defects registries	Collects information on newborns with birth defects
Diabetes registries	Collects cases of patients with diabetes for the purpose of assistance in managing care as well as for research
Implant registries	Tracks the performance of implants including complications, deaths, and defects resulting from implants, as well as implant longevity
Transplant registries	Maintains databases of cases of patients who need organ transplants
Immunization registries	Collects information within a particular geographic area on children and their immunization status and maintains a central source of information for a particular child's immunization history, even when the child has received immunizations from a variety of providers

methods of diagnosis and treatment. The data collected also may provide comparisons in survival rates and quality of life for patients with different treatments and at different stages of cancer at the time of diagnosis. In population-based registries, emphasis is on identifying trends and changes in the incidence (new cases) of cancer within the area covered by the registry.

The Cancer Registries Amendment Act of 1992 provided funding for a national program of cancer registries with population-based registries in each state. According to the law, these registries were mandated to collect data such as:

- Demographic information about each case of cancer

- Information on the industrial or occupational history of the individuals with the cancers (to the extent such information is available from the same record)

- Administrative information, including date of diagnosis and source of information

- Pathological data characterizing the cancer, including site, stage of the neoplasm (specifies the amount of metastasis, if any), incidence, and type of treatment (Public Law 102-515 1992).

Case Definition and Case Finding in the Cancer Registry

As defined previously, case definition is the process of deciding which cases should be entered in the registry. For example, in a cancer registry all cancer cases except skin cancer might meet the definition for the cases to be included. In addition to information on malignant neoplasms, data on benign and borderline brain or central nervous system tumors must be collected by the National Program of Cancer Registries (CDC 2013).

In the facility-based cancer registry, the first step is case finding. One way to find cases is through the discharge process in the HIM department. During the discharge procedure, coders or discharge analysts can easily earmark cases of patients with cancer for inclusion in the registry. Another case-finding method is using the facility-specific disease indexes to identify patients with diagnoses of cancer.

Additional methods may include reviews of pathology reports and lists of patients receiving radiation therapy or other cancer treatments to determine cases that have not been found by other methods.

Population-based registries usually depend on hospitals, physician offices, radiation facilities, ambulatory surgery centers (ASCs), and pathology laboratories to identify and report cases to the central registry. The administrators of a population-based registry have a responsibility to ensure that all cases of cancer have been identified and reported to the central registry.

Data Collection for the Cancer Registry

Data collection methods vary between facility-based and population-based registries. When a case is first entered in the registry, an accession number is assigned. This number consists of the first digits of the year the patient was first seen at the facility, and the remaining digits are assigned sequentially throughout the year. For example, the first case in the year might be 16-0001. The 16 indicates that the person was seen in the year 2016. The accession number may be assigned manually or by the automated cancer database used by the organization. An accession registry of all cases can be kept manually or provided as a report by the database software. This listing of patients in accession number order provides a way to ensure that all cases have been entered into the registry.

In a facility-based registry, data are initially obtained by reviewing and collecting them from the patient's health record. In addition to demographic information, data in the registry about the patient include:

- Type and site of the cancer
- Diagnostic methodologies
- Treatment methodologies
- Stage at the time of diagnosis

The stage provides information on the size and extent of spread of the tumor throughout the body. There are currently several staging systems. The American Joint Committee on Cancer (AJCC) has worked through its Collaborative Stage Task Force with other organizations with staging systems to develop a new standardized staging system—the Collaborative Stage Data Set. This system uses computer algorithms to describe how far a cancer has spread (Collaborative Stage 2014). After the initial information is collected at the patient's first encounter, data in the registry are updated periodically through the follow-up process (discussed in the following section).

Frequently, the population-based registry only collects information when the patient is diagnosed. Sometimes, however, it receives follow-up information from its reporting entities. These entities usually submit information to the central registry electronically.

Reporting and Follow-up for Cancer Registry Data

Formal reporting of cancer registry data is done through an annual report. The annual report includes aggregate data on the number of cases in the past year by site and type of cancer. It also may include information on patients by gender, age, and ethnic group. Often a particular site or type of cancer is featured with more in-depth data provided.

Other reports are provided as needed. Data from the cancer registry are frequently used in the quality assessment process for a facility as well as in research. Data on survival rates by site of cancer and methods of treatment, for instance, would be helpful in researching the most effective treatment for a type of cancer.

Another activity of the cancer registry is patient follow-up. On an annual basis, the registry attempts to obtain information about each patient in the registry, including whether he or she is still alive, status of the cancer, and treatment received during the period. Various methods are used to obtain this information. For a facility-based registry, the facility's patient health records may be checked for return hospitalizations or visits for treatment. Additionally, the patient's physician may be contacted to determine whether the patient is still living and to obtain information about the cancer.

When patient status cannot be determined through these methods, an attempt may be made to contact the patient directly using information in the registry such as the patient's address and telephone number. In addition, contact information from the patient's health record may be used to request information from the patient's relatives. Other methods used include reading newspaper obituaries for deaths and using the Internet to locate patients through sites such as the Social Security Death Index and online telephone books. The information obtained through follow-up is important and allows the registry to develop statistics on survival rates for particular cancers and different treatment methodologies.

Population-based registries do not always include follow-up information on the patients in their databases. However, those who follow up usually receive the information from the reporting entities such as hospitals, physician offices, and other organizations providing follow-up care.

Standards and Approval Processes for Cancer Registries

Several organizations have developed standards or approval processes for cancer programs. The American College of Surgeons (ACS) Commission on Cancer has an approval process for cancer programs. One of the requirements of this process is the existence of a cancer registry as part of the program. The ACS standards are published in the Cancer Program Standards (ACS 2011a). When the ACS surveys the cancer program, part of the survey process is a review of cancer registry activities.

The North American Association of Central Cancer Registries (NAACCR) has a certification program for state population-based registries. Certification is based on the quality of data collected and reported by the state registry. NAACCR has developed standards for data quality and format and works with other cancer organizations to align their various standards sets.

The Centers for Disease Control and Prevention (CDC) also has national standards regarding the completeness, timeliness, and quality of cancer registry data from state registries through the National Program of Cancer Registries (NPCR). NPCR was developed as a result of the Cancer Registries Amendment Act of 1992. The CDC collects data from the NPCR state registries.

Education and Certification for Cancer Registrars Traditionally, cancer registrars have been trained through on-the-job training and professional workshops and seminars. The **National Cancer Registrars Association (NCRA)** has worked with colleges to develop formal educational programs for cancer registrars. A cancer registrar may become credentialed as a **certified tumor registrar (CTR)** by passing an examination provided by the National Board for Certification of Registrars (NBCR). Eligibility requirements for the certification examination include a combination of experience and education (NCRA 2014b).

Trauma Registries

Trauma registries maintain databases on patients with severe traumatic injuries. A **traumatic injury** is a wound or other injury caused by an external physical force such as an automobile accident, a shooting, a stabbing, or a fall. Information collected by the trauma registry may be used for performance improvement and research in the area of trauma care. Trauma registries may be facility based or may include data for a region or state.

Case Definition and Case Finding for Trauma Registries The case definition for the trauma registry varies but frequently involves inclusion of cases with diagnoses from the trauma diagnosis codes from the ICD. To find cases with trauma diagnoses, the trauma registrar can access the disease indexes looking for cases with codes from this section of ICD. In addition, the registrar may look at deaths in services with frequent trauma diagnoses—such as trauma, neurosurgery, orthopedics, and plastic surgery—to find additional cases.

Data Collection for Trauma Registries After the cases have been identified, information is abstracted from the health records of the injured patients and entered into the trauma registry database. The data elements collected in the abstracting process vary from registry to registry. Abstracting can be either the process of extracting information from a document to create a brief summary of a patient's illness, treatment, and outcome, or extracting elements of data from a source document or database and entering them into an automated system. Data elements in the abstracting process include:

- Demographic information on the patient
- Information on the injury
- Care the patient received before hospitalization (such as care at another transferring hospital or care from an emergency medical technician who provided care at the scene of the accident or in transport from the accident site to the hospital)
- Status of the patient at the time of admission
- Patient's course in the hospital
- Diagnosis and procedure codes
- Abbreviated Injury Scale
- Injury Severity Score

The **Abbreviated Injury Scale (AIS)** reflects the nature of the injury and its threat to life by body system. It may be assigned manually by the registrar or generated as part of the database from data entered by the registrar. **The Injury Severity Score (ISS)** is an overall severity measurement calculated from the AIS scores for patients with multiple injuries (ACI 2016).

Reporting and Follow-up for Trauma Registries Reporting varies among trauma registries. An annual report is often developed to show the activity of the trauma registry. Other reports may be generated as part of the performance improvement process, such as self-extubation (patients removing their own tubes) and delays in abdominal surgery or patient complications. Some hospitals report data to the National Trauma Data Bank (ACS 2011b).

Trauma registries may or may not follow up on the patients entered in the registry. When follow-up is done, emphasis is frequently on the patient's quality of life after a period of time. Unlike cancer, where physician follow-up is crucial to detect recurrence, many traumatic injuries do not require continued patient care over time. Thus, follow-up is often not given the emphasis it receives in cancer registries.

Standards and Approval Process for Trauma Registries The ACS verifies levels I, II, III, IV and V trauma centers. As part of its requirements, the ACS states that the level I trauma center must have a trauma registry (ACS 2015). The ACS certifies levels I, II, III, IV, and V trauma centers. As part of its certification requirements, the ACS states that the level I trauma center, the type of center receiving the most serious cases and providing the highest level of trauma service, must have a trauma registry (ACS 2015). See table 7.2 for a description of each trauma center level.

Education and Certification of Trauma Registrars Trauma registrars may be registered health information technicians (RHITs), registered health information administrators (RHIAs), registered nurses (RNs), licensed practical nurses (LPNs), emergency medical technicians (EMTs), or other health professionals. Training for trauma registrars is through workshops and on-the-job training. The American Trauma Society (ATS) provides core and advanced workshops for trauma registrars and also provides a certification examination for trauma registrars who meet their education and experience requirements through its Registrar Certification Board. Certified trauma registrars

have earned the certified specialist in trauma registry (CSTR) credential.

Birth Defects Registries

Birth defects registries collect information on newborns with birth defects. Often population based, these registries serve a variety of purposes. For example, they provide information on the incidence of birth defects to study causes and prevention; monitor trends in birth defects; improve medical care for children with birth defects; and target interventions for preventable birth defects.

In some cases, registries have been developed after specific events have put a spotlight on birth defects. After the initial Persian Gulf War, for example, some feared an increased incidence of birth defects among the children of Gulf War veterans because of possible exposure to poisonous gases, pesticides, and other toxic substances (USA Today 2003) The Department of Defense subsequently started a birth defects registry to collect data on the children of these veterans to determine whether any pattern could be detected.

Case Definition and Case Finding for Birth Defects Registries Birth defects registries use a variety of criteria to determine which cases to include in the registry. Some registries limit cases to those with defects found within the first year of life. Others include those children with a major defect that occurred in the first year of life and was discovered within the first five years of life. Still other registries include only children who were live born or stillborn babies with obvious birth defects.

Cases may be detected in a variety of ways, including review of disease indexes, labor and delivery logs, pathology and autopsy reports, ultrasound reports, and cytogenetic reports. In addition to information from hospitals and physicians, cases may be identified from rehabilitation centers and children's hospitals and from vital records such as birth, death, and fetal death certificates.

Table 7.2 Trauma center levels and definitions

Trauma center level	Description
Level I	Able to provide total care for every aspect of injury from prevention through rehabilitation
Level II	Able to initiate definitive care for all injured patients
Level III	Able to provide prompt assessment, resuscitation, surgery, intensive care and stabilization of injured patients and emergency operations
Level IV	Able to provide advanced trauma life support (ATLS) prior to transfer of patients to a higher-level trauma center; provides evaluation, stabilization, and diagnostic capabilities for injured patients
Level V	Able to provide initial evaluation, stabilization, and diagnostic capabilities, and prepares patients for transfer to higher levels of care

Source: ATS 2015.

Data Collection for Birth Defects Registries   A variety of information is abstracted for the birth defects registry, including:

- Demographic information
- Codes for diagnoses
- Birth weight
- Status at birth, including live born, stillborn, aborted
- Autopsy
- Cytogenetics results
- Whether the infant was a single birth or one in a multiple birth
- Mother's use of alcohol, tobacco, or illicit drugs
- Father's use of drugs and alcohol
- Family history of birth defects

Diabetes Registries

Diabetes registries include cases of patients with diabetes for the purpose of assistance in managing care as well as for research. Patients whose diabetes is not kept under control frequently have numerous complications. The diabetes registry can keep up with whether the patient has been seen by a physician in an effort to prevent complications.

Case Definition and Case Finding for Diabetes Registries   There are two types of diabetes mellitus: type 1 and type 2 diabetes. Registries sometimes limit their cases by type of diabetes. In some instances, there may be further definition by age. Some diabetes registries, for example, only include children with diabetes.

Case finding includes the review of health records of patients with diabetes. Other case-finding methods include review of the following:

- Diagnostic codes
- Billing data
- Medication lists
- Physician identification
- Health plans

Although facility-based registries for cancer and trauma are usually hospital based, facility-based diabetes registries are often found in physician offices or clinics. The office or clinic is the main location for diabetes care. Thus, data about the patient to be entered into the registry are available at these sites rather than at the hospital. The health records of diabetes patients treated in physician practices may be identified through diagnosis code numbers for diabetes, billing data for diabetes-related services, medication lists for patients on diabetic medications, or identification of patients as the physician treats them.

Health plans also are interested in optimal care for their enrollees because diabetes can have serious complications when not managed correctly. The plans can provide information to the office or clinic on enrollees who are diabetics.

Data Collection for Diabetes Registries   In addition to demographic information about the cases, other data collected may include laboratory values such as glycated hemoglobin also known as HbA1c. This test is used to determine the patient's blood glucose for a period of approximately 60 days prior to the time of the test. Moreover, facility registries may track patient visits to follow up with patients who have not been seen in the past year.

Reporting and Follow-up for Diabetes Registries   A variety of reports can be developed from the diabetes registry. For facility-based registries, one report might keep up with laboratory monitoring of the patient's diabetes to allow intensive intervention with patients whose diabetes is not well controlled. Another report might concern patients who have not been tested within a year or have not had a primary care provider visit within a year.

Population-based diabetes registries might provide reporting on the incidence of diabetes for the geographic area covered by the registry. Registry data also might be used to investigate risk factors for diabetes.

Follow-up is aimed primarily at ensuring that the diabetic is seen by the physician at appropriate intervals to prevent complications.

Implant Registries

An implant is a material or substance inserted into the body, such as breast implants, heart valves, and pacemakers. Implant registries have been developed for the purpose of tracking the performance of implants including complications, deaths, and defects resulting from implants, as well as implant longevity. In the recent past, the safety of implants has been questioned. For example, there have been questions about the safety of silicone breast implants and temporomandibular joint implants. When such cases arise, it has often been difficult to ensure that all patients with the implants have been notified of safety concerns. A number of federal laws have been enacted to regulate medical devices, including implants. These devices were first covered under Section 15 of the Food, Drug, and Cosmetic Act. The Safe Medical Devices Act of 1990 was passed (GPO 1990). It was amended through the Medical Device Amendments of 1992 (GPO 1992). These acts required a sample of facilities to report deaths and severe complications thought to be due to a device to the manufacturer and the Food and Drug Administration (FDA) through its MedWatch reporting system. The MedWatch reporting system alerts health professionals and the public of safety alerts and medical device recalls (FDA 2014). Implant registries may help to assure compliance with legal reporting requirements for device-related deaths and complications.

Case Definition and Case Finding for Implant Registries
Implant registries sometimes include all types of implants but often are restricted to a specific type of implant. Examples of specific types of implants may be cochlear, silicone, or temporomandibular joint.

Data Collection for Implant Registries
Demographic data on patients receiving implants are included in the registry. The FDA requires that all reportable events involving medical devices include the following information: "User facility report number; name and address of the device manufacturer; device brand name and common name; product model, catalog, serial, and lot numbers; brief description of the event reported to the manufacturer or the FDA; where the report was submitted (for example, to the FDA, manufacturer, or distributor)" (FDA 2015).

Thus, these data items also should be included in the implant registry to facilitate reporting.

Transplant Registries

Transplant registries may have varied purposes. Some organ transplant registries maintain databases of patients who need organs. When an organ becomes available, allocation of the organ to the patient is based on a prioritization method. In other cases, the purpose of the registry is to provide a database of potential donors for transplants using live donors, such as bone marrow transplants. Post-transplant information also is kept on organ recipients and donors.

Because transplant registries are used to try to match donor organs with recipients, they are often national or even international in scope. Examples of national registries include the UNet of the United Network for Organ Sharing (UNOS) and the registry of the National Marrow Donor Program (NMDP).

Data collected in the transplant registry may be used for research, policy analysis, and quality control.

Case Definition and Case Finding for Transplant Registries
A physician will identify patients needing transplants. Information about the patient is provided to the registry. When an organ becomes available, information about it is matched with potential donors. For donor registries, donors are solicited through community information efforts similar to those carried out by blood banks to encourage blood donations.

Data Collection for Transplant Registries
The type of information collected varies according to the type of registry. Pre-transplant data about the recipient include:

- Demographic data
- Patient's diagnosis
- Patient's status codes regarding medical urgency
- Patient's functional status

- Whether the patient is on life support
- Previous transplantations
- Histocompatibility (compatibility of donor and recipient tissues)

Information on donors varies according to whether the donor is living. For organs harvested from patients who have died, the following information is collected:

- Cause and circumstances of the death
- Organ procurement and consent process
- Medications the donor was taking
- Other donor history

For a living donor, information includes:

- Relationship of the donor to the recipient (if any)
- Clinical information
- Information on organ recovery
- Histocompatibility

Reporting and Follow-up for Transplant Registries

Reporting includes information on donors and recipients as well as survival rates, length of time on the waiting list for an organ, and death rates.

Follow-up information is collected for recipients as well as living donors. For living donors, the information collected might include complications of the procedure and length of stay in the hospital. Follow-up on recipients includes information on status at the time of follow-up (for example, living, expired, lost to follow-up), functional status, graft status, and treatment, such as immunosuppressive drugs. Follow-up is carried out at intervals throughout the first year after the transplant and then annually after that.

Immunization Registries

Children are supposed to receive a large number of immunizations during the first six years of life. These immunizations are so important that the federal government has set several objectives related to immunizations in Healthy People 2020, a set of health goals for the nation. These include increasing the proportion of children and adolescents

that are fully immunized and increasing the proportion of children in population-based immunization registries (HHS 2015).

Immunization registries usually have the purpose of increasing the number of infants and children who receive the required immunizations at the proper intervals. To accomplish this goal, registries collect information within a particular geographic area on children and their immunization status. They also help by maintaining a central source of information for a particular child's immunization history, even when the child has received immunizations from a variety of providers. This central location for immunization data also relieves parents of the responsibility of maintaining immunization records for their children. This helps to ensure that there is immunization data on children.

Case Definition and Case Finding for Immunization Registries

All children in the population area served by the registry should be included in the registry. Some registries limit their inclusion of patients to only those seen at public clinics. Although children are usually targeted in immunization registries, some registries do include information on adults for influenza and pneumonia vaccines.

Children are often entered in the registry at birth. Registry personnel may review birth and death certificates and adoption records to determine which children to include and which children to exclude because they died after birth. In some cases, children are entered electronically through a connection with an electronic birth record system.

Data Collection for Immunization Registries

The National Immunization Program at the CDC has worked with the National Vaccine Advisory Committee (NVAC) to develop a core set of immunization data elements to be included in all immunization registries. These data elements include:

- Patient name (first, middle, and last)
- Patient birth date
- Patient sex
- Patient race

- Patient ethnicity
- Patient birth order
- Patient birth state and country
- Mother's name (first, middle, last, and maiden)
- Vaccine type
- Vaccine manufacturer
- Vaccination date
- Vaccine lot number (CDC 2012a)

Other items may be included as needed by the individual registry.

Reporting and Follow-up for Immunization Registries Because the purpose of the immunization registry is to increase the number of children who receive immunizations in a timely manner, reporting should emphasize immunization rates. Immunization registries also can provide automatic reporting of children's immunization to schools to check the immunization status of their students.

Follow-up is directed toward reminding parents that it is time for immunizations as well as seeing whether parents fail to bring the child in for the immunization after a reminder. Reminders may include a letter, email, automatic reminder generated from the EHR, or telephone calls. Autodialing systems may be used to call parents and deliver a prerecorded reminder. Moreover, registries must decide how frequently to follow up with parents who do not bring their children in for immunization. Maintaining up-to-date addresses and telephone numbers is an important factor in providing follow-up. Registries may allow parents to opt out of the registry if they prefer not to be reminded.

Standards and Approval Processes for Immunization Registries The CDC provides funding for some population-based immunization registries. In recognition of the growing importance of Immunization Information System (IIS) to the broader health information technology landscape, the 2001 IIS Minimum Functional Standards have been revised. The new standards are an attempt to lay the framework for the development of IIS through 2017 (CDC 2012b). The new program goals and standards include objectives from Healthy People 2020 and are listed in figure 7.2. The CDC also provides funding for population-based immunization registries.

Other Registries

Registries may be developed for any type of disease or condition. Other commonly kept types of registries are HIV/AIDS, cardiac registries, and registries for chronic disease management and gastroenterology.

Registries may be developed for administrative purposes also. The National Provider Identifier Registry is an example of an administrative registry. The NPI Registry enables users to search for a provider's national plan and provider enumeration system information, including the national provider identification number. The NPI number is a 10-digit unique identification number assigned to healthcare providers in the United States (CMS 2015). There is no charge to use the registry and it is updated daily (National Plan and Provider Enumeration System 2015).

Healthcare Databases

Databases are developed for a variety of purposes. For example, the federal government developed databases to carry out surveillance, improvement, and prevention duties. HIM managers may provide information for these databases through data abstraction or from data reported by a facility to state and local entities. They also may use these data to perform research or work with other researchers on issues related to reimbursement and health status.

National and State Administrative Databases

Some databases are established for administrative rather than disease-oriented reasons. Databases are developed, for example, for claims data submitted on Medicare claims. Other administrative databases assist in the credentialing and privileging of health practitioners. Some of these are addressed as follows.

Figure 7.2   Program standards and goals for Healthy People 2020

1. Support the delivery of clinical immunization services at the point of immunization administration, regardless of setting.
   1.1 The IIS provides individual immunization records accessible to authorized users at the point and time where immunization services are being delivered.
   1.2 The IIS has an automated function that determines vaccines due, past due, or coming due ("vaccine forecast") in a manner consistent with current ACIP recommendations. Any deficiency is visible to the clinical user each time an individual's record is viewed.
   1.3 The IIS automatically identifies individuals due or past due for immunization(s), to enable the production of reminder and recall notifications from within the IIS itself or from interoperable systems.
   1.4 When the IIS receives queries from other health information systems, it can generate an automatic response in accordance with interoperability standards endorsed by CDC for message content and format and transport.
   1.5 The IIS can receive submissions in accordance with interoperability standards endorsed by CDC for message content and format and transport.

2. Support the activities and requirements for publicly-purchased vaccine, including the Vaccines For Children (VFC) and state purchase programs.
   2.1 The IIS has a vaccine inventory function that tracks and decrements inventory at the provider site level according to VFC program requirements.
   2.2 The IIS vaccine inventory function is available to direct data entry users and can interoperate with EHR or other inventory systems.
   2.3 The IIS vaccine inventory function automatically decrements as vaccine doses are recorded.
   2.4 Eligibility is tracked at the dose level for all doses administered.
   2.5 The IIS interfaces with the national vaccine ordering, inventory, and distribution system (currently VTrckS).
   2.6 The IIS can provide data and produce management reports for VFC and other public vaccine programs.

3. Maintain data quality (accurate, complete, timely data) on all immunization and demographic information in the IIS.
   3.1 The IIS provides consolidated demographic and immunization records for persons of all ages in its geopolitical area, except where prohibited by law, regulation, or policy.
   3.2 The IIS can regularly evaluate incoming and existing patient records to identify, prevent, and resolve duplicate and fragmented records.
   3.3 The IIS can regularly evaluate incoming and existing immunization information to identify, prevent, and resolve duplicate vaccination events.

3.4 The IIS can store all IIS Core Data Elements.
3.5 The IIS can establish a record in a timely manner from sources such as Vital Records for each newborn child born and residing at the date of birth in its geopolitical area.
3.6 The IIS records and makes available all submitted vaccination and demographic information in a timely manner.
3.7 The IIS documents active or inactive status of individuals at both the provider organization or site and geographic levels.

4. Preserve the integrity, security, availability and privacy of all personally identifiable health and demographic data in the IIS.
   4.1 The IIS program has written confidentiality and privacy practices and policies based on applicable law or regulation that protect all individuals whose data are contained in the system.
   4.2 The IIS has user access controls and logging, including distinct credentials for each user, least-privilege access, and routine maintenance of access privileges.
   4.3 The IIS is operated or hosted on secure hardware and software in accordance with industry standards for protected health information, including standards for security and encryption, uptime, and disaster recovery.

5. Provide immunization information to all authorized stakeholders.
   5.1 The IIS can provide immunization data access to healthcare providers, public health, and other authorized stakeholders (for example, schools, public programs, payers) according to law, regulation, or policy.
   5.2 The IIS can generate predefined or ad hoc reports (for example, immunization coverage, vaccine usage, and other important indicators by geographic, demographic, provider, or provider groups) for authorized users without assistance from IIS personnel.
   5.3 With appropriate levels of authentication, IIS can provide copies of immunization records to individuals or parents and guardians with custodial rights.
   5.4 The IIS can produce an immunization record acceptable for official purposes (for example, school, child care, camp).

6. Promote vaccine safety in public and private provider settings.
   6.1 Provide the necessary reports and functionality to facilitate vaccine recalls when necessary, including the identification of recipients by vaccine lot, manufacturer, provider, and time frame.
   6.2 Facilitate reporting and/or investigation of adverse events following immunization.

Source: CDC 2012b.

Medicare Provider Analysis and Review File   The Medicare Provider Analysis and Review (MEDPAR) File is made up of acute care hospital and skilled nursing facility (SNF) claims data for all Medicare claims. It consists of the following types of data:

- Demographic data on the patient
- Data on the provider
- Information on Medicare coverage for the claim
- Total charges
- Charges broken down by specific type of service, such as operating room, physical therapy, and pharmacy charges
- ICD diagnosis and procedure codes
- Medicare severity diagnosis-related groups (MS-DRGs)

The MEDPAR file is frequently used for research on topics such as charges for particular types of care and MS-DRGs. The limitation of the MEDPAR data for research purposes is that the file contains only Medicare patients.

National Practitioner Data Bank   The National Practitioner Data Bank (NPDB) was mandated under the Health Care Quality Improvement Act of 1986 to provide a database of medical malpractice payments, adverse licensure actions, and certain professional review actions (such as denial of medical staff privileges) taken by healthcare entities such as hospitals against physicians, dentists, and other healthcare providers as well as private accrediting organizations and peer review organizations (NPDB 2010). A peer review organization performs review of medical records for medical necessity, quality, and appropriateness of healthcare services provided to Medicare beneficiaries. Peer review organizations are now called quality improvement organizations (AHIMA 2014b). The NPDB was developed to alleviate the lack of information about malpractice decisions, denial of medical staff privileges, or loss of medical license. Because these data were not widely available, physicians who lost their license to practice in one state or facility could move to another state or another facility and begin practicing again with the current state or facility unaware of previous actions against the physician.

Information in the NPDB is provided through a required reporting mechanism. Entities making malpractice payments, including insurance companies, boards of medical examiners, and entities such as hospitals and professional societies, must report to the NPDB. The information reported includes information about the practitioner, the reporting entity, and the judgment or settlement. Information about physicians and other healthcare providers must be provided (NPDB 2010). Entities such as private accrediting organizations and peer review organizations are required to report adverse actions to the data bank. In addition, adverse licensure and other actions against any healthcare entity must be reported, not just physicians and dentists. Adverse actions may include reporting incidents of license suspensions or revocations. It may also include issues related to professional competence, and malpractice payments. Monetary penalties may be assessed for failure to report.

The law requires healthcare facilities to query the NPDB as part of the credentialing process when a physician initially applies for medical staff privileges and every two years thereafter.

State Administrative Data Banks   States also frequently have health-related administrative databases. For example, many states collect either Uniform Hospital Discharge Data Set or UB-04/837 institutional data on patients discharged from hospitals located within their area.

National, State, and County Public Health Databases

Public health is the area of healthcare dealing with the health of populations in geographic areas such as states or counties. Publicly reported healthcare data vary from quality and patient safety measurement data to patient satisfaction results. The aggregated data range from a local to national perspective, such as state-specific public health conditions to national morbidity and mortality statistics. In addition, consumers are becoming more actively involved in their healthcare. Publicly reported data may be presented for consumer use through various star ratings on different quality measures via organizations such as The Leapfrog Group, HealthGrades, or Hospital Compare. The Leapfrog Group and Hospital Compare allow users to select various hospitals to compare data such as specific medical conditions, surgical procedures, or overall patient safety ratings. Based on the selections made, data is compared to the hospitals selected as well as to state and national averages. One of the duties of public health agencies is surveillance of the health status of the population within their jurisdiction.

The databases developed by public health departments provide information on the incidence and prevalence of diseases, possible high-risk populations, survival statistics, and trends over time. Data for the databases may be collected using a variety of methods, including interviews, physical examinations of individuals, and reviews of health records. Thus, the HIM manager may have input in these databases through data provided from health records. At the national level, the **National Center for Health Statistics (NCHS)** has responsibility for these databases. The NCHS provides statistical, accurate, relevant, and timely data that helps guide actions and policies to improve the health of the American people. The information or data obtained may be gathered through surveys.

National Health Care Survey One of the major national public health surveys is the National Health Care Survey. To a large extent, it relies on data from patients' health records. It consists of a number of parts, including:

- National Hospital Care Survey
- National Survey of Ambulatory Surgery
- National Nursing Home Survey
- National Home and Hospice Care Survey

Data in the National Hospital Care Survey is a combination of data from the National Hospital Discharge Survey (NHDS) and the National Hospital Ambulatory Medical Care Survey (NHAMCS). Information on the utilization of healthcare provided in inpatient settings, emergency departments, outpatient departments, and ambulatory surgery centers are collected in one place.

Data for the National Survey of Ambulatory Surgery are collected on a representative sample of hospital-based and freestanding ambulatory surgery centers. Data include patient demographic characteristics, source of payment, and information on anesthesia given, diagnoses, and surgical and non-surgical procedures on patient visits. It is a mailed survey about the facility and abstracts of patient data.

The National Nursing Home Survey provides data on each facility, current residents, and discharged residents. Information is gathered through an interview process. The administrator or designee provides information about the facility being surveyed. For information on the residents, the nursing staff member most familiar with the resident's care is interviewed. The staff member uses the resident's health record for reference during the interview. Data collected on the facility include information on ownership, size, certification status, admissions, services, full-time equivalent employees, and basic charges. Interviews about both current and discharged residents provide demographic information on the resident as well as length of stay, diagnoses, level of care received, activities of daily living (ADL), and charges.

For the National Home and Hospice Care Survey, data are collected on the home health or hospice agency as well as on their current and discharged patients. Data include referral and length of service, diagnoses, number of visits, patient charges, health status, reason for discharge, and types of services provided. Facility data are provided through an interview with the administrator or designee. Patient information is obtained from the caregiver most familiar with the patient's care. The caregiver may use the patient's health record in answering the interview questions.

Because of bioterrorism scares, the CDC developed the National Electronic Disease Surveillance System (NEDSS) that serves as a major part of the Public Health Information Network (PHIN). This system provides a national surveillance system by connecting the CDC with local and state public health partners. It allows the CDC to monitor trends from disease reporting at the local and state levels to look for possible bioterrorism incidents.

Other national public health databases include the National Health Interview Survey used to monitor the health status of the population of the United States, and the National Immunization Survey, which collects data on the immunization status of children between the ages of 19 months and 35 months living in the United States.

State and local public health departments also develop databases, as needed, to perform their duties of health surveillance, disease prevention, and research. An example of state databases is infectious or notifiable disease databases. Each state has a list of diseases that must be reported to the state—such as AIDS, measles, and syphilis—so that containment and prevention measures can be taken to avoid large outbreaks of these diseases. As mentioned previously, state and local reporting systems connect with the CDC through NEDSS to evaluate trends in disease outbreaks. There also may be statewide databases or registries that collect extensive information on particular diseases and conditions such as birth defects, immunizations, and cancer.

Vital Statistics Vital statistics include data on births, deaths, fetal deaths, marriages, and divorces. Responsibility for the collection of vital statistics rests with the states. The states share information with the NCHS. The actual collection of the information is carried out at the local level. For example, birth certificates are completed at the facility where the birth occurred and then are sent to the state. The state serves as the official repository for the certificate and provides vital statistics information to the NCHS. From the vital statistics collected, states and the national government develop a variety of databases.

One vital statistics database at the national level is the Linked Birth and Infant Death Data Set. In this database, the information from birth certificates is compared to death certificates for infants less than one year of age. This database provides data to conduct analyses for patterns of infant death. Other national programs that use vital statistics data include the National Mortality Followback Survey, the National Survey of Family Growth, and the National Death Index (CDC 2015a). In some of these databases, such as the National Maternal and Infant Health Survey and the National Mortality Followback Survey, additional information is collected on deaths originally identified through the vital statistics system.

Similar databases using vital statistics data as a basis are found at the state level. Birth defects registries, for example, frequently use vital records data with information on the birth defect as part of their data collection process. For additional information on vital statistics, see chapter 14.

Clinical Trials A clinical trial is a research project in which new treatments and tests are investigated to determine whether they are safe and effective. The trial proceeds according to a protocol, which is the list of rules and procedures to be followed. Clinical trials databases have been developed to allow physicians and patients to find clinical trials. A patient with cancer or AIDS, for example, might be interested in participating in a clinical trial but not know how to locate one applicable to his or her type of disease. Clinical trials databases provide the data that enables patients and practitioners to determine what clinical trials are available and applicable to the patient.

The Food and Drug Administration Modernization Act of 1997 mandated that a clinical trials database be developed. The National Library of Medicine (NLM) has developed the database, available on the Internet for use by both patients and practitioners. The NLM is a biomedical library that maintains and makes available a vast amount of print collections and produces electronic information resources on a wide range of topics (NLM 2015).

Health Services Research Databases Health services research is research concerning healthcare delivery systems, including organization and delivery and care effectiveness and efficiency. Within the federal government, the organization most involved in health services research is the

Agency for Healthcare Research and Quality (AHRQ). AHRQ looks at issues related to the efficiency and effectiveness of the healthcare delivery system, disease protocols, and guidelines for improved disease outcomes.

A major initiative for AHRQ has been the **Healthcare Cost and Utilization Project (HCUP).** HCUP uses data collected at the state level from either claims data or discharge-abstracted data, including the UHDDS items reported by individual hospitals and, in some cases, by freestanding ambulatory care centers. Which data are reported depends on the individual state. Data may be reported by the facilities to a state agency or to the state hospital association, depending on state regulations. The data then are reported from the state to AHRQ, where they become part of the HCUP databases (AHRQ 2015).

HCUP consists of a set of databases, including:

- Nationwide inpatient sample (NIS): inpatient database from a sample of hospitals

- State inpatient database (SID): hospital discharge database

- Nationwide emergency department sample (NEDS): database on emergency department (ED) state emergency department databases (SEDD): database from hospital emergency departments (EDs)

- Kids inpatient database (KID): database of inpatient discharge data on children (HCUP 2015).

These databases are unique because they include data on inpatients whose care is paid for by all types of payers, including Medicare, Medicaid, private insurance, self-paying, and uninsured patients. Data elements include demographic information, information on diagnoses and procedures, admission and discharge status, payment sources, total charges, length of stay, and information on the hospital or freestanding ambulatory surgery center. Researchers may use these databases to look at issues such as those related to the costs of treating particular diseases, the extent to which treatments are used, and differences in outcomes and cost for alternative treatments.

National Library of Medicine The National Library of Medicine (NLM) produces two databases of special interest to the HIM manager—MEDLINE and UMLS.

Medical Literature, Analysis, and Retrieval System Online (MEDLINE) is the best-known database from the NLM. It includes bibliographic listings for publications in the areas of medicine, dentistry, nursing, pharmacy, allied health, and veterinary medicine. HIM managers use MEDLINE to locate articles on HIM issues as well as articles on medical topics necessary to carry out quality improvement and medical research activities.

The **Unified Medical Language System (UMLS)** provides a way to integrate biomedical concepts from a variety of sources to show their relationships. This process allows links to be made between different information systems for purposes such as electronic health record systems. UMLS is of particular interest to the HIM manager because of medical vocabularies such as ICD-10-CM, CPT, and the Healthcare Common Procedure Coding System (HCPCS).

Health Information Exchange Health information exchange (HIE) initiatives were developed in an effort to move toward a longitudinal patient record with complete information about the patient available at the point of care. This is patient-specific rather than aggregate data and is used primarily for patient care. Some researchers have looked at the amount of data available through the health information exchanges as a possible source of data to aggregate for research. Since HIE is a fairly new concept, it is important that HIEs take the time to develop policies and procedures covering the use of data collected for patient care for other purposes. Special attention needs to be paid to whether patients included in the HIE need to provide individual consent to be included when the data is aggregated for research and other purposes. Aggregated data can be deidentified to add another layer of protection for the patient's identity. For additional information on HIE, see chapter 12.

Data for Performance Measurement The Joint Commission, CMS, and some health plans require healthcare facilities to collect data on core performance measures. These measures are secondary data because they are taken from patient medical records. Facilities must determine how to collect these measures and how to aggregate the data for reporting purposes. Whether a facility reports such measures will be used as a basis for pay for performance systems. It is, therefore, extremely important that the data accurately reflect the quality of care provided by the facility. More information can be found in chapter 6.

Check Your Understanding 7.2

Instructions: **Answer the following questions.**

1. Which of the following indexes is an important source of patient health record numbers?
   A. Physician index
   B. Master patient index
   C. Operation index
   D. Disease index

2. After the types of cases to be included in a registry have been determined, what is the next step in data acquisition?
   A. Case registration
   B. Case definition
   C. Case abstracting
   D. Case finding

3. What number is assigned to a case when it is first entered in a cancer registry?
   A. Accession number
   B. Patient number
   C. Health record number
   D. Medical record number

4. What are the patient data such as name, age, and address called?
   A. Demographic data
   B. Secondary data
   C. Aggregate data
   D. Identification data

5. What type of registry maintains a database on patients injured by an external physical force?
   A. Implant registry
   B. Birth defects registry
   C. Trauma registry
   D. Transplant registry

6. Why is the MEDPAR File limited in terms of being used for research purposes?
   A. It only provides demographic data about patients.
   B. It only contains Medicare patients.
   C. It uses ICD-10-CM diagnoses and procedure codes.
   D. It breaks charges down by specific type of service.

7. Which of the following acts mandated establishment of the National Practitioner Data Bank?
   A. Health Care Quality Improvement Act of 1986
   B. Health Insurance Portability and Accountability Act of 1996
   C. Safe Medical Devices Act of 1990
   D. Food and Drug Administration Modernization Act of 1997

8. I started work today on a clinical trial and need to familiarize myself with the rules and procedures to be followed. This information is called the:
   A. Protocol
   B. MEDPAR
   C. UMLS
   D. HCUP

9. An advantage of HCUP is that it:
   A. Contains only Medicare data
   B. Is used to determine pay for performance
   C. Contains data on all payer types
   D. Contains bibliographic listings from medical journals

 ## Real-World Case 7.1

Hundreds of hospitals, clinics, and health departments automatically report certain symptoms and diagnoses to the government each day. This practice of biosurveillance helps officials track the spread of flu, detect outbreaks, and watch for odd symptoms that might signal a brand new disease or bioterrorism. Although information is reported daily, doctors rarely know what their colleagues nearby are diagnosing. Instead they often call the health department to ask if anyone has heard of any outbreak of certain cases. Work is being done to create a mechanism to track diseases before they become outbreaks (CNS News 2011).

Researchers are now working on technology that will link local biosurveillance to electronic health records, and even mobile applications. Providing data on the amount of disease or infection that is spreading locally can improve diagnosis and treatment methods.

Federal health officials are working to create an easy-to-use web tool that will allow doctors and consumers to search for local surveillance information. Websites and mobile applications such HealthMap, CDC Influenza, and Flu Near You are tools used to track cases in specific areas (Arbiter Online 2015).

Real-World Case 7.2

Registries are an important and integral component of our healthcare system. Registries allow entities to collect data on real-world patient outcomes, create a feedback mechanism for health care providers, and facilitate changes in care based on the feedback received (Wheatley 2014).

A collaborative effort between Kaiser Permanente Institute for Health Policy, AcademyHealth, and The Pew Charitable Trust joined forces to highlight the benefits of registries and their impact on healthcare policy. Six clinical data registries were profiled: Kasier Permanente's Total Joint Replacement Registry (TJRR), Australian Orthopaedic Association (AOA) National Joint Replacement Registry (NJRR), Transcatheter Valve Therapy (TVT), National Surgical Quality Improvement Program (NSQIP), Get with the Guidelines-Stroke (GWTG-Stroke), and the Cystic Fibrosis Patient Registry (Wheatley 2014). The information generated allows stakeholders to make informed healthcare decisions.

As more and more registries are developed, such issues as de-identification, genetic testing, and standardization need to be addressed. The Surveillance, Prevention, and Management of Diabetes Mellitus DataLink (SUPREME-DM) holds nearly 1.1 million diabetic de-identfied patient records (Hall 2012). Additionally, the National Institute of Health has an online Genetic Testing Registry which allows users to search for genetic tests using the name of the test, the provider of the test or a condition or gene that could be detected via the test (Bowman 2012).

References

Agency for Clinical Innovation. 2016. Injury Scoring. http://www.aci.health.nsw.gov.au/get-involved/institute-of-trauma-and-injury-management/Data/injury-scoring.

Agency for Healthcare Research and Quality. 2015. Healthcare Cost and Utilization Project (HCUP). http://www.ahrq.gov/research/data/hcup/index.html.

American College of Surgeons. 2015. The Committee on Trauma. https://www.facs.org/quality-programs/trauma.

American College of Surgeons. 2011a. Commission on Cancer. https://www.facs.org/quality-programs/cancer.

American College of Surgeons. 2011b. National Trauma Data Bank. https://www.facs.org/quality-programs/trauma/ntdb.

American Health Information Management Association. 2014a. Health Data Analysis Toolkit. http://library.ahima.org/PdfView?oid=107504.

American Health Information Management Association. 2014b. *Pocket Glossary of Health Information Management and Technology*. Chicago: AHIMA.

American Health Information Management Association. 2008. Statement on Data Stewardship. http://library.ahima.org/doc?oid=100307#.Vw_QDPkrLDc.

American Trauma Society. 2015. Trauma Center Levels Explained. http://www.amtrauma.org/?page=traumalevels.

Arbiter Online. 2015. Phone Apps Track Influenza. https://arbiteronline.com/2015/01/23/phone-apps-track-influenza/.

Bowman, D. 2012. NIH's Genetic Testing Registry Up and Running. http://www.fiercehealthit.com/story/nihs-genetic-testing-registry-and-running/2012-03-05.

Centers for Disease Control. 2015a. National Notifiable Disease Surveillance System. http://wwwn.cdc.gov/nndss/.

Centers for Disease Control. 2015b. Survey and Data Collection Systems. http://www.cdc.gov/nchs/surveys.htm.

Centers for Disease Control. 2013. National Program of Cancer Registries Program Standards. http://www.cdc.gov/cancer/npcr/pdf/npcr_standards.pdf.

Centers for Disease Control. 2012a. Core Data Elements. http://www.cdc.gov/vaccines/programs/iis/core-data-elements.html.

Centers for Disease Control. 2012b. Immunization Information System Functional Standards. http://www.cdc.gov/vaccines/programs/iis/func-stds.html.

Centers for Medicare and Medicaid Services. 2015. National Provider Identifier Standard (NPI). https://www.cms.gov/Regulations-and-Guidance/HIPAA-Administrative-Simplification/NationalProvIdentStand/index.html?redirect=/NationalProvIdentStand/.

CNS News. 2011. Real-Time Tracking of Diseases Improves Diagnosis. http://cnsnews.com/news/article/real-time-tracking-diseases-improves-diagnosis-0.

Collaborative Stage Data Collection System. 2014. Collaborative Stage Transition Newsletter. https://cancerstaging.org/cstage/about/news/Documents/CS%20Transition%20Newsletter%20Issue%202%20-%206%2016%2014.pdf.

Department of Health and Human Services. 2015. Healthy People 2020. http://www.healthypeople.gov/2020/topics-objectives/topic/immunization-and-infectious-diseases.

Food and Drug Administration. 2015. Mandatory Reporting Requirements. http://www.fda.gov/MedicalDevices/DeviceRegulationandGuidance/PostmarketRequirements/ReportingAdverseEvents/ucm2005737.htm#3.

Food and Drug Administration. 2014. Reporting by Health Professionals. http://www.fda.gov/Safety/MedWatch/HowToReport/ucm085568.htm.

Government Publishing Office. 1992. Medical Device Amendments of 1992. http://www.gpo.gov/fdsys/pkg/STATUTE-106/pdf/STATUTE-106-Pg238.pdf.

Government Publishing Office. 1990. Safe Medical Devices Act of 1990. http://www.gpo.gov/fdsys/pkg/STATUTE-104/pdf/STATUTE-104-Pg4511.pdf.

Hall, S. 2012. Better Data Standards, Registries Key to Value-Based Healthcare. http://www.fiercehealthit.com/story/better-data-standards-registries-key-value-based-healthcare/2012-06-25.

Healthcare Costs and Utilization Project. 2015. Overview of HCUP. http://www.hcup-us.ahrq.gov/overview.jsp.

Mon, D. 2007. *Development of a National Health Data Stewardship Entity: Response to Request for Information.* Chicago: AHIMA. http://library.ahima.org/xpedio/groups/public/documents/ahima/bok1_044422.pdf.

National Cancer Registrars Association. 2014a. History. http://www.ncra-usa.org/i4a/pages/index.cfm?pageid=3873.

National Cancer Registrars Association. 2014b. Education. http://www.ncra-usa.org/i4a/pages/index.cfm?pageid=3865.

National Library of Medicine. 2015. About the National Library of Medicine. https://www.nlm.nih.gov/about/index.html#.

National Plan and Provider Enumeration System. 2015. https://npiregistry.cms.hhs.gov/.

National Practitioner Data Bank. 2010 (January 28). Adverse information on physicians and other health care practitioners: Reporting on adverse and negative actions. *Federal Register* 75.

Public Law 102-515. 1992. Cancer Registries Amendment Act. http://www.cdc.gov/cancer/npcr/pdf/publaw.pdf.

USA Today. 2003. Study: Gulf War Vets' Children Have Higher Death Rates. http://usatoday30.usatoday.com/news/health/2003-06-03-vets-birth-defects_x.htm.

Wheatley, B. 2014. Health Care Registries: Powerful Tool, Narcoleptic Name. http://thehealthcareblog.com/blog/2014/12/14/health-care-registries-powerful-tool-narcoleptic-name/.

Part III
Information Protection: Access, Disclosure, and Archival Privacy and Security

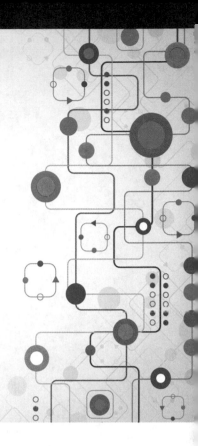

8

Health Law

Laurie A. Rinehart-Thompson, JD, RHIA, CHP, FAHIMA

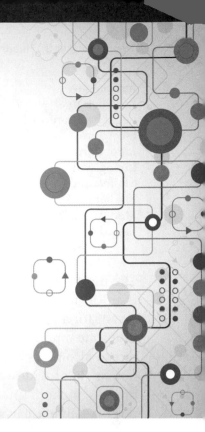

Learning Objectives

- Identify the types of laws that govern the healthcare industry
- Identify the steps in a legal proceeding
- Apply professional liability theories to situations of wrongdoing
- Report on the purpose and types of consents and advance directives
- Identify factors that govern the maintenance and content of the health record
- Identity legal issues related to ownership, control, and use and disclosure of health information
- Identify the content of the legal health record
- Adhere to legally sound health record retention and destruction principles
- Identify medical staff credentialing principles
- Demonstrate the differences among licensure, certification and accreditation

Key Terms

Accreditation
Administrative law
Admissibility
Alternative dispute resolution
Appeals
Appellate courts
Arbitration
Authentication
Bench trial
Breach
Breach of contract
Causation
Cause of action
Certification

Clinical privileges
Complaint
Consent
Constitutional law
Counterclaim
Courts of appeal
Credentialing
Cross-claim
Default
Defendant
Deposition
Designated record set (DRS)
Discovery
District court

Do-not-resuscitate (DNR) order
Durable power of attorney for healthcare decisions (DPOA-HCD)
Express contract
False Claims Act
General consent
Health Care Quality Improvement Act of 1986
Implied contract
Informed consent
Injury (harm)
Intentional tort
Joinder

Judicial law
Jurisdiction
Legal health record
Licensure
Litigation
Living will
Malfeasance
Mediation
Medical malpractice
Metadata

Misfeasance
National Practitioner Data Bank
  (NPDB)
Negligence
Nonfeasance
Personal health record (PHR)
Plaintiff
Private law
Privileged communication
Public law

Rules and regulations
Standard of care
Statute of limitations
Statutory law
Subpoena
Summons
Supreme courts
Tort
Trial court
Voir dire

The most important purpose of the health record is to document patient treatment and provide a means for a patient's healthcare providers to communicate among each other. However, the health record also plays an important role as a legal document. It provides critical evidence in the legal process, including medical malpractice and other personal injury lawsuits, criminal cases, healthcare fraud and abuse investigations and actions, and quasi-judicial proceedings such as workers' compensation determinations.

This chapter discusses legal issues associated with health information and includes an overview of sources of law and the legal system; patient healthcare decision making; health record creation, maintenance, and retention; ownership and control of the health record; the legal health record; licensure and certification of healthcare professionals; and licensure, certification, and accreditation of organizations.

Basic Legal Concepts

There are many federal and state statutes and regulations that provide a protective framework around the health record and also form its content. The most well-known is the federal Privacy Rule of the Health Insurance Portability and Accountability Act (HIPAA) and the American Recovery and Reinvestment Act (ARRA), which are discussed in chapter 9. However, those are only two of the laws with which the health information management (HIM) professional must be familiar.

In addition to federal and state laws, healthcare organizations may be subject to the standards of accrediting bodies such as the Joint Commission or the American Osteopathic Association (AOA), which also provide requirements related to the protection and the content of health records.

Sources of Laws

Law can be classified as public or private. **Public law** involves the government at any level and its relationship with individuals and organizations.

Its purpose is to define, regulate, and enforce rights where any part of a government agency is a party (Showalter 2012). The most familiar type of public law is criminal law, where the government is a party against an accused who has been charged with violating a criminal statute. In healthcare, the Medicare Conditions of Participation (COP)—the requirements set forth for healthcare providers who accept Medicare patients—are public law. Public law includes both criminal and civil actions.

Private law involves rights and duties among private entities or individuals. For example, private law applies when a contract for the purchase of a house is written between two parties. Normally, private law encompasses issues related to contracts, property, and **torts** (injuries). In the medical arena, it often applies when there is a breach of contract or when a tort occurs through malpractice. Private law includes civil actions.

There are four sources of public and private law: constitutions, statutes, administrative law, and judicial decisions, also known as common law or case law.

Constitutions

Constitutional law defines the amount and types of power and authority governments are given. The US Constitution defines and sets forth the powers of the three branches of the federal government. The legislative branch, which is the US Congress and is comprised of the House of Representatives and the Senate, creates statutory law (statutes). Examples include Medicare and HIPAA. The executive branch (the president and staff, namely cabinet-level agencies) enforces the law. For example, the Centers for Medicare and Medicaid Services (CMS), an agency within the cabinet-level Department of Health and Human Services (HHS), enforces the Medicare laws. The judicial branch (the court system) interprets laws passed by the legislative branch. This three-branch government structure is also found in state governments. Each state's constitution is the supreme law of that state, but it is subordinate to the US Constitution, the supreme law of the nation (Rinehart-Thompson et al. 2012).

Statutes

Statutes (which form statutory law) are enacted by legislative bodies. The US Congress and state legislatures are legislative bodies. Local bodies, such as municipalities, also can enact statutes, sometimes referred to as ordinances (Rinehart-Thompson et al. 2012).

Administrative Law

Administrative law is a type of public law. As previously noted, the executive branch of government is responsible for enforcing laws enacted by the legislative branch. Administrative agencies, which are part of the executive branch, develop and enforce rules and regulations that carry out the intent of statutes. For example, HHS developed rules and regulations to carry out the intent of the HIPAA statute, and it has the power to enforce them. These rules and regulations are administrative law. The federal Food and Drug Administration (FDA), another agency within HHS, has the power to develop rules that control the manufacture of drugs. The legislative branch of the federal government has given a number of administrative agencies the power to establish regulations (Rinehart-Thompson et al. 2012).

Judicial Decisions

The fourth major source of law is judicial law (that is, common law or case law), which is law created from court (judicial) decisions. Courts interpret statutes, regulations and constitutions, and resolve individual conflicts. Judicial decisions are the primary source of private law (Showalter 2012).

The traditional method of resolving legal disputes is through court systems. In the United States, one court system exists at the federal level. The 50 states, the US territories, and the District of Columbia have their own court systems. Although the court system is the most familiar method for resolving legal disputes, there is growing reliance on alternative dispute resolution to lighten court dockets and provide less costly and time-consuming alternatives for parties to settle their differences. Alternative dispute resolution includes arbitration (parties agree to submit a dispute to a third party to make a decision) and mediation (parties agree to submit a dispute to a third party facilitator, who assists the parties in reaching an agreed-upon resolution).

The US court system consists of state and federal courts. Both federal and state court systems have a three-tier structure: trial courts (called district courts in the federal system); courts of appeal (also called appellate courts) that hear appeals on final judgments of the trial courts; and supreme courts, the highest courts in a system that hear final appeals from intermediate courts of appeal. In many states, trial courts are divided into courts of limited jurisdiction and hear cases pertaining to a particular subject (for example, landlord and tenant or juvenile) or involve crimes of lesser severity or civil matters of lower dollar amounts. Courts of general jurisdiction hear more serious criminal cases or civil cases involving larger sums of money. Cases presented to courts of appeal or supreme courts are not trial reenactments. Legal documents are prepared by each party's attorney(s), who argue the merits of the case before a panel of appellate judges. Appeals are designed nearly exclusively to address legal errors or problems alleged to have occurred at the lower court, but they are not meant to address the facts of the case again.

In order to prepare for a judicial decision as the ultimate outcome of a legal proceeding (**litigation**), a **plaintiff** initiates a lawsuit against a **defendant** by filing a **complaint** in court, which outlines the defendant's alleged wrongdoing. After it is filed, a copy of the complaint is served to the defendant along with a **summons**. The summons and complaint give the defendant notice of the lawsuit and to what it pertains, and informs the defendant that the complaint must be answered or some other action taken. If the defendant fails to answer the complaint or take other action, the court grants the plaintiff a judgment by **default**.

Usually, the defendant answers the complaint in one of four ways: denying, admitting, or pleading ignorance to the allegations, or bringing a countersuit (**counterclaim**) against the plaintiff by filing a complaint. A defendant may file a complaint against a third party (**joinder**) or against another defendant (**cross-claim**). The defendant can ask the court to dismiss the plaintiff's complaint, but not without substantial reason.

The next stage of litigation is **discovery**, where parties use various strategies to obtain information about a case prior to trial and determine the strength of an opposing party's case. There are several types of discovery methods, but most likely to be encountered are the **deposition**, which obtains one's out-of-court testimony under oath; and an associated discovery tool, the **subpoena**, which compels a response in a legal proceeding. There are two types of subpoenas—the *subpoena ad testificandum* seeks one's testimony and the *subpoena duces tecum* seeks the documents one can bring with him or her.

After discovery is complete, the trial begins. A jury is selected through a process called **voir dire** or, if a jury is waived, a judge hears the case (**bench trial**). Evidence is then presented. The plaintiff's attorney is the first to call witnesses and present evidence. In turn, the defendant's attorney calls witnesses and presents evidence. Typically, in both health-related and non–health-related cases

that involve records as evidence, the record custodian is called as a witness by one party or the other to testify as to the authenticity of a record sought as evidence. Testifying as to a record's authenticity means the records custodian is verifying that it contains information about the individual in question, was compiled in the usual course of business, and is reliable and truthful as evidence. Because individuals who document in a health record do not typically falsify their entries, the truthfulness of a health record is generally not questioned. Parties to litigation often agree (stipulate) as to a record's authenticity and allow it to be entered into evidence without requiring the records custodian to appear in court and testify. The parties may also agree to allow a photocopy of the record or a printed version of the electronic health record (EHR) to be introduced into evidence rather than the original. This generally requires the records custodian to certify in writing that the copy is an exact duplicate of the original. State laws vary on the **admissibility**, or the court allowing consideration as evidence, of EHR printouts.

Many times, a case is settled before it reaches trial. This saves time, money, and emotional hardship on the parties. A settlement may be reached between or among parties and their attorneys with or without intervention from a third party.

After the court (either a jury or the judge) has rendered a verdict, the next stage in litigation is the appeal. If at least one of the parties disagrees with the verdict and has a legal argument on which to base its disagreement (for example, evidence was wrongfully considered at trial), a case may be appealed to the next court for review. The final stage of noncriminal litigation is collection of the judgment, which may be in equity (that is, the defendant is required to do or refrain from doing something) or monetary. Examples of judgments in equity include ordering the completion of a construction project (requiring the defendant to do something) or requiring that a construction project be stopped (requiring the defendant to refrain from doing something). Examples of collection of monetary judgments include single payments, garnishment of wages (by court order), seizure of property, or a lien on property. The final

Figure 8.1. Branches of the US government

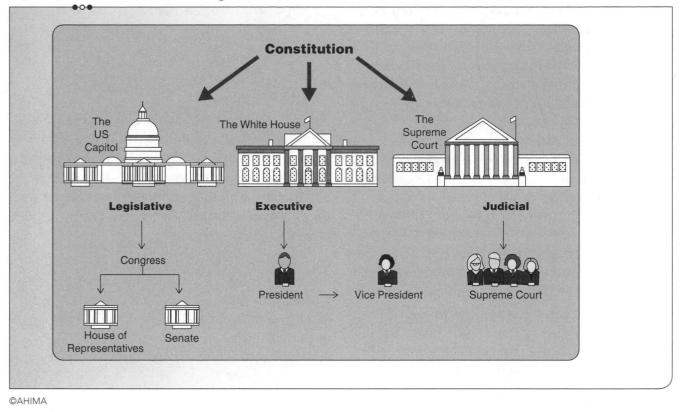

©AHIMA

stage of criminal proceedings is sentencing, which may include confinement and monetary penalties. Figure 8.1 provides a visual of the branches of the US government.

Professional Liability

Professionals in many fields, including healthcare, face potential liability for allegedly failing to meet the standards established in their fields of practice. **Medical malpractice** is the professional liability of healthcare providers—physicians, nurses, therapists, or others involved in the delivery of patient care. Breach of contract, intentional tort, and negligence are all **causes of action**, or theories under which lawsuits are brought that are related to professional liability. To understand how these causes of action apply, examine the elements of the physician–patient relationship.

A physician–patient relationship is established by either an **implied contract** or an **express contract**. Implied contracts are created by the parties' behaviors (for example, a patient's arrival at a physician's office). Express contracts are articulated, either in writing or verbally (a patient's written or verbal agreement to treatment). A contract is usually created by the mutual agreement of the parties involved—in this case, the patient and the physician or other healthcare provider. Termination of the contract usually occurs when the patient either gets well or dies, the patient and physician mutually agree to contract termination, the patient dismisses the physician, or the physician withdraws from providing care for the patient.

No medical liability for breach of contract can exist without a physician–patient relationship. However, when this relationship does exist, the physician's failure to diagnose and treat the patient with reasonable skill and care may cause the patient to sue the physician for **breach of contract**.

Healthcare providers also can be held responsible for professional tort liability when they harm another person. A tort is a wrongful act that results in injury to another. Tort law is broad and include non–healthcare-related acts (for example, a driver runs a red light and strikes another vehicle) or healthcare-related acts (a nurse administers the wrong medication). An intentional tort is where an individual purposely commits a wrongful act that results in injury. Usually, however, professional liability actions are brought against healthcare providers because of the tort of negligence, or unintentional wrongdoing.

Negligence occurs when a healthcare provider does not do what a prudent person would normally do in similar circumstances. There are three types of negligence:

- Nonfeasance: failure to act, such as not ordering a standard diagnostic test
- Malfeasance: a wrong or improper act, such as removal of the wrong body part
- Misfeasance: improper performance during an otherwise correct act, such as nicking the bladder during an otherwise appropriately performed gallbladder surgery

For a negligence lawsuit to be successful, the plaintiff must prove four elements:

1. The existence of a duty to meet a standard of care (degree of caution expected of an ordinary and reasonable person under given circumstances)
2. Breach or deviation from that duty
3. Causation, the relationship between the defendant's conduct and the harm that was suffered
4. Injury (harm), which may be economic (medical expenses and loss of wages) or non-economic (pain and suffering)

The causes of actions mentioned are not the only ones that can be brought against an individual healthcare provider or a healthcare organization. Other tort actions applicable to healthcare include battery, assault, false imprisonment, infliction of emotional distress, defamation, invasion of privacy, and wrongful disclosure of confidential information.

Patient Rights Regarding Healthcare Decisions

It is an established right in the United States that individuals generally have the right of autonomy over their own bodies. Included in this right is the right of individuals to make their own healthcare decisions provided that they are not legally incompetent (namely, incompetent by virtue of a mental disability or status as a minor). Consents play an important role in documenting individuals' wishes regarding the healthcare they will receive. Similarly, advance directives are important in documenting individuals' end-of-life decisions.

Consent is one's agreement to receive medical treatment. It can be written (preferable because it offers greater proof) or spoken; further, it can be express (communicated through words) or implied (communicated through conduct or a mechanism other than words, such as an unconscious person who is brought to the emergency

room). As a matter of practice, healthcare organizations obtain a general consent from a patient for routine treatment and failure to do so can result in a legal action; generally for battery, or harmful or offensive contact. When a treatment or procedure becomes progressively more risky or invasive, it is important that informed consent be completed to ensure the patient has a basic understanding of diagnosis and the nature of the treatment or procedure, along with the risks, benefits, alternatives (including opting out of treatment), and individuals who will perform the treatment or procedure. Informed consent is a process and it is the responsibility of the provider who will be rendering the treatment or performing the procedure to obtain the patient's informed consent and answer the patient's questions. Failure to obtain informed consent can result in legal action generally based on negligence (Klaver 2012).

Advance Directives

An advance directive is a special type of consent that communicates an individual's wishes to be treated—or not—should the individual become unable to communicate on his or her own behalf. Once created, it is important that advance directives become a part of an individual's health record.

By creating a **durable power of attorney for healthcare decisions (DPOA-HCD)** an individual, while still competent, designates another person (proxy) to make healthcare decisions consistent with the individual's wishes on his or her behalf. "Durable" means that the document is in effect when the individual is no longer competent.

A **living will** is executed by a competent adult, expressing the individual's wishes regarding treatment should the individual become afflicted with certain conditions (for example, a persistent vegetative state or a terminal condition) and no longer be able to communicate on his or her own behalf. Living wills often address extraordinary life-saving measures such as ventilator support and either the continuation or removal or nutrition and hydration.

A third type of document that always specifies an individual's wish *not* to receive treatment (specifically, cardiopulmonary resuscitation (CPR) is the **do-not-resuscitate (DNR) order**. Most often used by individuals who are elderly or in chronically ill health, it directs healthcare providers to refrain from performing the otherwise standing order of CPR should the individual experience cardiac or respiratory arrest. Prior to executing a DNR, the patient and physician should have a discussion, a consent form should be signed by the patient, and the physician writes an order in the patient's health record. State law provides the framework for completing DNR orders and forms. Joint Commission-accredited organizations are required to implement policies regarding advance directives and DNR orders (Klaver 2012).

The lack of advance directives can result in legal battles regarding the undocumented wishes of individuals who become legally incompetent. Highly publicized end-of-life cases include those of Karen Ann Quinlan, Nancy Cruzan, and Terri Schiavo (Klaver 2012). These cases had significant legal and ethical implications on how healthcare providers handle right-to-die situations.

Check Your Understanding 8.1

Instructions: **Answer the following questions.**

1. Law can be classified as which of the following?
   A. Public or private
   B. Public or criminal
   C. Criminal or medical malpractice
   D. Trial or appeal

2. Private law:
   A. Defines, regulates, and enforces rights where any government agency is a party
   B. Involves rights and duties among private parties
   C. Creates statutes
   D. Convicts individuals charged with crimes

3. Which of the following is a source of law?
   A. Standard
   B. Statute
   C. Accrediting body
   D. Guideline

4. Statutes are laws:
   A. Created by an administrative body
   B. Created between private parties
   C. Created by trial and appellate courts
   D. Created by legislative bodies

5. Administrative law is a type of which of the following?
   A. Criminal law
   B. Private law
   C. Public law
   D. Statutory law

6. Arbitration is the submission of a dispute to a:
   A. Mediator
   B. Third party
   C. Judge, without a jury
   D. Judge, with a jury

7. Medical malpractice:
   A. Refers to the professional liability of healthcare providers
   B. Is related to breach of contract actions only
   C. Excludes intentional torts
   D. Is synonymous with negligence

8. Mrs. Elfman has filed a medical malpractice lawsuit against Dr. Quinn. She accomplishes this by which of the following?
   A. Counterclaim
   B. Voir dire
   C. Cross-claim
   D. Complaint

9. If a defendant fails to answer a complaint or take other action, the courts grants the plaintiff a judgment by:
   A. Joinder
   B. Deposition
   C. Default
   D. Oral testimony

10. A tort is:
   A. A wrongful act that results in injury to another
   B. A purposeful wrongful act against another
   C. Mutual consent between two parties
   D. The professional liability of healthcare providers

11. Which of the following is an element of negligence?
   A. Consent
   B. Duty
   C. Summons
   D. Joinder

12. Which of the following is an element of consent?
   A. It is one's agreement to receive medical treatment
   B. It must only be obtained for invasive procedures
   C. It must be in writing to be legally valid
   D. It is an element of negligence

13. Which of the following is an advance directive?
    A. Tort
    B. Jurisdiction
    C. District court
    D. Living will

14. A physician–patient relationship:
    A. Is established by contract
    B. Is established by written agreement
    C. Is permanent
    D. Cannot be subject to a breach of contract legal action

15. A lawsuit by a defendant against a plaintiff is a:
    A. Cross-claim
    B. Joinder
    C. Summons
    D. Counterclaim

Overview of Legal Issues in Health Information Management

For the HIM professional, legal aspects of health records and health information include these topics addressed in the following sections:

- Compilation, maintenance, and retention of health records
- Ownership and control of health records, including use and disclosure
- Defining the legal health record

Additionally, the HIM professional may be involved in the medical staff credentialing process as well as organizational licensure, certification, and accreditation.

Compilation and Maintenance of Health Records

Requirements for compiling and maintaining health records are usually found in state rules and regulations. Typically developed by state administrative agencies responsible for licensing healthcare organizations, many often specify only that health records be complete and accurate.

However, others specify categories of information to be kept or outline the detailed contents of the health record.

In some circumstances, the federal government stipulates specific requirements for maintaining health records. For example, the Medicare Conditions of Participation contain specific requirements that must be satisfied by healthcare organizations that treat Medicare or Medicaid patients.

In addition to state and federal requirements, accrediting bodies have established standards for maintaining health records. Specifically, the Joint Commission's standards relate to information management through its Information Management (IM) and Record of Care, Treatment, and Services (RC) chapters. Acute care, long-term care, home health, and behavioral health providers, among others, must follow these standards if they are to be accredited by the Joint Commission. In addition to regulatory and accrediting bodies, professional organizations such as the American Health Information Management Association (AHIMA) publish best practice information.

Finally, third-party payers play an important role in the maintenance and content of health records. Payers often have specific requirements about content that must be present in the health record in order for reimbursement to occur. Failure to comply with requirements by external entities will likely result in some type of penalty such as loss of licensure or accreditation, nonpayment of claims, or fines. Thus, health information must be compiled and maintained appropriately and in compliance with all applicable requirements.

In addition to legal, accreditor, and payer requirements, best practice dictates that health record entries and health records in their entirety be complete, accurate, and timely. These characteristics contribute to high-quality patient care and contribute toward a legally defensible health record that can protect a healthcare organization in malpractice litigation. Because health records are frequently admitted into evidence in medical malpractice suits, the absence of complete, accurate, and timely documentation can result in a verdict against the healthcare organization.

Taking all of these factors into consideration, healthcare organizations establish their own requirements to ensure the uniformity of health record format and content. The healthcare organization does this in the form of organizational policies and procedures as well as medical staff rules and regulations. Each of the influential factors listed should be incorporated into policies and procedures, as well as professional practice standards such as those established by AHIMA.

In general, health record form and content should conform to the following guidelines.

- The health record should be organized systematically to facilitate the retrieval and compilation of data.
- The health record should only be documented by persons authorized by the hospital's policies and medical staff rules and regulations.
- Hospital policy and medical staff rules and regulations should specify who may receive and transcribe a physician's verbal orders.

- Health record entries should be documented at the time the treatment they describe is rendered.
- The authors of all entries should be clearly identifiable.
- Abbreviations and symbols should be used in the health record only when approved according to hospital and medical staff bylaws, and per regulation. The Joint Commission maintains a list of prohibited abbreviations that must be taken into consideration when the organization's approved list is created and updated. For example, "u" cannot be used to designate "unit" because it can be mistaken for a zero, four, or cc.
- All entries in the health record should be permanent.
- To correct errors or make changes in the paper health record, a single line should be drawn in ink through the incorrect entry. The word error should be printed at the top of the entry along with a legal signature or initials; date; time; and discipline of the person making the change. The existing entry should be left intact and corrections should be entered in chronological order. Late entries should be labeled as such. Error correction in EHR is particularly important because courts have historically viewed their integrity as suspect. Thus, procedures must be developed to control, check, and track changes made to data housed in the EHR. In particular, changes must be transparent so a court is satisfied that they cannot be done surreptitiously and without traceable evidence of the change.
- If a patient wishes to change information in his or her health record, the change should not be made to the original entry but, rather, should be made as an addendum (also known as an amendment). The information should be clearly identified as an additional document appended to the original health record at the request of the patient. The HIPAA Privacy Rule allows an individual to request an amendment to his or her health

record, although the provider may deny this request. HIPAA amendment requests are discussed in greater detail in chapter 9 (Odom-Wesley and Brown 2009).

Ownership and Control of Health Records, Including Use and Disclosure

HIM professionals must understand the concepts of health record ownership and control. The health record and its contents are owned by the organization that created and maintains it. As the legal custodian, the organization is responsible to ensure it maintains its integrity and the health record is kept secure. This is true regardless of whether the health record is paper or electronic. Although patients often believe they own their health record and do, in fact, own the information in it, ultimate responsibility for the physical health record still rests with the organization.

Control of the health record encompasses its *use* (how health information is used internally) and *disclosure* (how health information is disseminated externally). Although health records and other documents (for example, radiologic images) that relate to the delivery of patient care are owned by the healthcare organization, patients, and other legitimately interested third parties have the right to access them. Associated with control is the issue of patient access to one's own health records. HIPAA grants individuals the right to access their protected health information, with some exceptions that will be discussed in more detail in chapter 9. As patient portals become more available and encouraged by providers, this right is transforming into a patient expectation as well.

State Laws Involving Use and Disclosure

Most states have laws that protect patient confidentiality (Brodnik and Sharp 2012). Known as privileged communication statutes (for example, to protect information shared by a patient with his physician during an office visit), they generally prohibit medical practitioners from disclosing information arising from the parties' professional relationship and relating to the patient's care and treatment (Showalter 2012). If patients waive their privilege, the medical provider is not prohibited from making disclosures.

State law may specifically provide a patient with the right to access his or her health information. Even without state law, however, the federal HIPAA Privacy Rule grants an individual the right to access his or her health information for as long as it is maintained, with limited situations where access may be denied. It also establishes standards by which others may access an individual's health information.

Disclosure of health information without patient authorization may be required under specific state statutes. Examples include reporting vital statistics (for example, births and deaths) and other public health, safety, or welfare situations. For example, healthcare providers may be required to provide information to the appropriate state agency about patients who suffer from venereal and other communicable diseases, have been injured by knives or firearms, or have wounds that suggest some type of violent criminal activity. The treatment of suspected victims of child abuse or neglect also must be reported. Because requirements vary by state, HIM professionals must know the reporting requirements for the states in which they practice. Health information has a variety of purposes—from the provision of direct patient care to use by outside entities such as insurance and pharmaceutical companies—and those uses and disclosures must be appropriate. Compliance with legal requirements for appropriate use and disclosure must be ensured, as must adherence to the profession's ethical principles of practice.

Use of Health Records and Health Information in Judicial Proceedings

The health record of an individual who is a party to a legal proceeding is usually admissible in litigation or judicial proceedings provided it is material or relevant to the issue (Showalter 2012). Either a court order or subpoena is used to obtain health information for a court that has jurisdiction (legal authority to make decisions) over the pending litigation. These are discussed in more detail in chapter 9.

Responses to court orders and subpoenas depend on state regulations. In some instances, states allow copies of health records to be certified and mailed to the clerk of the court or other designated individuals. In other instances, however, original health records must be produced in person and the records custodian is required to authenticate them. **Authentication** affirms a record's legitimacy through testimony or written validation.

Legal Health Record

The **legal health record** is the record used for legal purposes, and is the "record released upon a valid request" (Rinehart-Thompson et al. 2012). It can be stored on any medium (paper, electronic, microfilm, or a hybrid combination). Its content is defined by the organization rather than by law.

Importance of Legal Health Record

The legal health record distinction is important for several reasons. First, it is important to an organization's business and legal processes (Rinehart-Thompson et al. 2012). Second, because the legal health record is the record that is produced upon request, including legal requests, it becomes important to ensure that the legal health record is legally sound and defensible as a valid document in legal situations (Rinehart-Thompson et al. 2012).

It is also important to differentiate the legal health record from other types of records that are integral to health information. These include the designated record set, the EHR, and the personal health record. The **designated record set (DRS)**, which is a term specific to HIPAA and described further in chapter 9, also includes other records (for example, billing records) and, as such, is more expansive than the legal health record. The EHR is also more expansive because it contains components (like metadata) that are not ordinarily included in legal health record content. **Metadata** are data about data and include information that track actions such as when and by whom a document was accessed or changed. The **personal health record (PHR)** is owned and managed by the individual who is the subject of the record. As such, it is not the legal business record of the organization. For more information on the PHR, refer to chapter 3.

Content of Legal Health Record

Determining the content of the legal health record can be challenging because of the myriad of documents that exist, the presence of documentation in multiple locations, and—for the EHR—the existence of documentation that does not exist with paper health records. Organizations should develop and maintain an inventory of all documents and data that could comprise the legal health record, considering all locations in the organization (for example, separate departments or servers) where such information could be housed. Electronic document considerations include e-mails, electronic fetal monitoring strips, diagnostic images, digital photography, and video (AHIMA 2011a). Organizations should also carefully consider whether to include data such as pop-up reminders, alerts, and metadata. Metadata are data about data and include information that track actions such as when and by whom a document was accessed or changed.

Retention of the Health Record

The HIM professional must consider multiple factors when developing health record retention policies that determine how long health records are to be kept. These factors include applicable federal and state statutes and regulations; accreditation standards; operational needs of the organization; and the type of organization.

Some state laws designate how long health records must be retained in their original form and specify whether they can be stored on other media, such as digitally or on microfilm. Additionally, state and local laws that require information to be maintained for reporting to public authorities (for example, vital statistics and public health data) must be adhered to.

The health record must be available as evidence in legal actions, as governed by statutes and regulations. Health records should be retained for at least the period specified by the state's **statute of limitations**, which is the period of time in which a lawsuit (such as medical malpractice) must be filed. In particular, the health record of a minor should be retained until the patient reaches the age of majority (as defined by state law) plus the period of statute of limitations, unless otherwise provided by state law. A longer retention period is prudent because the statute may not begin to run until a potential plaintiff learns of the causal relationship between an injury and the care received. Other claims must also be taken into consideration when determining how long to retain health records as evidence. For example, under the **False Claims Act**, claims of fraud may be brought for up to 10 years after the incident (31 USC 3729). Payer requirements must also be considered; for example, the Medicare Conditions of Participation, which is federal regulation, require five-year retention for hospital records.

The standards of accreditation bodies such as the Joint Commission and the AOA must be followed in developing a health record retention policy. In particular, the Joint Commission defers to state law (for example, it specifies that verbal orders must be authenticated within a time frame specified by law).

Health record retention also depends on how the healthcare organization uses the information contained in the record. For example, an acute-care facility may have very different retention policies than a long-term care facility providing geriatric nursing care. Further, an organization providing care exclusively to children may have different retention policies than a home health agency. Healthcare organizations with significant educational and research operations may need to retain health records for longer periods than other healthcare organizations.

Governing boards and medical staffs of every healthcare organization must analyze the organization's medical and administrative needs to ensure health records are available for peer review, quality assessment, and other activities. These needs must be considered in conjunction with legal and accreditation requirements. In many instances, healthcare organizations retain health records longer than the law requires.

AHIMA Retention Recommendations

AHIMA routinely publishes recommendations for the retention of health records (AHIMA 2013). HIM professionals should use these to determine how their organizations compare with industry-wide best practices. AHIMA recommends, at a minimum, that health record retention schedules:

- Are designed to meet an organization's needs so that health information is available for not only patient care, but also for research, education, and to meet the legal requirements that apply to the organization

- Should be specific about the retention of information, including a description of what information is to be kept, for how long it is to be kept, and the medium on which it will stored (that is, paper, microfilm, optical disk, magnetic tape)

- Clearly specify in its policies and procedures the destruction method that is to be used for each medium on which health information is housed (AHIMA 2013).

Further, table 8.1 shows AHIMA's retention recommendations for various types of health information.

Table 8.1   AHIMA retention standards

Health information	Recommended retention period
Diagnostic images (such as x-ray film) (adults)	5 years
Diagnostic images (such as x-ray film) (minors)	5 years after the age of majority
Disease index	10 years
Fetal heart monitor records	10 years after the age of majority
Master patient/person index	Permanently
Operative index	10 years
Patient health records (adults)	10 years after the most recent encounter
Patient health records (minors)	Age of majority plus statute of limitations
Physician index	10 years
Register of births	Permanently
Register of deaths	Permanently
Register of surgical procedures	Permanently

Source: AHIMA 2011b.

Destruction

Not all information must be kept forever. Just as the HIM professional must consider multiple factors when determining retention, many factors must also be taken into consideration with regard to health record destruction. These include applicable federal and state statutes and regulations; accreditation standards; pending or ongoing litigation; storage capabilities; and cost.

Any health record involved in investigations, audits, or litigation should not be destroyed, even if the record retention schedule would provide for destruction otherwise. Destruction procedures must ensure that health information is not inappropriately disclosed in the process. For paper health records, common destruction methods include shredding, burning, pulping or pulverizing (Rinehart-Thompson et al. 2012). For electronic health records, care should be taken to actually destroy them rather than merely deleting the pathway to access them. Destruction methods for electronic health records include overwriting; magnetic degaussing or demagnetizing (neutralizing the magnetic field to erase data); and physical destruction of the medium on which the health record resides, including pulverizing (laser discs) and shredding or cutting (DVDs) (AHIMA 2013). With electronic health records in particular, there is the risk of duplicate records remaining in circulation (Rinehart-Thompson et al. 2012).

Health record destruction may be accomplished by the organization that owns the records, or the process may be outsourced. In either case, a list of all destroyed health records and the manner of destruction must be documented. A certificate of destruction and an agreement that assures the protection of the information should both be obtained (AHIMA 2013; Rinehart-Thompson et al. 2012).

Medical Staff Appointments and Privileges

Another area with significant legal implications that the HIM professional may become involved in is medical staff appointments, also referred to as credentialing. A basic understanding of the legal issues and some of the functions in the credentialing process is important.

The healthcare facility is ultimately responsible for the quality of care it provides. This includes the quality of the medical staff—the physicians who have been given permission to provide a healthcare facility's clinical services. A healthcare facility's governing board (board of directors) is accountable to establish policies and procedures that ensure reasonable care in the appointment of medical practitioners to the facility's medical staff and the granting of clinical privileges. Clinical privileges are the defined set of services a physician is permitted to perform in that facility such as admitting patients, performing surgeries, or delivering infants.

Credentialing includes both the initial appointment and reappointment of individuals to the medical staff and determination of the extent of their privileges. The customary process by which an application for medical staff appointment and privileges is reviewed involves several levels. These include the appropriate clinical departments, credentials committee, medical staff executive committee, and board of directors. Although the board of directors relies on the advice and recommendations of the medical staff, ultimate responsibility for making appointments and reappointments and for ensuring the medical staff members are qualified to perform the functions for which they have been granted privileges rests with the board (Pozgar 2016).

An important part of the credentialing process is querying the National Practitioner Data Bank (NPDB), which was established by the federal Health Care Quality Improvement Act of 1986. One goal of the NPDB is to limit the movement of physicians throughout the United States where their negative histories such as medical malpractice lawsuits and loss of privileges at other healthcare facilities may go undetected. NPDB regulations include requirements for reporting information to the NPDB and querying information from the NPDB prior to granting medical staff privileges (Pozgar 2016). Penalties and liability can result from failure to use the NPDB.

The HIM professional may serve as the medical staff coordinator, involving the collection, organization, verification, and storage of all information associated with credentialing. This includes information about the individual staff member's professional background, credentials, previous professional experience, and quality profiles. All this information, including that obtained from the NPDB, is confidential. Therefore, policies and procedures must be in place to specify who may have access to what information and under what circumstances.

Licensure

Licensure is a designation given to an individual or an organization by a governmental agency or board that gives the individual permission to practice, or the organization to operate, within a certain field of practice. For example, physicians, nurses, and physical therapists must be licensed to practice. In many states, hospitals must be licensed in order to treat patients. Where licensure exists for a practice area, it is mandatory. Once an individual or organization becomes licensed, it is subject to further regulation by the governmental body to ensure that it is maintaining at least a minimal level of competence. For individuals, further regulation may include required continuing education. The legal significance of licensure in healthcare is that a government entity has deemed the individual or organization qualified to provide competent and safe patient care. HIM professionals are not licensed, but can be certified. However, they may serve a role in taking part in or coordinating licensure maintenance for their organizations. They may also assume the role of ensuring that licensure records of individual practitioners are updated and maintained by the organization in which they work.

Certification

Certification of individuals is a designation given by a private organization to acknowledge a requisite level of knowledge, competencies, and skills. Whether or not certification is required for an individual to practice (as is licensure) is an employer decision. Certification may either be entry level or mastery level. In the HIM profession, RHIA (Registered Health Information Administrator) and RHIT (Registered Health Information Technician) credentials signify entry-level generalist competency. AHIMA also offers mastery-level specialty certifications such as the CHPS (Certified in Healthcare Privacy and Security), CCS (Certified Coding Specialist), and CHDA (Certified Health Data Analyst). For information on these credentials, refer to chapter 1. In healthcare organizations, certification is a designation by the US Department of Health and Human Services that its Conditions of Participation have been met. Although certification is not required for a healthcare organization to operate, it is required for the organization to participate in (and thus reimbursed by) the Medicare and Medicaid programs.

Accreditation

The HIM professional will likely find herself or himself in a role that involves compliance with accreditation standards. This role may involve compliance with standards that relate to health information or coordinating an organization's overall compliance with the standards of the body by which they are accredited. Accreditation is a designation given to a healthcare facility by an accrediting organization, demonstrating that the healthcare facility has met the accrediting body's requirements for excellence. Accreditation is generally viewed as the highest level of competence or validation. In acute care, Joint Commission is the most prevalent accrediting body. Other accreditors include the AOA and the American Association for Ambulatory Health Care (AAAHC). A prevalent accreditor in rehabilitation is the Commission on Accreditation of Rehabilitation Facilities (CARF). By successfully completing the Joint Commission deemed status survey, an organization that is accredited by the Joint Commission is also deemed to have met the Medicare and Medicaid requirements. Via successful completion of the Joint Commission's accreditation survey, the organization is concurrently certified by Medicare and Medicaid.

✓ Check Your Understanding 8.2

Instructions: **Answer the following questions.**

1. The principal purpose of the health record is to:
   A. Serve as evidence in litigation
   B. Support statistical analysis and research
   C. Document patient treatment and allow providers to communicate
   D. Provide a record for reimbursement purposes

2. A health record is owned by which of the following?
   A. Patient who is the subject of the record
   B. Healthcare organization that created and maintains it
   C. Staff members who document in it
   D. Insurance company that pays for the patient's care

3. A court's legal authority to make decisions is called:
   A. Joinder
   B. Judicial law
   C. Jurisdiction
   D. Litigation

4. Which of the following actions by a health records custodian affirms the legitimacy of a health record?
   A. Testimony
   B. Authentication
   C. Jurisdiction
   D. Certification

5. Which of the following is a characteristic of the legal health record?
   A. It must be electronic
   B. It includes the designated record set
   C. It is the record disclosed upon request
   D. It includes a patient's personal health record

6. Which of the following determines health record content?
   A. Constitutional amendments
   B. Nursing licensure laws
   C. Accrediting body standards
   D. Record retention policies

7. AHIMA recommends that the operative index be retained for how long?
   A. 5 years
   B. 7 years
   C. 10 years
   D. Permanently

8. Which of the following is true about health information retention?
   A. Retention depends only on accreditation requirements.
   B. Retention periods differ among healthcare facilities.
   C. The operational needs of a healthcare facility cannot be considered.
   D. Retention periods are frequently shorter for health information about minors.

9. Which of the following is true regarding the development of health record destruction policies?
   A. All applicable laws must be considered.
   B. The organization must find a way not to destroy any health records.
   C. Health records involved in pending or ongoing litigation may be destroyed.
   D. Only state laws must be considered.

10. Which of the following is a characteristic of credentialing?
    A. It is ultimately the responsibility of the medical staff
    B. It is the hiring of qualified nurses in a hospital
    C. It applies to the granting of specific clinical privileges to medical staff members
    D. It grants one level of privileges to all medical staff members

11. Medical staff credentialing refers to which of the following?
    A. Rewarding physicians who have treated the most patients
    B. Appointing and granting clinical privileges to physicians
    C. Renewing physicians' medical licenses
    D. Establishing physicians' medical malpractice premiums

12. Erin is an HIM professional. She is teaching a class to clinicians about proper documentation in the health record. Which of the following is an example of improper teaching?
    A. Obliterate errors
    B. Leave existing entries intact
    C. Label late entries as being late
    D. Ensure the legal signature of an individual making a correction accompanies the correction

13. Which of the following gives an individual permission to practice or an organization to operate within a certain field of practice?
    A. Licensure
    B. Certification
    C. Accreditation
    D. Medicare Conditions of Participation

14. Which of the following describes the National Practitioner Data Bank?
    A. It allows an organization to be reimbursed by Medicare and Medicaid.
    B. It is a type of certification for healthcare providers.
    C. It limits movement of physicians with negative histories.
    D. It was repealed by Congress.

15. Certification is:
    A. granted only to individuals
    B. granted only to organizations
    C. synonymous with accreditation
    D. granted to both individuals and organizations

Real-World Case 8.1

Although medical malpractice is usually associated with physician liability, it actually applies to the professional liability of healthcare providers generally, including not only physicians but also nurses, therapists, and others involved in the delivery of patient care. For example, a patient filed a lawsuit against a physical therapist, alleging that he refused to stop treatment when she requested it. The patient alleged that the treatment caused physical injuries that were serious and permanent, and she also suffered mental injuries. The therapist had a very positive reputation, but co-workers testified as to his aggressiveness. The parties settled out of court for $400,000 with an additional $38,000 in legal expenses. It was estimated that a jury would have likely awarded the patient $800,000 had the case gone to trial (Healthcare Providers Service Organization 2006).

Real-World Case 8.2

Healthcare organizations develop record retention guidelines in accordance with applicable laws (for example, a state's statute of limitations for medical malpractice and Medicare Conditions of Participation retention requirements) and operational needs (for example, research, education, and strategic planning). As long as an organization follows its guidelines, and those guidelines conform to applicable laws, the organization is legally compliant. Further, there is no requirement that patients be notified of an organization's record retention periods. This, however, is not the case in California. California Senate Bill 1415 (2008) requires:

...physicians, podiatrists, dentists, optometrists, and chiropractors...who create patient records, at the time the initial patient record is created, to provide a statement to be signed by the patient, or the patient's representative, that sets forth...the intented retention period for the records, as specified in applicable law, or by the health care provider's retention policy." Further, the bill "requires a health care provider, if he or she plans to destroy patient records earlier than the period specified in the signed statement, to notify the patient.

In comments accompanying the bill, it was stressed that it is important for patients to be able to access their health records so that they can follow the patient's lifespan.

References

American Health Information Management Association. 2013. Retention and Destruction of Health Information (updated October 2013). http://library.ahima.org/doc?oid=107114.

American Health Information Management Association. 2011a. Fundamentals of the legal health record and designated record set. *Journal of AHIMA*. 82(2):expanded online version. http://library.ahima.org/doc?oid=104008#.Vw_Ty_krLDc.

American Health Information Management Association. 2011b. Retention and Destruction of Health Information. Appendix C: AHIMA's Recommended Retention Standards (updated August 2011). http://library.ahima.org/doc?oid=107114.

Brodnik, M.S. and M. Sharp. 2012. Access, Use, and Disclosure/Release of Health Information. Chapter 12 in *Fundamentals of Law for Health Informatics and Information Management*. Edited by M.S. Brodnik, L.A. Rinehart-Thompson, and R.B. Reynolds. Chicago: AHIMA.

California Senate Bill 1415 (2008). Patient Records: Maintenance and Storage. http://www.leginfo.ca.gov.

Healthcare Providers Service Organization. 2006. CNA HealthPro Physical Therapy Claims Study. http://www.hpso.com/ptclaimstudy.

Klaver, J.C. 2012. Evidence. Chapter 4 in *Fundamentals of Law for Health Informatics and Information Management*. Edited by M.S. Brodnik, L.A. Rinehart-Thompson, and R.B. Reynolds. Chicago: AHIMA.

Odom-Wesley, B. and D. Brown. 2009. *Documentation for Medical Records*. Chicago: AHIMA.

Pozgar, G.D. 2016. *Legal Aspects of Health Care Administration*. Sudbury, MA: Jones and Bartlett.

Rinehart-Thompson, L.A., R.B. Reynolds, and K. Olenik. 2012. The Legal Health Record: Maintenance, Content, Documentation, and Disposition. Chapter 8 in *Fundamentals of Law for Health Informatics and Information Management*. Edited by M.S. Brodnik, L.A. Rinehart-Thompson, and R.B. Reynolds. Chicago: AHIMA.

Showalter, J.S. 2012. *The Law of Healthcare Administration*. Chicago: Health Administration Press.

31 USC 3729: False Claims Act. 1986.

9

Data Privacy and Confidentiality

Laurie A. Rinehart-Thompson, JD, RHIA, CHP, FAHIMA

Learning Objectives

- Identify methods and tools used in the legal discovery process
- Identify discovery challenges associated with electronic information (e-discovery)
- Apply the HIPAA Privacy Rule, including American Recovery and Reinvestment Act (ARRA) requirements such as breach notification, with regard to health information use and disclosure

- Protect health information through use and disclosure policies and procedures that apply to both state law and HIPAA regulations
- Apply authorization requirements to the valid release of information
- Identify types of medical identity theft and actions required by the Red Flags Rule

Key Terms

Access report
Administrative simplification
Admissibility
American Recovery and Reinvestment Act (ARRA)
Authorization
Breach
Breach notification
Business associate (BA)
Business associate agreement (BAA)
Business records exception
Clinical Laboratory Improvement Amendments (CLIA) of 1988
Complaint

Confidentiality
Consent
Court order
Covered entity (CE)
Deidentified information
Department of Health and Human Services (HHS)
Deposition
Designated record set (DRS)
Disclosure
Discovery
E-discovery
Facility directory
Fair and Accurate Credit Transactions Act

Federal Rules of Civil Procedure (FRCP)
Federal Rules of Evidence (FRE)
Federal Trade Commission (FTC)
Fundraising
Health Information Technology for Economic and Clinical Health Act (HITECH)
Health Insurance Portability and Accountability Act (HIPAA)
Hearsay
Individual
Individually identifiable health information
Interrogatories

Legal hold
Marketing
Medical identity theft
Metadata
Minimum necessary standard
Notice of privacy practices
Office of the National Coordinator
    for Health Information
    Technology (ONC)
Personal representative
Preemption
Privacy

Privacy officer
Privacy Rule
Protected health information
    (PHI)
Red Flags Rule
Release of information (ROI)
Right of access
Right to request accounting of
    disclosures
Right to request amendment
Right to request confidential
    communications

Right to request restrictions
    of PHI
Sale of information
Spoliation
Subpoena
Subpoena ad testificandum
Subpoena duces tecum
Treatment, payment,
    and operations (TPO)
Use
Warrant
Workforce

The health record is used for many purposes but it is not a public document. The patient has the right to his or her privacy. **Privacy** is a social value and is the right "to be let alone" (Rinehart-Thompson and Harman 2017). The US Constitution does not grant a right of privacy, but courts have interpreted it to give privacy rights in certain areas such as religion and child-rearing. There is no constitutional right of privacy to one's health information, but this privacy protection has also been established through court cases as well as laws such as the **Health Insurance Portability and Accountability Act (HIPAA)**, discussed in great detail in this chapter.

Confidentiality is similar to privacy, but it stems from the sharing of private thoughts in confidence with someone else. Legally, such sharing is protected when the communication is between parties such as physician and patient, attorney and client, or clergy and parishioner. Laws define those communications that are protected (Brodnik 2012).

Use and Disclosure

Use is how an organization avails itself of health information internally. **Disclosure** is how health information is disseminated outside an organization. Use and disclosure are usually associated with the concepts of ownership and control of the health record because the organization that owns and controls the health record is also able to control the use and disclosure of its contents. Compliance with all applicable privacy and confidentiality laws and standards is important to avoid inappropriate use and disclosure of health information. Disclosure becomes very important when a healthcare organization is involved in litigation and health information becomes key evidence necessary for fact-finding during the discovery process and at trial.

Discovery

Discovery—which is both a process and a period of time—is a pretrial stage where parties to a lawsuit use numerous strategies to discover or obtain information that other parties hold. The purpose of discovery is to learn of each party's relative weaknesses and strengths in a case to avoid a surprise at trial and perhaps encourage pretrial settlement (Rinehart-Thompson 2012). There are several methods by which information can be discovered prior to trial. Additionally, there are tools used to facilitate discovery.

Deposition

A **deposition** is an important discovery method. It is a formal proceeding where the oral testimonies of parties to a lawsuit (plaintiff and defendant) and other relevant witnesses are obtained (Rinehart-Thompson 2012). Attendance is compelled via a **subpoena**, a legal document that instructs a person or entity to do something. The subpoena is issued for an individual to appear at an appointed time and place to testify under oath before a reporter who transcribes the testimony (that is, what the person is testifying about). Usually, the attorneys for both plaintiff and defendant are present. Health information management (HIM) professionals can be subpoenaed to testify as to the authenticity of the health records by confirming the records were compiled in the usual course of business and have not been altered in any way.

Interrogatories

Interrogatories are a discovery method used to obtain information from other parties in a lawsuit. Through interrogatories, parties are given questions to respond to in writing. Interrogatories may be answered by a party's legal counsel rather than by the party himself, but they require a confirmation regarding the truthfulness and accuracy of the answers (Rinehart-Thompson 2012).

Subpoena

One of the most important discovery tools is the subpoena. It is not a method of discovery that actually elicits information (such as depositions and interrogatories), but it facilitates discovery by compelling individuals to appear at certain times and places or to produce requested documents. A subpoena is initiated on behalf of one of the parties in the case, although it is issued through the court. There are two types of subpoenas. A subpoena that seeks testimony is a **subpoena ad testificandum**. More frequently, records custodians are served a **subpoena duces tecum**. *Duces tecum* means to bring documents and other records with oneself. These subpoenas may direct that originals or copies of health records, laboratory reports, x-rays, or other records be brought to a deposition or to court. In most instances, a subpoena for the disclosure of an individual's health information must be accompanied by an **authorization**, or permission, from that individual. (Authorization, a HIPAA requirement, is discussed in detail later in this chapter.) Each state has different rules governing the production of health records in litigation.

Court Order

Another type of discovery tool is the court order. A **court order** is a document issued by a judge. At times, a court order will be issued to compel the production of health records. If the recipient does not comply with the court order, he or she risks contempt-of-court (namely, failure to comply) sanctions, possibly including jail time. Although both are issued through the court, any legal document that requests a patient's health information must carefully be reviewed to determine which type it is, a court order or subpoena. As noted previously, a subpoena often requires an individual's authorization if health information is being sought.

Warrants

If health records are relevant to a criminal case, they may be obtained via a warrant. A specialized type of court order, a **warrant** is a judge's order that authorizes law enforcement to seize evidence and, often, to conduct a search as well. Criminal cases in which health records are most likely to be obtained via warrant involve healthcare fraud and abuse investigations (Rinehart-Thompson 2012).

E-Discovery

The concept of discovery as defined earlier seems relatively straightforward with paper records. However, it is changing as health records become hybrid (a combination of paper and electronic documents) or completely electronic. **E-discovery** is the same pretrial process as discovery, but parties now obtain and review electronically stored data. The **Federal Rules of Civil Procedure (FRCP)** incorporated electronic information through the creation of e-discovery rules. The FRCP applies only to cases in federal district courts, but many states have adopted similar e-discovery rules that apply to both civil and criminal cases.

Impact of Technology

While the role of the HIM professional in paper-based discovery was often limited to responding to a subpoena for records or testifying as to a record's authenticity, involvement begins much earlier with e-discovery. For example, attorneys for the parties in a lawsuit must agree on matters such as document discovery. Early interaction among an organization's health information professionals, information technology (IT) professionals, and legal counsel is very important. Electronic health records (EHR) allow massive volumes of information to be created and stored, subjecting much greater amounts of information to discovery than paper records. Not all information is discoverable. Whether it is discoverable or not depends on legal protections or the lack thereof.

Discoverable Data

Any electronically stored evidence may potentially be compelled as evidence. Discoverable data includes not only the EHR, but also e-mails, texts, voicemails, drafts of documents, electronic schedulers, websites, and information housed on mobile devices such as smartphones or flash drives (AHIMA 2012). Other information that must be considered as potentially discoverable includes information housed on ancillary systems and other databases throughout an organization because they may be relevant to a particular case. Discoverable data also include metadata, which are data about data, a concept that was unheard of in paper documents. Metadata provides information such as who accessed or attempted to access a system and when, which parts of the system were affected, and what operations (for example, creating, viewing, printing, editing) took place (Rinehart-Thompson 2013).

Because the e-discovery rule affects retention and destruction of health information, HIM professionals must be involved in those ongoing processes. To preserve discoverable data, they must also ensure that records involved in litigation or potential litigation are preserved through a legal hold, which is generally a court order to preserve a health record if there is concern about destruction. A legal hold supersedes routine destruction procedures. It also prevents spoliation—the act of destroying, changing, or hiding evidence intentionally (Klaver 2012).

Data That Is Not Discoverable

Rules and judicial law (court decisions) addressing discovery are broad, thus favoring discovery when it is in doubt. Information-sharing during discovery is encouraged so each party knows the relative strength of their case (which may lead to settlement) and to avoid surprises at trial. The federal rule permits discovery of any relevant non-privileged information (for example, information protected by attorney–client privilege) that may be limited by the court for reasons such as the request being unnecessary, duplicative, or too expensive for the party being asked to produce the requested information (FRCP 26(b)).

Testifying in Court

An individual may be compelled to testify in court. This may occur after an individual has provided testimony at a deposition, or it may be the first time an individual testifies in a particular case. Rules regarding admissibility, described in chapter 8, are much more stringent than discovery rules (Rinehart-Thompson 2012). Thus, much information can be shared during pretrial discovery that is not permitted to be admitted as evidence at trial. The Federal Rules of Evidence governs admissibility in the federal court system. Separate rules of evidence that often mirror the federal rules govern admissibility in each state.

Generally only relevant evidence—that which makes a purported fact either more or less probable—may be admitted at trial. However, even relevant evidence with probative value (that is, significant in providing something) may be excluded from admissibility if it is outweighed as unfairly prejudicial or if presenting the evidence would cause undue delay. Evidence may also be excluded if it is misleading or redundant (Klaver 2012). Hearsay is also often excluded. It is an out-of-court statement used to prove the truth of a matter, and it is inherently deemed untrustworthy because the maker of the statement was not cross-examined at the time the statement was made. Hearsay can be admitted into evidence if it meets one of the hearsay exceptions. The exception most common to the health record is the business records exception. This exception exists because business records are deemed inherently trustworthy and are admissible as long as they are made at or near the time of the event being recorded, are kept in the regular courses of business, and the record was created through the regular practice of business (Klaver 2012).

Testimony by HIM professionals is often focused on the authenticity of the health record (discussed in chapter 2) and refers to the document's baseline trustworthiness (Klaver 2012). HIM professionals must take care to present a professional decorum when testifying by dressing professionally, answering questions honestly and without becoming defensive, and responding to the questions asked rather than unnecessarily elaborating. If the questioning attorney poses a question that is outside the scope of the individual's expertise as an HIM professional (for example, eliciting information about a patient's condition or purpose for medical treatment), the HIM professional should respectfully decline to answer the question by stating that it is beyond his or her area of professional expertise.

State Laws—Privacy

Laws protecting the privacy of health information vary from state to state. Some are very prescriptive while others are general or even absent. Regardless of state laws, every person or organization that is subject to HIPAA, which is federal law, must comply with it. State laws must also comply with HIPAA or HIPAA will supersede them. This is the concept of preemption, which is discussed later in this chapter.

In addition to state laws that protect health information privacy, all states have laws that require the disclosure of health information, even without patient authorization. These include the reporting vital statistics (births and deaths) and other public health, safety, or welfare situations. For example, healthcare providers may be required to provide information to the appropriate state agency about patients who suffer from venereal and other communicable diseases, have been injured by knives or firearms, or have wounds that suggest some type of violent criminal activity. The treatment of suspected victims of child abuse or neglect also must be reported. These purposes are permitted by HIPAA and described later in the chapter.

Check Your Understanding 9.1

Instructions: Answer the following questions.

1. The right of privacy:
   A. Has been granted by the US Constitution
   B. Has been granted via court decisions
   C. Does not apply to health information
   D. Does not exist

2. Which of the following describes discovery?
   A. It is designed to limit access to information that other parties hold
   B. It is a type of deposition
   C. It is a pretrial process
   D. It is intended to result in surprises at trial

3. Which of the following is a discovery method?
   A. Subpoena
   B. Deposition
   C. Hearsay
   D. Legal hold

4. Which of the following compels a person to bring records to a deposition or trial?
   A. Subpoena ad testificandum
   B. Subpoena duces tecum
   C. Interrogatories
   D. E-discovery

5. Which of the following is an example of metadata?
   A. Text message
   B. Information that shows who accessed a record
   C. Voicemail message
   D. Printout of a patient's operative report

6. A subpoena requesting patient records:
   A. Is initiated by a judge
   B. Is also referred to as a court order
   C. Must usually be accompanied by patient authorization
   D. Can be ignored

7. Which of the following is an element of a deposition?
   A. Testimony is not transcribed because it cannot be used at trial
   B. An individual appears at an appointed time and place to testify under oath
   C. Only the testimony of the plaintiff and defendant can be obtained
   D. Attorneys for the plaintiff and defendant are prohibited from attending

8. A legal hold serves to:
   A. Confine a person in jail
   B. Subject records to a search warrant
   C. Preserve information
   D. Create information

9. Spoliation can be defined as which of the following?
   A. It is required after a legal hold is imposed
   B. It is the negligent destruction or changing of information
   C. It is destroying, changing, or hiding evidence intentionally
   D. It can only be performed on records that are involved in a court proceeding

10. State laws that protect the privacy of health information:
    A. Will not be preempted by HIPAA
    B. Are standard across all fifty states
    C. May be preempted by HIPAA
    D. Prohibit disclosure of information without patient authorization

HIPAA Privacy Rule and ARRA

The HIPAA **Privacy Rule** is one of the key federal laws that govern the protection of protected health information (PHI). This chapter provides an overview of HIPAA legislation (namely, the Privacy Rule) and the accompanying American Recovery and Reinvestment Act (ARRA) of 2009.

HIPAA and ARRA Overview

As shown in figure 9.1, HIPAA contains five titles. Title II is the most relevant title to the HIM professional. It contains provisions relating to the prevention of healthcare fraud and abuse and medical liability (medical malpractice) reform, as well as

Figure 9.1 HIPAA structure

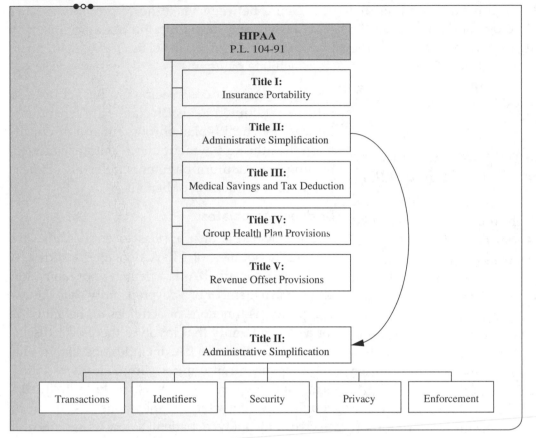

administrative simplification. The HIPAA Privacy Rule resides in the administrative simplification provision of Title II along with the HIPAA security standards, national provider identifiers, and transaction and code set standardization requirements. **Administrative simplification** is HIPAA's attempt to streamline and standardize the healthcare industry's nonuniform business practices, such as billing, including the electronic transmission of data.

Before HIPAA was enacted, no federal statutes or regulations generally protected the confidentiality of health information. Specific laws applied only in particular circumstances, such as to providers of Medicare services or to those receiving federal funds to provide substance abuse treatment.

Patient privacy protection laws governing access, use, and disclosure had largely resided with the individual states. They varied considerably, creating a patchwork of laws across the United States. Many states had passed laws to protect highly sensitive health records such as mental health and HIV/AIDS, but many states had no statutes or regulations to protect health information generally. If health information was wrongfully disclosed, individuals had to resort to lawsuits, often alleging negligence. With the Privacy Rule, protection was achieved uniformly across all the states through a consistent set of standards affecting providers, healthcare clearinghouses, and health plans.

The legal doctrine of **preemption** means that federal law (for example, the HIPAA Privacy Rule) may supersede state law. However, the Privacy Rule is only a federal floor, or minimum, of privacy requirements so it does not preempt or supersede stricter state statutes (or other federal statutes). *Stricter* means that a state or federal statute provides an individual with greater privacy protections or gives individuals greater rights with respect to their PHI. If a question arises, it is important to consult with legal counsel to determine which law prevails.

The **American Recovery and Reinvestment Act (ARRA)** provides significant funding for health information technology and other stimulus funding, and also made important changes to the HIPAA Privacy and Security Rules. These changes are located in the **Health Information Technology for Economic and Clinical Health Act (HITECH)**, which is a part of ARRA.

Office of the National Coordinator for Health Information Technology (ONC)

The **Office of the National Coordinator for Health Information Technology (ONC)** was first established by presidential executive order. It is now recognized by statute as an entity within the United States **Department of Health and Human Services (HHS)**. It is the primary federal entity with responsibility for coordinating national efforts to implement and use health information technology, and to promote the exchange of electronic health information. It includes 10 offices, including the Office of Policy, Office of Standards and Technology, and Office of the Chief Privacy Officer, which plays an important role in promoting electronic health information privacy and security (ONC 2014).

Applicability of the Privacy Rule

This section identifies, first, *to whom* the Privacy Rule applies. This includes persons or organizations (covered entities, business associates, and workforce). This section also discusses *what* the Privacy Rule protects, by defining protected health information (PHI).

Covered Entities

A **covered entity (CE)** is a person or organization that must comply with the HIPAA Privacy Rule. There are three types of covered entities:

- Healthcare providers that conduct certain transactions (financial or administrative) electronically. Healthcare providers include hospitals, long-term care facilities, physicians, and pharmacies.
- Health plans, which pay for the cost of medical care (for example, a health insurance company).

- Healthcare clearinghouses, which process claims between a healthcare provider and payer (for example, an intermediary that processes a hospital's claim to Medicare to facilitate payment).

Electronic transactions specified in the act include but are not limited to health claims and encounter information, health plan enrollment and disenrollment, healthcare payment and remittance advice, health plan premium payments, referral certification, and coordination of benefits.

Business Associates

The Privacy Rule also applies to entities that are business associates of HIPAA-covered entities. A **business associate (BA)** is a person or organization other than a member of a covered entity's workforce that performs functions or activities on behalf of or for a covered entity that involves the use or disclosure of PHI. Common BAs include consultants, billing companies, transcription companies, accounting firms, and law firms. ARRA also includes in the BA definition patient safety organizations (PSOs), which receive and analyze patient safety issues; health information organizations (HIOs); e-prescribing gateways and persons who facilitate data transmissions; as well as personal health record (PHR) vendors who, by contract, enable covered entities to offer PHRs to their patient as part of the covered entity's EHR (HHS 2010, 40872).

A BA's subcontractors are also BAs if they require access to an individual's protected health information, regardless of whether an agreement has actually been signed (HHS 2010, 40873). ARRA requires BAs and their subcontractors to comply with certain HIPAA provisions and subjects them to the same civil and criminal penalties that covered entities face for violating the law. In addition to the Privacy Rule, BAs and their subcontractors must also comply with the HIPAA security provisions (covered in chapter 10).

The Privacy Rule does not allow covered entities to disclose PHI to BAs unless the two enter into a written contract, or **business associate agreement (BAA)**, that meets HIPAA and ARRA requirements. However, if a person or organization meets the definition of a BA, they are a BA by law (even if the required agreement has not been signed) and are

Figure 9.2   Provisions to include in a BAA

- Prohibit the BA from using or disclosing the PHI for any purpose other than that stated in the contract, and pursuant to the Privacy Rule and minimum necessary standard, which limits the use and disclosure of information to only the amount that is needed

- Prohibit the BA from using or disclosing the PHI in a manner that would violate the requirements of the HIPAA Privacy Rule

- Require the BA to maintain safeguards, as necessary, to ensure that the PHI is not used or disclosed except as provided by the contract

- Require the BA to report to the covered entity any use or disclosure of the PHI that is not provided for in the contract

- Clarify that the BA is responsible to report breaches of unsecured PHI

- Clarify that the BA must adhere to policy and procedure, and documentation requirements imposed by the HIPAA Security Rule

- Establish how the covered entity would provide access to PHI to the individual whom the information is about when the BA has made any material alterations to the information

- Require the BA to make available its internal practices, books, and records relating to the use and disclosure of PHI received from the covered entity to HHS or its agents

- Establish how the entity would provide an individual access to his or her PHI in circumstances where the BA holds the information and the covered entity does not

- Require the BA to incorporate any amendments or corrections to the PHI when notified by the covered entity that the information is inaccurate or incomplete

- At termination of the contract, require the BA to return or destroy all PHI received from the covered entity that it still maintains and prohibit the associate from retaining it

- State that individuals who are the subject of disclosed PHI are intended third-party beneficiaries of the contract

- Authorize the covered entity to terminate the contract when it determines that the BA has repeatedly violated a term required in the contract

- State the BA is subject to the HIPAA Security Rule, including implementation of administrative, technical, and procedural safeguards, and procedural and documentation requirements

- State that the BA will receive satisfactory assurances from its subcontractors that the subcontractors will appropriately safeguard protected health information

- State that subcontractors of the BA are responsible for complying with HIPAA, and are directly liable for HIPAA violations, as is the BA even if the BA has not entered into a contractual agreement with the subcontractor

- Clarify that the BA is responsible to take action, possibly including termination, against a subcontractor if it violates HIPAA or provisions of the business associate agreement

- Clarify that the BA is subject to civil monetary penalties for violation of the Privacy Rule or the Security Rule

Source: Adapted from Cassidy 2000, updated 2010 per ARRA/HITECH requirements NPRM 40872-40874.

subject to HIPAA's penalties if they violate HIPAA. The BA may use or disclose PHI once it agrees to the covered entity's requirements to protect the information's security and confidentiality. Covered entities must respond to BA noncompliance, and ARRA requires BAs to respond to covered entity noncompliance. They do this by corrective action or severing the relationship with the covered entity.

Business associate agreements must be updated to comply with ARRA. There are a minimum number of provisions that an agreement between a covered entity and BA should contain. These are outlined in figure 9.2.

Workforce Members

Both covered entities and BAs (including their subcontractors) are responsible under the Privacy Rule for their **workforce** members. A workforce consists not only of employees, but also volunteers,

student interns, trainees, and even employees of outsourced vendors who routinely work on-site in the covered entity's facility.

To illustrate this, examine the following scenario. Ted is employed as a custodial worker by Tidy Team, a company that contracts with Mercy Hospital to provide janitorial services. Ted has been assigned to Mercy Hospital. As part of his duties, he routinely cleans the floors and empties the trash in the HIM department. What is Tidy Team's relationship with Mercy Hospital? What is Ted's relationship with Mercy Hospital? Does a BA relationship exist here?

In this example, Tidy Team was contracted to clean the hospital, not to use or disclose individually identifiable health information. The fact that Ted is in close proximity to such information on a regular basis does not make him (or Tidy Team) a BA. More appropriately, because he routinely works in Mercy

Hospital's HIM department, he would be treated as a workforce member and should be trained as such.

Protected Health Information

The Privacy Rule safeguards a category of information called **protected health information (PHI)**. PHI either identifies an individual or provides a reasonable basis to believe the person could be identified from the information given. PHI can be in any form including electronic, paper, and oral. Determining whether information is PHI or not requires meeting all parts of a three-part test. First, the information must be held or transmitted by a covered entity or a BA in any of the forms listed previously. Second, it must be **individually identifiable health information**. To be individually identifiable, the information must either identify the person or provide a reasonable basis to believe the person could be identified from the information. Third, it must relate to one's past, present, or future physical or mental health condition, the provision of healthcare, or payment for the provision of healthcare. Per a federal rule published subsequent to ARRA, PHI of deceased persons loses PHI status and is no longer protected by HIPAA after the individual has been deceased more than 50 years.

Deidentified Information

Not all patient information is PHI. This definition does not include **deidentified information**, which the Privacy Rule does not protect.

Deidentified information does not identify an individual because personal characteristics have been stripped from it in such a way that it cannot be later constituted or combined to reidentify an individual. It is commonly used in research.

Information technology is powerful in assisting with the collection and analysis of data, so it is possible to identify individuals by combining specific data. Therefore, the HIPAA Privacy Rule requires the covered entity to do one of the following things to ensure deidentification:

- The covered entity can strip certain elements to ensure that the patient's information is truly deidentified. These elements are listed in figure 9.3 (Rinehart-Thompson 2013).
- The covered entity can have an expert apply generally accepted statistical and scientific principles and methods to minimize the risk that the information might be used to identify an individual.

Figure 9.3   Data elements to be removed for deidentification of information

Eighteen identifiers must be removed for deidentification. They pertain to the individual, relatives, employers, and household members:

- Names
- Geographic identifiers including subdivisions smaller than a state, street addresses, city, county, precinct, and zip code if the geographic unit contains fewer than 20,000 people (the initial three digits of the zip code must be changed to 000 or zip codes with the same three initial digits may be combined to form a unit of more than 20,000 people)
- All elements of dates, except the year, directly related to an individual including birth, admission, discharge, and death dates; in addition, all ages over 89 and all elements of dates (including the year) that would identify such age cannot be used, but individuals over 89 can be aggregated into a single category of 90 and over
- Telephone numbers
- Fax numbers
- E-mail addresses
- Social Security numbers

- Medical record numbers
- Health plan beneficiary numbers
- Account numbers
- Certificate and license numbers
- Vehicle identifiers and serial numbers, including license plates
- Device identifiers and serial numbers
- Web universal resource locators (URLs)
- Internet protocol (IP) address numbers
- Biometric identifiers, including fingerprints and voiceprints
- Full-face photographic images and any comparable images
- Any other unique identifying number, characteristic, or code except for permissible reidentification to match information back to the person (code must not be derived from or related to information about the individual, cannot be translated to her or her identity, may not be used for any other purpose, and may not disclose the reidentification mechanism)

Other Basic Concepts

In addition to understanding *to whom* the Privacy Rule applies and *what* it protects, it is important to understand other basic HIPAA concepts, discussed as follows.

Individual

The Privacy Rule defines an **individual** as the person who is the subject of the PHI (45 CFR 160.103).

Personal Representative

A **personal representative** is a person who has legal authority to act on another's behalf. Per the Privacy Rule, a personal representative must be treated the same as an individual regarding use and disclosure of the individual's PHI.

Designated Record Set

A **designated record set (DRS)** includes the health records, billing records, and various claims records that are used to make decisions about an individual (45 CFR 164.501). HIPAA provisions apply to the DRS. The DRS is broader than the legal health record, which was discussed in chapter 8, because it contains more components than those that would ordinarily be produced upon request.

Minimum Necessary

The **minimum necessary standard** requires uses, disclosures, and requests must be limited to only the amount needed to accomplish an intended purpose. For example, for payment purposes, only the minimum amount of information necessary to substantiate a claim for payment should be disclosed. The minimum necessary standard does not apply to PHI used, disclosed, or requested for treatment purposes.

Policies and procedures should identify those persons or classes of persons who work for the covered entity who need to access PHI to perform their duties and should identify the PHI needed to perform their jobs. For example, employees working in the housekeeping department would not have the same level of access to PHI as a nurse working in critical care.

Until a final clarification of *minimum necessary* is made per ARRA, covered entities are to use the limited data set (PHI with certain specified direct identifiers removed) for using or disclosing only minimum necessary information, while reverting back to the *amount needed to accomplish the intended purpose* definition when the limited data set definition is inadequate (AHIMA 2009).

Treatment, Payment, and Operations

Treatment, payment, and operations (TPO) is an important concept because the Privacy Rule provides a number of exceptions for PHI that is being used or disclosed for TPO purposes. *Treatment* means providing, coordinating, or managing healthcare or healthcare-related services by one or more healthcare providers. For example, treatment includes caring for patients admitted to the hospital or coming for an appointment with a physician. Treatment also includes healthcare provider consultations and referrals of the patient from one provider to another.

Payment includes activities by a health plan to obtain premiums, billing by healthcare providers or health plans to obtain reimbursement, claims management, claims collection, review of the medical necessity of care, and utilization review.

The Privacy Rule provides a broad list of activities that are healthcare *operations*. They include quality assessment and improvement, case management, review of healthcare professionals' qualifications, insurance contracting, legal and auditing functions, and general business management functions such as providing customer service and conducting due diligence. Operations do not include marketing or fundraising activities.

Individual Rights

There are two key goals to the Privacy Rule: (1) to provide greater privacy protections for one's health information (this also serves to limit access by others) and (2) to provide an individual with greater rights with respect to his or her health information. HIPAA's individual rights further the latter goal. The individual rights include right of access, right to request amendment of PHI, right to accounting of disclosures, right to request restrictions of PHI, right to request confidential communications, and right to complain of Privacy Rule violations. These rights are described as follows.

Right of Access

The Privacy Rule's **right of access** allows an individual to inspect and obtain a copy of his or her own PHI contained within a designated record set, such as a health record (45 CFR 164.524). The right of access extends as long as the PHI is maintained, although HIPAA does not require that records be retained for a specified period. There are exceptions to the right of access. For example, psychotherapy notes; information compiled in reasonable anticipation of a civil, criminal, or administrative action or proceeding; or PHI subject to the Clinical Laboratory Improvements Act (CLIA) are all exceptions to the right of access. ARRA requires covered entities with EHRs to make PHI available electronically per individual request if it is readily producible or if the individual requests to send PHI to a designated person or entity electronically (Rinehart-Thompson 2013).

Grounds for Denial of Access

Per the Privacy Rule, there are times when a covered entity can deny an individual access to PHI. These are described as follows and are generally categorized as *no opportunity to review* or *opportunity to review.*

No Opportunity to Review   A covered entity can deny an individual access to PHI without providing him or her an opportunity to review or appeal the denial in these situations:

- PHI is in psychotherapy notes
- PHI was compiled in reasonable anticipation of, or for use in, civil or criminal litigation or administrative action
- The covered entity is a correctional institution or provider that has acted under the direction of a correctional institution, and an inmate's request for his or her PHI creates health or safety concerns

- PHI is created or obtained by a covered healthcare provider in research that includes treatment, and an individual receiving treatment as part of a research study agrees to suspend his or her right to access PHI temporarily, while the study is in progress
- PHI was obtained from someone other than a healthcare provider under a promise of confidentiality and the access requested would be reasonably likely to reveal the source of the information
- PHI is contained in records that are subject to the federal Privacy Act (5 USC. 552a) if the denial of access under the Privacy Act would meet the requirements of that law
- PHI is maintained by a covered entity that is subject to the **Clinical Laboratory Improvement Amendments (CLIA) of 1988**, which regulates the quality of laboratory testing, and CLIA would prohibit access
- PHI is maintained by a covered entity exempt from CLIA requirements (Rinehart-Thompson 2013)

Opportunity to Review   In two instances, the Privacy Rule requires a covered entity to give an individual the right to review a denial of access. These are situations where a licensed healthcare professional determines that access to requested PHI would likely endanger the life or physical safety of the individual or another person, or would reasonably endanger the life or physical safety of another person mentioned in the PHI.

When a denial is made, the covered entity must write the denial in plain language and include a reason. Second, it must explain that the individual has the right to request a review of the denial. Third, it must describe how the individual can complain to the covered entity and must include the name or title and phone number of the person or office to contact. Finally, it must explain how the individual can lodge a complaint with the secretary of HHS.

The individual has the right to have the denial reviewed by a licensed healthcare professional who did not participate in the original denial and is designated by the covered entity to act as the reviewing official. The covered entity must grant or deny access in accordance with the reviewing official's decision.

Requesting Access to One's Own PHI

HIPAA gives individuals the right to request access to their PHI, but the covered entity may require that requests be in writing. An individual's request for review of PHI must be acted on no later than 30 days after the request is made (or 60 days if the PHI is not on-site). This may be extended once by a maximum of 30 additional days if the individual is given a written statement (within the 30 days) explaining the reasons for the delay and the date by which the covered entity will respond. A covered entity must arrange a convenient time and place for an individual to inspect his or her PHI; otherwise, a copy of the PHI must be mailed if requested. HIPAA allows a reasonable cost-based fee when the individual requests a copy of PHI or agrees to accept summary or explanatory information. The fee may include the cost of:

- Copying, including supplies and labor of copying
- Postage, when the individual has requested that the copy or summary or explanation be mailed
- Preparing an explanation or summary, if agreed to by the individual (45 CFR 164.524)

HIPAA does not permit retrieval fees to be charged to patients. However, they are permitted for non-patient requests.

A covered entity must provide access to the PHI in the format requested if it is readily producible in such form or format. If not, it must be produced in a readable hard-copy form or other format agreed to by the covered entity and the individual.

Right to Request Amendment of PHI

The Privacy Rule allows an individual the **right to request amendment**. With this right, one may request that a covered entity amend PHI or a record about the individual in a designated record set (45 CFR

164.526). The covered entity may deny the request when it determines that the PHI or the record:

- Was not created by the covered entity
- Is not part of the designated record set
- Is not available for inspection as noted in the regulation of access (for example, psychotherapy notes, inmate of a correctional institution, and so on)
- Is accurate or complete as is (45 CFR 164.526)

A covered entity may require that the amendment request be in writing and include a rationale if that requirement was communicated in advance (usually in the Notice of Privacy Practices, discussed later in the chapter).

An individual's amendment request must be acted on no later than 60 days after receipt by allowing it or denying it in writing. The covered entity may extend its response once, by 30 days, if it explains the reasons for the delay in a written statement and gives a date by which it will act. If an amendment is granted, the Privacy Rule requires a covered entity to:

- Identify the records in the designated record set that are affected by the amendment and append the information through a link to the amendment's location. For example, if the diagnosis was incorrect, the amendment would have to appear and/or be linked to each record or report in the designated record set.
- Inform the individual that the amendment was accepted and have him or her identify the persons with whom the amendment needs to be shared and then obtain his or her agreement to notify those persons. The covered entity must make reasonable efforts to provide the amendment within a reasonable amount of time to anyone who has received the PHI (45 CFR 164.526).

Denials must be made within 60 days of the request, be written in plain language and contain:

- The basis for the denial
- The individual's right to submit a written statement disagreeing with the denial

- The process by which the individual can submit his or her disagreement

- A statement explaining how, when the individual does not submit a disagreement, he or she may request that both the original amendment request and the covered entity's denial accompany any future disclosures of the PHI that is the subject of the amendment

- A description of how the individual may complain to the covered entity, including the name or title and telephone number of the contact person or office (45 CFR 164.526)

The covered entity can prepare a written rebuttal if the individual submits a disagreement statement, but it must provide the individual with a copy of the rebuttal.

All requests for amendments, denials, the individual's statement of disagreement, and the covered entity's rebuttal (if one was created) must be appended or linked to the record or PHI that is the subject of the amendment request. Future disclosures of the subject information must include this material or a summary. If a request for amendment was denied and the individual did not write a statement of disagreement, the request for amendment and denial must accompany future disclosures only if the individual requests such action.

Right to Request Accounting of Disclosures

Maintaining some type of accounting procedure for monitoring and tracking PHI disclosures has been a common practice in HIM departments. However, the Privacy Rule has a specific standard with respect to such recordkeeping. Per the **right to request accounting of disclosures**, an individual has the right to receive an accounting of certain disclosures made by a covered entity (45 CFR 164.528). HIPAA originally required an accounting of all disclosures within the six years prior to the date on which the accounting was requested, with ARRA to decrease it to three years (AHIMA 2009). A covered entity may either account for the disclosures of its BAs or require the BA to make its own accounting. Per ARRA, BAs must respond to accounting requests that are made directly to them (AHIMA 2009).

The types of disclosures that must be accounted for are limited, but include those made erroneously (that is, breaches, which are discussed later in the chapter), for public interest and benefit activities (discussed later in this chapter) where patient authorization is not obtained, and pursuant to a court order. Disclosures for which an accounting is *not* required (that is, exceptions) are disclosures:

- For treatment, payment, and healthcare operations (although, per ARRA, this exception only applies to covered entities without EHRs)

- To individuals to whom the information pertains, or the individual's personal representative

- Incidental to an otherwise permitted or required use or disclosure (for example, a patient's name appears on a sign-in sheet at a physician office; this is a permitted use that may be seen by [disclosed to] the next patient who signs in)

- Pursuant to an authorization

- For use in the facility's directory, to persons involved in the individual's care, or for other notification purposes

- To meet national security or intelligence requirements

- To correctional institutions or law enforcement officials

- As part of a limited data set

- That occurred before the compliance date for the covered entity (45 CFR 164.528) (Rinehart-Thompson 2013)

A proposed rule published by HHS in 2011 would exclude use, as well as TPO, from an accounting for both paper and electronic records. Instead, individuals (upon request) would be able to receive a separate **access report** from covered entities with EHRs. This report would allow an individual to see a record of every person who viewed the individual's DRS during the previous three years. TPO disclosures would therefore be displayed in the access report rather than in the accounting of disclosures, as previously suggested. This proposal is pending (HHS 2011a).

The definition of healthcare operations is broad, but HIPAA has carved out exceptions to this definition so the following must be included in an accounting of disclosures. For example, mandatory public health reporting is not part of a covered entity's operations (this includes state requirements to report births [birth certificates]; communicable diseases; and incidents of abuse or suspected abuse of children, mentally disabled individuals, and the elderly). As a result, these must be included in an accounting of disclosures. For example, if a physician's office reports a case of tuberculosis to a public health authority, that disclosure must be included if the patient requests an accounting. If a covered entity provides PHI to a third-party public health authority to review, but the third party does not actually review it, the third-party's access must be included in an accounting of disclosures.

Disclosure pursuant to a court order (if without a patient's written authorization) is also subject to an accounting. However, disclosure pursuant to a subpoena that is accompanied by a patient's written authorization is not subject to an accounting because the authorization exempts the disclosure from the accounting requirement. The accounting requirement includes disclosures made in writing, by telephone, or orally. In some situations, an individual's right to an accounting of PHI disclosure may be suspended at the written request of a health oversight agency or law enforcement official indicating that an accounting would impede its activities and specify how long such a suspension is required. HIPAA has provided a list of exceptions to the accounting requirement, but has not included a list of which disclosures must be accounted for. ARRA provides that those items which are to be included are explicitly listed.

The following elements must be included in an accounting of disclosures:

- Date of disclosure
- Name and address (when known) of the entity or person who received the information
- Brief description of the PHI disclosed
- Brief statement of the purpose of the disclosure or a copy of the individual's written authorization or request be included (45 CFR 164.528).

A covered entity must act on a request for an accounting of disclosures no later than 60 days after receipt (extended by no more than 30 days if the covered entity notifies the individual in writing of the reasons for the delay and the date by which the accounting will be made available). ARRA proposes to limit the response period to 30 days, with one 30-day extension.

The first accounting within any 12-month period must be provided without charge. Additional requests within a 12-month period may be assessed a reasonable, cost-based fee if the individual is informed in advance and given an opportunity to withdraw or modify the request or avoid or reduce the fee.

The Privacy Rule requires documentation to be maintained on all accounting requests, including information included in the accounting, the written accounting that was provided to the individual, and the titles of persons or offices responsible for receiving and processing requests for an accounting. Policies and procedures must be developed to ensure that PHI disclosed from all areas of an organization, likely including departments outside HIM, can be tracked and compiled when an accounting request is received.

Right to Request Restrictions of PHI

An individual can request that a covered entity restrict the uses and disclosures of PHI to carry out treatment, payment, or healthcare operations (45 CFR 164.522(a)(1)). This is the **right to request restrictions of PHI**. In almost all cases, a covered entity can decline a restriction request. However, ARRA requires that restriction requests be complied with (unless otherwise required by law) if the disclosure would be made to a health plan for payment or operations purposes and the individual had paid for the healthcare service or item completely out of pocket (AHIMA 2009).

When a covered entity agrees to a restriction, whether voluntarily or as required by ARRA, it must live up to the agreement. To illustrate how difficult this can be, examine the following scenario. A patient, Mr. Smith, agrees to allow a hospital to tell callers that he has been admitted to the hospital and therefore is in the facility's patient directory. Such notification is a hospital operation. However, he requests that this information be restricted and withheld only from his Aunt Mary and Uncle Jack, if they should call. What would the responsible party for making the decision about a restriction such as this do?

In this scenario, the hospital is not required to agree to this request for a restriction. In fact, the hospital probably should not agree to this request because of the administrative difficulty of informing certain individuals, but not others, as well as the risk of accidentally violating the request. It would be difficult for every receptionist to recall this small restriction, particularly if other patients had similar restrictions on their information. The risk of violation simply becomes too great.

An agreed-upon restriction can be terminated by either the individual or the covered entity. When the covered entity initiates termination of the agreement, it must inform the individual that it is doing so. However, the termination is only effective with respect to the PHI created or received after the individual has been informed (45 CFR 164.522(a)).

Right to Request Confidential Communications

Healthcare providers and health plans must give individuals the opportunity to request that communications of PHI be routed to an alternative location or by an alternative method (45 CFR 164.522(b)(1)). This is the **right to request confidential communications**. Healthcare providers must honor such a request without requiring a reason if it is reasonable. Health plans must honor such a request if it is reasonable and if the requesting individual states that disclosure could pose a safety risk. However, providers and health plans may refuse to accommodate requests if the individual does not provide information as to how payment will be handled or an alternative address or method by which he or she can be contacted.

An example of a request for confidential communications would be a woman who requests that billing information from her psychiatrist, from whom she is seeking treatment because of a domestic violence situation, be sent to her work address instead of to her home.

Right to Complain of Privacy Rule Violations

A covered entity must provide a process for an individual to file a **complaint** or allegation about the entity's policies and procedures, its noncompliance with them, or its noncompliance with the Privacy Rule (45 CFR 164.530(d)(1)). The covered entity's notice of privacy practices, described later in this chapter, must contain contact information at the covered entity level and inform individuals of the ability to submit complaints to HHS. All complaints must be documented along with their disposition.

 ## Check Your Understanding 9.2

Instructions: **Answer the following questions**

1. The Privacy Rule establishes that a patient has the right of access to inspect and obtain a copy of his or her PHI:
    A. For as long as it is maintained
    B. For six years
    C. Forever
    D. For 12 months

2. HIPAA regulations:
    A. Never preempt state statutes
    B. Always preempt state statutes
    C. Preempt less strict state statutes where they exist
    D. Preempt stricter state statutes where they exist

3. The Privacy Rule applies to:
   A. Healthcare providers only
   B. Only healthcare providers that receive Medicare reimbursement
   C. Only entities funded by the federal government
   D. Covered entities and their business associates

4. The Privacy Rule extends to protected health information:
   A. In any form or medium, except paper and oral forms
   B. In any form or medium, including paper and oral forms
   C. That pertains to mental health treatment only
   D. That exists in electronic form only

5. Per the right to request confidential communications, if the individual does not provide information as to how payment will be handled:
   A. Health plans must still honor the request
   B. Only healthcare providers may deny the request
   C. Healthcare providers must still honor the request
   D. Both health plans and healthcare providers may deny the request

6. When an individual requests a copy of the PHI or agrees to accept summary or explanatory information, the covered entity may:
   A. Impose a reasonable cost-based fee
   B. Not charge the individual
   C. Impose any fee authorized by state statute
   D. Charge only for the cost of the paper on which the information is printed

7. Business associate agreements are developed to cover the use of PHI by:
   A. The covered entity's employees
   B. Organizations outside the covered entity's workforce that use PHI to perform functions on behalf of the covered entity
   C. The covered entity's entire workforce
   D. The covered entity's janitorial staff

8. The term *minimum necessary* means that healthcare providers and other covered entities must limit use, access, and disclosure to the minimum necessary to:
   A. Retain records needed for patient care
   B. Accomplish the intended purpose
   C. Treat an individual
   D. Perform research

9. Which of the following is part of Hillside Hospital's workforce?
   A. Information system firm staff
   B. Volunteers
   C. Employees who work on-site for a contractor of the hospital
   D. A business office employee at a competing hospital

10. Deidentified information:
    A. Does not identify an individual
    B. Is information from which only a person's name has been stripped
    C. Can be constituted later or combined to reidentify an individual
    D. Is subject to the HIPAA Privacy Rule

HIPAA Privacy Rule Documents

The Privacy Rule outlines three key documents that inform patients and give them a degree of control over their PHI. Two of the documents—the notice of privacy practices and the authorization—are required. HIPAA states that the consent document is optional.

Notice of Privacy Practices

Except for certain variations or exceptions for health plans and correctional facilities, an individual has the right to a notice explaining how his or her PHI will be used and disclosed (45 CFR 164.520). This is the **notice of privacy practices**. It also must explain in plain language the patient's rights and the covered entity's legal duties with respect to PHI. Healthcare providers with a direct treatment relationship with an individual must provide the notice of privacy practices by the first service delivery date (for example, first visit to a physician's office, first admission to a hospital, or first encounter at a clinic), including service delivered electronically. Notices must be available at the site where the individual is treated and must be posted in a prominent place where patients can reasonably be expected to read them. If the facility has a website with information on the covered entity's services or benefits, the notice of privacy practices must be prominently posted to it. Per ARRA, the notice of privacy practices must be updated to reflect material changes. It must state that uses and disclosures not described in the notice will require an authorization. It must also address marketing and the right to opt out of fundraising communications (both of which are explained later in this chapter). A covered entity's obligation to comply with a restriction request if the item or service is paid in full must also be included in the notice. AHIMA outlines the requirements for the content of the notice of privacy practices (McClendon and Rose 2013). In general, the notice is to include the following:

1. A header such as: "this notice describes how information about you may be used and disclosed and how you can get access to this information. Please review it carefully."

2. A description, including at least one example of the types of uses and disclosures that the covered entity is permitted to make for treatment, payment, and healthcare operations

3. A description of each of the other purposes for which the covered entity is permitted or required to use or disclose PHI without the individual's written consent or authorization

4. A statement that other uses and disclosures will be made only with the individual's written authorization and that the individual may revoke such authorization

5. When applicable, separate statements that the covered entity may contact the individual to provide appointment reminders or information about treatment alternatives and other health-related benefits and services that may be of interest to the individual

6. A statement indicating that most uses and disclosures of psychotherapy notes (where appropriate), uses and disclosures of protected health information for marketing purposes, and disclosures that constitute a sale of protected health information require authorization.

   CEs that do not record or maintain psychotherapy notes are not required to include a statement.

7. A statement regarding fundraising communications and an individual's right to opt out of receiving such communications, if a CE intends to contact an individual to raise funds for the CE.

   Note: If a CE does not make fundraising communications then this statement does not need to be included.

8. For health plans that perform underwriting activities only, a statement must be included indicating the health plan is prohibited from using or disclosing genetic information for underwriting purposes.

9. A statement of the individual's rights with respect to PHI and a brief description of how the individual may exercise these rights including:

   a. The right to request restrictions on certain uses and disclosures as provided by 45 CFR 164.522(a), including a statement that the covered entity is not required to agree to a requested restriction

   b. For healthcare providers only, a statement indicating the right to restrict certain disclosures of PHI to a health plan when the individual pays out of pocket in full for the healthcare item or service

   c. The right to receive confidential communications of PHI

   d. The right to access, inspect, and receive a copy of PHI on paper, including the right to have electronic copies if kept in electronic form

   e. The right to request electronic copies of PHI be forwarded to a third party

   f. The right to request an amendment of PHI

   g. The right to receive an accounting of disclosures

   h. The right to be notified of the CE's privacy practices

   i. The right to control PHI use for marketing, sales, and research

   j. The right to be notified of a breach to PHI

   k. The right to file complaints with the Office for Civil Rights

10. A statement that the covered entity is required by law to maintain the privacy of PHI and to provide individuals with a notice of its legal duties and privacy practices with respect to PHI

11. A statement that the covered entity is required to abide by the terms of the notice currently in effect

12. A statement that the covered entity reserves the right to change the terms of its notice and to make the new notice provisions effective for all PHI that it maintains

13. A statement describing how the covered entity will provide individuals with a revised notice

14. A statement that individuals may complain to the covered entity and to the Secretary of Health and Human Services if they believe their privacy rights have been violated, a brief description of how one files a complaint with the covered entity, and a statement that the individual will not be retaliated against for filing a complaint

15. The name or title and the telephone number of a person or office to contact for further information

16. An effective date, which may not be earlier than the date on which the notice is printed or otherwise published

Consent to Use or Disclose PHI

Under the Privacy Rule healthcare providers are not required to obtain patient **consent,** which is the patient's agreement to use or disclose personally identifiable information for treatment, payment, and healthcare operations (45 CFR 164.506(b)). However, some providers obtain consents as a matter of policy. Except for special circumstances such as emergencies (discussed in this section), patient consent is usually obtained at the time care is provided and has no expiration date (figure 9.4). However, it can be revoked by the individual as long as the revocation is in writing. Consents should be written in plain language. The covered entity must document and retain signed consents and revocations. A sample consent is provided in figure 9.4.

Authorization

Authorization by an individual for the use or disclosure of their health information is a long-standing legal requirement and health information practice. However, the authorization is a

Figure 9.4 Sample consent for the use or disclosure of individually identifiable health information

**Consent to the Use and Disclosure of Health Information
for Treatment, Payment, or Healthcare Operations**

I understand that as part of my healthcare, this organization originates and maintains health records describing my health history, symptoms, examination and test results, diagnoses, treatment, and any plans for future care or treatment. I understand that this information serves as:

- A basis for planning my care and treatment

- A means of communication among the many health professionals who contribute to my care

- A source of information for applying my diagnosis and surgical information to my bill

- A means by which a third-party payer can verify that services billed were actually provided

- A tool for routine healthcare operations such as assessing quality and reviewing the competence of healthcare professionals

I understand and have been provided with a Notice of Information Practices that provides a more complete description of information uses and disclosures. I understand that I have the right to review the notice prior to signing this consent. I understand that the organization reserves the right to change its notice and practices and prior to implementation will mail a copy of any revised notice to the address I've provided. I understand that I have the right to object to the use of my health information for directory purposes. I understand that I have the right to request restrictions as to how my health information may be used or disclosed to carry out treatment, payment, or healthcare operations and that the organization is not required to agree to the restrictions requested. I understand that I may revoke this consent in writing, except to the extent that the organization has already taken action in reliance thereon. Therefore, I consent to the use and disclosure of my healthcare information.

☐ I request the following restrictions to the use or disclosure of my health information.

Signature of Patient or Legal Representative

_____

Witness _____

Date Notice Effective _____

Date or Version _____

☐ Accepted   ☐ Denied

Signature _____

Title _____

Date _____

Source: HHS 2000. 82818.

key component of the HIPAA Privacy Rule. As a general requirement, the Privacy Rule states that an authorization for uses and disclosures must be obtained from an individual (45 CFR 164.508). However, there are a number of exceptions, outlined later in this chapter.

Authorizations are always required for the use or disclosure of psychotherapy notes except to carry out treatment, payment, or healthcare operations for treatment by the originator of the notes, in mental health training programs by the covered entity, to defend a legal action or other proceeding brought by the individual, or for oversight of the originator of the notes (45 CFR 164.508(a)).

An individual may revoke an authorization at any time if it is in writing. However, revocation does not apply to disclosures that have already been made.

The Privacy Rule requires that authorizations be obtained for uses and disclosures of PHI in research unless the covered entity obtains documentation that an Institutional Review Board

Table 9.1   Differences among notice of privacy practices, consent, and authorization

	Notice of privacy practices	Consent	Authorization
Required?	Required by HIPAA	Optional	Required by HIPAA
Requirements regarding TPO	Must explain TPO uses and disclosures, along with other types of uses and disclosures	Only obtains patient permission to use or disclose PHI for TPO purposes	Is used to obtain for a number of types of uses and disclosures, although it not required for TPO uses and disclosures
PHI this document addresses	Provides prospective and general information about how PHI might be used or disclosed in the future (and includes information that may not have been created yet)	Provides prospective and general information about how PHI might be used or disclosed in the future for TPO purposes (and includes information that may not have been created yet)	Obtains patient permission to use or disclose specific information that generally has already been created and for which there is a specific need
Required for treatment?	May not refuse to treat an individual because he or she declines to sign this form	May condition treatment on individual signing this form	May not refuse to treat an individual because he or she declines to sign this form
Time limit on document validity	No time limit on validity of the document	No time limit on validity of the document	Time limit on validity of document (specified by an expiration date or event)

Source: Adapted from Rinehart-Thompson 2012.

(IRB) or privacy board has approved an alteration or waiver. Where authorizations are required, the Privacy Rule requires that the authorization contains the required core elements, which are described later in this chapter.

Table 9.1 outlines differences among the three key HIPAA documents.

The Privacy Rule also provides other specifications for authorization, including those requested by a covered entity for its own uses and disclosures and those requested for disclosures by others. This section of the Privacy Rule also generally prohibits requiring an authorization as a condition of treatment and allows authorizations to be combined only in certain situations (45 CFR 164.508). Covered entities must document and retain signed authorizations and permit individuals to review what was disclosed.

Uses and Disclosures of Health Information

As table 9.2 shows, PHI may not be used or disclosed by a covered entity unless the individual who is the subject of the information authorizes the use or disclosure in writing or the Privacy Rule *requires or permits* such use or disclosure without the individual's authorization. The Privacy Rule *requires* such use or disclosure in only two situations: when the individual or individual's personal representative requests access to or an accounting of disclosures of the PHI (with the exceptions detailed earlier in this chapter), and when HHS is conducting an investigation, review, or enforcement action.

In addition to the two situations where use or disclosure is *required* without the individual's authorization (section A of table 9.2), there are many situations where the Privacy Rule *permits* a covered entity to use or disclose PHI without an individual's written authorization (45 CFR 164.510 and 164.512). These exceptions to the patient authorization requirement are summarized in section B of table 9.2.

Patient Has Opportunity to Agree or Object

As listed in table 9.2 (section B), the Privacy Rule lists two circumstances where PHI can be used

Table 9.2. Authorization requirements for use and disclosure of PHI

I. Patient authorization required:
All situations except those listed in Part II

II. Patient authorization not required:

    A. When use or disclosure is *required*, even without patient authorization
- When the individual/patient or individual's/patient's personal representative requests access or accounting of disclosures (with exceptions)
- HHS investigation, review, or enforcement action

    B. When use or disclosure is *permitted*, even without patient authorization
- Patient has opportunity to informally agree or object
  - Facility directory
  - Notification of relatives and friends
- Patient does not have opportunity to agree or object
  - Public interest and benefit
    1. As required by law
    2. For public health activities
    3. To disclose PHI regarding victims of abuse, neglect, domestic violence
    4. For health oversight activities
    5. For judicial and administrative proceedings
    6. For law enforcement purposes (six specific situations)
    7. Regarding decedents
    8. For cadaveric organ, eye, or tissue donation
    9. For research, with limitations
    10. To prevent or lessen serious threat to health or safety
    11. For essential government functions
    12. For workmen's compensation
  - Situations other than public interest and benefit
    13. TPO
    14. To the individual/patient
    15. Incidental disclosures
    16. Limited data set

or disclosed without the individual's authorization, although the individual must be informed in advance and given an opportunity to informally agree or object (45 CFR 164.510). The covered entity may inform the individual verbally and obtain his or her verbal agreement or objection.

The first circumstance is when the healthcare facility maintains a **facility directory** of patients for persons who ask for individuals by name and for clergy. The information may include the patient's name, location in the facility, condition described in general terms, and religious affiliation. Disclosure of an individual's religious affiliation is limited to members of the clergy.

The covered entity must inform the patient of the information to be included in the directory and to whom information may be disclosed. The patient must have the opportunity to prohibit all uses or disclosures from the facility directory

or request restrictions of some of the uses and disclosures.

When it is not possible to get the patient's agreement (for example, in emergencies), the organization can use and disclose PHI in the directory if the disclosure is consistent with the prior expressed preference of the patient or the organization believes it is in the patient's best interest. When it becomes possible after the emergency situation, the organization must inform the patient and give him or her the opportunity to object to use and disclosure from the facility directory.

The second circumstance is disclosing to a family member or a close friend PHI that is directly relevant to his or her involvement in the patient's care or payment. The patient's written authorization is not required but verbal agreement is, if it can be obtained. Likewise, a covered entity may disclose PHI, including the patient's location, general condition, or death, to notify or assist in the notification of a family member, personal representative, or some other person responsible for the patient's care (45 CFR 164.510(b)). Reasonably inferred from the circumstances that the patient does not object to the disclosure.

The covered entity may also use or disclose PHI to a public or private entity authorized by law or by its charter to assist in disaster relief efforts.

Patient Does Not Have Opportunity to Agree or Object

There are 16 circumstances where PHI can be used or disclosed without the individual's authorization, nor does the individual have the opportunity to agree or object. The first 12 circumstances are sometimes referred to as public interest and benefit circumstances because they are of benefit to society (45 CFR 164.512). Although the Privacy Rule permits the 12 public interest and benefit uses or disclosures without an individual's authorization, if it would violate a state law that otherwise protects the patient's information, the information cannot be legally used or disclosed. This is because, as a general rule, HIPAA does not preempt state laws that provide a greater level of privacy protection.

A use or disclosure may meet more than one of the 12 public interest and benefit situations. They are:

1. *As required by law*: Disclosures are permitted when required by laws that meet the public-interest requirements of disclosures relating to victims of abuse, neglect, or domestic violence, judicial and administrative proceedings, and law enforcement purposes (45 CFR 164.512(a)).

2. *Public health activities*: These include preventing or controlling diseases, injuries, and disabilities, and reporting disease, injury, and vital events such as births and deaths. Examples include the reporting of adverse events or product defects to comply with US Food and Drug Administration (FDA) regulations and, when authorized by law, reporting a person who may have been exposed to a communicable disease and

may be at risk for contracting or spreading it (45 CFR 164.512(b)). Per a federal rule published subsequent to ARRA, disclosure of students' immunization records may be considered a public health disclosure. Where applicable law requires that a school obtain a student's authorization records prior to enrollment, authorization is not required for the information to be disclosed to the school. An oral agreement from the student's legal guardian or the student (if age of majority has been reached) is, however, still required.

3. *Victims of abuse, neglect, or domestic violence*: An example is the reporting to authorities authorized by law to receive information about child or other abuse or neglect. In non–child abuse situations, the Privacy Rule requires the covered entity to promptly inform the individual or personal representative that a report has been or will be made unless it believes that doing so would place the individual at risk of serious harm or not be in his or her best interest (such as informing the personal representative, who is believed to be responsible for the abuse, neglect, or other injury) (45 CFR 164.512(c)).

4. *Healthcare oversight activities*: An authorized health oversight agency may receive PHI for activities authorized by law such as audits, civil or criminal investigations, licensure, and other inspections (45 CFR 164.512(d)).

5. *Judicial and administrative proceedings*: Disclosures of specified PHI are permitted in response to a court order or an administrative agency order. For subpoenas and discovery requests, the party seeking the PHI must assure the covered entity that it has made reasonable efforts to make the request known to the subject individual. The covered entity also must be assured that the time for the individual to raise objections to the court or administrative agency has elapsed and that either no objections have been filed, all objections have been resolved, or a qualified protective order has been secured (45 CFR 164.512(e)).

6. *Law enforcement purposes*: The Privacy Rule specifies six instances when disclosures to law enforcement do not require patient authorization or the patient has no opportunity to agree or object:

   ○ Pursuant to legal process or otherwise required by law: Examples of legal process include a court order, a court-ordered warrant, or a subpoena or a summons issued by a judicial officer. An example of "otherwise required by law" is a state law that requires certain types of wounds or other physical injuries to be reported to law enforcement.

   ○ In response to a law enforcement official's request for the purpose of identifying or locating a suspect, fugitive, material witness, or missing person. Only the following may be disclosed: name and address, date and place of birth, Social Security number, ABO blood type and Rh factor, type of injury, date and time of treatment, date and time of death (if applicable), and description of distinguishing physical characteristics including height, weight, gender, race, hair and eye color, and presence or absence of facial scars or tattoos.

   ○ In response to a law enforcement official's request about an individual who is, or is suspected to be, a victim of a crime (when the individual agrees to the disclosure or when the covered entity is unable to obtain the individual's agreement because of incapacity or other emergency circumstance). The law enforcement official must show the information is needed to determine whether a violation of law has occurred, that immediate law enforcement activity depends on the disclosure, and that disclosure is in the best interest of the individual as determined by the covered entity.

   ○ About a deceased individual when the covered entity suspects that the death may have resulted from criminal conduct.

   ○ To a law enforcement official when the covered entity believes in good faith that the information constitutes evidence of criminal conduct that occurred on the covered entity's premises.

   ○ To a law enforcement official in response to a medical emergency when the covered entity believes that disclosure is necessary to alert law enforcement to the commission and nature of a crime, the location or victims of such crime, and the identity, description, and location of the perpetrator of such crime. Further, it is permitted when the covered entity believes the medical emergency was the result of abuse, neglect, or domestic violence (45 CFR 164.512(f)).

7. *Decedents*: Disclosures to a coroner or medical examiner are permitted to identify a deceased person, determine a cause of death, or for other purposes required by law. In accordance with applicable law, disclosures to funeral directors are permitted, as necessary, to allow them to carry out their duties with respect to the decedent. This type of information also may be disclosed in reasonable anticipation of an individual's death (45 CFR 164.512(g)).

8. *Cadaveric organ, eye, or tissue donation*: PHI may be disclosed to organ procurement agencies or other entities to facilitate procurement, banking, or transplantation of cadaveric organs, eyes, or tissue (45 CFR 164.512(h)).

9. *Research*: Authorizations for the use of PHI in research are required except where an IRB or privacy board alters or waives the authorization requirement (in whole or in part) and documents it (45 CFR 164.512(i)). Table 9.3 provides a detailed analysis of the responsibilities of both the IRB and the researcher under the Privacy Rule requirements. Per a federal rule published subsequent to ARRA, a covered entity may combine conditioned authorizations (that is,

Table 9.3 Actions required for use of PHI in research

Type of information	IRB	Researcher	Research subject (patient or decedent)
PHI preparatory to research	None*	Representation that use is solely and necessary for research and will not be removed from covered entity	None
Deidentified health information	None*	Removal of safe-harbor data or statistical assurance of deidentification	None
Limited data set	None*	Removal of direct identifiers and data use agreement	None
Individually identifiable health information on decedents	None*	Representation that use is solely and necessary for research on decedents and documentation of death upon request of covered entity	None
PHI of human subjects (whether research is interventional or record review)	Waive authorization requirement if determined that risk to privacy is minimal	Representation that: 1. Privacy risk is minimal based on: • Plan to protect identifiers • Plan to destroy identifiers unless there is a health or research reason to retain • Written assurance that PHI will not be reused or redisclosed 2. Research requires use of specifically described PHI 3. Justify the waiver 4. Obtain IRB approval under normal or expedited review procedures	None
	Approve alteration of authorization (for example, to restrict patient's access during study) if determined that risk to privacy is minimal	Same as above	Sign altered authorization form
	Approve research protocol ensuring that there is an authorization for use either combined with consent for and disclosure of PHI research or separate		Sign authorization combined with consent for research or sign standard authorization for use and disclosure of PHI for research as described in authorization

* There may be requirements imposed by the IRB, but there are none imposed by HIPAA.
Source: Amatayakul 2003.

those that condition research-related treatment upon research participation) and unconditioned authorizations (that is, those that do not condition research-related treatment upon research participation) as long as the conditioned and unconditioned components are clearly distinguished and the individual is able to opt in to the unconditioned research activities. This provision does not apply to psychotherapy notes (Rinehart-Thompson 2013).

10. *Threat to health and safety*: Use or disclosure is allowed if thought necessary to prevent or lessen a serious and imminent threat to the health or safety of an individual or the public. Disclosure must be made to a person who can reasonably prevent or lessen the threat. Disclosures are permissible when law enforcement officials must apprehend an individual who may have caused harm to the victim being treated or when the individual appears to have escaped from a correctional institution or lawful custody. For correctional institutions or to a law enforcement official who has lawful custody of an inmate,

the Privacy Rule allows disclosures if the institution states that the information is necessary to provide continuing healthcare; to secure the health and safety of the individual or other inmates, officers, employees, transportation personnel, or law enforcement on the premises; or to ensure the administration and maintenance of the institution's safety, security, and good order (45 CFR 164.512(j)).

11. *Specialized government functions*: These include information regarding armed forces personnel for military and veterans activities, for purposes of national security and intelligence activities, for protective services for the President of the United States and others, and for public benefits and medical suitability determinations (45 CFR 164.512(k)).

12. *Workers' compensation*: The Privacy Rule permits the disclosure of PHI relating to work-related illness or injury or a workplace-related medical surveillance if the disclosure complies with workers' compensation laws (45 CFR section 164.512(l)).

The remaining four types of uses and disclosures that do not require patient authorization or an opportunity for the patient to agree or object are TPO, disclosure to the subject individual, incidental disclosures, and limited data set. The first two have been addressed in this chapter; the latter two are examined here.

- *Incidental uses or disclosures* occur as part of a permitted use or disclosure (CFR 164.502(a)(1)(iii)). For example, calling out patients' names in a physician office is an incidental disclosure because it occurs as part of office operations. It is permitted as long as the information disclosed is the minimum necessary (for example, the patient's name with no diagnostic information).

- A *limited data set* is PHI that excludes direct identifiers of the individual, the individual's relatives, employers, or household members without completely deidentifying it (45 CFR 164.514(e)(2)). Restrictions are lifted for items such as ages and dates, and parts of geographic subdivisions that are deemed not too specific (for example, city, state, or zip code) (Rinehart-Thompson 2013). Such PHI may be used or disclosed, provided it is used or disclosed only for research, public health, or healthcare operations.

✓ Check Your Understanding 9.3

Instructions: **Answer the following questions.**

1. Notices of privacy practices must be available at the site where the individual is treated and:
   A. Must be posted next to the entrance
   B. Must be posted in a prominent place where it is reasonable to expect that patients will read them
   C. May be posted anywhere at the site
   D. Do not have to be posted at the site

2. Calling out patient names in a physician's office is:
   A. An incidental disclosure
   B. Not subject to the minimum necessary requirement
   C. A disclosure for payment purposes
   D. An automatic violation of the HIPAA Privacy Rule

3. Janice is a well-informed patient. She knows that the Privacy Rule requires that individuals be able to:
   A. Be granted all requested restrictions on uses and disclosures of PHI
   B. Be granted all requested amendments to their PHI
   C. Receive a copy of the notice of privacy practices
   D. Receive free copies of their protected health information

4. Treatment of an individual can be conditioned on the signing of which of the following documents?
   A. Authorization
   B. Consent
   C. Notice of privacy practices
   D. Research waiver

5. Which of the following describes consents?
   A. They are the same as authorizations
   B. They expire 60 days after they are executed
   C. They are required under the HIPAA Privacy Rule
   D. They are not required to permit use and disclosure of PHI for treatment, payment, or operations

6. Disclosure in a facility's patient directory:
   A. Can occur only with the patient's written authorization
   B. Is automatic upon a patient's admission to a healthcare provider
   C. Is subject to the patient having had the opportunity to informally agree or object
   D. Can include all PHI in the patient's designated record set

7. An individual has a number of rights and prohibitions including:
   A. Revoking an authorization in writing
   B. Not being permitted to revoke a valid authorization
   C. Not being able to specify an expiration date on an authorization
   D. Restricting himself from being included in a facility directory

8. The Privacy Rule public interest and benefit purposes include provisions for all of the following except:
   A. Facilitating organ donations
   B. Information about decedents
   C. Information provided to law enforcement
   D. Information provided to a treating physician

9. Release of birth and death information to public health authorities:
   A. Is prohibited without patient consent
   B. Is prohibited without patient authorization
   C. Is a public interest and benefit disclosure that does not require patient authorization
   D. Requires both patient consent and authorization

10. An individual's authorization for research purposes:
    A. Is always required
    B. Is not required if the research involves a clinical trial
    C. Is never required
    D. Is not required if an IRB or privacy board alters or waives the authorization requirement

Breach Notification

As originally implemented, HIPAA required covered entities to mitigate (lessen the harmful effect) of the wrongful use or disclosure of PHI as much as possible. However, notification to the individual was optional (Rinehart-Thompson 2013). This changed with ARRA, which defined a breach.

ARRA also added **breach notification** requirements that specify victims of breaches be notified and, depending on the number of individuals affected, the federal government and media outlets also be notified. HIPAA-covered entities and BAs are subject to HHS-issued regulations, and noncovered entities and non-BAs (including PHR vendors) are subject to regulations issued by the **Federal Trade Commission (FTC)**. The FTC is a federal agency that promotes consumer protection.

Definition of Breach under ARRA

A **breach** is an "unauthorized acquisition, access, use or disclosure of PHI that compromises the security or privacy of such information" (ARRA 2009). There are three exceptions to the breach definition:

- Unintentional acquisitions made in good faith and within the scope of authority;
- Disclosures where the recipient would not reasonably be able to retain the information; and
- Disclosures by a person authorized to access PHI to another authorized person at the covered entity or BA (ARRA 2009).

A breach should be presumed following an impermissible use or disclosure unless the covered entity or BA demonstrates a low probability that the PHI has been compromised (Rinehart-Thompson 2013).

Breach notification requirements only apply to unsecured PHI that technology has not made unusable, unreadable, or indecipherable to unauthorized persons (Rinehart-Thompson 2013). This PHI is considered to be most at-risk. Covered entities should have mechanisms in place to identify incidents that meet the breach definition and determine whether any exceptions apply. Further, per their agreements BAs must notify covered entities of breaches. Finally, all workforce members must be educated to notify the appropriate contact person within the covered entity when they learn of a breach so the required notifications can be made.

Notification Requirements

Breaches by covered entities and BAs (both are governed by HHS breach notification regulations) are deemed discovered when the breach is first known or reasonably should have been known. All individuals whose information has been breached must be notified without unreasonable delay, and not more than 60 days, by first-class mail or a faster method such as by telephone if there is the potential for imminent misuse. If 500 or more individuals are affected they must be individually notified immediately and media outlets must be used as a notification mechanism as well. The Secretary of HHS must specifically be notified of the breach (AHIMA 2009). All breaches affecting fewer than 500 people must be logged by the covered entity in an HHS online reporting system and submitted annually as a report not later than 60 days after the end of the calendar year (AHIMA 2009).

Individuals who are notified that their PHI has been breached must be given a description of what occurred (including date of breach and date that breach was discovered); the types of unsecured PHI that were involved (such as name, Social Security number, date of birth, home address, account number); steps that the individual may take to protect himself or herself; what the entity is doing to investigate, mitigate, and prevent future occurrences; and contact information for the individual to ask questions and receive updates.

Companion breach notification regulations by the FTC provide protection to individuals whose information has been breached by noncovered entities and non-BAs that are PHR vendors, third-party service providers of PHR vendors, or other non-HIPAA covered entities or BAs that are affiliated with PHR vendors (AHIMA 2009). In addition to notifying the individuals affected by the breach, these entities must also notify the FTC of the breach. Third-party PHR service providers shall notify the PHR vendor or entity of the breach. Other notification requirements, such as the content and nature of breach notices, parallel HHS requirements (AHIMA 2009).

Requirements Related to Marketing, Sale of Information, and Fundraising

The Privacy Rule defines marketing as communication about a product or service that encourages the recipient to purchase or use that product or service (45 CFR 164.501). PHI use or disclosure for marketing requires an authorization from the individual except in certain cases. Marketing activities that do not require authorization are those that:

- Occur face to face between the covered entity and the individual, or
- Concern a promotional gift of nominal value provided by the covered entity

Some activities look like marketing but do not meet the Privacy Rule's definition of marketing. As a result, no authorization is required for:

- Communications to describe health-related products and services provided by, or included in the plan of benefits of, the covered entity itself or a third party
- Communication for treatment of the individual
- Case management or care coordination for the individual, or to direct or recommend alternative treatments, therapies, healthcare providers, or care settings (45 CFR 164.501)

Per ARRA, unless a communication fits one of these categories, it is not a healthcare operation and authorization is required. Additionally, even the categories here are not healthcare operations if the covered entity was paid for making the communication. There are exceptions, however. If a communication describes a currently prescribed drug, if the payment was reasonable (and the covered entity made the communication and received an authorization from the recipient), or the communication was made by a BA on behalf of a covered entity and is consistent with a business associate agreement, then the communication will be considered a healthcare operation despite payment (AHIMA 2009). If the covered entity has received—or will receive—direct or indirect payment in exchange for making a communication to an outside entity, this must be prominently stated.

In addition, when the communication is directed toward a specific target audience (for example, not a broad spectrum or cross-section of patients), it must instruct individuals how to opt out of future communications.

If a covered entity uses PHI to target an individual or group based on health status or condition, it must determine that the product or service being marketed may benefit the health of the type of individual being targeted before it makes the communication. Then, the communication must explain why the individual has been targeted and how the product or service relates to his or her health.

Related to the concept of marketing is the sale of information. This is addressed specifically by ARRA, which prohibits a covered entity or BA from selling (receiving direct or indirect compensation) in exchange for an individual's PHI without that individual's authorization. The authorization must also state whether the individual permits the recipient of the PHI to further exchange the PHI for compensation. Exceptions to this prohibition include public health and research data, treatment, and healthcare operations to a BA pursuant to a business associate agreement, to an individual who is receiving a copy of his or her own PHI, and for other exchanges deemed by the Secretary of HHS to be permissible (AHIMA 2009).

For fundraising activities that benefit the covered entity, the covered entity may use or disclose to a BA or an institutionally related foundation, without authorization, demographic information and dates of healthcare provided to an individual. However, the covered entity must inform individuals in its notice of privacy practices that PHI may be used for this purpose. It must also include in its fundraising materials instructions on how to opt out of receiving materials in the future.

If a fundraising activity targets individuals based on diagnosis (for example, patients with kidney disease are solicited in a capital campaign for a new kidney dialysis center), prior authorization is required. Per ARRA, fundraising communications that meet the definition of healthcare operations must clearly and conspicuously provide the opportunity to opt out of future communications. This opt-out is a revocation of authorization (AHIMA 2009).

HIPAA Privacy Rule Administrative Requirements

HIPAA provides standards regarding administrative requirements that are important to the health information professional, including:

- Designation of a privacy officer and a contact person for receiving complaints
- Requirements for privacy training
- Requirements for establishing privacy safeguards for handling complaints
- Standards for policies and procedures and changes to policies and procedures

Designation of Privacy Officer

The Privacy Rule requires covered entities to designate an individual as a chief **privacy officer** to be responsible for privacy practices within the organization. This position is ideally suited to the background, knowledge, and skills of the health information professional because the role includes developing and implementing privacy policies and procedures, facilitating organizational privacy awareness, performing privacy risk assessments, maintaining appropriate forms, overseeing privacy training, participating in compliance monitoring of BAs, ensuring that patient rights are protected, maintaining knowledge of applicable laws and accreditation standards, and communicating with the Office for Civil Rights (OCR) and other entities in compliance reviews and investigations of alleged privacy violations (AHIMA 2015).

Additionally, the covered entity must designate a person or office as the responsible party for receiving initial complaints about alleged privacy violations. This individual must be able to provide further information about matters covered by the entity's notice of privacy practices.

Privacy Training

Every member of the covered entity's workforce must be trained in PHI policies and procedures to include maintaining the privacy of patient information, upholding individual rights guaranteed by the Privacy Rule, and reporting alleged breaches and other Privacy Rule violations. Each new employee must be trained within a reasonable period of time after joining the workforce. When material changes are made to policies or procedures regarding privacy, employees must receive additional training. It is also recommended that refresher training be provided to all workforce members at least annually.

Further, the covered entity must maintain documentation showing that privacy training has occurred. Although not required, a signed acknowledgment of training by each workforce member is helpful to show compliance. It is also recommended that training be conducted for new employees, but as a refresher for all workforce members at least annually.

Privacy Safeguards

A covered entity must have safeguards and mechanisms in place to protect the privacy of PHI. This includes appropriate administrative, technical, and physical safeguards. These safeguards should work hand in hand with those specified in the HIPAA Privacy Rule. (Chapter 10 contains additional information on HIPAA security regulations.)

Standards for Policies and Procedures

The covered entity must implement policies and procedures to ensure compliance with the Privacy Rule. This process includes an ongoing review of privacy policies and procedures and ensuring that all policy changes are consistent with changes in the privacy and security regulations. Any regulatory changes that materially affect the covered entity's notice of privacy practices must be reflected in the notice; thus the notice may have to be updated. All revisions must be noted in the policies, procedures, or notice of privacy practices. Health information professionals are ideally qualified for developing and overseeing policies and procedures.

Enforcement of Federal Privacy Legislation and Rules

Per ARRA, legal responsibility for HIPAA privacy *and* security violations is not limited to covered entities. Employees or other individuals can be individually prosecuted. Civil and criminal penalties also apply to both BAs and covered entities.

Penalties

ARRA/HITECH established tiered penalties, with a range of $100 to $50,000 per violation for unknowing violations; $1,000 to $50,000 per violation if due to reasonable cause; $10,000 to $50,000 per violation for willful neglect that was corrected; and $50,000 per violation for willful neglect that was uncorrected. The nature and extent of both the violation and the harm determine the amount assessed within each statutory range. A method for compensating individuals harmed by HIPAA and ARRA provisions is to be recommended.

Legal Action by State Attorneys General

ARRA/HITECH also grants state attorneys general the ability to bring civil actions in federal district court on behalf of residents believed to have been negatively affected by a HIPAA violation. The OCR offered training to all state attorneys general in 2011. Topics included an introduction to the Privacy and Security Rules, investigative techniques to identify and prosecute alleged violations, a review of the relationship between HIPAA and state law, OCR's enforcement role, the roles and responsibilities of state attorneys general under both HIPAA and ARRA/HITECH, and available resources (HHS 2011b).

Audits

HIPAA enforcement does not occur solely based on complaints, as it did in the past (AHIMA 2009). Unannounced audits by OCR to detect Privacy and Security Rule violations are mandated for covered entities and BAs under ARRA/HITECH. Audits determine whether comprehensive policies and procedures are in place and whether they have been implemented to comply with the Privacy and Security Rules.

Release of Information

The release of information process has long been central to the health information professional's responsibilities. **Release of information (ROI)** is the process of providing PHI access to individuals or entities that are deemed to be authorized to either receive or review it (Brodnik and Sharp 2012).

Protecting the security and privacy of patient information is one of a healthcare organization's top priorities, and the HIM department is usually responsible for determining appropriate access to and ROI from patient health records. For example, ROI may take the form of a patient's request to mail copies of his or her records to a healthcare provider.

The ROI Function

The management of the ROI function includes the following steps:

1. *Enter the request in the ROI database*: Generally, information such as patient name, date of birth, health record number, name of requester, address of requester, telephone number of requester, purpose of the request, and specific health record information requested is entered in the computer. Figure 9.5 is an example of a computer screen used for entering ROI data.

2. *Determine the validity of authorization*: The HIM professional will compare the authorization form signed by the patient with organizational requirements for authorization to determine the validity of the authorization form. The organization's requirements are based on state and federal (for example, HIPAA) regulations. Certain

types of information such as substance abuse treatment records, behavioral health records, and HIV records require that specific components be included in the authorization form per state and federal regulations. If the request is valid, the HIM professional proceeds to the next step. If the authorization is invalid, the problem with the authorization is noted in the ROI database and it is returned to the requester with an explanation.

3. *Verify the patient's identity*: The HIM professional must verify that the patient has been a patient at the facility. This is done by comparing the information on the authorization form with information in the master patient index. The patient's name, date of birth, Social Security number, address, and phone number are used to verify the identity of the patient whose record is requested. The patient's signature in the health record is compared with the patient's signature on the authorization for release of information form.

4. *Process the request*: The record is retrieved and only the information authorized for release is copied and released.

Figure 9.5 ROI database screen

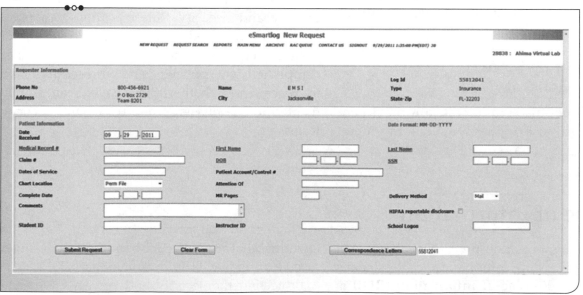

Source: AHIMA Virtual Lab HealthPort eSmart.

To comply with HIPAA, a healthcare organization must maintain a record that accounts for all disclosures from the health record.

ROI may also be a response to a subpoena duces tecum (discussed in chapter 8). It is necessary to verify that the subpoena is valid and the requested information can be released to the court in compliance with applicable state or federal law. In response to subpoenas, a representative from the HIM department may appear in person in court or at a deposition and give sworn testimony as to the health record's authenticity.

The ROI function has grown immensely in the past decade, due in part to HIPAA. Staffing has increased in some departments to address this growth. Other HIM departments outsource ROI to companies that specialize in this function. This may be done to keep pace with requests or to eliminate backlogs. Even with outsourcing, however, the HIM department remains ultimately responsible for ensuring that proper practices are followed and all laws are followed.

ROI Quality Control

Quality control in ROI includes both productivity (that is, turnaround time) and accuracy (namely, information released appropriately). The HIM department receives a high volume of requests and must prioritize the processing of ROI. Continuity of care requests are processed before other types of requests to align with the mission of most healthcare organizations. Turnaround time standards are established by the department. Productivity standards must be established in order to meet the expected turnaround time of various requests. With these standards, the average turnaround times for release of information may be tracked and delays in responding to requests for information may be addressed. While productivity information may be collected manually, electronic systems offer tools for data manipulation and can provide individual production statistics, departmental request volumes, and information regarding request turnaround times. The accuracy of ROI must also be monitored. The following examples illustrate how the timeliness and accuracy of ROI can be monitored.

To monitor timeliness, the date a request is received and the date that copies are sent are entered into an ROI database. This information can be used to generate a report that will determine whether the records are being sent in a timely manner.

To monitor accuracy of ROI, a sample of authorization is checked to verify authorization validity and to ensure compliance with federal and state regulations. A validation of the appropriate records released is also conducted. The error rate (or, alternatively, the accuracy rate) can be determined and compared against a set standard (Cerrato and Roberts 2013).

Authorizations

Authorizations have long been a key component of the release of information process, used as a tool to document and validate the legal use and disclosure of health information. While HIPAA generally requires authorization for the use and disclosure of PHI and specifies situations where authorization is not required (discussed earlier in this chapter), it also specifies requirements for a valid authorization form. Elements of the authorization form, such as patient name and signature, dates of service to be released, and names of the entities both disclosing and receiving the information, are well established in health information practice. However, with the passage of HIPAA many established health information practices have also become legal requirements.

Valid Authorization

The HIPAA Privacy Rule provides specific parameters regarding the content required for a valid authorization. Under the Privacy Rule, an authorization must be written in plain language. A valid authorization is one that contains at least the following elements:

- A description of the information to be used or disclosed that identifies the information in a specific and meaningful fashion
- The name or other specific identification of the person(s), or class of persons, authorized to make the requested use or disclosure

- The name or other specific identification of the person(s), or class of persons, to whom the covered entity may make the requested use or disclosure

- An expiration date or event that relates to the individual or the purpose of the use or disclosure

- A statement of the individual's right to revoke the authorization in writing and the exceptions to the right to revoke, together with a description of how the individual may revoke

- A statement that information used or disclosed pursuant to the authorization may be subject to redisclosure (subsequent release of information) by the recipient and no longer protected by this rule

- Signature of the individual and date

- When the authorization is signed by a personal representative of the individual, a description of the representative's authority to act for the individual (45 CFR 164.508(c))

An authorization is considered invalid when any one of the following defects exists:

- The expiration date has passed or the expiration event is known by the covered entity to have occurred.

- The authorization has not been filled out completely.

- The authorization is known by the covered entity to have been revoked.

- The authorization lacks a required element (for example, appropriate signature).

- The authorization violates the compound authorization requirements, if applicable.

- Any material information in the authorization is known by the covered entity to be false (45 CFR 164.508(b)).

Health information professionals must also ensure the validity of an authorization by confirming that the patient or patient's personal representative actually signed the form (through signature comparisons), the person who signed the form is legally competent, and whether there is evidence that the authorization form was signed involuntarily or without the patient's knowledge (Brodnik and Sharp 2012).

Who Can Authorize Release

Legally competent individuals have the right to authorize or refuse to authorize the disclosure of their own health information. As noted previously in this chapter, HIPAA provides many exceptions to the authorization requirement. Additionally, there are situations where an individual is not deemed legally competent, and authority to authorize release of their health information resides with someone else. For example, by law (and with exceptions), minors are deemed legally incompetent and a personal representative (a parent or guardian) will provide the authorization. Adults may also be legally incompetent by virtue of a permanent disability (such as a developmental disability) or a temporary condition (for example, incompetent to stand trial until restored to competency). A legal guardian then acts to handle the matters of the incompetent individual, including authorizing the release of health information. Table 9.4 highlights authorization authority based on the type of individual whose health information is involved. Where highly sensitive information is involved, such as

Table 9.4 Authorization authority for disclosure of health information

	Permitted to authorize disclosure?	If no, who can authorize disclosure?
Legally competent adult	Yes	N/A
Legally incompetent adult (permanent)	No	Personal representative (for example, guardian)
Legally incompetent adult (temporary)	No	Personal representative (until competency is restored) (for example, guardian)
Minor	No	Personal representative (for example, parent or guardian)

behavioral health, substance abuse, HIV/AIDS, or genetic information, the same principles apply regarding who has the legal authority to authorize the release of information. However, legal requirements and best practices also dictate that individuals specifically designate their permission and awareness of the fact that highly sensitive information will be released.

Medical Identity Theft

Medical identity theft is a crime that challenges healthcare organizations and the health information profession. A type of healthcare fraud that includes both financial fraud and identity theft, it involves either (a) the inappropriate or unauthorized misrepresentation of one's identity (for example, the use of one's name and Social Security number) to obtain medical services or goods, or (b) the falsifying of claims for medical services in an attempt to obtain money (Dixon 2006). Regardless of the purpose, the individual's health information is either created under the wrong name or altered, leading to potentially deadly consequences. Medical identity theft does not include the inappropriate change of patient information if the patient's identity has not been assumed or abused by someone else. Likewise, using a patient's financial information to purchase nonmedical goods or service is not medical identity theft because there are financial, but not medical, consequences.

Medical identity theft can be internal or external. Internal medical identity theft is committed by insiders in an organization, such as clinical or administrative staff with access to vast amounts of patient information. Culprits ranging from individuals to sophisticated crime rings may infiltrate an organization to commit internal medical identity theft. External medical identity theft is committed by individuals outside an organization who assume a person's identity, perhaps to utilize the victim's health insurance benefits. As a result, medical information about the culprit is created under the victim's name, and information about the two individuals may be intertwined (Olenik et al. 2012). The addition of information about another patient in the victim's record can result in improper medical treatment. The World Privacy Forum suggests that internal crimes occur more frequently than external ones (Dixon 2006). Further, there is concern that the evolution of the electronic health record may assist culprits by granting them broad access to patient information.

Patient Verification

It is important to verify a patient's identity at the beginning of a healthcare encounter by requiring presentation of a driver's license, taking a photograph of the patient for future reference, or even using biometric identifiers such as fingerprints. However, there are two caveats. Patient verification does not hinder internal medical identity theft. Further, the measures listed rely on valid baseline patient verification. If the information the organization relies upon is the culprit's information (for example, photo, signature, or fingerprint), all future encounters will be based on fraudulent information, decreasing the chances of detecting the fraud or causing the organization to wrongfully identify the true patient as the culprit if he later presents to that organization for treatment. Measures to combat internal medical identity theft include performing background checks on new hires and contractors (Olenik et al. 2012). The collection of Social Security numbers and staff access to them should be limited. Electronic health record access and access to other business records should only be given to the extent that people need information to complete their jobs. Technical measures also include routinely monitoring access or attempted access through audit trails and using features such as screen savers and automatic logoffs.

Fair and Accurate Credit Transactions Act (FACTA)

The federal **Fair and Accurate Credit Transactions Act (FACTA)** requires financial institutions and creditors to develop and implement written identity theft programs that identify, detect, and respond to red flags that may signal the presence of identity theft. Although this law does not specifically address medical identity theft, many healthcare organizations meet the definition of creditor, which is anyone who meets one of the three following criteria:

- Obtains or uses consumer reports in connection with a credit transaction
- Furnishes information to consumer reporting agencies in connection with a credit transaction
- Advances funds to—or on behalf of— someone, except for funds for expenses incidental to a service provided by the creditor to that person

The law includes the **Red Flags Rule**, which consists of five categories of red flags that are used as triggers to alert the organization to a potential identity theft (16 CFR Part 681). The categories are:

- Alerts, notifications, or warnings from a consumer reporting agency
- Suspicious documents
- Suspicious personally identifying information such as a suspicious address
- Unusual use of, or suspicious activity relating to, a covered account
- Notices from customers, victims of identity theft, law enforcement authorities, or other businesses about possible identity theft in connection with an account (16 CFR Part 681)

In addition to mandated red flags, healthcare providers must act to prevent, detect, and mitigate activities that address both external and internal incidents. Employee awareness and training, and implementation of organization-wide policies and procedures, are important.

Patient Advocacy

Over time, the role of the HIM professional has evolved. It continually becomes more multifaceted. Today, it includes the role of patient advocate. As a patient advocate, the HIM professional is a steward of the patient's record, ensuring not only its integrity, but also that it is safeguarded in accordance with all applicable laws, policies and procedures, and industry best practices. However,

as the healthcare industry has placed increasing emphasis on patient-centered healthcare, patient empowerment, and health literacy, the role of the health information professional must also prioritize the patient to ensure that patients gain needed and legal access to their health records and have the tools to understand the information documented about them.

Compliance

Compliance is an industry concept that means to conform to applicable laws. A culture of compliance within an organization is critical. Healthcare is a heavily regulated industry and there are many healthcare-specific laws as well as relevant non–healthcare-specific laws with which healthcare organizations must comply (for example, fair labor

standards and environmental regulations). This chapter has focused on laws that regulate the privacy of patient information, most notably the HIPAA Privacy Rule. HIPAA compliance is critical to safeguard individuals' health information and preserve their dignity while, at the same time, avoiding penalties that are assessed as the result of noncompliance.

Check Your Understanding 9.4

Instructions: **Answer the following questions.**

1. The use or disclosure of PHI for marketing:
   A. Always requires written authorization from the patient
   B. Does not require written authorization for face-to-face communications with the individual
   C. Requires written authorization from the patient when products or services of nominal value are introduced
   D. Never requires written authorization from the patient

2. Mary's PHI has been breached. She must be informed of all of the following except:
   A. Who committed the breach
   D. Date the breach was discovered
   C. Types of unsecured PHI involved
   D. What she may do to protect herself

3. The privacy officer is responsible for all of the following except:
   A. Handling complaints about the covered entity's violations of the Privacy Rule
   B. Developing and implementing privacy policies and procedures
   C. Providing information about the covered entity's privacy practices
   D. Encrypting all electronic PHI

4. Which of the following is a characteristic of breach notification?
   A. It is only required when 500 or more individuals are affected
   B. It applies to both secured and unsecured PHI
   C. It applies when one person's PHI is breached
   D. It only applies when 20 or more individuals are affected

5. A valid authorization must contain all of the following except:
   A. A description of the information to be used or disclosed
   B. A signature and stamp by a notary
   C. A statement that the information being used or disclosed may be subject to redisclosure by the recipient
   D. An expiration date or event

6. Medical identity theft includes which of the following
   A. Using another person's name to obtain durable medical equipment
   B. Purchasing an EHR
   C. Purchasing surgical equipment
   D. Using another healthcare provider's national provider identifier to submit a claim

7. Per the Fair and Accurate Credit Transactions Act (FACTA), which of the following is not a red flag category?
   A. An account held by a person who is over 80 years old
   B. Warnings from a consumer reporting agency
   C. Unusual activity relating to a covered account
   D. Suspicious documents

8. With regard to training in PHI policies and procedures:
   A. Every member of the covered entity's workforce must be trained
   B. Only individuals employed by the covered entity must be trained
   C. Training only needs to occur when there are material changes to the policies and procedures
   D. Documentation of training is not required

9. As a general rule, which of the following is a legally competent individual?
   A. A minor with a developmental disability
   B. An adult with a developmental disability
   C. A minor without a developmental disability
   D. A minor's personal representative

10. Per HIPAA requirements regarding fundraising:
   A. Fundraising materials do not have to include opt-out instructions
   B. Prior authorization is only required if individuals are not targeted based on diagnosis
   C. Individuals must be informed in the notice of privacy practices that their information may be used for fundraising purposes
   D. Authorization is never required for fundraising solicitations

 ## Real-World Case 9.1

HIPAA privacy breaches are of great concern and they occur too frequently. In April 2015, Cornell Prescription Pharmacy (CPP) reached a settlement with OCR to pay $125,000 and implement a corrective action plan following the disposal of PHI pertaining to 1,610 patients in an unlocked container on the premises. The information had not been shredded. No policies and procedures had been implemented, and no training had been conducted (HHS 2015).

This case highlights the fact that simple nontechnical measures (for example, shredding or burning PHI) can avoid a breach. Further, the role of an effective privacy officer (in this case, to implement policies and procedures and provide workforce training) would have been to raise awareness among staff that likely would have prevented this incident from occurring.

The fact that CPP is a small pharmacy with a single location demonstrates that breaches and penalties resulting from breaches do not occur in large organizations only. Covered entities and business associates of all types and sizes can commit breaches and be penalized for them.

 ## Real-World Case 9.2

Ronnie Bogle, a resident of San Jose, California, is a medical identity theft victim. He discovered this when he was rejected for a credit card application. He learned that he had multiple pages of unpaid medical treatments, emergency room visits, and hospital stays from around the country, none of which were his. Still battling hospitals over unpaid bills more than five years after he discovered that he was a victim of this crime, it is noted that the intertwining of the perpetrator's and victim's medical information makes it much more difficult to undo than simple financial identity theft cases. Further, because medical identity theft involves a person's health profile, it cannot be quickly shut down as a credit card number can. In 2014, damages related to medical identity totaled $20 billion and affected 2.3 million Americans (Nguyen et al. 2014).

References

Amatayakul, M. 2003. HIPAA on the job: Another layer of regulations: Research under HIPAA. *Journal of AHIMA.* 74(1):16A–16D.

American Health Information Management Association. 2015. Sample (Chief) Privacy Officer Job Description. http://library.ahima.org/doc?oid=107672#.Vw_3FPkrLDc.

America Health Information Management Association. 2012. Mobile Device Security (Updated). *Journal of AHIMA.* 83(4):50–55.

American Health Information Management Association. 2009. Analysis of health care confidentiality, privacy, and security provisions of the American Recovery and Reinvestment Act of 2009, Public Law 111-5. http://library.ahima.org/PdfView?oid=91955.

American Recovery and Reinvestment Act of 2009. Title XIII: Health Information Technology, Subtitle D: Privacy, Part 1: Improved Privacy Provisions and Security Provisions, Sections 13401-13411.

Brodnik, M.S. 2012. Introduction to the Fundamentals of Law for Health Informatics and Information Management. Chapter 1 in *Fundamentals of Law for Health Informatics and Information Management.* Edited by M.S. Brodnik, L. A. Rinehart-Thompson, and R.B. Reynolds. Chicago: AHIMA.

Brodnik, M. and M. Sharp. 2012. Access, Use, and Disclosure/Release of Health Information. Chapter 12 in *Fundamentals of Law for Health Informatics and Information Management.* Edited by M.S. Brodnik, L.A. Rinehart-Thompson, and R.B. Reynolds. Chicago: AHIMA.

Cassidy, B. 2000. HIPAA on the job: Update on business partner/associate agreements. *Journal of AHIMA.* 71(10):16A–16D.

Cerrato, L. and J. Roberts. 2013. Health Information Functions. Chapter 7 in *Health Information Management Technology: An Applied Approach.* Edited by N. Sayles. Chicago: AHIMA.

Dixon, P. 2006 (May 3). Medical identity theft: The information crime that can kill you. *World Privacy Forum.* http://www.worldprivacyforum.org.

Federal Rules of Civil Procedure (FRCP) 26: Duty to disclose; general provisions governing discovery.

Klaver, J.C. 2012. Evidence. Chapter 4 in *Fundamentals of Law for Health Informatics and Information Management.* Edited by M.S. Brodnik, L. A. Rinehart-Thompson, and R.B. Reynolds. Chicago: AHIMA.

McClendon, K. and A. D. Rose. 2013 (Update). Notice of Privacy Practices (2013 update). AHIMA Practice Brief. http://bok.ahima.org/doc?oid=107006#.Vtn_b_krJQI.

Nguyen, V., D. Paredes, and S. Pham. 2015 (March 30). 2.3 Million Americans Victims of Medical Identity theft. NBC Bay Area Investigative Unit. http://www.nbcbayarea.com/investigations/23-Million-Americans-Victims-of-Medical-Identity-298070211.html.

Office of the National Coordinator for Health Information Technology (ONC). 2014. Healthit.gov.

Olenik, K., R. Reynolds, and L. Rinehart-Thompson, Laurie. 2012. Security Threats and Controls. Chapter 11 in *Fundamentals of Law for Health Informatics and Information Management.* Edited by M.S. Brodnik, L.A. Rinehart-Thompson, and R.B. Reynolds. Chicago: AHIMA.

Rinehart-Thompson, L.A. 2013. *Introduction to Health Information Privacy and Security.* Chicago: AHIMA.

Rinehart-Thompson, L.A. 2012. Civil Procedure. Chapter 3 in *Fundamentals of Law for Health Informatics and Information Management.* Edited by M.S. Brodnik, L.A. Rinehart-Thompson, and R.B. Reynolds. Chicago: AHIMA.

Rinehart-Thompson, L. and L. Harman. 2017. Privacy and Confidentiality. Chapter 3 in *Ethical Health Informatics: Challenges and Opportunities,* 3rd ed. Edited by L. Harman and J. Glover. Sudbury, MA: Jones and Bartlett.

US Department of Health and Human Services. 2015. HIPAA Settlement Highlights the Continuing Importance of Secure Disposal of Paper Medical Records. http://www.hhs.gov/ocr/privacy/hipaa/enforcement/examples/cornell/cornell-press-release.html.

US Department of Health and Human Services. 2011a (May). HIPAA Privacy Rule accounting of disclosures under the Health Information Technology for Economic and Clinical Health Act. 45 CFR Part 164. *Federal Register.* 76(104):31426–31449.

US Department of Health and Human Services. 2011b. HIPAA Enforcement Training for State Attorneys General. http://www.hhs.gov/ocr/privacy/hipaa/enforcement/sag/sagmoreinfo.html.

US Department of Health and Human Services. 2010 (July). Modifications to the HIPAA Privacy, Security, and Enforcement Rules under the Health Information Technology for Economic and Clinical Health Act; Proposed Rule. 45 CFR Parts 160 and 164. *Federal Register.* 75(134):40868–40924.

US Department of Health and Human Services. 2000. *Federal Register.* 65(250):82818.

Walsh, T. 2015. tw-Security. http://www.tw-security.com/.

5 USC § 552a: Privacy Act (1974).

16 CFR Part 681: Identity Theft Rules. 2012.

45 CFR 160.103: Definitions. 2006.

45 CFR 164.501: Definitions. 2006.

45 CFR 164.502(a)(1)(iii): Uses and disclosures of protected health information: general rules. 2006.

45 CFR 164.506(b): Consent for uses and disclosures permitted. 2006.

45 CFR 164.508: Uses and disclosures for which an authorization is required. 2006.

45 CFR 164.508(a): Authorizations for uses and disclosures. 2006.

45 CFR 164.508(b): Implementation specifications: General requirements. 2006.

45 CFR 164.508(c): Implementation specifications: Core elements and requirements. 2006.

45 CFR 164.510: Uses and disclosures requiring an opportunity for the individual to agree or to object. 2006.

45 CFR 164.510(b): Uses and disclosures for involvement in the individual's care and notification purposes. 2006.

45 CFR 164.512: Uses and disclosures for which an authorization or opportunity to agree or object is not required. 2006.

45 CFR 164.512(a): Uses and disclosures required by law. 2006.

45 CFR 164.512(b): Uses and disclosures for public health activities. 2006.

45 CFR 164.512(c): Disclosures about victims of abuse, neglect or domestic violence. 2006.

45 CFR 164.512(d): Uses and disclosures for health oversight activities. 2006.

45 CFR 164.512(e): Disclosures for judicial and administrative proceedings. 2006.

45 CFR 164.512(f): Disclosures for law enforcement purposes. 2006.

45 CFR 164.512(g): Uses and disclosures about decedents. 2006.

45 CFR 164.512(h): Uses and disclosures for cadaveric organ, eye or tissue donation purposes. 2006.

45 CFR 164.512(i): Uses and disclosures for research purposes. 2006.

45 CFR 164.512(j): Uses and disclosures to avert a serious threat to health or safety. 2006.

45 CFR 164.512(k): Uses and disclosures for specialized government functions. 2006.

45 CFR 164.512(l): Disclosures for workers' compensation. 2006.

45 CFR 164.514(e)(2): Implementation specification: Limited data set. 2006.

45 CFR 164.522(a)(1): Right of an individual to request restriction of uses and disclosures. 2006.

45 CFR 164.522(b)(1): Confidential communications requirements. 2006.

45 CFR 164.524: Access of individuals to protected health information. 2006.

45 CFR 164.526: Amendment of protected health information. 2006.

45 CFR 164.528: Accounting of disclosures of protected health information. 2006.

45 CFR 164.530(d)(1): Complaints to the covered entity. 2006.

10
Data Security

Laurie A. Rinehart-Thompson, JD, RHIA, CHP, FAHIMA

Learning Objectives

- Demonstrate the elements of a data security program
- Identify threats to the security of data
- Organize components of a security program
- Identify methods to safeguard data from inappropriate access
- Apply disaster planning and disaster recovery mechanisms to a situation where data availability has been disrupted
- Identify the primary components of the security provisions of the Health Insurance Portability and Accountability Act and extensions by the HITECH Act and American Recovery and Reinvestment Act
- Demonstrate methods to detect inappropriate access or attempted inappropriate access to data

Key Terms

Access control
Access safeguards
Administrative safeguards
American Recovery and Reinvestment Act (ARRA)
Application control
Application safeguards
Audit control
Audit trail
Authentication
Authorization
Biometrics
Business continuity plan
Context-based access control (CBAC)
Contingency plan

Cryptography
Data availability
Data consistency
Data definition
Data dictionary
Data integrity
Data security
Decryption
Digital certificates
Digital signatures
Disaster recovery plan
Edit check
Emergency mode of operations
Encryption
External threats
Firewall

HIPAA Security Rule
Impact analysis
Implementation specifications
Incident
Incident detection
Information Technology Asset Disposition (ITAD)
Internal threats
Intrusion detection
Intrusion detection system (IDS)
Likelihood determination
Malware
Network controls
Password
Physical safeguards

Private key infrastructure
Public key infrastructure (PKI)
Risk analysis
Risk management
Role-based access control (RBAC)
Security

Security breach
Security program
Security threat
Single-key encryption
Single sign-on
Sniffers

Technical safeguards
Trigger events
Two-factor authentication
Unsecured electronic protected
    health information (e-PHI)
User-based access control (UBAC)

Chapter 9 described requirements for maintaining the privacy and confidentiality of data. This chapter examines the concept of data **security**, which encompasses measures and tools to safeguard data and the information systems on which they reside from unauthorized access, use, disclosure, disruption, modification, or destruction (NIST 2008). Maintaining data security begins with identification of the basic elements of a data security program.

An effective data **security program** embodies three basic elements to help prevent system or access errors from occurring:

- Protecting the privacy of data
- Ensuring the integrity of data
- Ensuring the availability of data

Protecting the Privacy of Data

Within the context of data security, protecting data privacy means defending or safeguarding access to information. This concept is at the center of information governance. In other words, only those individuals who need to know information should be authorized to access it. In the healthcare context, the protection of data privacy generally refers to patient-related data. However, the privacy of other information in the healthcare organization should

be protected as well. For example, the privacy of certain information about providers (physicians, nurses, therapists), employees, and the organization itself should be maintained. Information leaked to unauthorized individuals about providers, employees, or the organization can have as devastating an effect as information leaked about patients because it can affect an organization's reputation and lead to liability if such information was unlawfully disclosed.

Ensuring the Integrity of Data

Data integrity means that data are complete, accurate, consistent, and up-to-date so it is reliable. This concept is at the center of data governance. A discussion about data governance and information governance can be found in chapter 6. The Security and Privacy Rule defines data integrity as data that has not been altered or destroyed in an unauthorized manner (45 CFR 164.304). Ensuring the integrity of healthcare data is important because providers

use it in making decisions about patient care. For example, an error made while recording a prescribed drug dosage could cause the wrong amount of medication to be given to a patient, potentially resulting in significant injury or even death. Thus, one important aspect of any security program is the implementation of measures that protect the integrity of data.

Data integrity is critical. The Institute of Medicine (IOM) reports that correct medication administration increases when hospitals use well-designed, robust computerized drug ordering systems and barcodes, but poorly designed systems can create hazards (IOM 2011). Therefore, a security program is as much about ensuring data quality and accuracy as it is about maintaining informational privacy.

Ensuring the Availability of Data

Ensuring **data availability** means making sure the organization can depend on the information system to perform as expected, and to provide information when and where it is needed.

Problems with the retrieval of information can occur with both paper and electronic records. For example, paper records may be misfiled or used by another provider. Retrieval and access problems occur when the information system is unreliable or unavailable (for example, either planned or unplanned downtime). A good security program will ensure data are available seven days a week, 24 hours a day. To accomplish this effectively, organizations must have backup and downtime procedures in place. Data backup procedures may involve server redundancy or duplexing (duplicate information on one or more servers) and sending data to off-site contracted vendors or data warehouses for safe and secure storage and access. Backup policies and procedures for all systems (including non-networked computers such as laptops) should be in place. Backup procedures are necessary to ensure that the organization's business can continue in the event of a disruption. Backup procedures are also necessary to be in compliance with federal and state regulations.

Backup policies and procedures should specify what files and programs require backup, what type should be performed, how frequently it should occur, and how it is to be conducted. For example, a backup policy and procedure may require that all data, operating systems, and utility files be adequately and systematically backed up including all patches, fixes, and updates. The policy may also indicate whether a full procedure (all data at one time) or incremental procedure (partial data at one time) be performed and the frequency with which it should occur (such as daily or weekly).

Records should be kept of what is backed up and where the back-up data is maintained. Copies of backup media and records of backups should be stored at a secure off-site location. This action is taken so that if a disaster such as a fire or flood occurs at the main site, backup copies will be unaffected. There are many companies that specialize in digital off-site storage.

Backed up media is only useful if it can be used in the event of an emergency. Therefore, regular tests of restoring data and software from backed up copies should be performed to ensure that they work in an emergency.

Systems have both planned and unplanned downtimes that affect system availability. For example, planned downtime may occur when system upgrades are scheduled. Unplanned downtime may occur due to an unforeseen disruption such as an electrical outage. In either case, protocols should be developed to maintain data availability to the greatest extent possible. These protocols should be part of the regular IT infrastructure and incorporated into the security program.

Every organization is subject to **security breaches**, or unauthorized data or system access, by people from both inside and outside the organization. It is essential to recognize the scope of data security needs of the organization and to develop a systematic and comprehensive program to deal with them. Security breaches also can occur through hardware or software failures and when an intruder hacks into the system. More often, however, they occur when an employee within an organization either accesses information without authorization or deliberately alters or destroys information. Therefore, an organization's security program must have protections in place to monitor its employees and to keep outsiders from harming or accessing information resources. Effective data security does not just happen. It requires planning, training, and the implementation of realistic policies and procedures that address both internal and external threats.

Data Security Threats

Before implementing a security program, it is important to understand the potential threats to **data security**. Threats from a number of sources can cause the loss of data privacy, and compromise data integrity or the availability of data. All threats can be categorized as either **internal threats** (threats that originate within an organization) or **external threats** (threats that originate outside an organization) (Rinehart-Thompson 2013). Both internal threats and external threats can be caused by people or by environmental and hardware and software factors.

Threats Caused by People

Humans are the greatest threat to electronic health information (Olenik et al. 2012). Threats to data security from people can be classified into five general categories:

- *Threats from insiders who make unintentional errors.* Examples include employees who accidentally make a typographical error, inadvertently delete files on a computer disk, or unknowingly disclose confidential information. Unintentional error is one of the major causes of security breaches.

- *Threats from insiders who abuse their access privileges to information.* Examples include employees who knowingly disclose information about a patient to individuals who do not have proper authorization; employees with access to computer files who purposefully snoop for information they do not need to perform their jobs; and employees who store information on a thumb or flash drive, remove it from the facility on a laptop or other storage device, and subsequently lose the device or have it stolen.

- *Threats from insiders who access information or computer systems for spite or profit.* Generally, such employees seek information to commit fraud or theft. Identity theft—stealing information from patients, their families, or other employees—is on the rise and can result in prosecution of those employees who obtained that information unlawfully.

- *Threats from intruders who attempt to access information or steal physical resources.* Individuals may physically come onto the organization's property to access information or steal equipment such as laptop computers or printers. They also may loiter in the organization's buildings hoping to access information from unprotected computer terminals or to read or take paper documents, computer disks, or other information.

- *Threats from vengeful employees or outsiders who mount attacks on the organization's information systems.* Disgruntled employees might destroy computer hardware or software, delete or change data, or enter data incorrectly into the computer system. Outsiders might mount attacks that can harm the organization's information resources. For example, malicious hackers can plant viruses in a computer system or break into telecommunications systems to degrade or disrupt system availability.

Four of the threats listed can involve an organization's employees. Therefore it is important for an organization to remain vigilant to ensure that their employees and others with routine access to patient data appropriately use this data.

Threats Caused by Environmental and Hardware or Software Factors

People are not the only threats to data security. Natural disasters such as earthquakes, tornadoes, floods, and hurricanes can demolish physical facilities and electrical utilities.

In 2005, Hurricane Katrina devastated coastal Louisiana, Mississippi, and neighboring states. New Orleans was hit hard and damage was significant particularly due to flood waters after the hurricane passed. Included in the loss of life and property was damage to medical practices and hospitals and their patient records. Many of the facilities and practices had paper records that were completely destroyed and those that did exist on computer hard drives were destroyed by winds, water, and other forces. Patient care was severely compromised because of lost records that contained vital patient information.

Further, a devastating tornado ripped through Joplin, Missouri, literally decimating St. John's Regional Medical Center with a direct hit. The winds were so powerful that items from the hospital, like medications, x-rays, and health records, were found in neighboring counties.

While this kind of devastation is not ordinary, organizations must protect themselves against the loss caused by environmental factors. Facilities in California and other earthquake-prone areas send backup information to vaults that are located many miles off-site, perhaps in a distant state, to assist in the recovery of data should an earthquake or other catastrophic event destroy on-site computer systems. Organizations that are not in areas prone to natural disasters must nonetheless consider threats that can occur anywhere, such as fire. To recover from the devastation caused by natural, organizations must have backup and recovery procedures in place both for paper and electronic health records and other important organizational data.

Other causes of security breaches are utility, software, and hardware failures. These include hardware breakdowns and software failures that cause information systems to shut down or malfunction unexpectedly. Examples include a hard-disk crash that destroys or corrupts data; a program code that does not execute properly and alters or destroys information; a failed, weak, or poorly configured firewall; and unsecured browsers.

Electrical outages and power surges also can cause problems. When an electrical outage occurs, information is unavailable to the end user. In addition, data might be corrupted or even lost. Power surges also can destroy or corrupt information. Thus, organizations must have the appropriate equipment to protect information systems from power surges and backup equipment to keep them running during an outage.

Yet another type of threat is a hardware or software malfunction. Security breaches may be introduced when new software or hardware is added to the system or when it is not correctly tested.

While malfunctions of various software applications can corrupt data, another type of threat is caused by intentional software intrusions known as malicious software or **malware**. These software applications can take over partial or full control of a computer and can compromise data security and corrupt both data and hard drives.

Examples of malware include the following.

- *Computer virus*: A program that reproduces itself and attaches itself to legitimate programs on a computer. A virus can be programmed to change or corrupt data. Frequently viruses can slow down the performance of a computer system.

- *Computer worm*: A program that copies itself and spreads throughout a network. Unlike a computer virus, a computer worm does not need to attach itself to a legitimate program. It can execute and run itself.

- *Trojan horse*: A program that gains unauthorized access to a computer and masquerades as a useful function. A Trojan horse virus is capable of compromising data by copying confidential files to unprotected areas of the computer system. Trojan horses may also copy and send themselves to e-mail addresses in a user's computer.

- *Spyware*: A computer program that tracks an individual's activity on a computer system. Cookies are a type of spyware. These programs can store authentication information such as an individual's password.

- *Backdoor programs*: A computer program that bypasses normal authentication processes and allows access to computer resources, such as programs, computer networks, or entire computer systems.

- *Rootkit*: A computer program designed to gain unauthorized access to a computer and assume control over the operating system and modify the operating system.

Malware usually gains access to computers via the Internet as attachments in e-mails or through browsing a website that installs the software after the user clicks on a popup window. To prevent the intrusion of malware, organizations establish antivirus policies and procedures that establish the use of antivirus software and specify: (1) what devices should be scanned, such as file servers, mail servers, desktop computers; (2) what programs, documents, and files should be scanned; (3) how often scans should be scheduled; (4) who is responsible for ensuring that scans are completed; and (5) what action should be taken when malware is detected. In addition, filters can be used to filter both incoming and outgoing e-mail so that malware is quarantined.

In addition to an antivirus policy, organizations should have security awareness policies and training that deal with prevention of and identification of malware in place.

Strategies for Minimizing Security Threats

The first and most fundamental strategy in minimizing security threats is to establish a secure organization that is responsible for managing all aspects of computer security. This involves appointing someone in the organization to coordinate the development of security policies and to make certain that they are followed. Generally, this individual is called the security officer or chief security officer (CSO).

In addition to appointing someone to the CSO position, the organization appoints an advisory or policy-making group. This group is called the information security committee or a similar title. It works with the CSO to evaluate the organization's security needs, establish a security program, develop associated policies and procedures including monitoring and sanction policies, and ensure that the policies are followed. The development and enforcement of sanction policies and procedures, which impose penalties, are important so employees understand the consequences for noncompliance with security and privacy rules.

The HIPAA Security Rule does not specify the roles and composition of an information security committee, but the responsibilities extend well beyond the protection of data and involve human resources, which typically assists in workforce clearances (that is, granting appropriate data access levels to individuals), employee termination procedures (for example, eliminating an employee's access to data immediately upon severance or notice of severance from the organization), and applications of sanctions to employees who violate established policies (Miaoulis 2011). Other roles include executive-level managers who should have a high-level understanding of the data security policies and procedures and approve security budgets. In addition, the health information management (HIM) director or designee should sit on the information security committee to assist in determining levels of access, authorization, and audit trail reviews. (Audit trails are discussed later in the chapter.) Other management positions involved in the information security committee are the chief information officer (CIO), information technology system directors, network engineers, and representatives from clinical departments (lab, nursing, pharmacy, radiology) as appropriate.

Once the appropriate people and committees are in place, the next step is to establish a data security program. The components of a data security program are described in the next section.

Check Your Understanding 10.1

Instructions: **Answer the following questions.**

1. An effective data security program embodies three basic elements. Which of the following is one of the elements discussed in this chapter?
   A. State-of-the-art hardware
   B. Quick retrieval
   C. Availability
   D. Anti-virus software

2. Which of the following is true of internal security threats?
   A. They are caused by people
   B. They are caused by disgruntled employees
   C. They originate within an organization
   D. They are natural disasters

3. Intentional software intrusions are also known as which of the following?
   A. Hackers
   B. Criminals
   C. Internal threats
   D. Malware

4. Which term is defined as data that is complete, accurate, consistent, and up-to-date?
   A. Availability
   B. Confidentiality
   C. Integrity
   D. Security

5. The categories of security threats by people demonstrate an organization's greatest potential liability group consists of:
   A. Patients
   B. Visitors
   C. Employees
   D. Hackers outside the organization

6. Which computer program can copy and run itself without attaching itself to a legitimate program?
   A. Computer worm
   B. Backdoor program
   C. Trojan horse
   D. Spyware

7. In what way might an organization's human resources department be involved in information security?
   A. Processing weekly payroll
   B. Assisting in workforce data access clearances
   C. Writing job descriptions
   D. Installing systems for employees to clock in

8. A healthcare organization's data privacy efforts should encompass
   A. Patient information only
   B. Employee information only
   C. Patient and organizational information only
   D. Patient, employee, and organizational information

9. Data backup policies and procedures may include
   A. Server redundancy
   B. Ensuring all data is maintained on-site
   C. Maintaining one copy of all data
   D. Avoiding the use of power generators

10. External security threats can be caused by which of the following?
    A. Employees who steal data during work time
    B. A facility's water pipes bursting
    C. Tornadoes
    D. The failure of a facility's software

Components of a Security Program

An effective security program should contain the following components:

- Employee awareness including ongoing education and training
- Risk management program
- Access safeguards
- Physical and administrative safeguards
- Software application safeguards
- Network safeguards
- Disaster planning and recovery
- Data quality control processes (Carlon 2013)

Each component will be discussed as it relates to the establishment of an organization's security program. Some of these same elements will also be discussed in relation to the provisions of the Security Rule later in this chapter.

Employee Awareness

As discussed previously, employees are often responsible for threats to data security. Consequently, employee awareness is a particularly important tool to reduce security breaches by wrongdoers (either intentional or unintentional) and to make witnesses cognizant of security breaches so they can recognize, respond to them, and report them appropriately.

The organization should offer a formal program that educates every new employee on the confidential nature of patient and organizational data.

The program should inform employees about the organization's security policies and the consequences of failing to comply with them. The organization should give each employee a copy of its security policies as they relate to the employee's job function. It also should require every employee to sign a yearly confidentiality statement. Finally, because data security is such an important part of everyone's job, employees should receive periodic and ongoing security reminders.

Included in the employee awareness program should be policies and procedures regarding mobile devices, the use of e-mail and faxed information, and appropriate and inappropriate use of social media.

Risk Management Program

Another strategy in protecting the organization's data is to establish a risk management program. **Risk management** encompasses the identification, evaluation and control of risks that are inherent in unexpected and inappropriate events (Klaver 2012). Healthcare entities must take steps to prevent, detect, and mitigate both external and internal incidents. A well-conceived risk management program can aid prevention, detection, and mitigation of security breaches including identity theft.

Risk Analysis

The Security Rule requires an organization to implement security measures that are sufficient to reduce risk and vulnerabilities, but it may use a flexible and reasonable approach to do so (45 CFR 164.308).

Risk management begins with a **risk analysis**. This includes identifying **security threats**. It also includes identifying vulnerabilities, which are weaknesses in an organization's operations of which a threat can take advantage (Rinehart-Thompson 2013). Finally, it includes a determination of how likely it is that any given threat may occur, and estimating the impact of a catastrophic event (Walsh 2011). In addition to threats and vulnerabilities, an organization should also identify how electronic protected health information (e-PHI) is created, managed, stored, and transmitted within the organization and whether vendors or consultants use or maintain e-PHI. Of increasing importance is the threat created by the ubiquitous use of mobile devices (phones, tablets, laptops, and so forth).

Once threats are identified, it is important for an organization to make a **likelihood determination**, which is an estimate of the probability of threats occurring, and an **impact analysis**, which is what the impact of threats on information assets might be. For example, an organization may be located in a region with frequent tornadoes (high likelihood). It is known that tornadoes can be extremely destructive (high impact). For this organization, then, it would make sense to implement expensive safeguards to protect and back up its information assets against tornadoes. If a threat is low likelihood and low impact (for example, a tornado on the Pacific Coast), expenditure of time and money to protect against the threat is not a wise use of resources. The organization must conduct this type of analysis on every identified threat—manmade, environmental, and those caused by hardware and software factors—in order to prioritize those that should be addressed first and to which resources should be allocated.

Not all information is of equal importance, so it is essential to determine the value of information to the organization and the consequences of its loss when establishing a risk management program. For example, what impact would a security breach have on quality of care, revenue, service, or organizational image? Identification of an organization's information assets includes an inventory of application software, hardware, networks, and other information assets. Once information assets have been identified, their value to the organization is determined. Value is determined based on a number of factors such as criticality of the asset in daily operations, degree of harm resulting if the asset is not available, legal and regulatory requirements, and loss of revenue should the asset be lost or damaged.

Incident Detection

Once possible threats and vulnerabilities are known, it is important to be able to detect whether a threat or incident or intrusion has occurred. An **incident** is an occurrence or an event. **Incident detection** methods should be used to identify both accidental and malicious events. Detection programs monitor the information systems for abnormalities or a series of events that might indicate that a security breach is occurring or has occurred. There are a variety of analytic detection tools and intrusion prevention systems used for this purpose.

Incident Response Plan and Procedures

Once a security incident has been identified, there must be a coordinated response to mitigate the incident. An incident response plan includes management procedures and responsibilities to ensure a quick response is effectively implemented for specific types of incidents. For example, in some instances the plan may call for a "watch and warn" response that includes monitoring and notification of an incident but takes no immediate action. In other instances a "repair and report" response may be instituted. This type of response may be used in the case of a virus attack. A third type of response may be "pursue and prosecute," which would include the monitoring of an attack, the minimization of the attack, the collection of evidence, and the involvement of a law enforcement agency. This last example might be used in instances of suspected identity theft. Under the Health Information Technology for Economic and Clinical Health (HITECH) Act, breach notification requirements provide for those situations when affected individuals must be notified about an information security breach affecting their protected health information (PHI).

The HIPAA Security Rule requires that security incidents be identified, reported to the appropriate persons, and documented. Responses to an incident include workforce notification, preserving evidence, mitigating harmful effects caused by the breach, and evaluating the incident as a part of the organization's risk management process (Rinehart-Thompson 2013).

Access Safeguards

Establishing **access safeguards** is a fundamental security strategy. Basically, this means being able to identify which employees should have access to what data. The general practice is that employees should have access only to data they need to do their respective jobs. For example, a registrar in the admitting office and a nurse would not have access to the same kinds of data. By establishing access safeguards, an organization is taking steps to lessen its vulnerabilities, although it cannot prevent them altogether because of the security threats that humans present.

Determining what data to make available to an employee usually involves identifying classes of information based on the employee's role in the organization. So the organization would determine what information a registrar, for example, would need to know to do his or her job. Subsequently, every individual who works as a registrar would have access to the same information.

Every role in the organization should be identified, along with the type of information required to perform it. This is **role-based access control (RBAC)** and is the one used most often in healthcare organizations. Additionally, **user-based access control (UBAC)** grants access based on a user's individual identity. For example, every employee in the quality improvement department could potentially have a different degree of access if they have unique responsibilities in that department. **Context-based access control (CBAC)** limits a user's access based not only on identity and role, but also on a person's location and time of access (Rinehart-Thompson 2013). For example, two respiratory therapists may be given the same access based on their identical roles. However, with CBAC access, their access will be further refined (and may differ) based on the units to which they are assigned and the respective shifts they work.

Access control is the restriction of access to information and information resources (such as computers) to only those who are authorized, by role or other means. For access control to be effective, mechanisms must be in place that restrict access. There are a number of access control mechanisms that can be used (discussed later in this chapter). However, the sophistication of the method used should correspond with the value of the information being protected. In other words, the more sensitive or valuable the information, the stronger the control mechanisms need to be. For example, access to information about patients in a behavioral health unit will only be granted to staff who work in that unit. Identification, authentication, and authorization are the foundation upon which access control mechanisms are based.

Identification

The basic building block of access control is identification of an individual. Usually identification is performed through the username or user number. Identification methods must be robust so that imposters cannot successfully pose as a legitimate user and enter a system illegitimately.

Authentication

The second element of access control is **authentication**. Authentication is the act of verifying a claim of identity. There are three different types of information that can be used for authentication—something you know, something you have, or something you are. These are described in the following sections.

Passwords Examples of *something you know* include such things as a personal identification number (PIN), a **password**, or your mother's maiden name. Passwords are frequently used in conjunction with username. Policies and procedures should be in place to ensure passwords cannot be easily compromised. For example, passwords should be of a specific length, include special characters and numbers, should be case sensitive, and should not be words that are included in a dictionary or related to the user's ID or personal information. For example, "password" and "12345" are weak yet popular passwords if they are allowed by the system in which they are used. Password policies should include mandatory changes of passwords at specified intervals. These types of restrictions help to limit the chance of an intruder guessing a password or using a program called a password cracker to identify passwords. To help increase security, many computer operating systems will lock out a user after a specified number of unsuccessful attempts to gain access to a computer system. In addition, password policies should prohibit users from sharing passwords or writing or displaying passwords. While passwords provide the least amount of security compared to other methods, if properly managed and used, they can be an effective security strategy.

Smart Cards and Tokens   Smart cards and token cards are examples of *something you have*. A smart card is a small plastic card with an embedded microchip that can store multiple identification factors for a specific user. Usually a smart card is used in combination with a user identification or password. A one-time password (OTP) token is a small electronic device programmed to generate and display new passwords at certain intervals. An OTP token is usually used in combination with user identification or a password. To access a system, a user puts in an identification code and the OTP token generates a one-time password that is displayed on the token.

Biometrics   *Something you are* refers to biometrics. Examples of **biometrics** include palm prints, fingerprints, voice prints, and retinal(eye) scans.

Two-Factor Authentication   Strong authentication requires providing information from two of the three different types of authentication information. For example, an individual provides something he knows and something he has. This is called **two-factor authentication**. Examples of two-factor authentication include the use of smart cards or tokens with user identification. Two-factor authentication is a stronger method of protecting data access than user identification with passwords. An example of two-factor identification is being used at Walt Disney World in Florida. Guests insert their park tickets and also have their index finger scanned.

Single Sign-On   **Single sign-on** allows login to many separate, although related, software systems. Single sign-on allows a user to log in one time and be able to access the many systems. This prevents the user from having to log in again for each of them.

Different systems have different requirements for usernames and passwords. This requires the single sign-on to translate and store the user name and password for all of the systems involved. When the user is finished, then single sign-off is used to log out of all of the systems with one action.

Authorization

The third element of access control is authorization. **Authorization** is a right or permission given to an individual to use a computer resource, such as a computer, or to use specific applications and access specific data. It is also a set of actions that gives permission to an individual to perform specific functions such as read, write, or execute tasks.

Authorization to use a computer system is usually addressed through identification and authentication, described previously. Authorization to use specific applications (for example, order entry, coding, and registration) and specific data would be different for different individuals in an organization. For example, employees in the admitting and registration department would not be given the same authorization to computers, programs, and data as nursing care employees.

Usually authorization is managed through special authorization software that uses various criteria to determine if an individual has authorization for access, sometimes referred to as an access control matrix. For example, authorization may be based on not only the individual's identity but also the individual's role (role-based) and physical location of the resource (that is, access to only certain computers), and time of day (context-based).

Systems may require verification that a human, not a computer, is accessing a website or storage portal. A Completely Automated Public Turing test to tell Computers and Humans Apart (CAPTCHA) requires the user to respond to a question that is assumed could not be answered by a machine. A typical example of a CAPTCHA is when access to a site requires the user to type in a string of characters that appears skewed or distorted.

Physical and Administrative Safeguards

Physical safeguards refer to the physical protection of information resources from physical damage, loss from natural or other disasters, and theft. This includes protection and monitoring of the workplace, computing facilities, and any type of hardware or supporting information system infrastructure such as wiring closets, cables, and telephone and data lines.

Equipment should be located in secure locations and protected from natural and environmental hazards and intrusion. Environmental hazards include such things as fire, floods, moisture, temperature variations, and loss of electricity. To protect from natural or environmental hazards, equipment should be housed in structurally sound and safe areas. There should be smoke and fire alarms, fire suppression systems, heat sensors, and appropriate monitored heating and cooling systems in place. Appropriate backup power sources such as uninterruptable power supply (UPS) devices or power generators should be available if a power outage occurs.

To protect from intrusion, there should be proper physical separation from the public. Doors, locks, audible alarms, and cameras should be installed to protect particularly sensitive areas such as data centers. Identification procedures should be in place; for example, the use of badges to identify employees. Processes should be established for logging in and out of computer equipment or media. For example, if a data disk or device is being

transported or removed from one location to another, there should be a sign-out and sign-in procedure to track access and removal. Furthermore, sign-in and sign-out logs should be in place to track access to sensitive areas such as data centers.

Backup and recovery procedures are also a part of physical security. Backup and recovery procedures should specifically include server, data, and network policies and procedures.

Provisions must also be made to protect workstations that are more exposed to the public. For example, locking devices can be used to prevent removal of computer equipment and other devices. Automatic logouts can be used to prevent access by unauthorized individuals. Laptops and other mobile devices such as personal digital assistants (PDAs) pose significant threats because they can be easily lost or stolen. Documentation of the custody of such devices must be addressed. One such method is maintaining a custody log that documents who has had custody of the device, the time period of custody, and what files and data were on the laptop during the custody period. Policies and procedures should be in place that cover laptop or mobile device use. Other security mechanisms such as two-factor authentication (discussed previously) and full disk encryption should be used. (Encryption is discussed later in this chapter.) Global positioning systems (GPS) can also be installed on laptops as well as systems to remotely locate a computer to retrieve and delete data from it, should a computer be lost or stolen. With these features, a computer can be located quickly and appropriate law enforcement officials notified.

In any security program, employee education is one of the best defenses for protection of data and computer resources. Training programs on data security should be conducted at least annually for all employees and cover applicable security responsibilities, policies, and procedures.

Administrative safeguards include policies and procedures that address the management of computer resources. For example, one such policy might direct users to log off the computer system when they are not using it or employ automatic logoffs after a period of inactivity. Other policies include password security (inappropriate sharing, minimum password requirements, changing the frequency of updating passwords, and failed log-in monitoring) and timely removal of terminated employee's system access. Another policy might prohibit employees from accessing the Internet for purposes that are not work related.

Finally, an organization should have a policy on **Information Technology Asset Disposition (ITAD)** that identifies how all data storage devices are destroyed and purged of data prior to repurposing or disposal.

Software Application Safeguards

Another security strategy is to implement **application safeguards**. These are controls contained in application software or computer programs to protect the security and integrity of information. One common **application control** is authentication, as previously described. Through the use of passwords, tokens or biometrics, a system keeps a record of end users' identifications and authentication mechanisms and then matches the authentication mechanism to each end user's privileges. This ensures that end users can access only the information they have permission to access.

Another application control is the **audit trail**. The audit trail is a software program that tracks every single access or attempted access of data in the computer system. It logs the name of the individual who accessed the data, terminal location or IP address, the date and time accessed, the type of data, and the action taken (for example, modifying, reading, or deleting data). Audit trails are usually examined by system administrators who use special analysis software to identify suspicious or abnormal system events or behavior. Because the audit trail maintains a complete log of system activity, it can also be used to help reconstruct how and when an adverse event or failure occurred. This information helps to identify ways to avoid similar problems in the future. Depending on the organization's policy, audit trails are reviewed periodically, on predetermined schedules or relative to highly sensitive information.

Yet another application control is the **edit check**. Edit checks help to ensure data integrity by allowing only reasonable and predetermined values to be entered into the computer. For example, a system using this feature would disallow an International Classification of Disease, Tenth Revision, Clinical Modification (ICD-10-CM) code that does not exist. Application controls are important because they are automatic checks that help preserve data confidentiality and integrity.

Network Safeguards

Another important strategy used to guard against security breaches is to implement network safeguards. All kinds of networks are used to transmit healthcare data today, and the data must be protected from intruders and corruption during transmission within and external to the organization. With the widespread use of the Internet, **network controls** also are essential to prevent the threat of hackers. The following are some common safeguards.

Firewalls

A **firewall** (also called a secure gateway) is a part of a computer system or network that is designed to block unauthorized access while permitting authorized communications. It is a software program or device that filters information and serves as a buffer between two networks, usually between a private (trusted) network like an intranet and a public (untrusted) network like the Internet. Firewalls allow internal users access to an external network while blocking malicious hackers from damaging internal systems. All messages entering or leaving the private network pass through the firewall, which examines and evaluates each message and blocks those that do not meet predefined security criteria. For example, an e-mail message that is believed to contain a Social Security number may be prohibited from leaving the private network. An e-mail believed to contain a virus may be prohibited from entering the private network. It may control the size of the file that is allowed through the firewall. A firewall is configured to permit, deny, encrypt, or decrypt computer traffic.

Cryptographic Technologies

Cryptography is a branch of mathematics that is based on the transformation of data by developing ciphers, which are codes that are to be kept secret. Cryptography is used as a tool for data security. Strong cryptography improves the security of information systems and their data. There are several types of cryptographic technologies. Cryptographic technology—such as encryption, digital signatures, and digital certificates—are used to protect information in a variety of situations. This includes protecting data when they are in storage (data at rest), on portable devices such as laptops and flash drives, and while they are being transmitted across networks. Three of these technologies used in healthcare are discussed as follows.

Encryption   **Encryption** is a method of encoding data, converting them to a jumble of unreadable scrambled characters and symbols as they are transmitted through a telecommunication network so that they are not understood by persons who do not have a key to transform the data into their original form. Data are usually encrypted using some type of algorithm. Upon receipt, data can only be decoded and restored back to their original readable form (**decryption**) by using a special algorithm. Encryption takes the message from one computer and encodes it in a form that only the receiving computer can decode.

One type of encryption is called **private key infrastructure**, or **single-key encryption**. In this method, two or more computers share the same secret key and that key is used to both encrypt and decrypt a message. However, the key must be kept secret. If it is compromised in any way, the security of the data is likely to be eliminated. Because the key that decodes the information is transmitted with the data, it could be intercepted (Rinehart-Thompson 2013). The best known secret key security is called the data encryption standard (DES) published by the National Institute of Standards and Technology (NIST).

A common encryption method used over the Internet is a system called Pretty Good Privacy (PGP) or **public key infrastructure (PKI)**. This method uses both a public and a private key, which form a key pair. The sending computer uses a key to encrypt the data and it gives a key to the recipient computer to decrypt the data. With this type of

system there is a registry of public keys, called a certificate authority. If one user wants to send an encrypted message to another, the registry is consulted and the receiving user's public key is used to encrypt the data. Only the recipient, who knows the private key, can decrypt the message into its original form.

Digital Signatures   A **digital signature** or digital signature scheme is a public key cryptography method that ensures that an electronic document such as an e-mail message or text file is authentic. This means that the receiver knows who created the document and is assured that the document has not been altered in any way since it was created.

In this method data are electronically signed by applying the sender's private key to the data. The digital signature can be stored or transmitted to the data. The signature can then be verified by the receiving party using the public key of the signer.

Digital signatures are sometimes confused with e-signatures. E-signature usually means a system for signing or authenticating electronic documents by entering a unique code or password that verifies the identity of the person and creates an individual signature on a document. E-signatures do not necessarily use cryptography.

Digital Certificates   **Digital certificates** are used to implement public key encryption on a large scale. A digital certificate is an electronic document that uses a digital signature to bind together a public key with an identity such as the name of a person or an organization, address, and so forth. The certificate can be used to verify that a public key belongs to an individual. An independent source called a certificate authority (CA) acts as the middleman who the sending and receiving computer trusts. It confirms that each computer is who it says it is and provides the public keys of each computer to the other.

Web Security Protocols

Transmission protocols also provide data security. Transport Layer Security (TLS) and its predecessor Secure Sockets Layer (SSL) are based on public key cryptography. These protocols are the most common protocols used to secure communications on the Internet between a web browser and a web server. Versions of these protocols can be used for almost any application but are frequently used for electronic mail, Internet faxing, instant messaging, e-commerce transactions, and voice communications over the Internet (VoIP).

These protocols allow authentication of the server. Once authentication of the server is established, secure communication can begin using symmetric encryption keys. The user's message is encrypted in the user's web browser using an encryption key from the host website. The message is then transported to the host website in encrypted format. Once received by the website, the message is decrypted.

Intrusion Detection Systems

Intrusion detection is the process of identifying attempts or actions to penetrate a system and gain unauthorized access. Intrusion detection can either be performed in real time or after the occurrence of an intrusion. The purpose of intrusion detection is to prevent the compromise of the confidentiality, integrity, or availability of a resource.

Intrusion detection can be performed manually or automatically. Manual intrusion detection might take place by examining log files, audit trails, or other evidence for signs of intrusions. A system that performs automated intrusion detection is called an **intrusion detection system (IDS)**. Procedures should be outlined in the organization's data security plan to determine what actions should be taken in response to a probable intrusion. For example, typical actions to be taken might include notification of appropriate individuals, generating an e-mail alert, and so on.

Disaster Planning and Recovery

As discussed, facilities have to prepare for emergencies such as natural disasters. Further, organizations must prepare both for events that cause minimal disruption (for example, short-term power outages) and for large-scale events such as tornadoes. A contingency plan and its component disaster recovery plan will guide an organi-

zation through undesirable nonroutine events. In healthcare organizations, the continuation of medical services to patients is the highest priority. An important element of medical services is the protection and continued availability of health information (Rinehart-Thompson 2013).

Disaster Planning

Disaster planning occurs through a **contingency plan**—a set of procedures, documented by the organization to be followed when responding to emergencies. It encompasses what an organization and its personnel need to do both during and after events that limit or prevent access to facilities and patient information. It typically includes policies and procedures to help the business continue operations during an unexpected shutdown or disaster. It also includes procedures the business can implement to restore its computer systems and resume normal operation after the disaster.

The contingency plan is based on information gathered during the risk assessment and analysis discussed previously. The risk assessment includes the probability that an unexpected shutdown will occur. Using this information, the contingency plan is developed based on the following steps:

1. Identifying the minimum allowable time for system disruption
2. Identifying alternatives for system continuation
3. Evaluating the cost and feasibility of each alternative
4. Developing procedures required for activating the plan (Johns 2008)

Disaster Recovery

An immediate component of a contingency plan is the **disaster recovery plan**, which addresses the resources, actions, tasks, and data necessary to restore those services identified as critical, as soon as possible, and to manage business recovery processes. The **business continuity plan** is a set of policies and procedures that directs the organization how to continue its business operations during a computer system shutdown. Similarly, an **emergency mode of operations** prescribes processes and controls to be followed until operations are fully restored. For health information, an important part of the disaster recovery plan is ensuring the availability and accuracy of data as soon as possible after a disaster. As described earlier in the chapter, ongoing data backup is critical for this reason. Restoring system integrity and ensuring that all data are recovered requires that all parts of the system be verified after the disaster has occurred. Usually one system or one component of a system is brought up at a time and processes are verified to ensure that they are working correctly. These processes are required by the HIPAA Security Rule.

A plan is only as good as its implementation. It must be tested periodically to ensure that all parts of the plan—from disaster identification to backup and recovery—work as expected (Johns 2008).

Data Quality Control Processes

Ensuring data quality is an essential part of any data security program. Responsibility for ensuring data quality is shared by many organization stakeholders. For example, data accuracy begins with any individual who enters or documents data or systems that capture and provide data such as intensive care unit monitoring systems. Monitoring and tracking systems that ensure data quality are part of a data security program.

Data availability, consistency, and definition are three data quality dimensions that are often addressed using computer tools. As described earlier, data availability means that the data are easily obtainable. Computer tools are used to monitor unscheduled computer downtime, determine why failures occurred, and provide data to help minimize future problems. **Data consistency**, a component of data integrity, means that data do not change no matter how often or in how many ways they are stored, processed, or displayed. Data values are consistent when the value of any given data element is the same across applications and systems. Procedures are usually developed to monitor data periodically to ensure that they are consistent as they move through computer processes or from one system to another.

Data definition is describing the data. Every data element should have a clear meaning and a range of acceptable values. Data definitions and their values are usually stored in a **data dictionary**, which is discussed in chapter 6.

 Check Your Understanding 10.2

Instructions: **Answer the following questions.**

1. Which of the following is a threat to data security?
   A. Cryptographic technologies
   B. People
   C. Intrusion detection systems
   D. Access controls

2. An HIM professional using her password can access and change data in the hospital's master patient index. A patient accounting representative, using his password, cannot perform the same function. Limiting the class of information and functions that can be performed by these two employees is managed by which of the following?
   A. Network controls
   B. Audit trails
   C. Administrative controls
   D. Access controls

3. Which of the following is the process that encodes material, converting it to scrambled data that must be decoded?
   A. An audit trail
   B. Encryption
   C. A password
   D. A physical safeguard

4. Training programs on data security should be conducted at least:
   A. Semi-annually
   B. Annually
   C. Every two years
   D. Quarterly

5. Password policies should do which of the following?
   A. Include mandatory scheduled password changes
   B. Permit password sharing only between good friends
   C. Require that passwords consist of numbers only
   D. Require that passwords be changed every 30 days

6. A firewall:
   A. Is an administrative safeguard
   B. Filters information between networks
   C. Only limits incoming information
   D. Only limits outgoing information

7. Which of the following is the identification of an organization's security threats and vulnerabilities?
   A. Risk analysis
   B. Likelihood determination
   C. Impact analysis
   D. Authentication

8. Which of the following is an example of an administrative safeguard?
   A. Placing heat sensors near computer equipment
   B. Writing a policy regarding automatic computer logoffs
   C. Locking data center doors
   D. Placing computer monitors to face away from public areas

9. Which of the following is the strongest type of authentication?
   A. Single-factor
   B. Biometric
   C. Two-factor
   D. Smart card

10. Which of the following is a software application safeguard?
    A. Firewall
    B. Impact analysis
    C. Edit check
    D. Contingency plan

Coordinated Security Program

How can the different threats to data security be managed in a coordinated security program? First, and most importantly, someone from inside the organization must be given responsibility for data security. This individual should be someone at the middle or senior management level. As mentioned earlier, he or she is frequently called the chief security officer (CSO). Figure 10.1 lists some of the CSO's functions.

When the data security program with policies and procedures is in place, the CSO is responsible for ensuring that everyone follows them. This is done using monitoring and evaluation systems, typically on an annual basis. Many organizations use outside

Figure 10.1 Common functions of the chief security officer

- Conduct strategic planning for information system security
- Develop a data and information systems security policy
- Develop data security and information systems procedures
- Manage confidentiality agreements for employees and contractors
- Create mechanisms to ensure that data security policies and procedures are followed
- Coordinate employee security training
- Monitor audit trails to identify security violations
- Conduct risk assessment of enterprise information systems
- Develop a business continuity plan

Source: Carlon 2013.

information systems auditing firms to conduct their security policy evaluations. In addition to the yearly audit, the CSO might establish procedures to audit and evaluate current processes randomly.

All data security policies and procedures should be reviewed and evaluated at least every year to make sure they are up-to-date and still relevant to the organization.

HIPAA Security Provisions

The Health Insurance Portability and Accountability Act (HIPAA) of 1996 includes provisions for insurance reform and administrative simplification. Included in the administrative simplification provisions was a requirement for setting standards to protect health information. The Department of Health and Human Services established the HIPAA Privacy Rule (discussed in chapter 9) and the HIPAA Security Rule (which will be discussed in this chapter). These standards apply to every health plan, healthcare clearinghouse, and healthcare provider processing financial or administrative transactions electronically. Additional changes to the Privacy and Security Rules were created as a result of the **American Recovery and Reinvestment Act (ARRA)**.

ARRA moved the enforcement for HIPAA security compliance from the Centers for Medicare and Medicaid Services' Office of Electronic Standards and Security to the Department of Health and Human Services Office for Civil Rights (OCR). The HITECH Act under ARRA mandated improved enforcement of the Privacy Rule

and Security Rule. Covered entities are subject to privacy and security audits if they are subject of a complaint or they experienced a high-profile incident, or via random audits. Enforcement of HIPAA security must be taken seriously by covered entities and others who must follow the HIPAA Security Rule. Penalties are severe.

Security Rule standards are grouped into five categories. These include:

- Administrative safeguards
- Physical safeguards
- Technical safeguards
- Organizational requirements
- Policies and procedures and documentation requirements

Essentially, the HIPAA security provisions follow the established best practices for the development and implementation of effective security policy. The requirements of the HIPAA Security Rule enforce the tenet of information governance, which is the protection of information and access by authorized individuals only.

General Rules

The General Rules provide the objective and scope for the **HIPAA Security Rule** as a whole. They specify that covered entities must develop a security program that includes a range of security safeguards to protect individually identifiable health information maintained or transmitted in electronic form. The General Rules include the following:

- Covered entities must demonstrate and document that they have done the following:
  - Ensure the confidentiality, integrity, and availability of all electronic protected health information (e-PHI) that is created, received, maintained, or transmitted by the covered entity
  - Protect e-PHI against any reasonably anticipated threats or hazards to the security or integrity of e-PHI
  - Protect e-PHI against any reasonable or anticipated uses or disclosure that are not permitted under the HIPAA Privacy Rule
  - Ensure compliance with HIPAA Security Rule by workforce members
- The Security Rule is flexible, scalable, and technology neutral. Regarding flexibility, HIPAA allows a covered entity to adopt security protection measures that are appropriate and reasonable for its organization. For example, security mechanisms will be more complex in a large healthcare organization than in a small group practice. In determining which security measures to use, the following must be taken into account:
  - Size, complexity, and capabilities of the covered entity
  - Technical infrastructure, hardware, and software capabilities
  - Security measure costs
  - Probability and criticality of the potential risks to e-PHI

Scalable means that the Security Rule is written so that it accommodates organizations of any size. Technology neutral means that specific technologies are not prescribed, allowing organizations to develop as their technological capabilities evolve (Rinehart-Thompson 2013).

- Standards: The General Rules specify which HIPAA Security Rule standards covered entities must comply with. Business associates, hybrid entities, and other related entities (discussed in chapter 9) are also required to comply with these standards.
- **Implementation specifications** define how standards are to be implemented. Implementation specifications are either required or addressable. Entities must apply all implementation specifications that are required. Addressable does not mean optional. For those implementation specifications that are labeled addressable, the covered entity must conduct a risk assessment and evaluate whether the specification is appropriate to its environment. After conducting a risk assessment, if the covered entity finds that the specification is not a reasonable and appropriate safeguard for its environment (for example, a small organization may decide not to encrypt PHI because it deems it too expensive to do so), then the covered entity must:

  1. Document why it is not reasonable and appropriate to implement the specification as written.
  2. Implement an equivalent alternative method if reasonable and appropriate.

- Maintenance: HIPAA requires covered entities and business associates to maintain their security measures. Maintenance requires review and modification, as needed, to comply with the provision of reasonable and appropriate protection of e-PHI (45 CFR 164.306).

Administrative Safeguards

Administrative safeguards, as introduced earlier in the chapter, are documented, formal practices to manage data security measures throughout the organization. They require the facility to establish a security management process similar to the concepts discussed earlier in this chapter.

The administrative safeguards detail how the security program should be managed from the organization's perspective. Policies and procedures should be written and formalized in a policy manual. The organization should issue a statement of its philosophy on data security. Further, it should outline data security authority and responsibilities throughout the organization. There are a number of ways that an organization can control the use of terminals, including user limitations such as maximum allowed login attempts, screen savers, and the timing out of terminals when a determined period of inactivity has been reached. Physically, terminals should be able to be locked when not in use, and an organization should maintain an inventory such that all terminals used within the organization can be identified.

The administrative safeguards include the following standards that must be implemented by covered entities:

- *Security management process:* An organization must have a defined security management process. This means that there is a process in place for creating, maintaining, and overseeing the development of security policies and procedures; identifying vulnerabilities and conducting risk analyses; establishing a risk management program; developing a sanction policy; and reviewing information system activity.

- *Assigned security responsibility:* Each covered entity must designate a security official who has been assigned security responsibility for the development and implementation of the policies and procedures required by the HIPAA Security Rule. Frequently, this individual is given the title of chief security officer (CSO) or security officer.

- *Workforce security:* The covered entity must ensure appropriate clearance procedures to grant access to individually identifiable information to workforce members who need to use e-PHI to perform their job duties and must maintain appropriate oversight of authorization and access. Likewise, covered entities must prevent access to information to those who do not need it and have clear procedures of access termination for employees who leave the organization. Sanction policies must also be in place.

- *Information access management:* This standard requires covered entities to implement a program of information access management. It includes specific policies and procedures to determine who should have access to what information.

- *Security awareness and training:* This standard requires entities to provide security training for all staff. They must address security reminders, detection and reporting of malicious software, login monitoring, and password management.

- *Security incident procedures:* This standard requires the implementation of policies and procedures to address security incidents, including responding to, reporting, and mitigating suspected or known incidents.

- *Contingency plan:* This standard requires the establishment and implementation of policies and procedures for responding to emergencies or failures in systems that contain e-PHI. It includes a data backup plan, disaster recovery plan, emergency mode of operation plan, testing and revision procedures, and applications and data criticality analysis to prioritize data and determine what must be maintained or restored first in an emergency.

- *Evaluation:* A periodic evaluation must be performed in response to environmental or operational changes affecting the security of e-PHI and appropriate improvements in policies and procedures should follow.

- *Business associate contracts:* This standard requires business associates to appropriately safeguard information in their possession and covered entities to receive satisfactory assurances that the business associates will do so (45 CFR 164.308).

Each of these standards contains required elements as well as those that are addressable.

Physical Safeguards

Physical safeguards include the protection of electronic systems from natural and environmental hazards and intrusion. They encompass related buildings and equipment. Physical safeguards consist of the following:

- *Facility access controls:* This includes establishing safeguards to prohibit the physical hardware and computer system itself from unauthorized access while ensuring that proper authorized access is allowed. Similar safeguards are also required to protect the computer system from catastrophic physical events (for example, fire, flooding, and electrical malfunctions).

- *Workstation use:* Policies and procedures must relate to workstations that access e-PHI and include proper functions to be performed, how they are to be performed, and the physical environment in which those workstations exist.

- *Workstation security:* Provisions under workstation security require that physical safeguards be implemented for workstations with access to e-PHI.

- *Device and media controls:* This standard requires the facility to specify proper receipt and removal of hardware and media with e-PHI and to address items as they move within an organization. The entity must also address procedures for removal or disposal including reuse or redeployment of electronic media, data backup, and the identity of persons accountable for the process. Information technology asset disposition (ITAD) policies are required under this standard. These policies should address end of life cycle hard drives, laptops, servers, and other media that have contained sensitive data. Because such equipment is often redeployed in an organization, all e-PHI and any other sensitive data must be removed. Before hard drives, servers, or laptops are disposed of, appropriate data destruction must be carried out (45 CFR 164.310).

Technical Safeguards

The **technical safeguards** consist of five broad categories. These provisions include those things that can be implemented from a technical standpoint using computer software. These provisions include:

- *Access controls:* The access controls standard requires implementation of technical procedures to control or limit access to health information. The procedures would be executed through some type of software program. This requirement ensures that individuals are given authorization to access only the data they need to perform their respective jobs. The implementation specifications include unique user identifications, emergency access procedures (for example, a break-the-glass capability that allows nonstandard access), automatic logoff after a predetermined period of workstation inactivity, and encryption and decryption, discussed earlier in the chapter.

- *Audit controls:* The **audit control** standard requires procedural mechanisms be implemented to record activity in systems that contain e-PHI and that the output be examined to determine appropriateness of access. Audit trails were discussed earlier in this chapter.

- *Integrity:* The data integrity standard requires covered entities to implement policies and procedures to protect e-PHI from being improperly altered or destroyed. In other words, this standard requires organizations to provide corroboration that their data have not been altered in an unauthorized manner. Data authentication can be substantiated through audit trails and system logs that track users who have accessed or modified data via unique identifiers.

- *Person or entity authentication:* This standard requires that those accessing e-PHI must be appropriately identified and authenticated as discussed earlier in this chapter.

- *Transmission security:* This standard requires the guarding of data against unauthorized access (interception) or improper modification without detection when they are in transit, whether via the open networks such as the Internet or private networks such as those internal to an organization. The two implementation specifications—integrity controls and encryption—are addressable. The Security Rule itself does not require encryption unless the organization deems it appropriate, but the security of e-PHI transmitted over public networks or communication systems must be accomplished. Data encryption that provides protection for data across transmission lines is important because eavesdropping is easily accomplished using devices called sniffers. **Sniffers** can be attached to networks for the purpose of diverting transmitted data. Protecting data during transmission is only one role of encryption. Data at rest can also be encrypted. Passwords stored in a database may also be encrypted. Thus, if a hacker breaks into the password database, the data will be unusable (45 CFR 164.312).

Organizational Requirements

This section includes just two standards—one addresses business associates and similar entities and the other addresses group health plan requirements.

- *Business associate or other contracts:* Covered entities must obtain a written contract with business associates or other entities (hybrid or other) who handle e-PHI. The written contract must stipulate that the business associate will implement HIPAA administrative, physical, and technical safeguards and procedures and documentation requirements that safeguard the confidentiality, integrity, and availability of the e-PHI that it creates, receives, maintains, or transmits on behalf of the covered entity. The contract must ensure that any agent, including a subcontractor, agrees to implement reasonable and appropriate safeguards. Specifically, HIPAA requires a business associate to report to the covered entity any security incident or breach of e-PHI of which it becomes aware. The covered entity must authorize termination of

the contract if it determines that the business associate has violated a material term of the contract.

- *Group health plan requirements:* Group health plans must ensure their plan documents provide that the plan sponsor (an entity that provides a health plan for its employees) will reasonably and appropriately safeguard e-PHI that is created, received, maintained, or transmitted by or to plan sponsors on behalf of the health plans (45 CFR 164.314).

Policies and Procedures and Documentation Requirements

The Security Rule requires that covered entities and business associates have policies and procedures and that they be documented in writing. Other information about any actions, assessments, or activities associated with the HIPAA Security Rule also must be in writing.

- *Policies and procedures:* Entities must implement reasonable and appropriate policies and procedures to comply with the HIPAA security standards, implementation specifications, and other requirements. Policies and procedures should be developed and implemented, taking into account the section on flexibility outlined in the rule.

- *Documentation:* Entities must maintain their security policies and procedures in writing (this includes electronic format). Any actions, assessments, or activities related to the HIPAA Security Rule also must be documented in writing. Documentation must be retained for six years from the date of its creation or the date when it last was in effect, whichever is later. It must be made available to those individuals responsible for implementing security procedures. Further, it must be reviewed periodically and updated as needed, in response to environmental or organizational changes that affect the security of e-PHI (45 CFR 164.316).

American Recovery and Reinvestment Act of 2009 Provisions

The HITECH Act, a portion of ARRA, broadened privacy and security provisions including greater individual rights and protections when third parties handle individually identifiable health information. These changes had a significant impact on the security provisions. (Chapter 9 addresses the HITECH changes affecting the privacy standards.)

The single most important change was the requirement that business associates of HIPAA-covered entities must comply with most of the same rules as covered entities. As noted in chapter 9, business associates (BAs) perform functions or activities on behalf of or for a covered entity that involve the use or disclosure of protected health information. Common BAs include consultants, billing companies, transcription companies, accounting firms, and law firms.

With the implementation of the ARRA, potential business associate liability increased. Business associates are now directly responsible for, and can now be held directly responsible for not complying with, the administrative, physical, and technical safeguards of the HIPAA Security Rule, as well as the policies and procedures and documentation requirements.

Another important change per the HITECH Act was defining breach and adding breach notification requirements. Breaches only apply to **unsecured e-PHI**, which is e-PHI that has not been made unusable, unreadable, or indecipherable to unauthorized persons (AHIMA 2013a). Thus, the need for encryption is clear. With regard to security, breach notification has implications for the protection of data in all phases:

- Data at rest—for example, data contained in databases, file systems, or flash drives
- Data in motion—for example, data moving through a network or wireless transmission
- Data in use—for example, data in the process of being created, retrieved, updated, or deleted
- Data disposed—for example, discarded paper records or recycled electronic media. It is critical to use appropriate data destruction methods to ensure disposed data cannot be read, retrieved, or reconstructed in any way (AHIMA 2009).

Forensics

With appropriate policies and procedures in place, it is the responsibility of the organization and its managers, directors, CSO, and employees with audit responsibilities to review access logs, audit trails, failed logins, and other reports generated to monitor compliance with the policies and procedures. These types of events are usually called **trigger events** and include employees viewing:

- Records of patients with the same last name or address of the employee
- VIP records (celebrities, board members, political figures)
- Records of those involved in high-profile events in the community

- Records with little or no activity for 120 days
- Other employee's records
- Files of minors
- Files of those treated for infectious diseases or sensitive diagnoses such as HIV/AIDS or sexually transmitted diseases
- Records of patients for which the viewing employee did not care
- Records of a spouse (without the same surname)
- Records of terminated employees
- Portions of records of a discipline not consistent with employee's expertise (AHIMA 2013b)

The organization should have specific policies and monitoring procedures in place to track employee's access via sign-ons and password and periodically audit all reports, especially when high-profile incidents occur or VIPs are treated. HIPAA does require a regular review of system activity such as monitoring new user access, reviewing system access by users in general, and testing the access of recently terminated employees to assure they have, in fact, been removed from access roles. There have been numerous cases where the hospital records of high-profile individuals have been inappropriately accessed by employees. These actions have led to discipline, including termination and fines, after audit trails revealed unauthorized access.

 Check Your Understanding 10.3

Instructions: **Answer the following questions.**

1. Which of the following is an example of a technical safeguard?
   A. A policy that states that passwords cannot be shared
   B. A policy that states that only authorized people can access the data center
   C. Locking the door of the data center
   D. Assigning passwords that limit access to computer-stored information

2. Covered entities must retain documentation of their security policies for at least:
   A. Six years
   B. Five years
   C. Two years
   D. Ten years

3. Which of the following is true regarding a coordinated security program?
   A. The CSO must hold a lower level position so as not to create controversy
   B. All security policies and procedures should be updated every six months
   C. This type of program should only be established if an organization has sufficient funds to support it
   D. Someone inside the organization must be responsible for data security

4. An employee views a patient's electronic health record. It is a trigger event if:
   A. The employee and patient have the same last name
   B. The patient was admitted through the emergency room
   C. The patient is over 89 years old
   D. A dietitian views a patient's nutrition care plan

5. The patient's address is the same in the master patient index, electronic health record, laboratory information system, and other systems. This means that the data values are consistent and therefore indicative of which of the following?
   A. Data availability
   B. Data accessibility
   C. Data privacy
   D. Data integrity

6. Which of the following provides the objective and scope for the HIPAA Security Rule as a whole?
   A. Administrative safeguards
   B. Documentation requirements
   C. General rules
   D. Physical safeguards

7. According to HIPAA standards, the designated individual responsible for data security:
   A. Must be identified by every covered entity
   B. Is only required in large facilities
   C. Is only required in hospitals
   D. Is not required in small physician office practices

8. The following type of data must be protected against breaches:
   A. Data at rest
   B. Only data at rest and data in motion
   C. Data disposed
   D. Data at rest, in motion, and disposed

9. If an implementation specification is addressable:
   A. It is optional
   B. If not implemented, the organization must document why it is not reasonable and appropriate to do so
   C. If not implemented, the organization does not have to account for its absence
   D. It must be carried out as written

10. According to American Recovery and Reinvestment Act revisions:
    A. No changes were made to the HIPAA standards
    B. Potential business associate liability was increased under HIPAA
    C. Business associate liability was decreased under HIPAA
    D. Breaches apply to both secured and unsecured PHI

Real-World Case 10.1

In 2014, the Department of Health and Human Services reported on its website a $4.8 million HIPAA settlement with New York and Presbyterian Hospital (NYP) and Columbia University following the 2010 breach of thousands of patients' e-PHI. A Columbia University physician, who was an attending physician at NYP, tried to deactivate a computer server that he owned on the network that contained NYP patient e-PHI. The e-PHI became accessible to the public on Internet search engines because technical safeguards were lacking. A patient's loved one found e-PHI about the patient on the Internet and filed a complaint.

In addition to the impermissible disclosure, both entities were noncompliant in other ways: (1) no attempts had been made to assure the server was secure; (2) a thorough risk analysis had never been completed that identified all systems able to access the e-PHI of NYP patients and therefore no plan to address potential threats and hazards existed; (3) no appropriate policies and procedures existed regarding authorizing access to its databases; and (4) they did not follow their own policies on information access management (HHS 2014).

This costly mistake, both monetarily and from a reputation standpoint, highlights the negative outcomes that can happen when both technical and administrative safeguards are not followed. It also emphasizes the importance of inventorying all systems and devices that can access an organization's e-PHI to address threats and an organization's vulnerabilities. This is not an easy task given the number of personal and mobile devices that access e-PHI, but it is critical.

Real-World Case 10.2

Riverside Health System in Virginia announced in 2014 that the e-PHI of nearly 1,000 patients was breached by a nurse who accessed Social Security numbers and EHRs. The violation was discovered during a random organizational audit. Riverside described its compliance program as robust with ongoing monitoring (McCann 2014). This case raises numerous issues; for example, the fact that humans present one of the greatest threats to data security. When this human threat is internal to the organization, it is heightened by the ability to access information in the course of doing business. The article did not describe what type of access was given to employees; however, a nurse role is likely to result in broad access. The inappropriate access had occurred over a four-year period, which raises the issue of monitoring adequacy. Nonetheless, monitoring was taking place. The nurse was terminated after the breach was discovered. When the perpetrator of the breach was identified, all electronic access for that person should have been terminated immediately as well.

References

American Health Information Management Association. 2013a. Analysis of Modifications to the HIPAA Privacy, Security, Enforcement, and Breach Notification Rules Under the Health Information Technology for Economic and Clinical Health Act and the Genetic Information Nondiscrimination Act; Other Modifications to the HIPAA Rules. http://library.ahima.org/PdfView?oid=106127.

American Health Information Management Association. 2013b. Privacy and security audits of electronic health information. *Journal of AHIMA.* 88(3):54–59. http://library.ahima.org/doc?oid=300276.

American Health Information Management Association. 2009. Analysis of the Interim Final Rule, August 24, 2009: Breach Notification for Unsecured Protected Health Information. http://library.ahima.org/PdfView?oid=100232.

Carlon, S. 2013. Information Security. Chapter 17 in *Health Information Management Technology: An Applied Approach.* Edited by N.B. Sayles. Chicago: AHIMA.

Institute of Medicine. 2011. Health IT and Patient Safety: Building Safer Systems for Better Care. Consensus Report. http://www.iom.edu/Reports/2011/Health-IT-and-Patient-Safety-Building-Safer-Systems-for-Better-Care.aspx.

Johns, M.L. 2008. Privacy and Security in Health Information. In *Electronic Health Records: A Guide for Clinicians and Administrators,* 2nd ed. Edited by J. Carter. Philadelphia: American College of Physicians.

Klaver, J.C. 2012. Risk Management and Quality Improvement. Chapter 14 in *Fundamentals of Law for Health Informatics and Information Management.* Edited by M.S. Brodnik, L.A. Rinehart-Thompson, and R.B. Reynolds. Chicago: AHIMA.

McCann, E. 2014 (January 2). 4-Year Long HIPAA Breach Uncovered. HealthITNews. http://www.healthcareitnews.com/news/four-year-long-hipaa-data-breach-discovered.

Miaoulis, W.M. 2011. *Preparing for a HIPAA Security Compliance Assessment.* Chicago: AHIMA.

National Institute of Standards and Technology (NIST). 2008. An Introductory Resource Guide for Implementing the Health Insurance Portability and Accountability Act (HIPAA) Security Rule. http://csrc.nist.gov/publications/nistpubs/800-66-Rev1/SP-800-66-Revision1.pdf.

Olenik, K., M. Brodnik, R. Reynolds, and L. Rinehart-Thompson. 2012. Security Threats and Controls. Chapter 11 in *Fundamentals of Law for Health Informatics and Information Management.* Edited by M.S. Brodnik, L.A. Rinehart-Thompson, and R.B. Reynolds. Chicago: AHIMA.

Public Law 104-91: Health Insurance Portability and Accountability Act of 1996. https://www.congress.gov/104/plaws/publ91/PLAW-104publ91.pdf.

Rinehart-Thompson, L.A. 2013. *Introduction to Health Information Privacy and Security.* Chicago: AHIMA.

US Department of Health and Human Services (HHS). 2014 (May 7). Data Breach Results in $4.8 million HIPAA Settlements. http://www.hhs.gov/news/press/2014pres/05/20140507b.html.

Walsh, T. 2011 (January). Practice Brief: Security Risk Analysis and Management: An Overview (updated). http://bok.ahima.org/doc?oid=300266#.VxEP7fkrK9I.

45 CFR 164.304: Security and privacy definitions. 2006.

45 CFR 164.306: Security standards: General rules. 2006.

45 CFR 164.308: Administrative safeguards. 2006.

45 CFR 164.310: Physical safeguards. 2006.

45 CFR 164.312: Technical safeguards. 2006.

45 CFR 164.314: Organizational requirements. 2006.

45 CFR 164.316: Policies and procedures and documentation requirements. 2006.

Part IV
Informatics, Analytics, and Data Use

11

Health Information Technologies

Margret K. Amatayakul, MBA, RHIA, CHPS, CPHIT, CPEHR, FHIMSS

Learning Objectives

- Demonstrate understanding of the scope of health information technology (health IT) and how it has evolved to its current state of implementation in hospitals, ambulatory care, and other settings
- Apply the systems development life cycle in the planning, selection, implementation, and ongoing management of health IT

- Utilize a systems approach to achieve systems integration so that health IT supports the national mission to improve health and healthcare, and reduce healthcare costs

Key Terms

Accredited Standards Committee X12 (ASC X12)
Adoption
Alert fatigue
American Recovery and Reinvestment Act (ARRA)
Analytics
Ancillary systems
Application service provider (ASP)
ASTM International
Auto-analyzer
Automated drug dispensing machines
Barcode medication administration record (BC-MAR)

Best of breed
Best of fit
Big data
Billing system
Biometrics
Business intelligence (BI)
Certificate authority
Certification
Change control program
Charge capture
Chart conversion
Chart tracking
Chief medical informatics officer (CMIO)
Claim

Claim attachment
Claims data
Claims status inquiry and response
Client/server system
Clinical data repository (CDR)
Clinical data warehouse (CDW)
Clinical decision support (CDS)
Clinical decision support system (CDSS)
Clinical Document Architecture (CDA)
Clinical documentation system
Clinical transformation
Closed-loop medication management

Cloud computing
Computerized provider order entry
 (CPOE)
CONNECT
Consent directive
Consent management systems
Consolidated Clinical Document
 Architecture (C-CDA)
Continuity of care document (CCD)
Continuity of care record (CCR)
Contraindication
Core measures
Data
Data conversion
Data dictionary
Data model
Data quality
Data Use and Reciprocal Support
 Agreement (DURSA)
Diagnostic studies
Digital certificate
Digital Imaging and Communica-
 tions in Medicine (DICOM)
Direct Project
Discrete reportable transcription
 (DRT)
Document imaging
Drug knowledge database
Due diligence
eHealth Exchange
Electronic clinical quality measures
 (eCQM)
Electronic health record (EHR)
Eligibility verification
Encoder
End user
e-Prescribing (e-Rx)
e-Prescribing for Controlled
 Substances (EPCS)
Evidence-based medicine
e-visits
Federal Health IT Strategic Plan
 2015–2020
Go-live
Health information exchange (HIE)
Health information organization
 (HIO)
Health Information Technology for
 Economic and Clinical Health
 (HITECH)
Health Insurance Portability and
 Accountability Act of 1996
 (HIPAA)

Health IT
Health Level Seven (HL7)
Health reform
Hospital information system (HIS)
Identity management
Identity matching algorithm
Identity proofing
Implementation
Information
Interface
Interoperability
Issues management
Kiosk
Knowledge
Laboratory information system
 (LIS)
Learning health system
Logical Observations, Identifiers,
 Names, and Codes (LOINC)
Meaningful Use
Meaningful Use (MU) program
Medical device integration
Medication five rights
Medication reconciliation
Message format standards
Metadata
National Council for Prescription
 Drug Programs (NCPDP)
National Drug Codes (NDC)
Natural language processing (NLP)
Nursing information system
Office of the National Coordinator
 (ONC) for Health Information
 Technology
Online analytical processing
 (OLAP)
Online transaction processing
 (OLTP)
Operating rules
Optimization
Opt in/opt out
Patient acuity staffing
Patient financial system (PFS)
Patient portal
Patient safety
Personal health record (PHR)
Personalized medicine
Pharmacy information system
Physician champion
Physician Quality Reporting
 System (PQRS)
Picture archiving and communica-
 tions system (PACS)

Point-of-care (POC)
 charting
Portals
Power user
Primary care physician (PCP)
Prior authorization
Protocol
Provider
Radio-frequency identification
 (RFID)
Radiology information system
 (RIS)
Record locator service (RLS)
Registration-Admission, Discharge,
 Transfer (R-ADT)
Registry
Remittance advice
Requirements specification
Results management
Revenue cycle management
 (RCM)
RxNorm
SCRIPT
Semantic interoperability
Shared Nationwide Interoperability
 Roadmap
SMART goals
Software as a Service (SaaS)
Source systems
Speech dictation
Steering committee
Storage management
Structured data
Sunsetting
System
System build
System configuration
System integration
Systems development life cycle
 (SDLC)
Telehealth
Template
Transaction
Two-factor authentication
Unintended consequence
Unstructured data
Use
Value
Value-based purchasing (VBP)
Vendor selection
Virtual private network (VPN)
Web services architecture (WSA)
Workstations on wheels (WOWs)

The **Federal Health IT Strategic Plan 2015–2020**, issued by the **Office of the National Coordinator (ONC) for Health Information Technology**, the agency within the federal government tasked to be a resource to the nation, describes a vision and mission for US use of health information technology (typically referenced by the federal government as health IT):

> Vision: High-quality care, lower costs, healthy population, and engaged people.
> Mission: Improve the health and well-being of individuals and communities through the use of technology and health information that is accessible when and where it matters most (ONC 2015a).

Prior to completion of the Federal Health IT Strategic Plan, the focus of federal government efforts in health IT was promoting use of the **electronic health record (EHR)** by organizations and providers. The **Health Information Technology for Economic and Clinical Health (HITECH)** component of the **American Recovery and Reinvestment Act (ARRA)** of 2009 provided eligible hospitals and professionals with financial incentives, in terms of healthcare payment adjustments, to make meaningful use of EHRs. This incentive program is commonly referred to as the **Meaningful Use (MU) program** and describes a qualified EHR as one that:

> includes patient demographic and clinical health information, such as medical history and problem lists; and has the capacity to provide clinical decision support, support physician order entry, capture and query information relevant to healthcare quality, and exchange electronic health information with and integrate such information from other sources (HealthIT.gov 2016).

As the vast majority of hospitals and healthcare professionals are expected to have implemented an EHR within their organizations, the MU program is expected to wind down starting in 2016. Beyond that, requirements for using an EHR may be incorporated in alternative payment models. Therefore, the Federal Health IT Strategic Plan focuses more broadly on outcomes of using health IT. The Federal Health IT Strategic Plan goals, shown in figure 11.1, illustrate how the nation's health IT infrastructure supports advancing patient-centered

Figure 11.1   Federal Health IT Strategic Plan 2015–2020

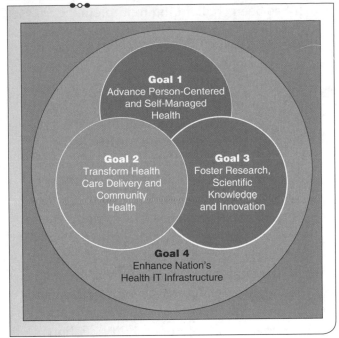

Source: ONC 2015a.

and self-managed health, transforming healthcare delivery and community health, and fostering research, scientific knowledge, and innovation (ONC 2015a).

The supporting health IT infrastructure envisioned by ONC was described in an earlier version of its strategic plan as one that supports collection, sharing, and use of health information. These principles remain important considerations for health IT:

- *Collection* emphasizes the importance of EHRs as a primary source of **data** (raw facts and figures) and **information** (facts and figures processed into usable form). The intent of the Federal Health IT Strategic Plan is to expand use of the EHR beyond hospitals and healthcare professionals to other providers—such as long-term care and behavioral health—potentially through allowance of the MU program to these providers.

- *Sharing* refers to the fact that the EHR, "has created a strong demand for the seamless sharing of information across technology systems, information platforms, location, provider, or other boundaries" (ONC 2015b). It has been challenging to implement EHRs. Typically they are costly and require significant workflow and process changes that impact healthcare professionals who have traditionally not used computers on the job. However, the goal of interoperability may be even more challenging than implementing EHRs. **Interoperability** is sharing information across EHRs and other health IT systems and the capability of different information systems and software applications to communicate and exchange data. A systems perspective (taking into account all systems) must be taken to achieve interoperability. **System** refers to all the components (technology, standards, people, policy, and process) that must work together to achieve a desired goal (interoperability). Following the release of the Federal Health IT Strategic Plan, the ONC published its **Shared Nationwide Interoperability Roadmap**, laying out a three stage vision for interoperability:

- o 2015–2017: Nationwide ability to send, receive, find, and use a common clinical data set
- o 2018–2020: Expand interoperable data, users, sophistication, and scale
- o 2021–2024: Broad-scale learning health system (ONC 2015c)
- *Use*, within the context of the Federal Health IT Strategic Plan, is linked to a number of subtle but powerful factors. These factors ultimately lead to the **learning health system**,

defined as "the alignment of science, informatics, incentives, and culture for continuous improvement and innovation, with best practices seamlessly embedded in the delivery process and new knowledge captured as an integral by-product of the delivery experience" (IOM 2011).

Dissemination of knowledge is stated as a goal in the Federal Health IT Strategic Plan. Knowledge is more than information; **knowledge** is the application of experience to information and provides value to information beyond only serving as evidence of actions taken. **Value** refers to the combination of quality and cost. For instance, when making a purchase it is desirable that what is purchased is of the highest possible quality at the lowest possible cost. The value in knowledge helps healthcare professionals learn from experience. In order to create knowledge, health IT needs to be used not only to collect and share information, but used in ways that will help professionals improve health, healthcare, and reduce costs. Health IT implies much more sophisticated forms of data and information management, processing, analysis, reporting, and presentation.

This chapter describes the scope of health IT, the importance of standards, and the need to take a systems approach to planning, selecting, implementing, and managing health IT so that the ultimate result meets the national vision and mission for healthcare and the goals for each **provider** (hospital, physician, nursing home, and others). Also discussed is the role health information management (HIM) professionals play in acquiring, implementing, gaining adoption, and optimizing use of health IT.

Health IT

The term **health IT** may be defined narrowly or broadly. Narrowly, health IT refers to computer hardware and software to enable collection and processing of data into useful information; as well as the communication and network technologies that enable data and information to be exchanged across various computers. More broadly, many use the term *health IT* to refer to all of the components just described in addition to the people, policy, and process elements that must be in place for healthcare professionals to learn how to use and make the most effective use of the hardware, software, communications, and network technologies. This broader definition may be referred to as a health information system or health IT system in order to convey the full scope of the system components.

Health information systems may also be considered narrowly or broadly. For example, a laboratory information system (LIS) would be one that includes:

- Hardware (computers, printers, laboratory devices)

- Software (computer programs designed to process requests for lab tests, produce specimen collection lists for hospitalized patients, produce labels for specimen container, and ultimately producing test results)

- Communications and network technologies (connections between a **computerized provider order entry system [CPOE]**, used by providers to enter orders for medications, lab tests, and other procedures, and the destination systems, such as pharmacy for medications, LIS for lab tests, billing system to capture charges for the medications and lab tests)

- Operational and cultural adaptations necessary to use the technologies in performing **diagnostic studies** on various specimens collected from patients and applying professional judgment in evaluating the quality of the data representing the results

- Policies and standards from the local organization in which the system is housed as well as accrediting and licensing bodies that must be followed for design of the technology and its use; policies and standards for LIS may include use of certain terminologies, such as the **Logical Observations, Identifiers, Names, and Codes (LOINC)**, which is mandated under the MU program to order and report lab results; as well as a policy that patients may have direct access to their test results, even prior to review by their ordering provider (per resent CLIA changes [*Federal Register* 2014])

- Workflow and process designs ensure the most efficient and effective use of the technology

It is almost impossible to describe any health information system without describing its broader reaches. In the past, the LIS required a lab technician to manually enter an order for a lab test into the system using a paper physician's order form, resulting in generated output in the form of a paper test result. Today that type of LIS is almost unheard of. An LIS not only receives an order for a lab test from a CPOE system, but communicates with other information systems. Some of these other information systems include a billing system that captures the charge for a lab test and the EHR that can alert the provider to availability of the new test result and plot a graph illustrating changes in test results over time. An LIS might also connect with a **barcode medication administration record (BC-MAR)** system. The BC-MAR is used by nurses to manage drug administration for patients and other procedures performed on the patient. If lab results may be impacted by medication the patient is receiving, the lab staff will want to know this in order to provide accurate lab test results.

An EHR system is large in scope. An EHR system not only supports physicians, nurses, and other healthcare professionals in their documentation and communication across the healthcare spectrum, but has connection points to many other applications in a healthcare organization. These connections are with other healthcare and related organizations, such as payers, public health departments, immunization registries, ambulance services, and many others. Healthcare organizations are also using health IT to connect with patients in multiple ways. Connections are available through **portals** (windows into information systems), personal health records (PHRs), personal medical devices, and **telehealth** services that assist in providing remote diagnosis and treatment.

There are many health IT systems and they are periodically updated and expanded. The following sections describe the current state of health IT systems and their scope—including source systems, core EHR applications, specialty systems and automated medical devices, supporting infrastructure, and connectivity systems.

Current State of Health IT Systems

Health IT systems for lab, pharmacy, and other ancillary services are not new, but they may be new to physicians and nurses. The degree to which technology is used by providers varies significantly.

As a result, the systems are continuously being updated and improved to meet the needs of the new users. The following terms and definitions help describe the various stages in which these new systems exist in healthcare.

- **Implementation** refers to technology having been installed, configured to meet the basic requirements of the healthcare organization, and demonstrated to users. **End users**, are those persons who will use the system for their daily processes.

- **Use** refers to the fact that those who are supposed to apply the technology to their daily work have been trained and are starting to apply the technology at a simple level. For example, nurses may enter data into nurse assessment **templates** (a guide for documentation) and document medication administration using the technology. Physicians may review lab results and other information collected by other healthcare professionals. Often "use" has not addressed workflow and process changes that enable intended users to seamlessly incorporate the technology into their everyday operations. Simple usage should begin immediately after implementation, but within a few months users should be moving to adoption.

- **Meaningful Use** is a term used by the federal government for the program designed to incentivize use of EHRs. The term *meaningful* was chosen to reflect the purposeful desire to get to the next stage of use beyond simply using the EHR as a search tool. There are two components to the MU program. One component is managed by the ONC and specifies the functionality an EHR must have in order for meaningful users to earn the incentives. The other component of the MU program is specified by CMS (CMS 2014). CMS establishes the percent of use that providers should make of the EHR. The MU program was implemented in three stages. Stage 1 was initiated in 2011; stage 2 in 2014; and stage 3 is expected to be implemented in 2016. Each stage requires increasing usage of the EHR. In stage 1, physicians were only required to use CPOE for

30 percent of medication orders in order for an eligible hospital to qualify for the incentives. This functionality, however, required clinical decision support that exceeded merely entry and retrieval of information to supplying alerts and reminders, such as indicating that a certain drug is contraindicated for a patient with an allergy. While many hospitals and physician practices have made progress toward true meaningful use, others are still at the "use" stage. Some hospitals completed stage 1 of the incentives by physicians using scribes or had enough users only in the emergency services department that they could meet stage 1. Still others found that physicians entered orders into CPOE, but ignored the clinical decision support alerts and reminders. Many hospitals and physicians are struggling with stage 2, and there are calls for delays of stage 3.

- **Adoption** is a term frequently associated with the intent of MU. Adoption reflects that the organization has implemented all of the major components of technology, although there may be some available technology that is more specialized, costly, and time-consuming to implement that has not yet been implemented. Adoption also requires that users rely on the technology to enter and retrieve most information, and where decision support is included to use it when appropriate. Adoption demonstrates effective integration into the daily routines of healthcare. Adoption of the system indicates it generally takes no more time to use than paper charting systems, and generally yields greater value to the user than paper systems.

- **Optimization** is the final state that demonstrates not only effective adoption for all routine operations, but also an understanding and appropriate use of the technology's features. At this state, the healthcare organization implements all or almost all of the technology available to it. The user who optimizes health IT has fully embraced the standard vocabularies supported by the technology, pays attention to alerts and reminders, is able to generate various reports that meet unique needs, frequently tailors the system to further take advantage of documentation aids, and may be considered a power user. **Power users** are able to use technology to significantly improve their productivity, and will likely see healthcare quality and cost benefits as well.

Scope of Health IT Systems

Health IT systems have evolved over time to automate more functions. The diagram in figure 11.2 summarizes health IT in the sequence in which it has generally been adopted within hospitals. This sequence started with various administrative and financial systems, then departmental clinical systems, and subsequently some or all specialty clinical systems and "smart" peripherals (such as clinical equipment with electronic components that support information collection and alerting). Collectively these are referred to as source systems because they are the source of basic data for the core clinical systems that comprise the EHR. Core clinical systems are currently being implemented with the help of the MU program. Both source systems and core clinical systems are applications that depend on supporting infrastructure technology (various types of databases) and connectivity systems (networks and standards). Following the diagram in figure 11.2, each of the major types of health IT is summarized in more depth and variations between hospitals and physician practices are described.

Source Systems

Source systems supply the EHR and other applications with data. Source systems may include administrative, financial, ancillary, or departmental systems.

Administrative and Financial Applications

Administrative and financial applications are usually managed by specific departments, such as admitting, patient financial services, and health information management. However, they are not considered departmental systems because they manage patient-specific data needed for all other applications, and do not process data that aid in management of the departments as do ancillary, or departmental, systems (see the next section). Administrative and financial systems, collectively and especially in the past when they were stand-alone systems, may be called **hospital information systems (HIS)** and include registration-admission, discharge transfer (R-ADT) systems, patient financial systems (PFS), and form creation systems.

Registration, Admission, Discharge, Transfer Systems Registration-admission, discharge, transfer (R-ADT) systems in hospitals that register patients for inpatient admission or outpatient services. The R-ADT captures demographic and insurance data and supplies this data to other applications as needed. An R-ADT system tracks when patients are admitted to the hospital and opens an account for them. It also tracks all transfers within the hospital, such as a patient moving from an intensive care unit to a cardiac unit. Finally, the R-ADT system closes the account when a patient is discharged. Other related systems keep track of the organization's census, track who is in what bed, compile length of stay information, and maintain a master person index. In a physician practice, an equivalent system might be a practice management system (PMS), although in some cases only a scheduling system is in place.

Patient Financial Systems Patient financial systems (PFSs), frequently called **billing systems** in a physician practice, serve to check patient insurance eligibility, capture charges for services (including codes for office visits), compile and send claims to payers, receive payment and remittance advice, and identify unpaid or denied claims for which other collections efforts must be made. The term **revenue cycle management (RCM)** refers to the entire process of creating, submitting, analyzing, and obtaining payment for healthcare services (Wolfskill 2014). RCM starts within a provider setting with:

- **Eligibility verification** systems to determine if a patient's health plan will provide reimbursement for services to be performed

Figure 11.2 Overview of health IT systems in hospitals

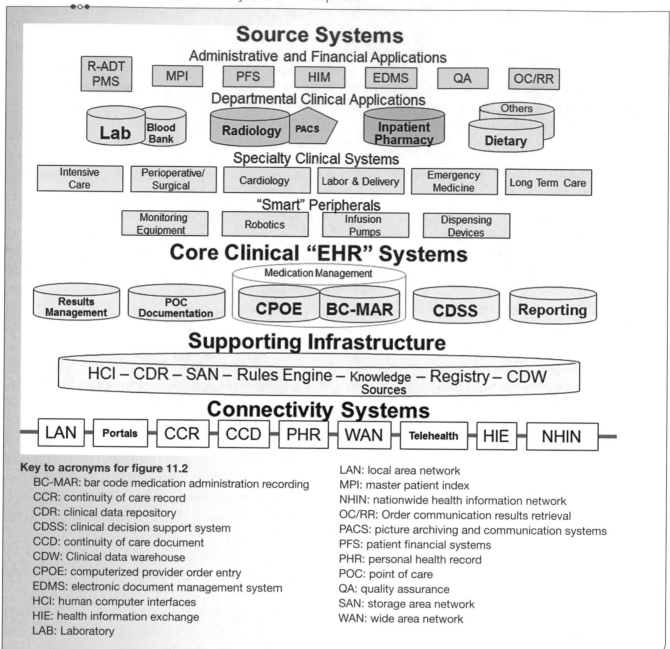

© Margret\A Consulting, LLC. Reprinted with permission.

- **Prior-authorization** management systems where a health plan requires review and approval of a procedure prior to its performance

- **Claim** generation systems for reimbursement by a health plan (and patient) that relies on **charge capture** to collect information about services performed from **ancillary** systems and **encoder** systems (ancillary systems support the department in which they exist, for example pharmacy and support coding diagnoses and procedures)

- **Claim attachment** systems where additional information required by the health plan to pay the claim can be sent electronically

- **Claims status inquiry and response** to determine if a health plan has a claim pending for additional information or is processing the claim, posting **remittance advice** reflecting actual fees reimbursed to the organization, and receiving electronic funds transfers (EFTs)

- Other related processes, such as collections and bad debt management (more information on revenue management is found in chapter 15)

The RCM functions that exchange data between providers and health plans are referred to as **transactions**. Each transaction, such as eligibility verification, claims status inquiry, and so forth have mandated standards for use under the **Health Insurance Portability and Accountability Act of 1996 (HIPAA)**. The standards specify in what format the data should be compiled and what data should be exchanged with payers. These standards are developed by the American National Standards Institute **Accredited Standards Committee (ASC) X12**. For example, the ASC X12 837 standard specifies the data and format for a claim. These standards have been or are being updated and revised under the Affordable Care Act (ACA).

ACA also requires standard **operating rules** that further explain the standards so their use is consistent across health plans. ACA also imposes penalties for health plan noncompliance with the standards.

Increasingly there is the need to integrate **claims data** (that is, data documented for reimbursement purposes) with clinical data (namely, the data documented about a patient's health status and treatment) for **health reform** initiatives or steps taken to make major policy changes in how providers are reimbursed for healthcare services. Figure 11.3 illustrates the HIPAA transactions and their relationship to clinical data. As claims data and clinical data (found in chapter 4) are used together, healthcare quality and cost improvements can be made. This integration of financial and clinical data provides **business intelligence (BI)** that helps support business decisions by both the administrative and clinical leadership of healthcare organizations. For example, with more complete clinical information available at the time of admission, a hospital is better able to verify a patient's eligibility for health plan benefits so that it is not faced with a denied claim later. Information that shows the hospital how many and what type of

Figure 11.3 HIPAA transactions and clinical data

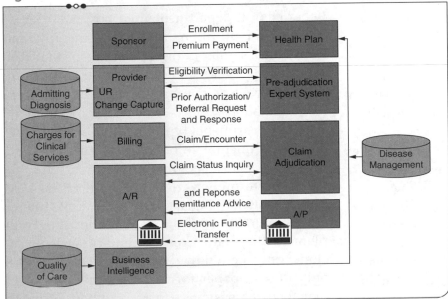

patients are readmitted within 30 days of discharge for the same condition is another example of BI that will enable a hospital to take proactive measures to monitor these patients more closely after discharge. Physicians are also starting to use integrated claims data and clinical data to evaluate medical necessity for repeat diagnostic studies, assess the value of costly drugs, and help patients make informed decisions about their healthcare options.

Form Creation Systems   Form creation systems automate some of the authorization, consent, advance directive, and other administrative forms used to manage healthcare administrative processes (McKenzie and Karnstedt 2010). These systems provide information to the patient, capture an electronic signature from the patient, and supply the patient with a copy of the signed form if requested.

Departmental Clinical Applications

Clinical departmental applications, also called ancillary systems, serve primarily to manage the department in which they exist, while at the same time providing key clinical data for the EHR. There are three main departmental systems that are necessary for an EHR to function in a hospital. These include:

- **Laboratory information system (LIS):** The LIS will receive an order for a lab test; generate a work list for specimen collection, labels for specimen containers, and accession numbers to track specimens; retrieve results from an **auto-analyzer** (device that analyzes the specimen); perform quality control; maintain an inventory of equipment and supplies needed to perform lab tests; and manage information on departmental staffing and costs. The LIS supplies the lab results to the user, either as a paper copy printout or an electronic print file, which is **structured data** (data able to be processed by the computer) to an EHR. The blood-banking and clinical pathology systems are often separate from the LIS.

- **Radiology information system (RIS):** The RIS performs functions similar to LIS—receiving an order for a procedure; scheduling it; notifying hospital personnel or the patient if performed as an outpatient; tracking the performance of the procedure and its output (that is, images in analog or digital form); tracking preparation of the report; performing quality control; maintaining an inventory of equipment and supplies; and managing departmental staffing and budget.

- **Pharmacy information system:** This system receives an order for a drug in a hospital; aids the hospital's pharmacist in checking for **contraindications** (situations that should be avoided as potentially harmful to a patient); directs staff in compounding any drugs requiring special preparation; assists in dispensing the drug in the appropriate dose and for the appropriate route of administration; maintains inventory (documenting medications in stock using the **National Drug Code**, the terminology maintained by the Food and Drug Administration [FDA] for use in identifying FDA-approved drugs); supports staffing and budgeting; and performs other departmental operations.

Other clinical departments in a hospital, such as dietary and nutrition, respiratory therapy, and others have similar information systems that both receive orders and supply results (or services) to users, as well as manage the respective department operations.

HIM departments typically do not have a specific departmental information system because they have many separate applications that assist in performing various different tasks. HIM departments may manage some of the RCM systems and support some of the applications that complement the EHR. Complementary systems include **document imaging** systems (when used only to scan paper forms), electronic document management systems (EDMS) (when scanning is coupled with workflow tools), or electronic document/content management (ED/CM) systems (when both documents and content in an XML-tagged document are managed). Also included are **speech dictation** systems that enable speech to be translated directly into a narrative document and **discrete reportable transcription (DRT)** systems that combine speech dictation with **natural language processing** (namely, the ability for a computer to not only convert speech to words, but apply sophisticated computer processes to put the words into appropriate context). Today, DRT is able to populate predefined templates with structured data. **Consent management systems** are those that help maintain patient preferences about who may have access to their health information. These may also be managed by the HIM or nursing department. HIM applications vary by how far the organization has progressed in implementing its EHR applications. For example, if the organization continues to retain some paper charts, the HIM department may have a **chart tracking** system to manage location of paper records (or to manage archived paper records). Many organizations do not yet have all the EHR components to be completely paperless, so they must complement the EHR components with systems to support dictation, transcription, and electronic document and content management. There are HIM functions unable to be fully addressed by the EHR. As a result, chart deficiency systems, release of information systems, coding and abstracting systems, and others are not likely to disappear soon, although there may be a transition in how they are managed. Additional information on HIM systems can be found in chapter 3.

Core Clinical EHR Systems

There are generally five main systems or applications necessary to consider when an organization has an EHR. These include the following and are illustrated in figure 11.4, a closer look at a section of figure 11.2.

- Results management
- Point-of-care (POC) clinical documentation
- Medication management encompassing CPOE and BC-MAR systems
- Clinical decision support (CDS) systems (CDSS) (of various types)
- Analytics and reporting

EHR applications include the basic functionality required for earning incentives in the MU program and, in some cases, additional functionality. The MU program requires that the EHR technology have **certification** from an ONC-designated certifying body that the EHR meets all of the basic functionality criteria for the MU program. The criteria, however, do not require all possible EHR functionality be available. For example, MU does not include support for charge capture despite the fact that most provider organizations find this an essential part of their EHR.

It is also important to note there are some variations in the core EHR applications as they are used in a hospital or physician practice. One main difference is that in a hospital, the EHR applications are often implemented separately; whereas in a physician practice EHR applications tend to be more integrated. Other differences are noted as each of these core applications is described more fully in the following sections.

Figure 11.4 Core clinical EHR systems

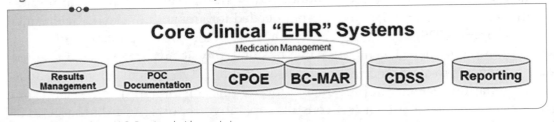

Results Management

Results management is an EHR application that enables diagnostic study results (primarily lab results) to be both reviewed in a report format and the data within the reports to be processed. Users can compare, trend, and graph the results. Depending on their level of sophistication, results management systems may also be able to compare lab results with other clinical data. For example, a graphic display could depict lab results as a function of medications administered, or be compared with a patient's vital signs. Lab results can also be extracted directly from the EHR for use in quality measurement studies, clinical research, and BI systems, not requiring a person to manually abstract the results from the chart; in order for a healthcare organization to have results management, all data to be processed must be in structured format and ideally stored together in one data repository.

The importance of results management cannot be emphasized enough. 70 percent of the ability to reach a diagnosis for a patient depends on lab results (Wians 2009). Similarly, as medications are increasingly powerful in their impact on the human body, monitoring vital signs and lab results in association with medication administration is critical to appropriate medication management. In fact, in one widely-publicized hospital incident, not taking appropriate action when a baby's blood test showed an extraordinarily high level of sodium chloride from a drug being administered resulted in the baby's death (Graham and Dizikes 2011).

Clinical Documentation

Another EHR component is clinical documentation. These systems are also called **point-of-care (POC) charting** systems. The intent of these applications is to inform the user what data needs to be recorded for the patient and to use that data to supply clinical decision support (CDS), including alerts and reminders, at the time when the clinician is able to be most responsive to alerts and reminders. **Clinical documentation systems** supply templates to the user to be completed primarily via point-and-click, drop-down, type-ahead, and

other data-entry tools. Usually the EHR has a library of templates. The user may choose the appropriate template, or the user's dashboard may display the appropriate template based on the user's profile as indicated via the login or by the patient's admitting diagnosis or chief complaint at the time of a physician's office visit. Some templates are extremely sophisticated and as the user enters data, the data fields adjust accordingly. As a simple example, a template for conducting a history and physical exam for a male patient would not display data fields applicable to females. If the system detects that the patient's condition involves heart disease, additional data fields may be displayed for associated signs, symptoms, and potential complications. The result is structured data that the computer is essentially processing into clinical documentation. More information on dashboards can be found in chapter 12.

Clinical documentation systems in a hospital may include only those for nursing staff, such as for nurse admission assessments, nursing problem lists, nurses' notes, vital signs (which may also be captured directly from patient monitoring systems), intake and output records, and other nursing documentation. Medication administration is also a nursing documentation requirement, but such systems are typically grouped under medication management systems, as described in the next section.

A **nursing information system** is generally considered a departmental system, not a clinical documentation system. Similar to LIS, RIS, and pharmacy information systems, a nursing information system manages the nursing department, including staffing, credentialing, training, budgeting, and other managerial functions. Clinical data may be combined with department operations data in a nursing information system to provide **patient acuity staffing** levels, where the number of staff needed for any shift or day is determined by how acutely ill the current patients are.

In a hospital, physicians are expected to document orders in a CPOE system. Physician documentation of the history and physical exam, consults, operative reports, and discharge summary in a hospital are still largely dictated and electronically fed as an image into the EHR. Progress notes may be handwritten and scanned into the EHR. The problem list may be handwritten, although is increasingly managed through a combination of sources including the admission order for the admitting diagnosis and directly from a drop-down menu for discharge diagnoses and procedures. The MU program requires that the problem list ultimately be automated and coded with either ICD or SNOMED-CT codes (see chapter 16).

In physician practices, clinical documentation is often entered directly as structured data into the EHR by both physicians and nurses. Structured data refer to data elements that are uniquely captured by the computer in fields that can then be processed. An example is drug–lab checking, where it may be necessary to have lab data (such as the results of a liver function study) before ordering a certain type of drug that may adversely affect the liver. Drug–lab checking can be performed in a CDS system, however such CDS depends on the selection of a specific drug programmed into the computer and lab data results also programmed into the computer that are available to the CDS system. The CDS system then can compare what drug is ordered against a patient's lab values to determine if there are contraindications. Structured data is contrasted with **unstructured data**, or narrative information not able to be uniquely processed by a computer. For example, a lab value posted to a specific field can be compared with other such lab values. A lab value simply documented in a note, comment field, or as a scanned image of paper cannot be processed by the computer in the same way as structured data.

Closed-Loop Medication Management

Closed-loop medication management refers to the use of certain systems that help assure **patient safety**, or preventing harm to patients, learning from errors, and building a culture of safety (Hughes 2008), from the point a drug is ordered to the point it is administered. These systems include CPOE, **e-prescribing (e-Rx)** as a special type of CPOE, BC-MAR, **medication reconciliation**

systems that compare drugs ordered against drugs dispensed and administered, and automated drug dispensing machines, as well as the policies, procedures, and workflows associated with ensuring proper drug ordering, dispensing, administering, and monitoring of reactions. Although there is no recommended sequence for implementing these systems, many hospitals in the past implemented CPOE last because it is difficult to get physicians to use such systems in the hospital. This is changing as MU incentives require use of a CPOE system first, then medication administration record systems. In the ambulatory setting, e-Rx has sometimes been implemented as a standalone system before an EHR (and its CPOE functionality) because some insurers and Medicare were providing incentives for its use. Physicians also found great value in the CDS for drug choices and in managing prescription refills and renewals.

CPOE Systems as written   CPOE systems can be used for entering all orders such as patient admission, laboratory tests, x-rays and other diagnostic studies, dietary and nutrition, therapies, nursing services, consults, discharge of patient, referrals, and even building personal task lists, as well as entering orders for medications. In the past, these orders were usually handwritten by the physician and were either internally faxed to various departments as applicable or transcribed by nursing personnel (such as ward secretaries or unit clerks) into an order communication system. This type of system, however, only enabled transmission of the order to various departments' information systems. There was no CDS in the order communication system. In fact, one of the issues physicians have with CPOE today is that they view themselves as now having to perform clerical data entry tasks. As a result, some hospitals have eased in implementation of CPOE, requiring its use—at least initially—only for medication ordering. The CPOE functionality in an ambulatory EHR is much more likely to be used by physicians, because the scope of the types of orders placed is more limited.

Other concerns from physicians include rudimentary CDS built into these systems so that providers are alerted to drug–allergy and drug–drug contraindication (situations that should be avoided as potentially harmful to a patient) as checked against a **drug knowledge database** (namely, a subscription service that provides current information about drugs and is accessible to users and CDS). Alerts and reminders about medication issues can be useful, if set up properly. If not, the alerts and reminders can be annoying and often ignored. For example, an alert that reminds a physician that aspirin should not be given to patients with gastrointestinal bleeding or uncontrolled hypertension is an alert that many physicians believe is unnecessary unless such a drug has been entered into the CPOE system for the patient who has one of these conditions already documented in the EHR. In fact, CDS that is not specific to the patient has become such a problem in some CPOE systems that the term **alert fatigue** is used to describe this issue. Another concern with CPOE systems is that they are often based on standard order sets. Standard order sets are lists of specific diagnostic studies and treatments as appropriate for specific diagnoses or procedures to be performed. These order sets reflect the current knowledge about patient care from research, experts, and other sources of **evidence-based medicine (EBM)**. A standard order set is frequently used for patients with common conditions. For example, a standard order set is often used for admissions for normal pregnancies, where the obstetrician only needs to approve of the standard items or make applicable changes rather than having to document the entire set of items normally required. However, despite that EBM may reflect the best scientific evidence on how to treat a patient with a specific condition, one size does not always fit all human beings. Even a woman with a normal pregnancy may have certain preferences, allergies, or additional conditions that have to be taken into account when using the standard order set for normal pregnancy. As a result, most standard orders sets need to be modified for each patient. In haste a physician may accept the standard orders or may make an error in modifying them—which may result in **unintended consequences** (AHRQ 2011). An unintended consequence is an unanticipated and undesired effect of implementing and using an EHR (Rollins 2012). These are often attributed to the EHR software even though they reflect that a user may not have applied professional judgment or due diligence in using the system (Campbell et. al 2006)

CPOE systems also generate the patient's medication list. The medication list is required under the MU program to be coded using one of the code sets standardized under **RxNorm** (a system maintained by the National Library of Medicine to normalize drug names across disparate vocabularies). Caution must also be applied here, as the medication list will only be as accurate and complete as all systems contributing information to it. For instance, if a medication is ordered prior to surgery, suspended during surgery, reinstated after surgery but then changed before administration, not only must the CPOE and BC-MAR contribute correct medication information, but the surgery information system may also need to be linked to the medication management systems, which is not always the case.

E-Rx E-Rx is a special type of CPOE used exclusively to write a prescription and transmit it electronically to retail pharmacies. The format and content of the prescription transmitted is standardized by the **National Council for Prescription Drug Programs (NCPDP)**, a standards development organization that sets standards for the pharmacy industry. The NCPDP **SCRIPT** standard is the standard developed for electronically transmitting a prescription. As such, the SCRIPT standard is used in ambulatory settings, including not only the physician practice but when a patient is discharged from the hospital or emergency service with a prescription and in hospital outpatient departments or clinics. The e-Rx system includes medication alerts and reminders just as the hospital-based CPOE system, but also includes formulary information that identifies whether the patient's health plan covers the cost of a drug and what co-pay may be required. Physicians can then work with their patients to find the most cost-effective as well as clinically-suitable drug. Because e-Rx systems are able to transmit prescriptions directly to retail pharmacies, physicians benefit from fewer calls from pharmacies not able to read their handwriting or needing to advise the physician that a drug ordered is not going to be covered by the patient's insurance because it is not on the list (formulary) of covered drugs, that is, it is considered "off formulary." Physicians are also able to receive electronic communications from retail pharmacies, such as for renewal approvals that can significantly save time in a practice. In 2010, the Drug Enforcement Administration (DEA), which previously banned use of **e-prescribing for controlled substances (EPCS)** such as narcotics, set special requirements allowing for use of EPCS. These requirements include use of a product that provides **identity proofing** (authentication credentials used to electronically sign such prescriptions) and **two-factor authentication**—a signature type that includes at least two of the following three elements: something known, such as a password; something held, such as a token or digital certificate; and something that is personal, such as **biometrics** (fingerprints, retinal scan, or other) to enable such use. **Digital certificates** are issued by a **certificate authority**, an organization that verifies a person's credentials (such as the provider's DEA number for EPCS) and can revoke the certificate if the credentials are revoked.

BC-MAR   Medication administration recording is a function performed by nurses in a hospital. The frequency and care that must be taken to assure that a nurse administers the right drug, in the right dose, through the right route, at the right time, and to the right patient (the **medication five rights**) is critical to avoid medication errors. As a result, computerized systems have been created. Early medication administration systems were simply electronically generated paper lists of medications from the pharmacy information system after it processed physician orders. Later, the lists were retained on the computer and nurses were expected to post the date and time of medication administration to the computer. Any exceptions or issues with medication administration, however, were still included in handwritten nurses' notes. Most importantly, these systems, while providing a legible list of medications did not fully address the medication five rights.

Today, most hospitals use BC-MAR systems. BC-MAR systems require the hospital to have each patient identified with a barcode (usually on a wrist band) and to package (or buy prepackaged) drugs in unit dose form, each with a barcode or **radio-frequency identification (RFID)** tag that identifies the drug, dose, and intended route of administration. (An RFID tag serves the same function as a barcode, but enables wireless transmission of the data rather than requiring a barcode to be read with a scanner.) At the time the drug is to be administered to a patient, the nurse logs into the BC-MAR system and scans the patient's wrist band and unit dose package. The system automatically dates and time-stamps the entry made through this process. As a result, the medication five rights have been followed. Most BC-MAR systems also enable notes to describe exceptions; for example, that the patient was in surgery at the time the next dose was to be administered. BC-MAR systems provide some CDS as do CPOE systems, often including links to additional information about drugs. BC-MAR systems also generate reports on timely administration of drugs.

There are some issues with using BC-MAR systems. One is that the bags that contain specially compounded drugs administered intravenously require special labels, which not all hospital pharmacy information systems can accommodate. In this case, special care must be taken to manually check and enter the medications being administered. The other important issue associated with using BC-MAR systems is bringing the computer, barcode wand, and medication to the patient bedside. Some hospitals use wireless **workstations on wheels (WOWs)**. Because WOWs can become heavy with their various devices plus a long life battery, an alternative is to carry (sometimes by wearing a sling) a tablet computer that may be outfitted with a wand device and the medication. Walking around all day with such equipment, however, is also not comfortable. Finally, it is important for the hospital to fully define what constitutes a medication administration error—a wrong time, for instance, may or may not be due to an error but rather the availability of the patient.

Medication Reconciliation The medication reconciliation process also can be automated, although not as easily as the other elements of medication management. Each time a patient is transferred across levels of care, such as when admitted, transferred into an intensive care unit, or sent to surgery, the medications the patient should be taking need to be reviewed. Often certain medications must be discontinued or a dose altered as a result of the change in level of care. In addition, the clinicians who work with the patient are different at each different level of care. Connecting all the systems at the different levels of care has been a challenge in which only a few hospitals have been successful.

Automated Drug Dispensing Machines Finally with respect to medication management, **automated drug dispensing machines** are available that both secure and make drugs more readily available to nursing staff. These machines are typically filled by pharmacy department staff based on the physician orders.

Clinical Decision Support

Clinical decision support (CDS) is a key component of the EHR system and sets it apart from simply automating paper documents. CDS functionality in the EHR system helps physicians, nurses, and other clinical professionals—collectively referred to as clinicians—as well as patients themselves make decisions about patient care. Some examples of CDS as previously discussed include alerts about potential drug contraindications, out-of-range lab results, and standard order sets in CPOE. In addition, CDS templates can help determine what documentation of clinical findings is necessary; provide suggestions for prescribing less expensive but equally effective drugs; supply **protocols** (specification of appropriate processes, based on expert best practices and clinical research findings) for certain health maintenance procedures; and alert that a duplicate lab test is being ordered. There are countless other decision-making aids for all stakeholders in the care process.

CDS may be built into each of the core EHR applications. However, CDS is also acquired as separate systems that work in conjunction with the EHR applications. In general, the CDS found in the core EHR applications is fairly rudimentary because they typically are able to only process data within the given application. More sophisticated CDS requires the convergence of different types of data from the various EHR components. As a result, separate applications are used to help integrate and analyze these data.

Separate CDS applications may be fully integrated with the core EHR applications or employed in a standalone fashion. An example of a separate CDS application is one that provides drug–lab checking, such as whether a drug is contraindicated for a patient with poor liver function. This is not a routine function of CPOE or LIS, but requires the combination of data from both sources and the ability to deliver the alert back to the appropriate system(s). This is commonly referred to as a separate **clinical decision support system (CDSS)**, even though it may be fully integrated into the core EHR applications through supporting infrastructure. Other examples of separate CDSSs that are integrated into the EHR system include the templates used in clinical documentation, standard order sets used in CPOE, and clinical pathways that guide nursing services. While some EHR products build a basic set of templates directly into their clinical documentation systems, others require a separate CDSS to generate the templates, or provide more sophisticated and customizable templates than exist in the basic clinical documentation applications.

CDSSs that are used in a standalone fashion are often those specific to a unique function. For example, a CDSS that is used in a standalone fashion in a hospital includes a system to alert infection control nurses of a potential hospital-acquired infection. It provides advice on which medication may be most effective in combating the infection given the causative agent. Such a system compiles data from clinical documentation (such as documentation of a high temperature), lab results (such as the strain of bacteria that is causing the infection), x-ray results (such as a finding of pneumonia), and other sources processed against automated clinical reference information to produce the specific findings.

An example of a CDSS used in a standalone fashion by physicians is a differential diagnosis system. This system may compare diagnostic images against a library of images and their known conditions, which is especially useful for radiologists, dermatologists, pathologists, and others. Other differential diagnosis CDS systems compare data from clinical documentation, especially the history of present illness and review of

systems, with a library of known signs and symptoms for specific diagnoses. Some of these are used only when the differential diagnosis is obscure. Others may be a routine part of a protocol, such as for assessing a patient presenting to the emergency service with chest pain. Still another CDS system can aid in identifying whether a patient's symptoms are due to a new condition or are the result of an adverse reaction to a medication. Figure 11.5 summarizes the different forms of CDS and CDSS.

Despite the advantages CDS can offer, many clinicians are still resistant to entering data into the computer system at the point of care, especially when the system requires a lot of structured data. This is both a workflow issue for which many clinicians have not been trained to overcome as well as a system design issue. As a result, in a number of both hospitals and physician practices, clinical

Figure 11.5 Types of clinical decision support

Data display
Data always available
Flow sheets (for example, problem list, medication list)
- Maintain longitudinally
- Across continuum
Dynamic displays
- Flow sheet, graphic, table, narrative—helps review data
- Clinical imaging integration
- Search tools
- Query support
Summaries or abstracts
- Quickens access, supports continuity of care
- Flags problems

Workflow
In-basket
- Reminders in support of timeliness, compliance
Schedule and patient list
- Patient status continuously
Workgroup tools
- Easy handoffs
Refills choice lists
Integrated clinical and financial
- Medical necessity checking
- Overcomes inability to pay for treatment
Telephony (the process of connecting a telephone to an electronic device), e-mail and visits, instant messaging
- Quick response

Data retrieval
Single sign-on (for multiple applications)
- Overcomes interface versus integration (through one system or repository) issues
Ease of navigation aids adoption
Density of screen
- "Flip-ability"
- Avoids getting lost in "drill downs"
Specialized formats focus information
Customized screens
- Standards versus personal preference

Data entry
Context-sensitive templates and order sets guide documentation
Provides immediate access to active decision support
- Alerts and reminders
- Clinical calculations
- Therapy critiquing and planning
Patient self-assessment and PHR
Medication list maintenance (by patient or claims consolidator)
Structured data and registry support
- Contributes to downstream knowledge
- Wellness or disease management reminders, interventions due, recalls
Access to reference information
- Context-insensitive, portal
- Context-sensitive, direct links

information is still dictated and turned into typed reports or handwritten and scanned into a document imaging system. However to take advantage of CDS, the data required for the system to work must be captured in or converted to structured data at some point.

Another example is social history of smoking, where use of a template to indicate whether a patient smokes and perhaps the number of cigarettes smoked per day are unique data points. When these data are entered as structured data they can then generate an alert that smoking cessation counseling should be given, which is one of the clinical quality measures for earning MU incentives. Another example might be the ability of the system to calculate the patient's body mass index (BMI), also required in the MU program, and recommend weight counseling. Many ambulatory EHR systems include reminders for preventive or chronic care services, such as dates when a vaccine, cancer screening, diabetes care, or other services are due.

Analytics and Reporting

Analytics and reporting are the final core EHR application. Analytics refers to statistical processing of data to reveal new information. Reporting is the supplying of the results of analytics to the intended recipient.

Analytics goes beyond the simple use of descriptive statistics, such as how many patients were seen for a specific condition, to questions such as which form of treatment for the specific condition had the best outcomes. The ability to produce such reports is increasingly important as there is ever more pressure to improve quality and reduce the cost of healthcare. Analytics, however, entail sophisticated processes to be performed on data—such as data mining, forecasting, neural networks (mathematical modeling that makes connections between data to discover relationships), and others.

In healthcare, analytics has been primarily performed in academic and research institutions, by health plans, at pharmaceutical manufacturers, and for public health departments. Analytics has produced many clinical benefits

for the healthcare industry, such as in genomic research and personalized medicine (also known as precision medicine) that tailors treatment to the specific individual, given not only co-morbidities but genomic characteristics and predispositions (SAS n.d.). Analytics are also used to create business intelligence, such as in predicting prescribing patterns of physicians or the impact of a disaster on local emergency services (Strome 2013).

Although most information systems are able to generate some data for analysis and reporting, there has been strong interest for the EHR system to provide more robust analysis of data. Unfortunately, the nature of the type of database required for POC charting and CDS, referred to as a clinical data repository (CDR), does not support complex analytics and reporting. The purpose of a CDR is primarily online transaction processing (OLTP), where each access, entry, or other process performed on data is a transaction. Often it is necessary to move data from the CDR to a separate database that has been optimized to perform analytics and reporting (online analytical processing [OLAP]). This type of database is referred to as a clinical data warehouse (CDW). In addition, healthcare organizations that want to perform sophisticated analytics need staff highly skilled in such statistical techniques. It may be that a given hospital or physician practice cannot perform the analytics and reporting itself, but sends data to a vendor who performs the analytics. An increasing number of EHR vendors are supplying such services, often aggregating data from many customers to enlarge the pool of data, making the results of analysis on the data more valid and reliable. When this data pool has a large volume of data it is referred to as big data. Big data offers greater reliability and validity. Big data analytics implies massive amounts of data that can be analyzed quickly in near real time to return new information to users at the POC. When collecting data from active patient health records, the data reflects current experience and analytics is then able to not only produce new information but new knowledge.

Another trait of big data in addition to its volume and velocity (speed at which it is transformed into knowledge) is that all of the data do not need to be structured. It is still important to ensure the quality of the data being captured in health information systems so that the results of analysis can be as accurate as possible. **Data quality** refers to adherence to standard data definitions and **metadata** (that is, data about data) requirements. **Data models** that organize data to depict relationships among data help ensure the quality of data collected by health IT systems. Standard vocabularies (the compilation of terms formally adopted for use in health IT systems) all for data exchange across different health IT systems. This exchange capability is referred to as **semantic interoperability**, or the ability to share common meanings for data across systems. Another important element that improves data quality in health IT systems is a **data dictionary** that lists all data elements used in a health IT system with their definitions and characteristics. For example, a data dictionary for a given health IT system would include the term *temperature* and specify that is must be documented in centigrade. The American Health Information Management Association (AHIMA) developed a data quality management model to illustrate these characteristics (AHIMA 2015).

Health plans have analyzed data from healthcare claims for a long time, and now they are receiving additional data from commercial labs, claims attachments, patient-entered data, and other sources to perform even more sophisticated analytics. Such information may impact whether the hospital or physician practice receives a favorable discount rate on its fees for services. Quality benchmarking depends on analytics. (Benchmarking is discussed in chapter 18.) Consumers are beginning to look at which hospital excels in cardiac care or has a center of excellence for orthopedics. Having aggregated data to understanding why one healthcare organization is ahead in its quality metrics over another can help poorer performers improve. Analytics and reporting are not only used for retrospective quality or research studies; an important set of reports include rule-based lists

for patient follow-up. Patient follow-up lists have not been easy to generate in the past, as much of the data had to be manually abstracted from paper records, transcription, or scanned images of documents. However, the ability to identify all patients requiring follow-up after discharge, for chronic disease care, to notify them of a drug or device recall, to send preventive care reminders, or any of many other similar types of reports or lists is integral to quality patient care.

Most analytics implementations are still retrospective. However, it can be anticipated that the use of big data analytics in near real time will help providers at the POC improve clinical decision making. Examples of such improved decision making include the ability to select affordable therapies (Chaiken 2011) and make earlier diagnoses of complex conditions such as rheumatoid arthritis and multiple sclerosis (Kalatzis et al. 2009).

Today, the federal government is putting increased emphasis on using EHR for quality improvement. For a number of years hospitals have been required to report quality measures to the Joint Commission to retain accreditation; and to the Centers for Medicare and Medicaid Services (CMS) in order to earn full reimbursement for their services under Medicare. These measures were consolidated and referred to as **core measures** for both programs. They are reported to the public by CMS on its HospitalCompare website. Physician quality reporting to earn incentives under the federal government's **Physician Quality Reporting System (PQRS)** was started more recently (CMS 2015). Reporting **electronic clinical quality measures (eCQM)** is also a requirement for earning MU incentives. However, going forward, it is anticipated that not only must quality measures be *reported*, but there must be the ability to demonstrate *improvement* in the measures over time. As health reform legislation encourages new and risk-based forms of reimbursement structures, such as accountable care organizations, bundled payments, and patient-centered medical homes (PCMH), the ability to predict patient volumes, outcomes, and improve quality will directly impact a healthcare organization's bottom line.

✓ Check Your Understanding 11.1

Instructions: **Answer the following questions.**

1. Which of the following is a source system?
   A. Clinical decision support system
   B. Laboratory information system
   C. Results management system
   D. Medication reconciliation system

2. Which of the following is considered a core EHR component?
   A. Computerized provider order entry
   B. Pharmacy information system
   C. Document imaging
   D. Registration-admission, discharge, transfer system

3. Dr. Smith always orders the same 10 things when a new patient is admitted to the hospital in addition to some patient-specific orders. What would assist in ensuring that the specific patient is not allergic to a drug being ordered?
   A. Clinical decision support
   B. Pharmacy information system
   C. Electronic medication administration record system
   D. Standard order set

4. What provides alerts and reminders to clinicians?
   A. Clinical decision support system
   B. Electronic data interchange
   C. Point-of-care charting system
   D. Workflow system

5. E-prescribing systems are used to do which of the following?
   A. Inventory and dispense drugs in retail pharmacies
   B. Write orders for drugs to be administered in hospitals
   C. Send prescriptions to retail pharmacies
   D. Report adverse drug events

6. True or false: BC-MARs supports medication five rights.

7. True or false: Medication reconciliation is the most difficult function of closed-loop medication management systems to implement.

8. True or false: When the EHR is said to be in the adoption state, not all of the available functionality is being used.

9. True or false: Templates utilize free text but not data-entry tools like drop-down lists.

10. True or false: The EHR itself does not have to perform analytics for complex analysis of data to be available to the healthcare organization.

Specialty Systems and Automated Medical Devices

In addition to source systems and core clinical EHR systems, specialty systems (see figure 11.2) support documentation of patient care in specialty areas such as intensive care units, emergency medicine, cardiology and perioperative services, and many others. These systems might be like a mini-EHR for the specialty area, although ideally should not replicate information collection and services provided by other source systems in the organization. Finally, some specialty applications are found in locations not integrated with general medical services. For example, most dentists practice in offices or clinics separate from their medical colleagues. It is only in the small percentage of federal qualified health centers, for example, where dental services are integrated with medical services.

Picture archiving and communications systems (PACSs) are another form of specialty information system for use in radiology modalities. They capture digital images from the various modalities, such as x-ray, ultrasound, and others and provide special viewing capabilities of these images via a computer. Standardization for PACS is established by the **Digital Imaging and Communications in Medicine (DICOM)** organization. Some PACS also have the ability to connect directly with a RIS, thereby providing the ability to integrate images with data.

Automated medical devices, until recently, have generally not been considered information systems, even though they have generated information—sometimes only in the form of blood pressure on a display screen and other times in the form of a continuous feed of data such as a fetal monitoring strip. Other examples of such medical devices include vital signs monitors, cardiac output monitors, defibrillators, electrocardiographs, infusion pumps, physiologic monitors, and ventilators (HIMSS Analytics 2010). Today many healthcare organizations would like to connect these devices to their EHR, but the technology to do so—**medical device integration**—requires special technical infrastructure. Hospitals and other healthcare provider settings are just beginning to prioritize integration of these medical devices into their EHR infrastructures (ECRI Institute 2014).

Supporting Infrastructure

Supporting infrastructure (see figure 11.2) refers to the technology that allows the various applications to work. This includes hardware, software, networks, and telecommunications capability. Hardware includes human computer interfaces (HCI) which are any form of input device used by humans. Hardware also includes all of the computer servers for processing and storage, as well as network devices. Many of the servers used for processing

have specific functions. For example, there may be an LIS or an EDMS server. There are also special servers, called rules engines, which process clinical decision support. Such servers also need to have access to knowledge sources, such as knowledge about the properties of drugs, or knowledge about surgical procedures that support standard order sets. These knowledge sources may be on a separate server locally, or more commonly, on a remote server that a vendor operates through a subscription service. A computer with its own software that processes data retained in the computer is no longer a viable structure for even a solo practitioner's office. Data must be exchanged, at a minimum between the solo practitioner and a nurse, and usually a receptionist, plus one or more payers to whom claims are sent. Computers must be networked together, whether via physical cabling or wireless services. When exchanging data within the organization, the network is referred to as a local area network (LAN), and when exchanging data across organizations, such as from a provider to a payer, the network is referred to as a wide area network (WAN). WANs need a secure connection, which is often a **virtual private network (VPN)**, an encrypted private connection over the Internet.

Infrastructure also must consider the policies for using the applications, address workflow changes, and provide training and support to users. For example, medical device integration requires not only special hardware and software, but inventory controls on the devices, identification of associated IP addresses, policies on how long the data may be retained, and changes to processes people use to review the results. A supporting infrastructure is vital to manage the different applications necessary for today's health information needs. Large hospitals may have nearly a thousand applications, with hundreds of applications being common in medium-sized hospitals. Physician practices may have only one combined PMS and EHR system, but frequently have some ancillary and specialty systems—potentially accumulating 10 to 20 or more systems. Increasingly, both hospitals and physicians not only exchange information among providers and with patients for treatment and payment, but also exchange information for operational functions. These operational functions may include supplying quality data to a **registry** (a specialized database for a predefined set of data and its processing), or various data storage management (archiving data organized for retrieval) techniques. These may include a clinical data repository (CDR) which is a special form of database for integrating all data from the source systems and EHR systems or a clinical data warehouse (CDW) that is a database used for aggregating data for analysis. A storage area network (SAN) may support the ability to retrieve data from any storage location for use in the EHR. Some SANs may be local to the healthcare organization. Others may use **cloud computing**, which uses a vendor to archive data and in some cases also provides application software (including an EHR) on multiple, disparate servers.

Connectivity Systems

Connectivity systems (see figure 11.2) help support the exchange of data across separate information systems both within a healthcare organization and across organizations and also with individuals.

Essentially health IT systems contain data in incompatible formats. Even within one healthcare organization that uses a single vendor to supply all applications, there is not necessarily true interoperability. The vendor most likely did not develop all applications itself. If some applications have been acquired from other vendors, it is necessary to have a translation process that hardwires the applications together in order to interoperate and exchange data seamlessly across the different applications. This hardwiring is referred to as **system integration**, and software that provides the hardwiring is referred to as an **interface**. The interface depends on each application using a common **message format standard** to structure the format of the data that are processed by the application. Even when newer systems utilize a **web services architecture (WSA)** that offers web-based forms of interfaces—such as XML structures—to accomplish this translation process, Internet protocols and other standards to achieve interoperability and make the exchange work are still required.

Interfaces may also be used to exchange data between one organization and another, such as between a physician's office and a commercial laboratory. Interfaces are commonly used when the office uses the same commercial laboratory frequently. Interfaces, however, are costly to write and maintain. Anytime one system is upgraded or modified in some way, the interface must be adjusted.

As a result, interfaces are not effective when attempting to exchange data across many different organizations. For example, a physician's office likely needs to exchange prescription information with many different retail pharmacies. In order for the exchange to occur in such cases, there needs to be a go-between that can manage the translation process. In addition, there are not only issues of data formatting differences but a number of other factors that must be in place for such exchange to occur. These include patient identification, directory services (for example, Which retail pharmacy is on Main Street?), security, and patient consent management.

There are essentially three forms of go-between processes used today in healthcare—telehealth, patient-exchanged information, and health information exchange.

Telehealth

The oldest form of exchanging health information is telehealth—a process that uses telecommunications to send voice, still pictures, and video between a remote location (where the patient is) and a base location (such as a hospital) for the purposes of diagnosis and, in some cases, treatment. Some might not consider telehealth to truly be a form of health IT because the information is only conveyed in sound or picture and not as structured data, though most telehealth conducted today does include some exchange of health information.

Connectivity is a challenge because telehealth is so often used to reach remote parts of the country, on a battlefield, or across the world. Telecommunications technology is not always the best in such areas. Broadband, for example, is still not available in all parts of the United States. Physician licensure has been another major challenge, where a physician may not be licensed to practice in another state, hence precluding the ability to cross state lines when conducting telehealth. Reimbursement for telehealth is not always provided by health plans, or only under certain, limited conditions. Specialized equipment must also be brought to the site where the patient is located. All of these challenges are being addressed where there is high need. For example, robots have been developed to reach injured soldiers. The VA has constructed all of its telehealth services to rely solely on dial-up telephone connections because many veterans needing telehealth are in remote areas. Telehealth is experiencing increasing interest to reach prison inmates, inner city communities where there are safety issues, and in various care coordination activities where patients have transportation limitations. Medicare is increasing its reimbursement for telehealth.

Patient-Exchanged Health Information

Another form of exchanging health information is to use the patient as the go-between. This might be considered even older than telehealth when considering the patient—or patient's family member or caregiver—has always been the knowledge base for history of present illness and other information. However, from a technology perspective portals, electronic personal health records, and the continuity of care document are technologies that are newer than telehealth.

A **patient portal** is special software that enables patients to log on to a website from home or a **kiosk** (special form of input device geared to people less familiar with computers) in a provider's waiting room to have access to some of their health information and other services. In many cases, the portal is used primarily for administrative functions, such as to request an appointment and even directly schedule an appointment, pay bills, obtain patient educational material, sign informed consents, exchange email with a provider, and request release of information. Under the MU program, the portal has been a common way for patients to access their health summary information. In some cases, the portal only provides

health summary information. In other cases it may provide a view into parts of the EHR or even the entire EHR. A portal may also be a way to access a personal health record supplied by a provider. (However, the MU program does not require a PHR.) In some cases, patients are starting to enter their own health history using a template that directs them to enter specific information via the portal that is then available to providers during the visit. Some providers are supporting **e-visits** through a portal, where existing patients can exchange e-mail in lieu of visiting the physician's office for follow-up or recurring care needs. E-visits are now reimbursable by some insurance companies.

The **personal health record (PHR)** has been defined by AHIMA as an electronic or paper health record maintained and updated by an individual for himself or herself; a tool that individuals can use to collect, track, and share past and current information about their health or the health of someone in their care. Although use of an electronic system for PHRs is encouraged by AHIMA, many more patients use a paper-based file folder as their PHR rather than an electronic offering. Whether electronic or paper-based, patients are expected to own and manage the information in the PHR, which comes from both healthcare providers and the individual. The PHR is maintained in a secure and private environment, with the patient determining rights of access. It is separate from and does not replace the legal health record of any provider or their EHR AHIMA has taken an active role in promotion of PHR. AHIMA maintains a PHR website (MyPHR) that provides the public with free educational resources about personal health information and PHRs (AHIMA e-HIM Personal Health Record Workgroup 2005).

Today, PHRs are in a transition state. The PHR may be provided through a portal offered by a provider or may be a standalone system offered via a vendor, employer, or affinity group. A PHR offered by a provider is an excellent tool if there is only one PHR for all who treat the patient, and especially if it enables more than minimal functionality. If a patient has multiple providers, however, it is likely that the patient will also have multiple PHRs. Today, there is little connectivity between these records. The patient might as well have a paper-based record system of their own if they wish to have any integration of data across these PHRs. PHRs offered by many providers also do not allow the patient to enter data, rather he or she can only view lab results and other summary health information. This somewhat defeats the purpose of having a centralized place that can be used to document changes in personal health status or communicate in real time with providers about changes in a patient's health status, such as high blood sugars, or weight gain in a patient with congestive heart failure.

PHRs have been most popular with patients who have chronic illnesses or with caretakers of elderly patients having to manage multiple providers, many drugs, and other data.

The **continuity of care document (CCD)** is yet another effort to supply patients with more information about their healthcare. The CCD is a combination of two standards.

The first standard that comprises the CCD is the **continuity of care record (CCR)** standard created by physicians from the Massachusetts Medical Society and other organizations working under the auspices of the **American Society for Testing and Materials (ASTM) International** standards development organization. The initial purpose of the CCR was to eliminate data inconsistencies when patients were referred from one provider to another. In the past when a patient was referred to another provider, the originating provider would dictate a letter describing the patient's case. There was no consistency across physicians as to what might be included in this referral letter. To eliminate this problem, the CCR standard recommends specific categories of information to include in referral letters. The developers of the standard emphasize that the CCR is not an EHR. Rather, it is a subset of data from an EHR. Many PHR vendors picked up on the CCR and have incorporated it into their commercial offerings, even though it is not considered a PHR standard.

The second standard that comprises the CCD is the **Clinical Document Architecture (CDA)** standard developed by the **Health Level Seven (HL7)** standards development organization that aids the exchange of XML documents between health IT systems. When the CCR is rendered as an XML document, the CDA provides structure (including a description of document content for users and discrete data for computer processing), vocabulary standards (such as SNOMED-CT and LOINC), and codes (to represent the vocabulary and other concepts, like a code structure for representing dates and units of measure) for sharing clinical documents in XML format. Subsequently, HL7 has created a transport mechanism not only for the CCR, but for a number of other healthcare documents. These document templates are collectively referred to as the **Consolidated Clinical Document Architecture (C-CDA)**.

The C-CDA may be transmitted electronically via HL7 standard messages, in attachments to e-mail, or via standard Internet file transfer protocols, such as file transfer protocol (FTP).

Health Information Exchange

Health information exchange (HIE) is another way to exchange information across multiple organizations and individuals. HIE is most often managed by an organization referred to as a **health information organization (HIO)**. The HIO typically provides governance, fee structure, and policies and procedures for exchanging health information; it is a business associate under HIPAA. HIOs have struggled financially, as paying for exchanging health information when generally provider-to-provider exchange has been free of charge—albeit a slow process—has not been accepted as well as expected.

In general, an HIO provides several key services, shown in figure 11.6. These include:

- Patient identification, usually using an **identity matching algorithm** in which specified patient demographic information is compared to select the patient for whom information is to be exchanged. The algorithmic

Figure 11.6   HIO services

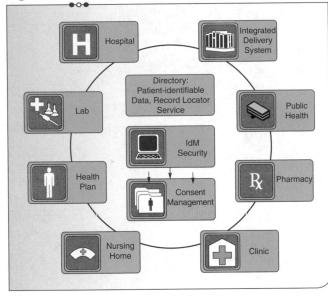

© Margret\A Consulting, LLC. Reprinted with permission.

process is determined by the vendor supplying the service, but uses sophisticated probability equations to identify patients.

- The **record locator service (RLS)** is a process that seeks information about where a patient, once identified, may have a health record available to the HIO.

- **Identity management** (not to be confused with patient identification) provides security functionality, including determining who (or what information system) is authorized to access information, authentication services, audit logging, encryption, and transmission controls.

- Consent management is yet another HIO service. In consent management, patients have **opt in/opt out** privileges for having their health information exchanged. As noted previously, the patient will often provide a **consent directive** for this purpose.

In addition to these basic services, each HIO establishes what type of data exchange it will support. For example, there are some that only conduct e-prescribing—exchanging prescriptions between providers who write prescriptions and retail pharmacies. Some states sponsor an HIO; if so, the HIO helps support public health activities (for example,

immunization registry reporting) and often some basic exchange of emergency information. Because such HIOs must help exchange information across many disparate types of health IT systems, usually only a limited amount of information is able to be exchanged through such an HIO. In an attempt to exchange more comprehensive information (and perhaps also to gain market share), EHR vendors have started to support exchange of health information across all organizations using the same EHR vendor.

HIE is developing across the nation. Initially referred to as the nationwide health information network (NHIN), the federal government wants such a network to be grounded in both federal and private sector needs. Today this is referred to as the **eHealth Exchange**. It includes federal agencies involved in healthcare and nonfederal organizations coming together (with assistance from a federal contractor) to offer a secure, trusted, and interoperable health information exchange service (The Sequoia Project 2015). Today, the eHealth Exchange connects all 50 states and includes use by the Department of Defense, VA, CMS, and Social Security Administration as well as 30 percent of all US hospitals, 10,000 medical groups, 8,200 pharmacies, and more than 900 dialysis centers—essentially connecting more than 100 million patients. Participants sign a **Data Use and Reciprocal Support Agreement (DURSA)**, participant agreement, and testing agreement. There are both testing and exchange fees for use.

There are two ways to connect using the eHealth Exchange.

- Direct exchange uses an initiative called the **Direct Project** for securely *pushing* patient health information to a known, trusted receiver using secure email technology (HIMSS 2013).

- CONNECT is an alternative way to connect with the eHealth Exchange. **CONNECT** is open-source software that implements health exchange specifications. It enables discovery of where there may be information as well as directly retrieving it from the source (HIMSS 2012).

Check Your Understanding 11.2

Instructions: **Answer the following questions.**

1. Software that is written to help exchange data between two applications is:
   A. Interoperability
   B. Interface
   C. e-Health Exchange
   D. System integration

2. Which of the following describes telehealth?
   A. It is a diagnosis or treatment of a patient who is not physically present with the provider
   B. It is an exchange of email for routine clinic visits
   C. It is a call center services for disease management
   D. It is remote monitoring

3. The Consolidated Clinical Document Architecture is:
   A. A summary health record
   B. Collection of healthcare document templates in XML format
   C. A standard for formatting structured data in healthcare
   D. Specification for the content of an EHR

4. An HIO provides identity management in order to:
   A. Help locate a specific patient
   B. Assure appropriate security services
   C. Validate a patient's consent for sharing information
   D. List all providers participating in the exchange

5. True or false: Cloud computing is a process where a vendor houses data (and software) on remote servers.

6. True or false: PHRs are required by the federal government to support the Continuity of Care Document.

7. True or false: In order to locate where a patient has health information, the Direct Project is used in a health information exchange environment.

8. True or false: A patient must access a PHR via a portal.

9. True or false: The eHealth Exchange is a free service available to all healthcare providers.

Systems Development Life Cycle

As described, health information systems include both technology (hardware and software) and operational elements addressing the needs of people (users), required policies, and process improvement. In addition to health information systems being comprised of a number of components that work together to accomplish a purpose, health information systems also reflect a life cycle. This life cycle demonstrates the need to manage changes so the system continues to produce the desired results.

The **systems development life cycle (SDLC)** refers to the steps taken from an initial point of recognizing the need for a desired result, through the steps taken to ensure that all components needed for the system to achieve the desired result are addressed. This cycle is repeated whenever the result of the system fails to continue to produce the desired result (NIST 2008). Failure of a system to produce the desired result may be due to internal or external changes. For example, if a health information system was acquired a number of years ago and there is a new federal mandate for a change in a code system such as the need to transition from ICD-9-CM to ICD-10-CM, or there is an operating system software change (for example, Windows XP is no longer supported), the healthcare organization must address needed changes in the system, or obtain a replacement, to continue to produce desired results. The general nature of an SDLC is illustrated in figure 11.7.

There may be variations in how the steps in the SDLC are described depending on the context in which it is used. For example, a hardware or software developer may go through an SDLC when creating a new product. The vendor may identify need for a new product, then determine the feasibility of creating the new product with specifications that would satisfy the new product needs, design the product, develop it for mass production, maintain the product as small changes in the environment may impact it, and monitor sales to justify continued maintenance or **sunsetting** (that is, no longer selling or supporting) the product. In a provider setting, the SDLC helps identify a need for health information systems support. The provider will then specify requirements needed to achieve the need, acquire a new system, implement the new system, maintain it, and monitor that it continues to meet needs over time. Sometimes a health information system may need to be replaced, in which case the SDLC of acquiring a new product is repeated.

While the SDLC is most often applied when information systems are being developed or acquired, it can be applied as part of a continuous improvement process to ensure that any system meets ongoing and new needs. For example, taking a systems view and applying the SDLC can be a useful process when planning any new service offerings. A hospital may be considering developing a center of excellence in orthopedics, or acquiring small community hospitals. A physician's office may be considering a merger, or expansion of services into retail offerings. An integrated delivery network may be evaluating the usefulness of spinning off long-term care facilities it operates. The key value of the SDLC is to apply a formal logical process to ensure all components needed for a system to optimally achieve its value are in place. Each of the components in the SDLC is discussed next.

Identify Needs

Needs for a healthcare organization that a health information system should address arise from various activities conducted by the organization or may be mandated by the federal government, health plans with which the organization contracts, or other external sources. Commonly referred to as needs identification, a healthcare organization may periodically conduct strategic planning that identifies a need; for example, more timely data available to infection control nurses, or that the surgical suite needs to improve communications with other departments. A hospital may find that its major commercial health plan has decided to promote **value-based purchasing (VBP)**, a specific health reform strategy of enhanced payment to deliver care that takes into consideration access, price, quality, efficiency, and alignment of incentives, rather than volume alone that has been the hallmark of fee-for-service payment mechanisms (NBCH 2011). This will necessitate significantly more integration of financial and clinical data.

Figure 11.7 Systems development life cycle

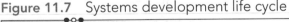

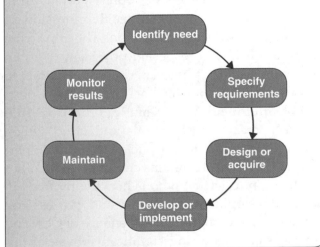

Needs are most commonly expressed as goals. Goals for what and how health information systems will achieve desired results reflect current and anticipated needs and should drive all elements of planning for the systems. Ideally, these should be written as **SMART goals**, or statements that identify results that are:

- Specific
- Measurable
- Attainable
- Relevant
- Time-based

Figure 11.8 is an example of a SMART goal for a hospital performing strategic planning for a health information system.

Any given organization will have several SMART goals for its health information system. For example, a clinic may include the following goal in its planning:

> Physicians will help reduce unnecessary diagnostic studies tests by 10 percent (measurable) over the next two years (time-based) using the interoperability capability of the system (realistic) that, when a test order is placed, makes available (attainable) the results from previous tests performed across the continuum of care for the patient specific to type of test and patient needs (specific).

SMART goals should address all system components, including desired functionality, specific technology requirements to support the desired

Figure 11.8 Example of a SMART goal

© Margret\A Consulting, LLC. Reprinted with permission.

functions, and the expectations for people to adopt new policies and processes to ensure achievement of goals and, therefore, provide value back to the organization for its investment (Amatayakul 2013).

Specify Requirements

Once needs are identified, a healthcare organization will want to specify detailed requirements for how the needs can be met. For health information systems, most organizations convene a **steering committee** that will identify and document a detailed set of specifications, often referred to as a **requirements specification**.

A steering committee may be an overarching committee comprised of key stakeholders to health information systems in general, or, less commonly, a steering committee will be convened for each specific health information system project and include only stakeholders associated with that project. The latter is normally not advisable because of the systems nature of health IT. For example, a BC-MAR will be impacted by CPOE and a pharmacy information system. Ultimately, it will also need to be integrated with a medication reconciliation system and may need to interoperate in the future with a home medication administration system.

The broadest possible set of stakeholders in a steering committee will ensure that all needs for a specific health information system are met. Members of the steering committee for health IT systems should include heavy representations from physicians, nurses, and other health professionals, including a physician champion. The **physician champion** is a well-respected physician who can informally help the physician community adapt to and ultimately adopt health IT. Recently, a position of **chief medical informatics officer (CMIO)** has been created in hospitals and large clinics. The CMIO is a salaried physician (most often part time so that he or she retains credibility with other practicing physicians) who is heavily involved in policy development, workflow and process improvement, and ongoing maintenance of CDS and other systems requiring significant physician input. Both the physician champion and CMIO help achieve a **clinical transformation**—a fundamental change in how medicine is practiced using health IT systems to aid in diagnosis and treatment.

In addition to the healthcare professional representation, IT representatives, the health information management professional, key operational staff, the procurement officer, and potentially others will round out the steering committee membership.

Guided by the SMART goals that define the overall need, the steering committee will seek input from the specific health information system's key stakeholders to enumerate specific requirements. For example, when planning for a BC-MAR system, nurses, pharmacists, IT staff, physicians, and quality assurance professionals may be the key stakeholders. They will review the literature, consult with peers in other facilities, and perhaps attend a trade show or visit another facility with a BC-MAR system to understand more about it and what users like and do not like.

Design or Acquire

Today, most healthcare organizations acquire health information systems from a commercial vendor. There are few healthcare organizations left in the United States that have and continue to support a home-grown, or self-designed information system—these are gradually being discarded in favor of commercial systems.

Commercial systems have several important advantages. First, they are generally cheaper in the long term because they offer economies of scale by selling the same product to many others. Second, they can be more interoperable. Vendors know they will have to do some integration with systems from other vendors in any given healthcare organization. In addition, with federal goals for interoperability, vendors know they will not survive in the marketplace if their systems are not at least standards-based, if not fully interoperable without interfaces. Third, the unique configurations that are often the hallmark of home-grown systems are feasible with many commercial products. These products offer toolkits that allow a user organization to tailor the systems to their needs, while not impacting the underlying product's architecture—thus assuring both customizations for users and interoperability with other systems. Finally, vendor longevity in the marketplace is more assured than that of the custom programmer hired for a specific job for one organization who then moves on to another custom job for another organization—leaving the first organization without ongoing support for maintenance of the system.

Acquiring a health information system may be performed in one of two ways. If a healthcare organization already has many health information system components from one vendor (often described as a **best-of-fit** environment), the organization likely will acquire additional components from the same vendor. A small amount of **due diligence** (that is, steps taken to confirm various facts about the product) may be performed to assure the organization that it does not need to go to another vendor to acquire the product, thus moving toward a **best-of-breed** environment where different components are acquired from different vendors. Much like home-grown systems, the best-of-breed environment is rapidly disappearing for essentially all the same reasons.

However, if a healthcare organization is just starting to acquire health information systems, if the desired system is not offered by the existing vendor, or if the organization has decided to replace the entire set of components with new components, the organization will want to conduct a formal **vendor selection** (HealthIT.gov 2014). With the exception of an unusual component not available from the existing vendor, organizations beginning the vendor selection process or reselecting a system will likely be small providers (for example, critical access hospitals or physician's offices) or specialty providers who were not able to take advantage of the MU program. Such specialty providers include home health agencies, nursing homes, mental health facilities, prisons, public health departments, and others.

The steps in vendor selection include:

1. *Needs identification:* This steps entails understanding and documenting the goals for the system being acquired.

2. *Requirements specification:* This involves determining and documenting the detailed features and functions desired in the system in order to meet the organization's specific goals.

   Requirements specification must also describe the manner in which the healthcare organization will acquire the health information system. **Client/server systems** are those where commercial software is installed on servers housed and maintained within the organization itself, housed within the organization and managed by an outsourced company, or housed and maintained by a contractor for the healthcare organization. The benefit to client/server systems is the extent to which the software can be configured to meet special needs of the healthcare organization. The primary disadvantage is that the healthcare organization must manage the IT infrastructure or a contractor to do so. An alternative is an **application service provider (ASP)** or **software as a service (SaaS)** arrangement. There are both similarities and differences between these two. Both essentially offer health information systems on a subscription basis, with the software and servers housed remotely. In an ASP arrangement, only a moderate amount of custom configuration is feasible and pays for 100 percent usage time, but the healthcare organization does not have responsibility for managing the technology infrastructure. Functionality is delivered to the user via dedicated communications technology. The SaaS arrangement is similar to the ASP, but there is generally less custom configuration ability. The SaaS also offers a pay as you go model, where you only pay for the actual time using the system. This may work well for physician's offices, but generally not for hospitals that have 24-hours a day, seven days a week, 365 days a year use requirements. The SaaS model may be delivered via dedicated communications technology or cloud computing.

3. *Request for Proposal (RFP):* An RFP includes developing and disseminating a description of the organization, its goals for the system, its requirements specification, and a statement of how the vendor should respond to the request for proposal. In recent years, an RFP was considered too much work both for organizations to compile and vendors to respond to. Many healthcare organizations were so new to health IT that they did not know what requirements they wanted met. However, with more experience many are coming to realize that it is probably the only way to ensure a comprehensive understanding of requirements and their availability in a product. Dissemination of the RFP was also challenging in the past with so many vendors. Small providers often relied on their specialty society recommendations or "friends," who may have been biased and too narrow in scope should the practice expand beyond the one specialty. Today, the consumer is more informed and has had an opportunity to learn about a variety of vendors. Sending the RFP to four to six vendors is realistic and doable.

4. *Analysis of RFP responses:* This is a formal review of the responses to the RFPs against the requirements specification. This process should be done as objectively as possible. Often the requirements analysis is used as a score sheet to help identify gaps or potential issues. While it cannot be expected that any one vendor will be able to fully address every requirement, prioritizing the requirements and determining which vendors should be further considered is a key step. At this point the four to six vendors should be narrowed to three or four at the most.

5. *Due diligence:* This involves requesting a product demonstration, checking references, and potentially conducting site visits to see the product in actual use. Depending on the size and location of the organization, a product demonstration might be conducted on-site or via a webinar. However it is conducted, there should be plenty of time set aside to fully put the product through its paces. Because most vendors will spend a lot of time before the actual product demonstration discussing the

values and history of the company, the healthcare organization needs to take charge of the demonstration and set timelines for how much time should be spent on such introductory information, how much should be spent with the vendor conducting a demonstration, and how much time should be allowed for further discussion and even more in-depth review of certain features and functions. Demonstrations may range from a two-hour webinar to a full day or even longer on-site for large organizations. At least half of the time allotted should be spent with detailed review of features and functions. At the conclusion of all forms of due diligence, a vendor of choice and one back-up vendor should result.

6. *Contract negotiation:* This may be the most critical, and often not well-performed, step in the entire vendor selection process. If money is to be spent on the vendor selection process, hiring a consultant who knows the marketplace as well as a review by legal counsel should be conducted. Vendor contract offerings are notoriously one-sided. Recently, many small providers have come to realize that they did not negotiate that federally regulated updates to systems must occur on a timely basis and at no cost to the healthcare organization. Many contracts also include payment schedules that require between 50 percent and 90 percent of the cost upfront—which should be dialed back considerably. Contracts must also recognize the responsibilities of the vendor under HIPAA. The best form of contract negotiation is for the healthcare organization or organization representative to prepare a list of issues to be addressed, present it to the vendor, and then hold a series of conversations to address each issue satisfactorily. Price should be the final negotiation step. An important caveat in contract negotiation, however, is that the result should be a win-win situation, not a win-loss, where the vendor loses so much money on the deal that they are unwilling or become unable to deliver on their promises. Implementation should not begin with an adversarial relationship between the vendor and the organization.

Develop and Implement

Once a commercial product has been acquired, there are both development and implementation steps to be taken by both the healthcare organization and vendor. A large part of acquiring a commercial product is associated with the implementation of the product. The vendor installs the software on specified hardware. Usually the vendor is also contracted for managing the implementation and appoints a project manager to do so. During implementation, **system configuration** (sometimes called **system build**) is conducted. This process provides customization of templates, review and customization of decision support, and other functions; in addition, master files and directories are loaded, and potentially some **data conversion** is performed. For example, a physician's office would want to have their logo displayed on the system, a list of all their patients made available to the application, fee schedules loaded, and data conversion to move their current accounts receivables to the new system. Depending on whether or not there was a previous EHR system, either EHR data must be moved to the new system (data conversion), typically by a vendor or other contractor; or key parts of the paper chart content must be entered (**chart conversion**). This entry may be done by staff, a contractor, or new users as patients are seen. While new users usually do not want to do this, it is an excellent way to learn the system and reduce unnecessary chart conversion steps.

Training is also a critical element of implementation. Some vendors will include, or sell for a separate price, training on using the system and may use a contractor for this. Other vendors supply a CD or webinar as their training option. This is usually insufficient for most new users, even when the user has experience with a different system. In addition, training is not a one-time event—there needs to ongoing orientation, introduction to principles, training, reinforcement, sometimes certification of users, and re-training or focused training. When the system is upgraded, modified, or enhanced, training is needed again. Most of such training is left to the provider organization. For additional information on training, see chapter 20.

Other implementation steps for which the healthcare organization is responsible are management of the vendor and elements of implementation related to people, policy, and process. Most healthcare organizations find it necessary to also appoint a project manager who is responsible for managing vendor relations, including **issues management** where any issues that arise during the implementation are documented, brought to the attention of the vendor, and hopefully resolved or escalated so that resolution is accomplished. Most (but not all) vendors typically do not perform change management that helps new users become acclimated to the significant change in not only documentation but the practice of medicine that results from using health IT, (additional) training, **go-live** (first use of the system in actual practice) support, monitoring usage post implementation, workflow and process analysis and redesign, and policy development. Experience has shown that these elements may be more critical to the success of a health information system than the hardware and software. Change management is discussed in chapter 17.

Workflow, process analysis, and redesign are often acknowledged by a vendor as important, but most vendors do not have time to provide such services. Those vendors who are at the top of the pricing scale do provide workflow and process analysis and redesign—and their results demonstrate the value of this. Unfortunately, many healthcare organizations are so overwhelmed by the amount of effort required in an implementation that they either do not have the energy or even overlook this critical step. As noted previously, unintended consequences can occur from use of health IT and most have been related to lack of training, lack of policy surrounding appropriate use of the systems, and lack of attention to workflow and process changes (Amatayakul 2011).

Testing of the software to guarantee it works with the hardware selected, it has been configured properly, and users understand how to use the system is also challenging. Many vendors will claim that their system has already been tested by virtue of their numerous customers, –but each customer will have a unique system build so this argument is not fully valid. Testing is often left to either super users using the system in advance of go-live and finding issues the vendor must address, or by the end users themselves as they start to use the system. The latter is not desirable, as the end users are already fearful of the change. Unfortunately, time often runs out and users want to begin using the system before it can be fully tested by super users.

Maintain

System maintenance refers to numerous tasks that keep the health information system running smoothly. Some tasks are routine in nature, such as preventive maintenance including the application of security patches or upgrades as delivered by vendors; others are corrective, modifying, or enhancing and performed based on calls to the help desk with issues or change requests for a modification or enhancement. Any changes to the fundamental system should be documented in a formal **change control program**. A change control program assures that there is documented approval for the change to be made and evidence that all elements of implementation, testing, rollout, training, and such are performed.

In a client/server environment, routine and some corrective system maintenance is left to the healthcare organization's staff or contractors; while other corrective, modifying, or enhancing maintenance may require consultation or direct work performed by the original vendor. Whoever performs system maintenance should provide regular reports on what maintenance has been done and this should be compared with policy, issues logs, and change requests. In an ASP or SaaS environment, most system maintenance will be performed by the vendor with the exception of maintenance on local hardware and any software not covered by the ASP or SaaS vendor. Healthcare organizations are advised to keep track of issues they report to the ASP or SaaS vendor and confirm they are appropriately addressed.

Monitor Results

To complete the SDLC, monitoring results is an essential element that ensures health information systems continue to meet the organization's goals, and identify when there are new needs. A formal monitoring program should begin immediately after go-live. The project manager or a compliance officer (or both) may be responsible for monitoring. The monitoring program should include formal processes such as user surveys, observations, benefits realization studies, and results analysis, as well as informal processes like the proverbial bagel breakfasts, pizza lunches, or milk and cookie breaks. During and immediately after go-live, it is helpful to have a break room set up where new users can unwind and talk about the system. Food is always inviting and often eases tensions when there are issues. Other forms of celebration for getting through the go-live day and reaching other milestones are also helpful. As time passes to more routine use, informal feedback mechanism may move to weekly, monthly, or quarterly opportunities, but should continue indefinitely. Feedback from both formal and informal methods should be documented and addressed. Users must see that their concerns are given attention.

Although monitoring results is improving, many healthcare organizations do not monitor results well. Staff complaints, technology issues, and low levels of use are often known, but not tracked in any formal manner. Often changes are not made until a crisis occurs or the next federal mandate is enforced. Monitoring use, however, can result in achieving full adoption and even optimization, which leads to goals achieved more quickly and comprehensively.

Check Your Understanding 11.3

Instructions: **Answer the following questions.**

1. Which of the following is a characteristic of the systems development life cycle?
   A. It lists the components of a health information system so that organizations do not have gaps in their strategic planning
   B. It describes the steps to ensure that all components needed for a system to achieve its desired results are addressed
   C. It is a roadmap for vendor selection of any products needed to meet an organization's vision, mission, and goals
   D. It serves as a guide for strategic planning for health IT

2. The systems development life cycle is cyclical because:
   A. There are six steps that are repeated continuously
   B. Feedback from monitoring results initiates repetition of the steps in the cycle
   C. It varies with the stages in which an organization has adopted health IT
   D. System theory reinvents itself periodically

3. In the systems development lifecycle, desired outcomes may be best specified as:
   A. Requirements specifications
   B. Steps in product selection
   C. SMART goals
   D. Request for proposal

4. A health IT steering committee that best guides an organization's technology plans includes:
   A. Physician leadership
   B. All information technology staff that will work on the project
   C. Legal counsel
   D. EHR vendor

5. Steps taken to confirm various facts about a product are referred to as:
   A. Vendor selection
   B. Systems development lifecycle
   C. Certification
   D. Due diligence

6. Which of the following is true in contract negotiation?
   A. Price is the most important thing to negotiate
   B. It is best to use an attorney who can ensure the product acquired will work
   C. All issues with terms of the contract must be negotiated
   D. Vendors should take charge of payment schedules to ensure payback

7. Moving data from an old system to a new system requires which of the following?
   A. Data conversion
   B. Chart conversion
   C. Loading master files
   D. System build

8. Steps taken to help new users acclimate to the new technology is:
   A. Change control
   B. Change management
   C. Training
   D. Testing

9. A situation in which a healthcare organization has multiple different vendors represented in its applications is referred to as:
   A. Best of breed
   B. Best of fit
   C. Application service provider
   D. Legacy environment

10. In implementing health IT, the step most often not performed or not performed well is:
    A. Contract negotiation
    B. Issues management
    C. Maintenance
    D. Workflow and process analysis and design

Real-World Case 11.1

A diabetic patient, John, moves to a new city and uses the Internet to select a local **primary care physician (PCP)**, who is a generalist physician and will coordinate his overall care. He is able to select a PCP who appears to have strong outcomes in diabetes and positive patient satisfaction scores. John schedules an appointment via the physician's website and is set up with a user ID and password to link the PCP with John's PHR, which is a record he maintains himself by uploading copies of records from various providers he has seen over the years. This enables the PCP to view and retrieve pertinent information from other providers and information John has recorded about his diet, over-the-counter medications taken, and other information relating to compliance with his diabetic treatment regimen.

John also asks his former hometown physician to send information to this new PCP. This physician does so using standard content and format specifications for exchanging referral information between providers. With the information supplied by the PHR and his former PCP, the new PCP's EHR is prepopulated with a current problem list, recent laboratory results, and other data. Additionally, John's medication history can be directly supplied to his new PCP's EHR by the PCP linking to information available from John's health plan.

When John visits the new PCP, information from these various sources will be validated and updated. The new PCP is able to document all components of John's visit at the time of the visit, including demonstrating medical necessity for lab work by applying ICD diagnosis codes and generating appropriate evaluation and management (E/M) codes for the level of service provided. The PCP decides to put John on a strict smoking-cessation program and exercise routine, with plans to adjust medications according to John's vital signs and blood sugar levels, which will be monitored remotely through a medical device.

All is going well until John has an accident at work that requires a visit to the emergency room, subsequent admission to the hospital, and outpatient physical therapy. All his providers, however, are members of a health information organization (HIO). As a result, each provider has immediate access to the specific information needed to treat John throughout his care and for which John has provided a consent directive enabling him to opt-in to the sharing of such information with all participants in the HIO.

At the hospital, the physician providing care is able to reconcile all of John's medications in accordance with the Joint Commission requirements and to select medications that have been screened against John's known allergies. The hospital is also part of a health reform mechanism that ties reimbursement to quality metrics. This improves the quality of healthcare and reduces costs in an assigned population of patients. As a result, the hospital has access to John's previous lab and x-ray results, so repeating these lab tests is not necessary—saving John time and potential health risks, and reducing overall costs. In selecting the physical therapy referral, the hospitalist has access to John's health plan benefits information, so no time is wasted in arranging for physical therapy to begin.

John's PCP also continuously monitors the impact of the accident on John's diabetes during his hospitalization and makes appropriate adjustments. After John is discharged and in physical therapy, the health plan can monitor whether he is following the prescribed exercise routine and can notify the PCP to follow up if necessary. John can access tailored discharge instructions that superimpose his picture on the exercise instructions so that it is clear how to avoid further injury. In addition, each provider John encountered throughout this episode of care follows up with him on the smoking-cessation program he started with his PCP, motivating him to keep from smoking.

Real-World Case 11.2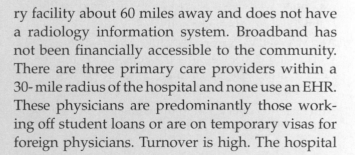

Rural Hospital is a 15-bed critical access hospital that has had a hospital information system (HIS) that provides typical administrative information systems services for a number of years. It also has had an LIS system from a different vendor. It does not have a full time pharmacist, so it has not had a pharmacy information system. Except for basic radiology procedures, it refers patients to a tertia-

ry facility about 60 miles away and does not have a radiology information system. Broadband has not been financially accessible to the community. There are three primary care providers within a 30-mile radius of the hospital and none use an EHR. These physicians are predominantly those working off student loans or are on temporary visas for foreign physicians. Turnover is high. The hospital decided to acquire an EHR system when the MU program started. Believing its options were limited, it contracted with a vendor who catered to critical access hospitals. The vendor implemented a stage 1 certified EHR.

The hospital subsequently found that because of its old and incompatible HIS, manual entry or re-entry of data was often required to register a patient into the EHR, to post discharges to the HIS, and such. Without a pharmacy information system, the physicians' orders for medications had to be printed for the traveling pharmacist to use in stocking the medication cabinet for the nurses. The lack of other physician and nurse documentation not required in stage 1 resulted in the hospital printing all contents of the EHR to paper and continuing to file a paper chart. The result was significantly more time required to use the EHR system than with the paper chart alone. Finally, when stage 2 criteria for certification were released, the vendor struggled to respond and ultimately was sold to another company with no experience servicing small hospitals.

Since incentives in the MU program were front loaded (the majority of the incentives were delivered for demonstrating meaningful use of stage 1) and the critical access hospital is presently reimbursed on a cost rather than fee-for-service basis (HealthIT.gov 2015), it made the decision to delay further deployment of health information systems. It wants to hire a health information management professional, contract for more comprehensive IT support, and engage physicians and community leaders in more thoroughly evaluating both health IT options and the state of reimbursement for critical access hospitals. It recognizes that whatever the future holds, it will need to move to a best-of-fit health IT environment, probably utilizing a SaaS provider through cloud computing, requiring affordable and reliable broadband services.

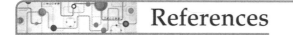 # References

Agency for Healthcare Research and Quality. 2011 (August). Guide to Reducing Unintended Consequences of Electronic Health Records. http://psnet.ahrq.gov/resource.aspx?resourceID=23191.

Amatayakul, M. 2013. *Electronic Health Records: A Practical Guide for Professionals and Organizations*, 5th ed. Chicago: AHIMA.

Amatayakul, M. 2011. *A Stepwise Approach to Workflow and Process Management for Health Information Technology and Electronic Health Records*. Boca Raton, FL: Productivity Press.

American Health Information Management Association. 2015 (update). Data quality management model. *Journal of AHIMA*. 86(10): expanded web version. http://bok.ahima.org/PB/DataQualityModel#.Vje-S53nZkh.

AHIMA e-HIM Personal Health Record Workgroup. 2005. Defining the Personal Health Record. http://library.ahima.org/doc?oid=59377#.VxEjKPkrK9I.

American Recovery and Reinvestment Act of 2009, Title XIII Health Information Technology.

Campbell, E.M., D.F. Sittig, J.S. Ash, K.P. Guappone, and R.H. Dykstra. 2006 (September–October). Types of unintended consequences related to computerized provider order entry. *Journal of the American Medical Informatics Association*. 13(5):547–556.

Centers for Medicare and Medicaid Services (CMS). 2015. Physician Quality Reporting System. https://www.cms.gov/Medicare/Quality-Initiatives-Patient-Assessment-Instruments/PQRS/index.html?redirect=/pqri/.

Centers for Medicare and Medicaid Services (CMS). 2014. EHR Incentive Programs. *Federal Register*. https://www.federalregister.gov/articles/2014/09/04/2014-21021/medicare-and-medicaid-programs-modifications-to-the-medicare-and-medicaid-electronic-health-record.

Chaiken, B.P. 2011. Web 3.0 Data-mining for comparative effectiveness and CDS. *Patient Safety & Healthcare Quality*. 8(5):10–11.

ECRI Institute. 2014 (January). EMR Integration Vendors and You: Hearing Each Other Loud and Clear. The Bench: ECRI Institute. http://www.ecri.org.

Graham, J. and C. Dizikes. 2011 (June 27). Baby's Death Spotlights Safety Risks Linked to Computerized Systems. *Chicago Tribune.* http://articles.chicagotribune.com/2011-06-27/news/ct-met-technology-errors-20110627_1_electronic-medical-records-physicians-systems.

HealthIT.gov. 2016. Glossary. https://www.healthit.gov/policy-researchers-implementers/about-onc-health-it-certification-program.

HealthIT.gov. 2015. Benefits for Critical Access Hospitals and Other Small Rural Hospitals. http://www.healthit.gov/providers-professionals/benefits-critical-access-hospitals-and-other-small-rural-hospitals.

HealthIT.gov. 2014 (March 20). Step 3: Select or Upgrade to a Certified EHR. https://www.healthit.gov/providers-professionals/ehr-implementation-steps/step-3-select-or-upgrade-certified-ehr.

Healthcare Information and Management Systems Society. 2013. HIMSS HIE in Practice Series, Frequently Asked Questions: eHealth Exchange, the Direct Project, and CONNECT. http://www.himss.org/ResourceLibrary/ResourceDetail.aspx?ItemNumber=11657.

Healthcare Information and Management Systems Society. 2012. The eHealth Exchange and CONNECT Overview. http://www.himss.org/ResourceLibrary/ResourceDetail.aspx?ItemNumber=10555.

HIMSS Analytics. 2010 (December 1). Medical Devices Landscape: Current and Future Adoption, Integration with EMRs, and Connectivity. A HIMSS Analytics White Paper. http://www.lantronix.com/wp-content/uploads/pdf/Medical-Devices-Landscape_Lantronix_HIMMS_WP.pdf.

Hughes, R.G., ed. 2008 (April). *Patient Safety and Quality: An Evidence-Based Handbook for Nurses.* Rockville, MD: Agency for Healthcare Research and Quality.

Institute of Medicine. 2011. *Digital Infrastructure of the Learning Health System: The Foundation for Continuous Improvement in Health and Health Care.* Washington, DC: National Academies Press.

Kalatzis, F.G., N. Giannakeas, T.P. Exarchos, L. Lorenzelli, A. Adami, M. Decarli, S. Lupoli, F. Macciardi, S. Markoula, I. Georgiou, and D.I. Fotiadis. 2009. Developing a genomic-based point-of-care diagnostic system for rheumatoid arthritis and multiple sclerosis. *Proceedings for Engineering in Medicine and Biology Society (EMBC), Annual International Conference of the IEEE*, pp. 827–830.

McKenzie, K. and P. Karnstedt. 2010 (September–October). Automated informed consent: Patients and institutions benefit alike. *Patient Safety & Quality Healthcare.* 7(4):38–45.

National Business Coalition on Health. 2011. Value-based Purchasing: A Definition. http://www.nbch.org/Value-based-Purchasing-A-Definition.

National Institute of Standards and Technology (NIST). 2008. Special Publication (SP) 800-64, Revision 2, Security Considerations in the System Development Life Cycle. http://csrc.nist.gov/publications/PubsSPs.html.

Office of the National Coordinator for Health Information Technology (ONC). 2015a. Federal Health IT Strategic Plan: 2015–2020. https://www.healthit.gov/sites/default/files/9-5-federalhealthitstratplanfinal_0.pdf.

Office of the National Coordinator for Health Information Technology (ONC). 2015b. Federal Health IT Strategic Plan: 2015–2020. Draft for Public Comment. https://www.healthit.gov/sites/default/files/federal-healthIT-strategic-plan-2014.pdf.

Office of the National Coordinator for Health Information Technology (ONC). 2015c. A Shared Nationwide Interoperability Roadmap, Version 1.0. https://www.healthit.gov/sites/default/files/hie-interoperability/nationwide-interoperability-roadmap-final-version-1.0.pdf.

Rollins, G. 2012 (January). Unintended consequences: Identifying and mitigating unanticipated issues in EHR use. *Journal of AHIMA.* 83(1):28–32.

SAS. N.d. Analytics in Healthcare. SAS White Paper. http://www.sas.com/en_us/whitepapers/analytics-healthcare-102465.html.

Strome, T.L. 2013. Chapter 1 in *Healthcare Analytics for Quality and Performance Improvement.* Hoboken, NJ: Wiley & Sons, Inc.

The Sequoia Project. 2015. eHealth Exchange. http://sequoiaproject.org/ehealth-exchange/about/.

Wians, F.H. 2009 (February). Clinical laboratory tests: Which, why, and what do the results mean? *LabMedicine* 40(2):105–113. http://labmed.ascpjournals.org/content/40/2/105.full.

Wolfskill, S. 2014. KEYS to Revenue Cycle Improvements: HFMA's Approach, Healthcare Financial Management Association. http://nepahfma.org/images/2_21_14_presentation_3.pdf.

12

Healthcare Information

Kathy Giannangelo, MA, RHIA, CCS, CPHIMS, FAHIMA

Learning Objectives

- Justify the importance of healthcare information to the healthcare industry
- Explain the role of data analytics in healthcare information
- State the strategic uses of healthcare information
- Define consumer informatics
- Explain the connection between consumer information access and navigation tools and healthcare information
- Differentiate between the benefits and challenges of sharing healthcare information

Key Terms

Clinical data analytics
Clinical data repository
Clinical data warehouse
Clinical decision support system
Dashboard
Database
Data abstraction
Data analytics

Data capture
Data mining
Decision support system
Discrete data
eHealth Exchange
Executive information system
Healthcare data analytics
Health informatics

Health information exchange
Key indicator
Natural language processing
Patient portal
Personal health record
Point-of-care charting
Scorecards
Structured data
Unstructured data

Healthcare information is important to patient care, research, reimbursement, and many more functions. Healthcare information is based on personal health data about individuals primarily for provider use in the management of care. Collection techniques include traditional methods such as paper health records as well as eHealth tools such as documentation templates. The sources of health information include the provider and the individual through the use of a personal health record (PHR). A **personal health record** is a record created and managed by an individual in a private, secure, and confidential environment. In addition, the federal incentives for the adoption of the electronic heath record (EHR) have progressed healthcare information exchange, including returning a patient care summary to the person whose information is discussed. Databases of healthcare information collected or maintained by healthcare providers, institutions, payers, and government agencies are of great importance to those who use them; for example, researchers or public health

agencies. Typically these secondary uses of healthcare information include those for administrative purposes, including determination of payment for services provided, measurement of quality performance indicators, and research.

In order for the government to achieve the desired benefits of electronic health information, it developed a strategy that requires the collection, sharing, and use of electronic health information. This strategy is illustrated in figure 12.1.

The health information management (HIM) professional's role is growing. These roles include data analytics, consumer engagement, and health information exchange (HIE). This chapter discusses HIE information from the perspective of data analytics and explores the strategic uses of health information. In addition, the consumers' link to healthcare information—specifically their needs for information, ease of access, navigational tools, and PHRs—is described. The various aspects of sharing and exchanging healthcare information are also addressed.

Figure 12.1 Strategies to achieve health IT goals

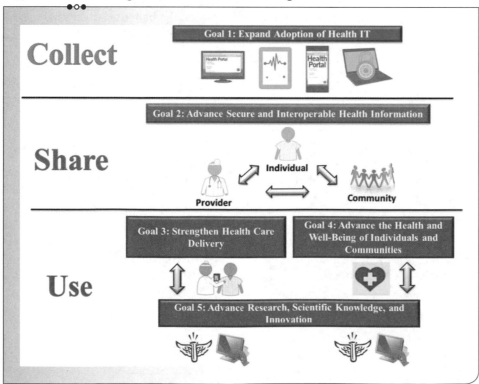

Source: ONC 2014a.

Role of Data Analytics in Healthcare Information

Data are needed to arrive at information. Health data are not health information until it is interpreted, evaluated, and appropriately displayed (RWJF 2015). The difference between data and information is described in chapter 3. **Data analytics** is the science of examining raw data with the purpose of drawing conclusions about that information. The role of data analytics depends on the type of data being captured, reviewed, and used for the purpose of turning it into healthcare information. Multiple types of data exist, two of which—healthcare and clinical—are further explained in the next section. If the data are of a clinical nature, then the analytics revolve around the contents of the health record. One use for this healthcare information is clinical decision support (CDS). "Clinical decision support provides clinicians, staff, patients or other individuals with knowledge and person-specific information, intelligently filtered or presented at appropriate times, to enhance health and healthcare" (ONC 2013).

Clinical data about an individual can also be combined with clinical data from other individuals to form population-based healthcare data. The resulting information may be used to improve the health of the public. Analytics also plays a role in leveraging data to improve healthcare quality and patient outcomes. The following is an introduction to analytics, its tools, and the knowledge areas for HIM professionals interested in data analytics.

Introduction to Analytics

There are different types of analytics. Descriptive analytics answers the question "what happened," diagnostic analytics answers the question "why did it happen," predictive analytics answers "what will happen," and prescriptive analytics answers "how can we make it happen" (Gartner 2012).

Analytics involves acquiring, managing, studying, interpreting, and transforming data into useful information for a variety of reasons. Types of data include clinical, financial, and operational data and the types of analytics include healthcare data analytics and clinical data analytics. **Healthcare data analytics** is the practice of using data to make business decisions in healthcare, whereas **clinical data analytics** is the process by which health information is captured, reviewed, and used to measure quality of care provided. What data are involved, the consumer of the information, and the decision the analysis supports influences the analytic process and choice of tools. However, there are certain steps that occur in order to prepare healthcare data for data analysis. The first step is data capture, which helps ensure the data needed is available and that the data is correct. The second is data provisioning, which ensures that the data is in a format that can be manipulated for data analysis. Data analysis, where data is interpreted, is the final stage of transforming raw data into meaningful analytics. These stages of transforming data into meaningful analytics are shown in figure 12.2.

Analytics Tools

The amount and type of data available for analysis has increased as more of it is available electronically. In addition, as technology advances, the various tools available to perform the analytics allow for new ways to study and present the data. A few of the more common tools are those used for visualization, to report on process measures, to capture the data, and for extracting and examining data from a database.

Data Visualization

The graphic display of data can help the viewer understand the data trends so it is easier to identify areas that need action, such as addressing a decline in the number of patients or an increase in the infection rate. Types of data visualization tools include tables, charts, and graphs. Choosing one over another can mean the difference between correct or incorrect data representation and drawing an accurate or erroneous conclusion. For example, tables display exact values whereas graphs show trends.

Figure 12.2 Three stages of transforming raw data into meaningful analytics

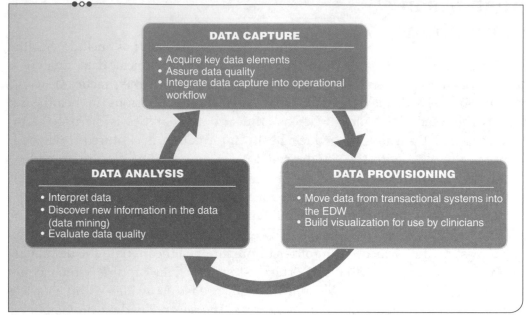

Source: Staheli 2014.

Following established guidelines for data visualization results in the delivery of a clear message. Overall when creating any visual presentation:

- Comprehend the data to be visualized, including intent and size.

- Evaluate the information to communicate and the way it should be visualized.

- Define your audience and examine how they process visual information.

- Display the intended information to the appropriate audience in the clearest, simplest form (SAS 2014).

Tables are used to organize quantitative data or data expressed as numbers. Charts (such as pie and bar charts) and graphs (such as line graphs) are appropriate when presenting relationships. Each tool has specific features to keep in mind when depicting the data. For additional information on tables, charts, and graphs, see chapter 13.

Figure 12.3 provides an example of poor and improved data display using a pie chart.

Dashboard

Another data analytics tool is the **dashboard**, which is a management report of process measures.

A dashboard is different from a **scorecard**, which reports outcomes measures. Both may involve key indicators. A **key indicator** is a quantifiable measure used over time to determine whether some structure, process, or outcome in the provision of care to a patient supports high-quality performance measured against best practice criteria. For example, a key indicator could monitor death rates or infections. For information on scorecards see chapter 18.

HIM professionals use dashboards to monitor a number of indicators to improve performance and meet the quality goals such as reducing infection rate. In order to track the process measure over time, metrics or benchmarks are established. (Metrics are discussed in chapter 18.) The results are displayed using the red, yellow, and green stoplight scheme. Dashboards provide early warnings signals and alerts the manager of areas in need of attention so organizational performance is improved.

For example, a recent HIM trend is instituting a clinical documentation improvement (CDI) program. Since this is not a small undertaking, dashboards can assist in measuring whether or not the program is successful. A monthly dashboard might show the number of clarifications requested by a

Figure 12.3   Poor and improved data display

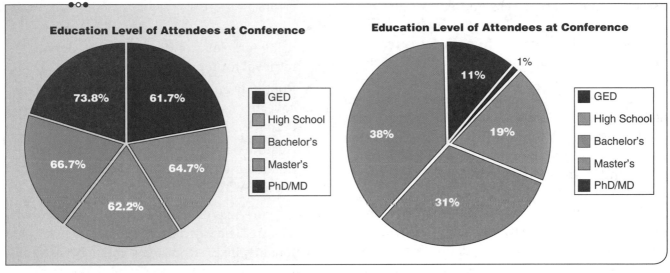

Source: AHIMA 2014.

CDI specialist that impacted a diagnosis-related group based on a benchmark. The dashboard would show green if the metric is met, yellow if it is in progress or halfway met, and red if the metric is below standard.

Dashboards are also used to manage revenue cycle management performance. For example, the Healthcare Financial Management Association (HFMA) has a web-based application called MAP App for use by healthcare providers to check revenue cycle performance and evaluate against provider peer groups (HFMA 2015). HFMA's key performance indicators can be used to track, monitor, and improve revenue cycle performance.

Data Capture Tools

Data capture is the process of recording data in a health record system or database. A database is an organized collection of data, text, references, or pictures in a standardized format, typically stored in a computer system for multiple applications. One of the most common healthcare databases is the relational database, which stores data in predefined tables consisting of rows and columns. Healthcare providers as well as patients may be the source of the data. There are several tools available for acquiring health-related data. Historically, data capture into a health record was via written notes or traditional voice dictation that was transcribed

and typed into a paper report. Another method for data capture is scanning documents into electronic document management systems that create a picture of the scanned document, making it accessible electronically. Devices also include traditional keyboard or touch screen handheld computers or patient-generated health data devices (discussed later in this chapter). When the software application is run on a mobile platform such as a tablet or cellular phone, system and application software (often referred to as apps) is needed in order for the device to function and perform the desired tasks.

Electronic healthcare data capture is a fundamental function of the electronic health record (EHR) (Amatayakul 2013, 6). The EHR is a system with a number of components and data capture is an element in each component. The components include source systems (such as the laboratory information system), core clinical EHR systems (such as point-of-care charting), supporting infrastructure such as human–computer interfaces, and connectivity systems such as personal health records (Amatayakul 2013, 16–19). In point-of-care charting the information is entered into the health record at the time and location of service. Nurses entering data using a tablet as they conduct patient assessments while at the bedside is an example of point-of-care charting.

A human–computer interface is the device used by humans to access and enter data into a computer system. A number of mobile devices are used for data entry into point-of-care charting systems. These handheld devices include tablet computers, laptop computers, and smartphones. They often contain built-in methods to facilitate the capture of structured data such as predefined or custom-built templates or forms with drop-down menus and point and click fields and word macros. All exist to make data collection easier.

The outcome of point-of-care charting can be unstructured or structured data. **Unstructured data** are nonbinary, human-readable data, whereas **structured data** are binary, machine-readable data in discrete fields. An example of unstructured data is free text that describes the patient's description of his or her condition. An example of structured data is using checkboxes to indicate patient symptoms. Structured data has many advantages over unstructured data when it comes to data analytics and health information exchange. For additional information structured and unstructured data, refer to chapter 6.

The structured data's entry fields and the potential entries in those fields are controlled, defined, and limited resulting in discrete data. **Discrete data** represent separate and distinct values or observations; that is, data that contain only finite numbers and have only specified values. Stored in databases and data warehouses, this standardized data are available in a usable and accessible form. However, physicians and other healthcare providers may express frustration when limited to recording only certain data in specific fields. While a set format ensures consistency and provides standard meaning, it may limit details considered important by clinicians.

When considering methods for EHR data capture, follow these best practices:

- Consider what data needs to be captured and customize available tools to collect it.
- Evaluate the data and determine its placement in the record to determine what rules or procedures are needed to upload

the information most efficiently and without errors.

- Collect the data in a standardized format using templates or discrete fields to make retrieval for reporting easier.
- Routinely audit a sample of records that are collected using the data capture methods described.
- Acquire primary and secondary data from existing internal or external data sources (AHIMA 2014).

Data capture may also occur with word processing software. The word processing copy and paste functionality in EHR systems must be carefully monitored, and limited or prohibited to prevent data quality issues. Measures for preventing data quality problems include the following.

- Clearly label the information as copied from another source
- Limit the ability for data to be copied and pasted from other systems
- Limit the ability of one author to copy from another author's documentation
- Allow a provider to mark specific results as reviewed
- Allow only key, predefined elements of reports and results to be copied or imported
- Monitor a clinician's use of copy and paste (AHIMA Work Group 2015)

For additional information on the copy and paste function and risks associated with it, refer to chapter 3.

Two other technologies—speech recognition (speech-to-text) and **natural language processing (NLP)**—provide yet another way to acquire health data. NLP is a technology that converts human language (structured or unstructured) into data that can be translated and then manipulated by computer systems. Integration of these technologies with the EHR system can result in the provision of clinical information needed by providers to inform decision making.

Back-end speech recognition (BESR) is a specific use of speech recognition technology (SRT) in an environment where the recognition process occurs after the completion of dictation by sending voice files through a server. In BESR, an employee edits or corrects the dictation. Front-end speech recognition (FESR) is a process where the provider speaks into a microphone or headset attached to a PC and upon speaking, the words are displayed as they are recognized. The physician corrects misrecognitions at the time of dictation. Use of FESR integrated with an EHR provides the best outcome, as the provider is able to respond to prompts from the EHR resulting in more complete, accurate, and timely documentation (AHIMA 2013). Templates and macros are also tools used with SRT to capture data. As the output of SRT is digital text, combining it with NLP results in the conversion of the text, or any free text narrative into data that can be translated and then manipulated by computer systems. Once transformed it becomes searchable along with other structured data.

Data Mining

Data mining is the process of extracting and analyzing large volumes of data from a database for the purpose of identifying hidden and sometimes subtle relationships or patterns and using those relationships to predict behaviors. It is a key piece of analytics and of the knowledge discovery process. There are several knowledge discovery process models such as the Knowledge Discovery in Databases (KDD), Sample, Explore, Modify, Model, Assess (SEMMA), and CRoss-Industry Standard Process for Data Mining (CRISP-DM) as well as hybrid models. Each has defined steps with data mining being one of them.

The available data for analytics strategy and mining can come from EHRs and various databases such as a clinical data repository and clinical data warehouse. A **clinical data repository** is a central database that focuses on clinical information. The **clinical data warehouse** allows access to data from multiple databases and combines the results into a single query and reporting interface. Specific applications of data mining methods are customized for certain uses of the extracted data. For example, data mining may be used to extract clinical data directly from the EHR for the purpose of compiling content for reporting clinical quality measures. The clinical data warehouse lends itself to data mining as it encompasses multiple sources of data. Systematically analyzing the data uncovers hidden patterns or trends for use in predicting behaviors. The information discovered from data mining databases aids clinical research. For example, data mining could be used to detect early signals of potential adverse drug events. Other data mining applications are used for the evaluation of treatment effectiveness, management of healthcare, customer relationship management, and detection of fraud and abuse (Koh and Tan 2005).

HIM Professionals and Analytics

Analytics start with data and HIM professionals, with their understanding of healthcare data, can help ensure that correct and accurate data are captured. HIM professionals are also proficient in business operations and clinical processes. However, data analytics require going beyond these into competencies such as business intelligence, database administration, inferential and descriptive statistics, health information technology, and project management (Sandefer et al. 2015).

AHIMA lists the following knowledge topics as important for data analytics.

- Clinical, financial, and operational data
- Understanding of database queries (such as structured query language [SQL])
- Understanding statistical software
- Data mining
- Quality standards, processes, and outcome measures
- Risk adjustment
- Business practices (for example, workflow or payer guidelines)
- Medical terminology
- Healthcare reimbursement methodologies
- Classification systems
- Source data
- Qualitative and quantitative analysis (AHIMA 2015a)

Strategic Uses of Healthcare Information

There are many reasons to collect data and turn it into information including administrative uses such as claims submission, meeting quality measurement reporting requirements, assessing health status and outcomes, and performing clinical research. As health information technology (IT) systems evolve, the ability to aggregate the collected data improves and the information from it better supports strategic analytics and organizational decision making. Through interpretation and evaluation of aggregated data from a variety of sources, development of strategies to improve patient care outcomes, reduce costs, and plan the future are possible through decision support, quality measurement, and clinical research, which are addressed in the following sections.

Decision Support

Information systems in healthcare are adopted for a variety of reasons. One of these is to improve the outcome in decision-making tasks. A **decision support system (DSS)** is a computer-based system that gathers data from a variety of sources and assists in providing structure to the data by using various analytical models and visual tools in order to facilitate and improve the ultimate outcome in decision-making tasks associated with nonroutine and nonrepetitive problems. A DSS is primarily used by management for operational as well as strategic decisions. A **clinical decision support system (CDSS)** is a "special subcategory of clinical information systems designated to help healthcare providers make knowledge-based clinical decisions" (Fenton and Biedermann 2014, 39). More information on clinical information systems can be found in chapter 11. In DSS and CDSS, typically the problem in need of solving is unstructured or the circumstances are unknown. For example, a CDSS could deliver targeted clinical decision support by supplying clinical reminders and alerts impacting the quality and efficiency of care. For example, within an EHR the clinician may receive a reminder that it is time for the patient's annual gynecological exam. In the case of a DSS, a manager could identify operational areas in need of improvement such as resource allocation, improving the cost efficiency of patient care delivery, or the need for an additional exam room.

The DSS offers potential to the user when strategic decisions are needed. With data, analytical models, and visual tools at their disposal, the user can perform simulations of patterns based on various assumptions, monitor and assess key indicators, or perform data comparisons to look for trends. For example, to evaluate the success or failure of interventions, track trends, and identify opportunities for improvement, a manager may monitor readmission rates using a scorecard generated by the DSS.

An **executive information system (EIS)** is a system that facilitates and supports senior managerial decisions. Given that information is an enterprise strategic asset, an EIS is required to consider the broad needs of the healthcare organization. An EIS can transcend the organizational structure, transform the business by standardizing and describing solutions throughout the enterprise, and drive information-centric decision making (3e Services LLC 2015).

The EIS is the source for identifying high-level strategic, operational, financial, or clinical issues. Rather than managing at the individual departmental level, an EIS can pull together financial, operational, and clinical information, with enterprise-wide policies and guidelines, to help the executive find actionable insights to drive enterprise performance. Organization-wide operational and informational processes improve with an EIS because business problems can be exposed or business opportunities discovered. Examples of organization-wide operational and information processes key indicators executives may monitor include surgical volume and patient satisfaction. Figure 12.4 provides an example of an executive healthcare dashboard regarding patient satisfaction.

Figure 12.4 Executive healthcare dashboard

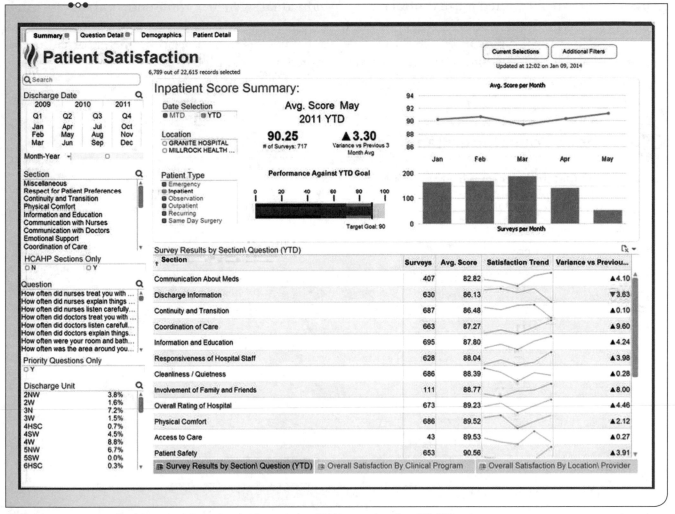

Quality Measurement

Using healthcare information to improve the quality of healthcare is not a new strategic initiative. What has changed, however, is the health IT available to collect and analyze the data for the purpose of turning it into healthcare information. For example, instead of manual data abstraction, or the identification of data elements by an individual through health record review, using standards and guidelines data mining can extract clinical data directly from the EHR to compile content for reporting clinical quality measures. Healthcare information can also be used to improve care effectiveness; for example, alerts can be sent to administrators and physicians when measures related to quality and patient safety fall outside a normal range along with notifications of what may be causing these abnormalities. Also, health system effectiveness (for example, knowing which intervention was ineffective) could result in better healthcare outcomes for patients based on standards of care.

Clinical Research

Besides patient care, one of the original reasons for collecting data and analyzing its information is to research and study diseases and interventions. Information systems can support research by supplying the health data needed to inform clinical research programs and population and public health surveillance. In these cases, multiple sources of data are integrated into a central repository where it is possible to find early markers of disease, and historical data can be used to simulate and model trends in long-term care needs.

For example, healthcare information such as an individual's genetic profile and local trends in disease prevalence may be used in patient-centered outcomes research. For additional information on research, see chapter 13.

 Check Your Understanding 12.1

Instructions: **Match the term with the definition.**

1. _____ Scorecard

2. _____ Data mining

3. _____ Dashboard

4. _____ Data capture

5. _____ Speech recognition
   A. Reports outcomes measures
   B. Reports process measures
   C. Speech-to-text conversion
   D. Extraction and analysis of data
   E. Process of recording data

Consumers and Healthcare Information

In recent years, consumers have become the focus when it comes to healthcare as a result of healthcare reform initiatives and the growth of digital technology. The Office of the National Coordinator for Health Information Technology (ONC) envisions that by 2020, "the power of each individual is developed and unleashed to be active in managing their health and partnering in their health care, enabled by information and technology" (Daniel et al. 2014). Terms such as *patient-centered care*, *patient-centric care*, and even *person at the center* have emerged to indicate the shift to the individual as the focal point when it comes to healthcare.

What follows is a brief introduction to consumer health informatics, and an overview of information access and navigation tools such as patient portals. Information sharing specific to personal health records (PHRs) is then discussed.

This section concludes with a review of HIM roles in consumer informatics.

Introduction to Consumer Health Informatics

Health informatics is the field of information science concerned with the management of all aspects of health data and information through the application of computers and computer technologies (Fenton and Biedermann 2014, 2). Adding consumers to health informatics makes them the focus for the technology that acquires, manages, maintains, and uses the data and information. Thus, "consumer informatics is the field devoted to informatics from multiple consumer or patient views" (AMIA n.d.). Consumer health informatics is a subtype of health informatics. A patient portal to a provider's website where a PHR can be developed and maintained is an example of consumer health informatics. Clinical email communication is another example of consumer health informatics.

With any number of computer technologies available to the consumer, such as mobile health (mhealth), health information is only a click away. Engaging patients in their care can be done by any number of health IT technologies designed for information access and navigation as well as those that allow the sharing of information. These health IT technologies improve patient–provider communication, allow for closer patient monitoring, and increase information access, all of which facilitate patient involvement with care providers. For example, through social networking sites consumers can connect with others who have the same condition and learn about their experiences.

Information Access and Navigational Tools

The Medicare and Medicaid EHR Incentive Programs funded by the American Recovery and Reinvestment Act of 2009 stimulated the healthcare industry to adopt EHRs. One of the objectives to achieve Meaningful Use (MU) for certified EHR technology is to provide patients with the ability to electronically view, download, and transmit their health information within a certain number of days of the information being available to the eligible professionals. By providing patients access to an electronic copy of their health information they, and their caregivers, can be more engaged in their care. For an explanation of MU, refer to chapter 11.

Consumer health IT applications for information access and navigation include hardware, software, and web-based applications. Tools such as mobile devices, patient portals, and social networking allow consumers to not only manage their health information electronically but also participate in their own healthcare via electronic means.

Mobile Devices

Portable, wireless computing devices or mobile devices include tablet computers, laptop computers, and smartphones. These devices combined with mobile medical apps can help consumers gain access to useful information wherever they may be and whenever it is needed. Apps for smartphones include pharmaceutical references with information about side effects and dosage amounts, access to licensed healthcare professionals allowing video chats about a medical problem, and guides providing step-by-step first aid instructions.

According to the US Food and Drug Administration (FDA), a mobile medical app is a mobile app that meets the definition of device in the Federal Food, Drug, and Cosmetic Act (FD&C Act) and either is intended "to be used as an accessory to a regulated medical device; or to transform a mobile platform into a regulated medical device" (FDA 2015).

The FDA considers the mobile app's intended use in determining whether the definition of a device has been met. The FDA guidance states a mobile app intended for use in performing a medical device function (such as for diagnosis of disease or other conditions) is a medical device, regardless of the platform on which it is run (FDA 2015). An example would be mobile apps intended to run on smart phones to analyze and interpret EKG waveforms to detect heart function irregularities.

Patient Portals

A **patient portal** is a system that allows consumers to log in to a secure online website to gain access to personal health information and navigate around it once inside the system. The type of patient portal and the modules implemented will offer different functionalities, such as:

- Accessing a subset of the patient's health records (for example, medical history, health issues, medication list, test results, care plans, allergy list)
- Sending a secure message to the patient's healthcare provider(s)
- Uploading clinical information and telemetry (for example, blood pressure, blood glucose values, and weight measured at home)
- Completing forms electronically instead of on paper (e-forms)

- Accessing a child or elderly parent's records with appropriate authorization (proxy access)
- Scheduling appointments
- Requesting medication refills
- Accessing billing records
- Paying bills online (Carayon et al. 2015)

The National Learning Consortium recommends implementing features that support engagement such as a portal that has a problem-solving orientation, interactive decision tools, and personalized messages and tools rather than one with an administrative slant with functionality such as scheduling appointments (NLC 2013). Each of these functions is geared toward encouraging patient involvement in his or her healthcare. For example, a patient may come to the portal wanting to know more about symptoms he or she is experiencing. An interactive decision tool would assist patients with assessing the symptoms through a series of questions. If the patient visits the portal to better understand a current diagnosis, a link to education material about the condition is available. Either scenario may result in communication with the provider via secure messaging about what was learned.

Social Media

A number of healthcare-focused social networks are available to consumers as individuals come together to interact and receive support from others with similar interests. Online communities specific to a condition or disease provide the consumer with information about the condition and which treatments may have greater success than others.

Providers use social media to inform consumers about diseases, conditions, and treatments. For example, Mayo Clinic's website contains patient care and health information on many diseases and conditions. In addition, the site has a symptom checker; a list of tests and procedures that includes a definition of each, how the test or procedure is performed, and how to prepare; risks and results; and details about drugs and supplements. Large well-known healthcare institutions such as the Cleveland Clinic and Johns Hopkins Medicine

publish photo videos. For example, the Cleveland Clinic provides patient education videos that contain actual surgery images.

Even government agencies use social media to inform consumers about healthcare. The Centers for Disease Control and Prevention (CDC) lists a number of mobile social activities including apps, a CDC video streaming station, and infographics. The Department of Health and Human Services Office of Disease Prevention and Health Promotion has initiatives aimed at healthcare consumers, which contain evidence-based health information and tools to help consumers make informed health choices along with their healthcare providers.

Information Sharing: Personal Health Records

An important piece of patient-centered healthcare is information sharing. Patients generate data outside of the provider settings. Sharing it with their providers expands the depth, breadth, and continuity of information resulting in the potential of improved healthcare outcomes.

Health IT tools connect patients and providers allowing the sharing of information, which strengthens the consumer engagement experience. Patient portals discussed previously are one such tool. Another tool is the personal health record, described as follows.

Introduction to Personal Health Records

A personal health record (PHR) is a record created and managed by an individual in a private, secure, and confidential environment. It differs from an EHR, which is created and managed by the healthcare provider. A PHR can be about the individual's health or the health of someone in his or her care and be used as a tool to collect, track, and share past and current information. Sharing the contents of a PHR with providers can enhance existing data, fill in information gaps, and provide a more complete picture of a patient's health. Other benefits of a PHR are improved patient engagement and enhanced provider–patient communication. It is projected that "within five years, the majority of clinically relevant data … will be collected outside of clinical settings" (Abowd 2011).

Data from a PHR is patient-generated health data (PGHD). ONC identified PGHD as an important issue for advancing patient engagement because patients may become more involved with their own care when patient–provider communication includes the use of the patient-generated data as part of healthcare decision making. According to ONC, PGHD are "health-related data created, recorded, or gathered by or from patients (or family members or other caregivers) to help address a health concern" (ONC 2015a). Examples of PGHD include health and treatment history and data from a wearable monitor, such as an exercise-tracking device. Figure 12.5 illustrates the patient-generated health data flow.

Information in Personal Health Records

PHRs can contain information from a number of sources including those from patients themselves as well as healthcare providers. While there is not a standard set of data and reports to include in a PHR because specific content depends on the type of healthcare received, the following reports are common to most health records.

- Identification sheet: form originated at the time of registration that contains demographic information
- *Problem list:* list of significant illnesses and operations
- *Medication record:* list of medication listing those prescribed or administered
- *History and physical:* past and current illnesses and surgeries, current medications and family history as well as a physical exam performed by the physician
- *Progress notes:* notes made by the doctors, nurses, therapists, and social workers that reflect their observations, the patient's response to treatment, and plans for continued treatment

Figure 12.5 Patient-generated health data flow

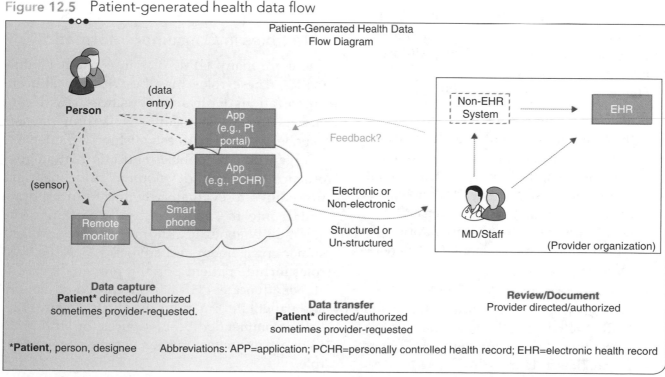

Source: Shapiro et al. 2012, 3.

- *Consultation:* opinion about the patient's condition made by a physician other than the attending physician

- *Physician's orders:* physician's directions to nurses and other members of the healthcare team regarding medications, tests, diets, and treatments

- *Imaging and x-ray reports:* findings of x-rays, mammograms, ultrasounds, and scans

- *Lab reports:* results of tests conducted on body fluids

- *Immunization record:* documentation of immunizations given for diseases such as polio, measles, mumps, rubella, and the flu

- *Consent and authorization forms:* consents for admission, treatment, surgery, and release of information (AHIMA 2015b)

Other health information such as exercise and diet plans, health goals, and home monitoring system results such as blood pressure levels may also be a part of the PHR.

Models of Personal Health Records

PHRs can be as simple as paper documents placed into a folder. However, an electronic PHR is better because of the accessibility factor and to gather, update, integrate, and manipulate the information more easily.

The two main types of electronic PHRs are:

- *Standalone:* Patients fill in information they want to share with their healthcare provider. The information is stored on patients' computers or through an online system. Some standalone PHRs accept data from external sources, such as healthcare providers and laboratories. Patients choose with whom they share the information.

- *Tethered or connected:* A type of PHR that is linked to a specific healthcare organization's EHR. A tethered PHR allows patients to access their own records through a secure portal. (HealthIT 2014).

There are many sources of PHRs. In addition to those listed, employers, and independent vendors offer PHRs. Connecting the PHR to the patient's legal health record protects it under the Health Insurance Portability and Accountability Act (HIPAA) Privacy Rule (ONC n.d.). For additional information on HIPAA, refer to chapter 9.

Patient Safety

Sharing the contents of a PHR with providers can enhance existing data, fill in information gaps, and provide a more complete picture of a patient's health, creating an opportunity to improve patient safety. For example, a PHR with information about allergies, medications, and adverse drug reactions complied from multiple sources can be used by a provider to reconcile the information against what is contained in the EHR, thus preventing medication errors or adverse events leading to patient harm. PHRs also support telehealth capabilities where access to the health information could impact clinical decision making. In an emergency situation, a PHR may provide information when the patient cannot. For additional information on telehealth see chapter 11.

HIM Roles in Consumer Informatics

There are many HIM roles in consumer informatics. These roles may be within healthcare organizations or physician practices or with consumers directly. For example, HIM professionals may be involved with establishing a framework of organizational policies and information governance practices, developing guidelines and procedures to evaluate whether to incorporate PGHD into the patient records, educating the community about health information, and consumer engagement and advocacy. Specific HIM roles include patient portal representative, consumer advocate, PHR liaison, care coordination, and patient information coordinator. Figure 12.6 lists recommended best practices for HIM practitioners in a consumer or patient engagement role.

Figure 12.6 Recommended best practices for consumer or patient engagement

- Establish or participate in an organizational committee, council, or information governance board whose charge is to address facilitation of patient engagement. This group should review all existing and proposed policies and procedures related to health information access with an eye toward gaps and barriers to patient engagement.

- When health information is accessed electronically by patients through portals, ensure that requests for clarifications, corrections, or amendments can be supported by automated workflow that confirms receipt of the request and routes the requests to the appropriate place and person.

- Reach out to community groups as a speaker on patient engagement.

- Work with clinicians to include a comprehensive set of clinical information, including physicians' notes and other forms of documentation, within the patient portal that goes beyond limited information such as appointment dates and lab results.

- Take on a leadership role with the patient portal managing portal processes.

- Establish a central and convenient (to patients) location for receiving and processing requests for all types of health information regardless of media, department, or source. This means establishing a one-stop shop for archived paper records, compact discs, diagnostic imaging media, pathology slides, and such.

- Create policies and design workflows for accepting and managing patient-generated health information

- Eliminate fees to patients for providing them with electronic copies of their health information.

- Stay up-to-date with public policy proposals and standards development that addresses and supports consumer engagement.

Source: Washington 2014.

Check Your Understanding 12.2

***Instructions:* Answer the following questions**

1. True or false: One type of electronic PHRs is tethered.

2. True or false: Scheduling appointments is a required functionality for a patient portal.

3. True or false: Home monitoring system results such as blood pressure levels are part of a PHR.

4. True or false: Consumer health IT applications for information access and navigation include smartphones.

5. True or false: PHRs can contain information from the patients themselves but not from healthcare providers.

Health Information Exchange

Health information exchange is an important part of the healthcare industry ecosystem. While there are several definitions of HIE, all of them note that the exchange of information is done electronically and the capacity exists for different information systems and software applications to exchange data.

- HIE is the exchange of health information electronically between providers and others with the same level of interoperability, such as labs and pharmacies.

- HIE "allows doctors, nurses, pharmacists, other healthcare providers, and patients to appropriately access and securely share a patient's vital medical information electronically—improving the speed, quality, safety and cost of patient care" (ONC 2014b).

- HIE "provides the capability to electronically move clinical information among disparate healthcare information systems, and maintain the meaning of the information being exchanged" (HIMSS 2014).

Determining a course of treatment having only the information contained in a single health record or encapsulated by a single provider of care is shortsighted and could result in duplicative treatments. While not an easy task, moving away from an ownership view of health data to a continuity of care perspective facilitates coordinated patient care. Successfully exchanging and integrating the information into clinical work practice fills information gaps and provides a more complete picture of a patient's health situation resulting in more informed clinical decisions by the healthcare team.

The remaining portion of this chapter provides an introduction to HIE, lists its forms, describes the benefits and users of HIE, explains eHealth exchange, states the challenges with sharing healthcare information, and identifies HIE roles for HIM professionals.

Introduction to Health Information Exchange

Health Information Technology for Economic and Clinical Health (HITECH) legislation and MU regulations mandate health information exchange (HIE) functionality and its use. A qualified EHR under HITECH includes, as one of the criteria, that the EHR has the capacity to exchange electronic health information with and integrate such information from other sources (45 CFR 170.102). A health information exchange organization is one that supports, oversees, or governs the exchange of health-related information among organizations according to nationally recognized standards. These organizations provide the means for HIE to occur. The health information exchange organization compiles data from a number of healthcare providers so that the physician currently treating the patient has a complete picture of the patient's

medical history and treatment including all current medications.

Health information exchange and health information interoperability are not the same. An interoperable health IT environment is one in which seamless health information exchange is possible across diverse EHR systems and the information is understood and shared with those in need of it at the time it is needed. There needs to be some exchange in order for interoperability to occur. What happens to the information after it is exchanged determines whether interoperability materializes. If the information is accepted—for example, an email is sent from one computer to another—then there was an exchange. However, if the information exchanged is understood by both computer systems and no meaning is lost when exchanged resulting in seamless use of it, this series of events meets the definition of interoperability. For additional information on interoperability, see chapter 6.

Forms of Health Information Exchange

Listed as follows are three key forms of health information exchange. Standards, policies and information technology serve as the foundation for all three forms.

- *Directed exchange* is the "ability to send and receive secure information electronically between care providers to support coordinated care" (ONC 2014b). Examples of patient information include ancillary test orders and results, patient care summaries, or consultation reports. The encrypted patient information is electronically sent securely between parties with an established relationship. For example, directed exchange is used to report public health data.
- *Query-based exchange* is the "ability for providers to find and/or request information on a patient from other providers, often used for unplanned care…. Query-based exchange is used to search and discover accessible clinical sources on a patient" (ONC 2014b). For example, a query-based exchange can assist a provider

in obtaining a health record on a patient who is visiting from another state, resulting in more informed decisions about the care of the patient.

- *Consumer-mediated exchange* is the "ability for patients to aggregate and control the use of their health information among providers" (ONC 2014b). For this form the patient is the driver, not the provider. For example, a patient portal may allow personal health information to be uploaded for provider access.

Benefits of Health Information Exchange

There are many benefits to HIE. One of the primary benefits is enhanced patient care coordination. Other potential benefits for patients, providers, payers and communities include the following.

- Reduction of duplicative treatments
- Elimination of redundant or unnecessary testing
- Less medication and medical errors, which can be costly and have a negative impact on the patient
- Increased patient safety
- Achievement of a basic level of interoperability
- More informed decision making for more effective care and treatment
- Improved public health reporting and monitoring
- Improved transitions of care
- Improved population health
- Improved efficiency in the healthcare system
- Reduction in paperwork, allowing more time for discussions about health concerns and treatments

Users of Health Information Exchange

Essential to changing from a fragmented provider-centric healthcare system to a patient-centered one are the users of the health information. Physicians, laboratories, hospitals, pharmacies, consumers, health plans, payers, and communities are all examples of users of electronically exchanged information. For example, a primary care provider electronically sends a clinical summary that includes basic clinical information regarding the care provided such as medications, problems, upcoming appointments, or other instructions to the patient portal.

HIE is a team effort and requires many groups to be successful. Technologically capable and willing exchange partners need to exist. Functionality within the EHR needs to exist so a conversation with the vendor is necessary to determine HIE capability or the timeframe for availability. Even if the functionality is there, a lack of cooperation among EHR vendors can hinder exchange. In addition, how the data are integrated into existing records and workflow can be challenging for providers. There may also be state laws blocking access to patient data. Other barriers to HIE users are competing priorities, financial concerns, issues related to data ownership, and privacy and security. Also, there must be a mechanism to allow patients to opt-in or opt-out of participating in HIE.

eHealth Exchange

HIE can occur at the local, state, regional, and national levels. The **eHealth Exchange** is a nationwide community of exchange partners. The community of federal and state agencies, care delivery organizations, consumer organizations, pharmacies, technology vendors, payers, and others agree to securely share information via the Internet using a common set of standards and specifications. Examples of components of the eHealth Exchange include one unified trusted, operational, and legal framework; governance model; operating policies and procedures; technical services; and operational support. Products are validated through the eHealth Exchange Product Testing Program. The eHealth Exchange has been successful in interoperable sharing of clinical information such as care summaries and quality data.

Challenges with Sharing Healthcare Information

ONC's principal objective for electronic health information exchange is for "information to follow a patient where and when it is needed, across organizational, health IT developer and geographic boundaries" (ONC 2015a). While this is a creditable goal, there are challenges to sharing health information among stakeholder groups from a cultural as well as technical standpoint. Two such challenges are patient identity and data standards.

Patient Identity

Maintenance of data integrity is a key aspect of data quality management. When it comes to patient identity and HIE, integrity is of prime importance to linking the patient to the correct information. Three events must occur in order to maintain patient identity data integrity. The data must be accurately collected, entered, and queried (AHIMA 2012).

Because of its complexity, establishing and maintaining patient identity integrity is fraught with challenges, some of which include:

- Not requiring proof of identification at the time data are collected

- Not making accurate registration a priority in the emergency department

- Data quality issues with patient identification data stored and managed in siloed legacy systems

- Not correcting data errors in a timely and comprehensive manner (AHIMA Work Group 2014).

Data Standards

A critical piece of enabling the exchange of information beyond groups of healthcare providers who subscribe to specific services or organizations is the adoption of standards. Data standards are "documented agreements on representations, formats, and definitions of common data" (PHDSC 2015). Several types are needed including vocabulary, code sets, and terminology; content and structure; transport; and services. Vocabulary, code set, and terminology standards represent the meaning of the clinical data. For example, LOINC is a data

standard for representing lab tests. Content and structure standards define the syntax conventions such as the Clinical Document Architecture (CDA), which specifies the structure and semantics of a care plan. Transport standards define the way in which information is moved from one location to another. An example of a transport standard is the Hypertext Transfer Protocol (HTTP). Digital Imaging and Communications in Medicine (DICOM) is an example of a services standard or the infrastructure components used to achieve specific interoperability requirements. In the case of DICOM, this standard is for exchanging imaging documents.

ONC is harmonizing the standards and specifications, and guiding implementation. Harmonization involves the identification of candidate standards, evaluation of the standards against specific criteria, and selection of a standard. An example of a specific criterion developed by ONC in the data standard selection process is whether the standard is used by federal agencies to electronically exchange health information with organizations engaging in the eHealth Exchange. An outcome of this work is the publication of best available lists. Table 12.1 shows examples from these lists.

HIM Roles in Health Information Exchange

The roles for HIM professionals in HIE include defining the data exchange model, developing guidelines for data stewardship and data governance, developing data integrity and quality standards, identifying strategies to ensure accurate patient identity, ensuring that privacy and security requirements are met, and performing provider and patient education about why HIE is important. A study conducted on trends in HIE organizational staffing found the data integration and master patient and client index roles as the primary staffing challenge and top jobs in demand (AHIMA and HIMSS 2012). Figure 12.7 lists additional HIM skills of value to HIE leadership.

Table 12.1   Best available standards and implementation specifications

	Purpose	Standard(s)	Implementation specification(s)
Vocabulary, code set, and terminology	Lab tests Patient "problems"	LOINC SNOMED CT	
Content and structure	Care plan Data element based on query for clinical health information	HL7 Clinical Document Architecture (CDA) Release 2.0, Normative Edition Fast Healthcare Interoperability Resources (FHIR)	HL7 Implementation Guide for CDA Release 2: Consolidated CDA Templates for Clinical Notes (US Realm) Draft Standards for Trial Use Release 2
Transport	Simple way for participants to push health information directly to known, trusted recipients Data sharing through service-oriented architecture (SOA) that enables two systems to interoperate together	Simple Mail Transfer Protocol (SMTP) RFC 5321 For security, Secure or Multipurpose Internal Mail Extensions (S/MIME) Version 3.2 Message Specification, RFC 5751 Hypertext Transfer Protocol (HTTP) 1.1, RFC 723X (to support RESTful transport approaches) Simple Object Access Protocol (SOAP) 1.2 For security, Transport Layer Security (TLS) Protocol Version 1.2, RFC 5246	
Services	Data element based query for clinical health information Image exchange	Fast Healthcare Interoperability Resources (FHIR) Digital Imaging and Communications in Medicine (DICOM)	

Source: ONC 2015c.

Figure 12.7   HIM contributions to HIE

HIM professionals can bring a variety of much-needed skills to HIEs. HIE leadership can look to HIM principles to provide support and guidance in the following areas:

- Drafting data governance and stewardship policies, including data ownership, data integrity, and data quality
- Managing master patient index and enterprise master patient index data conversions, development, and maintenance
- Developing and implementing HIPAA privacy and security rule requirements
- Developing and implementing HITECH privacy and security rule requirements

- Creating release of information policies, procedures, and practices
- Addressing state and federal requirements for patient confidentiality
- Meeting breach notification requirements
- Integrating data elements from multiple systems, organizations, and providers
- Identifying best practices in information management and records retention

Source: AHIMA 2010.

Check Your Understanding 12.3

Instructions: Answer the following questions.

1. Which of the following is a form of HIE?
   A. Provider-mediated exchange
   B. Data exchange
   C. Consumer-mediated exchange
   D. Collected exchange

2. Which events must occur in order to maintain patient identity data integrity?
   A. The data must be accurately queried
   B. The data must be accurately analyzed
   C. The data must be accurately normalized
   D. The data must be accurately coded

3. All definitions of HIE mention which of the following?
   A. The exchange of information is manual or done electronically
   B. The exchange of information is manual
   C. The exchange of information is done electronically
   D. The exchange of information maintains the meaning of the information being exchanged

4. Which of the following is an example of a service standard?
   A. DICOM
   B. FHIR
   C. CDA
   D. SNOMED CT

5. Which of the following is a benefit of HIE?
   A. A basic level of interoperability is met
   B. An advanced level of interoperability is met
   C. Billing records are accessible
   D. Medication refills can be electronically sent

Real-World Case 12.1

ONC funds research on approaches to capturing and using data directly from patients. The following is an example.

A research project conducted by Geisinger Health System, an integrated delivery system, looked at the interaction between patients and their providers and pharmacists when medication lists were made available through a patient portal. Prior to an upcoming appointment, patients were able to review their medication lists and submit changes if the content was inaccurate as well as ask questions about their medications. A pharmacist, who subsequently followed up with the patient either by phone or secure messaging, reviewed the information, revised the medication record, and informed the patient's provider. The revision was also documented in the EHR along with its source.

The study revealed patients were interested in being involved in the monitoring of medication data and they saw value in this knowledge during office visits with their provider. Revisions to the medication data suggested by the patients were found to be worthwhile to the point that in 80 percent of the cases, pharmacists made the patient-suggested changes. A benefit to providers was significant time savings in medication reconciliation (Deering 2013).

Real-World Case 12.2

The ONC-maintained Health IT Dashboard is a platform to distribute a broad range of health system and grant program performance measures tracking the adoption and meaningful use of various health information technologies (health IT), including EHRs and others enabling HIE.

The interactive tool provides the user with several ways to parse and examine the data visually. The data are derived from ONC programs, research, and the open government datasets. For example, under the category of exchange and interoperability are two choices—one for nonfederal acute-care hospital health IT adoption and another for office-based physician health IT adoption. Each one visualizes measures—14 for hospitals and 9 for physicians—of health IT adoption, which include adoption of EHRs, HIE, and patient engagement. Figure 12.8 is the dashboard showing the percent of physicians with the capability to electronically send orders for lab results.

Figure 12.8 Percent of physicians with the capability to electronically send orders for lab results

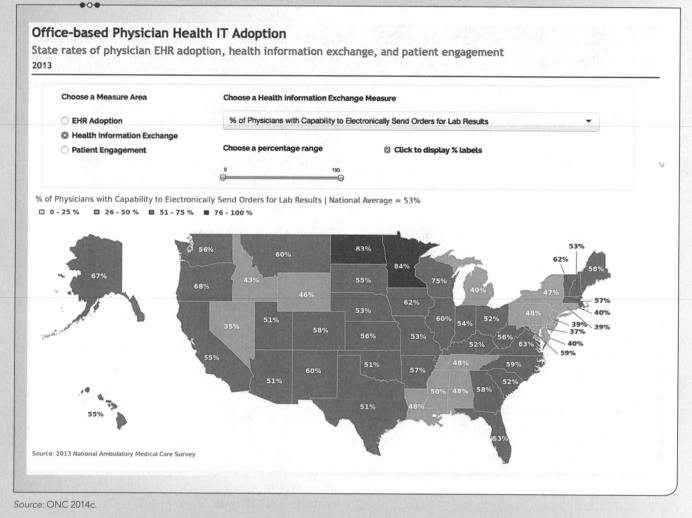

Source: ONC 2014c.

References

Abowd, G. 2011 (Oct. 24). Keynote Address to American Medical Informatics Association Annual Conference on Biomedical and Health Informatics. http://www.amia.org/amia2011/keynotes.

AHIMA Work Group. 2015. Assessing and Improving EHR Data Quality (updated). *Journal of AHIMA*. 86(5):58–64.

AHIMA Work Group. 2014. Managing the Integrity of Patient Identity in Health Information Exchange (updated). http://library.ahima.org/doc?oid=300436#.VxE0rPkrK9I.

Amatayakul, M.K. 2013. *Electronic Health Records: A Practical Guide for Professionals and Organizations*, 5th ed. Chicago: AHIMA.

American Health Information Management Association. 2015a. Certified Health Data Analyst (CHDA). http://www.ahima.org/certification/chda.

American Health Information Management Association. 2015b. myPHR. https://www.myphr.com/StartaPHR/what_is_a_phr.aspx.

American Health Information Management Association. 2014. *Health Data Analysis Toolkit*. Chicago: AHIMA. http://library.ahima.org/PdfView?oid=107504.

American Health Information Management Association. 2013. Speech recognition in the electronic health record (updated). *Journal of AHIMA*. 84(9):expanded web version. http://library.ahima.org/doc?oid=300181#.VxE1Y_krK9I.

American Health Information Management Association. 2012. Ensuring Data Integrity in Health Information Exchange. http://library.ahima.org/PdfView?oid=105612.

American Health Information Management Association. 2010. Understanding the HIE landscape. *Journal of AHIMA*. 81(9):60–65.

American Health Information Management Association (AHIMA) and Healthcare Information and Management Systems Society (HIMSS). 2012. Trends in Health Information Exchange Organizational Staffing. http://www.himss.org/ResourceLibrary/genResourceDetailPDF.aspx?ItemNumber=31182.

American Medical Informatics Association (AMIA). n.d. Consumer Health Informatics. https://www.amia.org/applications-informatics/consumer-health-informatics.

Carayon P, P. Hoonakker, R. Cartmill, and A. Hassol. 2015. Using Health Information Technology (IT) in Practice Redesign: Impact of Health IT on Workflow. Patient-Reported Health Information Technology and Workflow. (Prepared by Abt Associates under Contract No. 290-2010-00031I). AHRQ Publication No. 15-0043-EF. Rockville, MD: Agency for Healthcare Research and Quality.

Daniel, J., M. Deering, and M. Murray. 2014 (Jan. 10). Issue Brief: Using Health IT to Put the Person at the Center of Their Health and Care by 2020. http://www.healthit.gov/sites/default/files/person_at_thecenterissuebrief.pdf.

Deering, M.J. 2013. Issue Brief: Patient-Generated Health Data and Health IT. http://www.healthit.gov/sites/default/files/pghd_brief_final122013.pdf.

Fenton, S.H. and S. Biedermann. 2014. *Introduction to Healthcare Informatics*. Chicago: AHIMA.

Gartner. 2012 (Dec. 14). Predicts 2013: Information Innovation. http://insight.datamaticstech.com/dtlsp/rna_Presales/knowledgeHub/Gartner/predicts_2013_information_in_246040.pdf.

Healthcare Financial Management Association (HFMA). 2015. HFMA's MAP. http://www.hfma.org/Map/MapApp/.

Healthcare Information and Management Systems Society (HIMSS). 2014. *HIMSS Dictionary of Healthcare Information Technology Terms, Acronyms and Organizations*, 3rd ed. Chicago: HIMSS.

HealthIT. 2014. Are there different types of personal health records (PHRs)? https://www.healthit.gov/providers-professionals/faqs/are-there-different-types-personal-health-records-phrs.

Koh, H.C. and G. Tan. 2005. Data mining applications in healthcare. *Journal of Healthcare Information Management*. 19(2):64–72.

National Learning Consortium (NLC). 2013. How to Optimize Patient Portals for Patient Engagement and Meet Meaningful Use Requirements. http://www.healthit.gov/sites/default/files/nlc_how_to_optimizepatientportals_for_patientengagement.pdf.

Office of the National Coordinator for Health Information Technology (ONC). n.d. Personal Health Records: What Providers Need to Know. http://www.healthit.gov/sites/default/files/about-phrs-for-providers-011311.pdf.

Office of the National Coordinator for Health Information Technology (ONC). 2015a. Consumer eHealth. https://www.healthit.gov/policy-researchers-implementers/patient-generated-health-data.

Office of the National Coordinator for Health Information Technology (ONC). 2015b. Health Information Exchange Governance. http://www.healthit.gov/policy-researchers-implementers/health-information-exchange-governance.

Office of the National Coordinator for Health Information Technology (ONC). 2015c. The 2015 Interoperability Standards Advisory. http://www.healthit.gov/policy-researchers-implementers/2015-interoperability-standards-advisory.

Office of the National Coordinator for Health Information Technology (ONC). 2014a. Federal Health IT Strategic Plan. http://www.healthit.gov/sites/default/files/federal-healthIT-strategic-plan-2014.pdf.

Office of the National Coordinator for Health Information Technology (ONC). 2014b. Health Information Exchange (HIE). http://www.healthit.gov/providers-professionals/health-information-exchange/what-hie.

Office of the National Coordinator for Health Information Technology (ONC). 2014c. Office-Based Physician Health IT Adoption, Health IT Dashboard. http://dashboard.healthit.gov/dashboards/physician-health-it-adoption.php.

Office of the National Coordinator for Health Information Technology (ONC). 2013. Clinical Decision Support. http://www.healthit.gov/policy-researchers-implementers/clinical-decision-support-cds.

Public Health Data Standards Consortium (PHDSC). 2015. Health Information Technology Standards. http://www.phdsc.org/standards/health-information/d_standards.asp.

Robert Wood Johnson Foundation (RWJF). 2015. Data for Health: Learning What Works. http://www.rwjf.org/en/library/research/2015/04/data-for-health-initiative.html.

Sandefer, R., D. Marc, D. Mancilla, and D. Hamada. 2015. Survey predicts future HIM workforce shifts: HIM industry estimates the job roles, skills needed in the near future. *Journal of AHIMA*. 86(7):32–35.

SAS. 2014. Data Visualization Techniques: From Basics to Big Data with SAS® Visual Analytics. http://www.sas.com/content/dam/SAS/en_us/doc/whitepaper1/data-visualization-techniques-106006.pdf.

Shapiro, M., D. Johnston, J. Wald, and D. Mon. 2012. Patient-Generated Health Data White Paper. http://www.healthit.gov/sites/default/files/rti_pghd_whitepaper_april_2012.pdf.

Staheli, R. 2014. Best Practices for Analyzing Healthcare Data. Health Catalyst. https://www.healthcatalyst.com/healthcare-analytics-best-practices.

US Food and Drug Administration (FDA). 2015 (Feb. 9). Mobile Medical Applications: Guidance for Industry and Food and Drug Administration Staff. http://www.fda.gov/downloads/MedicalDevices/DeviceRegulationandGuidance/GuidanceDocuments/UCM263366.pdf.

Washington, L. 2014. Enabling consumer and patient engagement with health information. *Journal of AHIMA*. 88(2):56–59.

3e Services LLC. 2015. Developing an Enterprise Information Strategy: A Pillar of Success in Building the Future of Healthcare. http://static1.squarespace.com/static/53c98477e4b0985ac7917c0d/t/54c13ffce4b0c7e0a73a3be5/1421950972341/3eServices_EIS+HealthCare+Whitepaper_01_21_15.pdf.

45 CFR 170.102: Health information technology standards, implementation specifications, and certification criteria and certification programs for health information technology. 2012.

13

Research and Data Analysis

Valerie Watzlaf, PhD, RHIA, FAHIMA

Learning Objectives

- Apply graphical tools for data presentation using spreadsheets and statistical software
- Utilize descriptive statistics in healthcare decision making
- Understand the normal distribution and how it affects the use of certain types of statistics
- Analyze data to identify trends in quality, safety, and outcomes of care
- Explain common research methodologies
- Explain how the research methodologies are used in healthcare to include examples from the Institutional Review Board, Centers for Disease Control and Prevention (CDC), World Health Organization (WHO), and Agency for Healthcare Research and Quality (AHRQ)

Key Terms

Aggregate data
Agency for Healthcare Research and Quality (AHRQ)
Bar chart
Bubble charts
Centers for Disease Control and Prevention (CDC)
Chart
Comparative data
Continuous variable
Correlational studies
Descriptive statistics
Descriptive studies
Discrete variable

Ethnography
Experimental study
Frequency
Frequency polygon
Graph
Grounded theory
Healthcare research organizations
Histogram
Incidence rate
Independent variable
Individual data
Inferential statistics
Institutional Review Board (IRB)
Interval variables

Line graph
Mean
Measures of central tendency
Measures of variability
Median
Mixed-methodology
Mode
Nominal variables
Normal distribution
Ordinal variables
Pareto chart
Percentile
Pie chart
Presentation software

Proportion
Prospective study
Qualitative research
Qualitative variables
Quantitative study
Quantitative variables
Quasi-experimental study

Randomization
Range
Ratio variables
Research methodologies
Retrospective study
Scatter charts
Standard deviation

Stem and leaf plots
Statistical packages
Table
Variability
Variance
World Health Organization
(WHO)

Data are more abundant and important than ever before. Creating data and collecting it for business health intelligence, data analytics, and data use is vital for healthcare facilities to remain competitive. However, since healthcare data are so abundant, methods to analyze the data and present it in an understandable and useful fashion are desperately needed. Healthcare providers are inundated with healthcare data and struggle to find the meaning of that data in a quick and efficient manner. Health information management (HIM) professionals are the bridge between data and information. HIM professionals take data, present it clearly, and provide it to those who will use it to make important decisions. Data and information are defined and discussed in detail in chapter 6.

This chapter discusses ways to present statistical data clearly through tables, charts, and graphs using spreadsheets and statistical packages. Descriptive statistics and the normal distribution are also discussed to demonstrate methods of quantifying data using frequencies and percentiles, measures of central tendency (mean, median, mode) and measures of **variability** (range, variance, standard deviation). Analysis of data are also described using examples that relate to quality and safety. Finally, research methodologies that include quantitative, qualitative, and mixed-methods approaches are reviewed to demonstrate how data can be used within each type of study. The Institutional Review Board (IRB) and other healthcare research organizations are discussed as they relate to all areas of research and data analysis.

Presentation of Statistical Data

The key to presenting data is to make it clear, concise, and understandable. This can be done by using different types of presentation methods such as tables, charts, and graphs. How one determines what table, graph, or chart to use is determined by the type of data or variables that are being presented. **Quantitative variables** are numerical variables that can be classified as discrete or continuous. In healthcare, **discrete variables** are variables that can take on a finite number of values, usually whole numbers, or numbers that can be counted such as 204, 65, and 534. **Continuous variables** include any numerical value that goes from one whole number to the next whole number, such as $30, 567.32, 62.596, and 18.65. Examples of a discrete variable may include 204 coded medical records, 65 patients who receive a colonoscopy,

or the 534 physicians who provide generic-based medications to their patients. Examples of a continuous variable may include the cost of a patient's hospital stay ($30,567.32), a patient's height (62.596 inches), or a patient's weight (18.65 lbs). Quantitative variables can be further broken down into interval and ratio variables. **Interval variables** are those that have equal units with an arbitrary zero point. An example is temperature on the Fahrenheit scale. The temperature difference between 45 degrees and 50 degrees is the same as the temperature difference between 30 degrees and 35 degrees. Zero does not equal absence of temperature. **Ratio variables** are the most common quantitative variables used in healthcare. These include numbers that can be compared meaningfully with one another (four grapefruits are twice as many as two grapefruits). Zero is truly zero on

Table 13.1 Examples of types of variables: quantitative and qualitative

Quantitative or numerical variables	
Continuous	Discrete
Interval: Temperature	Number of medical records coded
Ratio: Height, weight, costs, charges	Number of patients who receive a colonoscopy
Qualitative or categorical variables	
	All discrete variables
Nominal (discrete categorical variables)	Gender (1 = male, 2 = female), race (1 = Caucasian, 2 = African-American, and such), smoking status (1 = nonsmoker, 2 = smoker)
Ordinal (discrete ordered variables)	Patient satisfaction scores (1 = not satisfied to 5 = very satisfied), quality of life scores (1 = not healthy to 5 = very healthy), pain scales (0 = no pain, 5 = moderate pain, 10 = worst pain)

the ratio scale. Examples include height (inches or meters) and weight (pounds or kilograms).

Qualitative variables are categorical; are all discrete and include both nominal and ordinal variables. **Nominal variables** are those in which a number is assigned to a specific category such as a 1 = male and 2 = female. **Ordinal variables** are ranked variables in which a number is assigned to rank a category in an ordered series but does not indicate the magnitude of the difference between any two data points. An example of a ranked variable is a response for a question on a patient satisfaction questionnaire such as: Your wait time to see your doctor was appropriate, where 1 = strongly agree, 2 = agree, 3 = disagree, 4 = strongly disagree. Table 13.1 summarizes the different types of variables and gives examples of each. Electronic spreadsheets and spreadsheet software can be used to construct nearly all of the charts graphs and tables explained in this chapter.

Tables

Tables are one type of tool to use to display data and can include both numbers and text. Tables are excellent ways to organize and categorize data and can be useful to examine the detail of a specific concept, category, or response. Table 13.2 is an example of a table that demonstrates the demographic characteristics of physicians who were part of a focus group to discuss ICD-10-CM/PCS (International Classification of Diseases, 10th revision, Procedure Coding System) and its effect on their physician practice. It can be easily seen from the table that 75 percent of the physicians have not been exposed to using ICD-10-CM/PCS in their practice during the time of the focus group.

The key to building a table is to make it able to stand alone so anyone reading it can understand the information displayed. Every table should be composted of certain elements including the table legend or title, column titles, the body of the table that includes the actual data, lines that divide certain parts of the table, and a footnote or reference citation if the table text was taken from an article or other source.

When presenting test results from electronic health records (EHRs), tables can be a more burdensome format to use and should be reconsidered when presenting data for clinicians using patient test results (Brewer et al. 2012). Alternatives are presented in the following sections.

Charts and Graphs

Charts and **graphs** are informative because they provide a picture of the numerical data being processed into information. Sometimes it can be difficult to succinctly describe what is happening with large amounts of data. Charts and graphs can be the perfect choice when trying to present a picture of the data. There are many different types of charts and graphs to use when transforming data into information. Each one has some rules or guidelines to follow when deciding to use a particular chart or graph. Bar charts, pie charts, line graphs, histograms, frequency polygons, scatter charts, bubble charts, and stem and leaf plots are some of the charts and graphs explained in the following sections.

Bar Charts

Bar charts are simple charts used to describe qualitative, categorical, or discrete variables such as

Table 13.2 Demographic characteristics of physician participants in a focus group study on the ICD-10-CM/PCS system and its effect on their practice

Respondents (N = 12) N = number of physicians responding		
Demographics		
	Mean	Standard deviation
Age	54.67	12.71
Years of experience	23.42	12.48
Gender	#	%
Male	9	75
Female	3	25
Setting	#	%
Hospital (or other facility) only	5	41.6
Private practice only	2	16.7
Both	5	41.6
Medical specialty	#	%
Emergency medicine	2	16.7
Ophthalmology	1	8.3
Internal medicine, geriatrics	1	8.3
Plastic or reconstructive surgery	1	8.3
General surgery	1	8.3
Obstetrics and gynecology	1	8.3
Psychiatry	2	16.7
Family medicine	1	8.3
Hematology and oncology	1	8.3
Physical medicine	1	8.3
Previous use of EHR	#	%
Yes	10	83.3
No	2	16.7
Exposure to ICD-10-CM/PCS	#	%
Yes	3	25
No	9	75

Source: Watzlaf et al. 2015.

nominal or ordinal data. The bars may be drawn vertically in which the value represents the height of the bar drawn or horizontally in which the value represents the length of the bar drawn. There are several types of bar charts. The easiest bar chart to build is the one-variable bar chart, which displays a bar to represent the amount of the specific category. For example, figure 13.1 presents a hypothetical example of a one-variable bar chart for the number of healthcare facilities located in an urban, suburban, or rural setting in a specific region.

Two-variable bar charts can also display an important summary of healthcare data. Figure 13.2 demonstrates a two-variable chart and includes not only the number of healthcare facilities in the region but also the number of trauma units in each of those settings. The two-variable bar chart can further distinguish or classify additional variables. Figures 13.3 through 13.5 demonstrate other examples of bar charts. The horizontal bar chart is used when label titles are long and therefore more difficult to read and also when sorting the data from the smallest amount at the top to the largest amount at the bottom.

The stacked bar chart can also be used when one is demonstrating a comparison of the proportion of two things. Shown below in figure 13.4, the stacked bar chart demonstrates the proportion of the number of trauma units in relation to the number of healthcare facilities. The stacked bar chart can help visualize the proportion.

When titles get longer or if data is shown from the smallest at the top to the largest at the bottom as well as showing proportions of two areas, the horizontal stacked bar chart can be used. Figure 13.5 provides an example.

When constructing bar charts it is important to know the audience, keep it simple, and make it clear, colorful, and concise. When using a bar chart the main goal is to succinctly provide clear and easy to understand data, as this data is often displayed to clinicians and other healthcare executives who do not have time to spend deciphering what the chart means. Therefore, if it takes too long to interpret the information from the chart, reconstruct it so it is clear and easy to understand. This includes providing a title, axes labels, legend, a number within or above the bars, percentages if it helps to clarify an aspect of the data, and appropriate colors to distinguish between groups. Everyone is different and sometimes what is clear to one person may not be to another, so knowing the audience ensures the appropriate type of bar chart is constructed to meet the audience's preferences.

Figure 13.1   Example of a one-variable bar chart

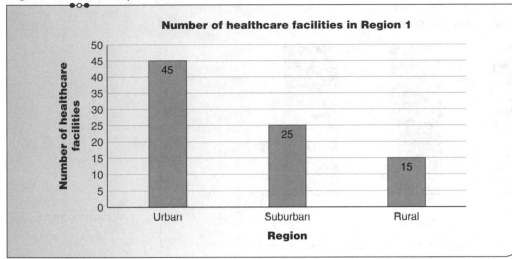

Figure 13.2   Example of a two-variable bar chart

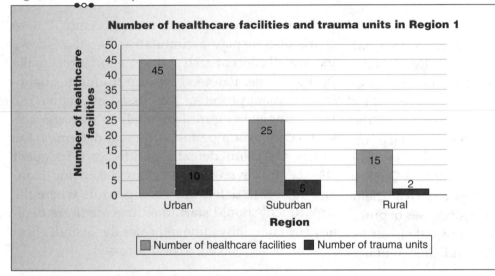

Figure 13.3   Example of a horizontal bar chart

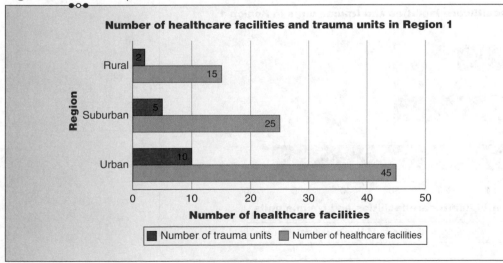
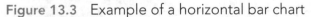

Figure 13.4   Example of a stacked bar chart with percentage of the whole

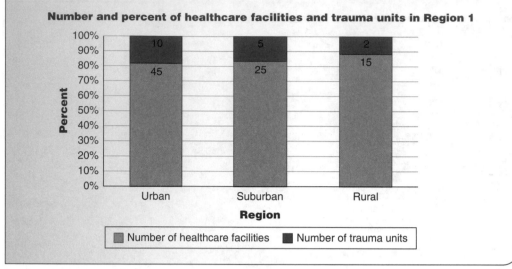

Pareto Chart

A **Pareto chart** is similar in appearance to a bar chart but the highest ranking value is listed as the first column and the next highest ranking is second, and so on, to the lowest ranking. Created by Vilfredo Pareto and based on his theory that "the significant few things will generally make up 80 percent of the whole, while the trivial many will make up about 20 percent" (Productivity-Quality Systems 2015). In healthcare this chart can help analyze data about the frequency or causes of problems in a process. Pareto charts show data in terms of arranging it into categories and then ranking each category according to its importance. Pareto charts also display a cumulative line that shows the overall effect of each of the categories that make up the whole. Pareto charts are useful in quality improvement processes (discussed in chapter 18). For example, in figure 13.6, a billing manager collected data over a period of time to determine the causes for claim denials for Medicare inpatient stays. After reviewing the chart the billing manager is able to determine coding errors where the department should start to reduce Medicare denials. The cumulative line indicates the overall effect if all of the areas were to be addressed.

Figure 13.5   Example of a horizontal stacked bar chart

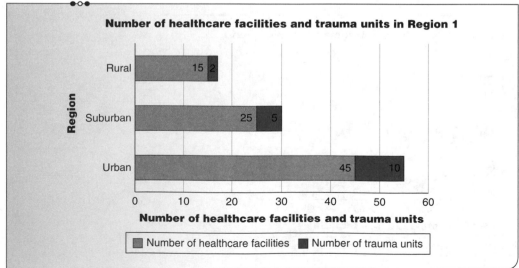

Figure 13.6 Example of a Pareto chart

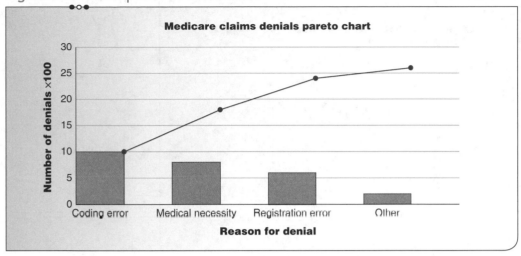

©AHIMA

Pie Charts

Pie charts are simple graphs that use the slices of the pie to explain numerical **proportion**. Pie charts are used a great deal in healthcare because they can depict a breakdown of numerical data elements by percentages. However, they are not the best to use when comparing data elements or when using many data elements because the slices of the pie can become too small to interpret. When explaining simple types of data, broken down into percentages, the pie graph may be a good statistical graphic to use. Using the same numbers that were used in figure 13.1, figure 13.7 provides not only the slices of the pie but also the individual percentages within each slice for easier reading and interpretation.

Line Graph

A **line graph** is a graphical device used to display continuous data and to show changes or trends of

Figure 13.7 Example of pie chart

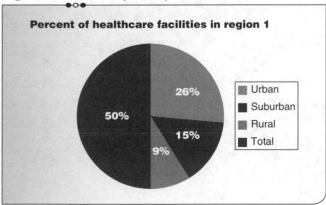

©AHIMA

the data over time. The x-axis on the line graph from left to right, designates time (such as month, day, or year) and the y-axis shows the quantity of the plotted data. A line graph looks similar to a frequency polygon although their purpose is different and is explained later in this chapter. A line graph is best to use when one has many different data points to plot or more than one set of data to be plotted; multiple lines can be put on one graph for very useful comparisons. The data to create the line graphs in figures 13.8 and 13.9 is in table 13.3.

Histograms

A **histogram** is a graph that represents the frequency distribution of numerical data. A frequency distribution is a distribution of data that demonstrates where data falls. For example, table 13.4 is a frequency distribution table. It provides the number of patients that fall into each of the weight categories listed. It also provides the percent of the total number of patients that fall within each weight category.

A histogram should be used with continuous data that is part of a frequency distribution. It differs from a bar graph because histograms use continuous data, there are no spaces between the bars, and each bar has a class interval at its base and the frequency or percentage of cases in that class interval at its height. See figure 13.10 for an example of a histogram with six groups of body mass index (from underweight to extremely obese) on the x-axis and percentage of population on the y-axis.

Figure 13.8 Example of a line graph

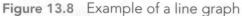
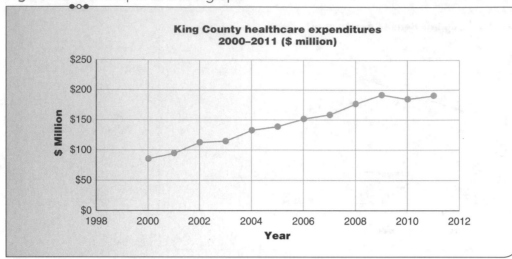

Source: CMS 2016.

Figure 13.9 Example of a line graph comparing two types of data

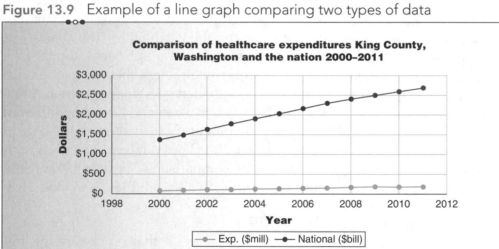

Source: CMS 2016.

Table 13.3 Data used to build line graphs for figures 13.8 and 13.9

Year	Expenditures ($ million)	National ($ billion)
2000	$86	$1,377.20
2001	$95	$1,493.40
2002	$113	$1,638.00
2003	$115	$1,778.00
2004	$133	$1,905.70
2005	$139	$2,035.40
2006	$152	$2,166.70
2007	$159	$2,302.90
2008	$177	$2,411.70
2009	$192	$2,504.20
2010	$185	$2,599.00
2011	$191	$2,692.80

Table 13.4 Example of a frequency distribution table

		Frequency	Percent
Valid	123.00	1	10.0
	125.00	1	10.0
	145.00	1	10.0
	155.00	2	20.0
	165.00	1	10.0
	176.00	1	10.0
	187.00	1	10.0
	201.00	1	10.0
	233.00	1	10.0
	Total	10	100.0

Figure 13.10 Example of a histogram that shows the distribution of body mass index in adults with diagnosed diabetes in the United States, 1999–2002

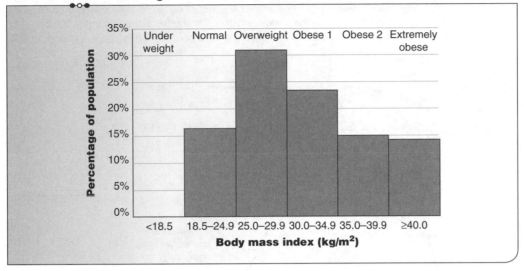

Source: CDC 2004.

Frequency Polygon

A **frequency polygon** is another graphical means to display a frequency distribution using continuous data in a line form. A single data point placed at the midpoint of the interval is used to mark the specific number of observations within that interval. Each point is then connected by a line. Figure 13.11 shows a frequency polygon over an outline of a histogram for the same data. The frequency polygon makes it easier to see the peak of the epidemic. This is important when examining epidemics over a four-week time period as in this example from the Centers for Disease Control and Prevention (CDC). Frequency polygons differ from line graphs in that frequency polygons (or histograms) display the entire frequency distribution (counts) of the continuous variable; a line graph plots only the specific data points over time.

Scatter Charts

A **scatter chart**, scatter plot, scatter diagram, or scatter graph is used to demonstrate a relationship between two variables. One of the two variables is plotted on the x-axis, and the other is plotted on the y-axis. A strong relationship between the two variables is seen as the data come closer to forming a straight line. Figure 13.12 demonstrates a strong positive relationship between age and income. When both variables increase and decrease at the

same time, the scatter chart will show a positive relationship. When one variable increases and the other variable decreases, the scatter chart will display a negative relationship. Figure 13.13 shows a negative relationship between age and physical activity, demonstrating that as age increases physical activity decreases. In Figure 13.12 physical activity was ranked from 0 = no physical activity to 5 = high level of physical activity. In the next hypothetical example, a scatter chart shows no relationship between age and the number of pets a person has in their household (figure 13.14). The main goal of the scatter plot is to illustrate nonlinear relationships between variables. Therefore, researchers can use it to determine quickly whether further calculations are needed—if the scatter plot demonstrates nonlinear relationships, then no further calculations, such as correlation or regression statistics, are needed.

Bubble Charts

A **bubble chart** is similar to a scatter chart except that it compares three data variables. Figure 13.15 takes the same data on personal income and adds two variables—cost of hospital admission and the percent of the cost of hospital admission in relation to personal income. The bubble chart shows that the larger the bubble the more that patient had to pay for the hospital admission in relation to personal income. Due to the size of

Figure 13.11 Example of a frequency polygon and histogram

The histogram shows number of cases as columns. The frequency polygon shows number of cases as data points connected by lines. The midpoints of intervals of the histogram intersect the frequency polygon. For the frequency polygon, the first data point is connected to the midpoint of the previous interval on the x-axis. The last data point is connected the midpoint of the following interval.

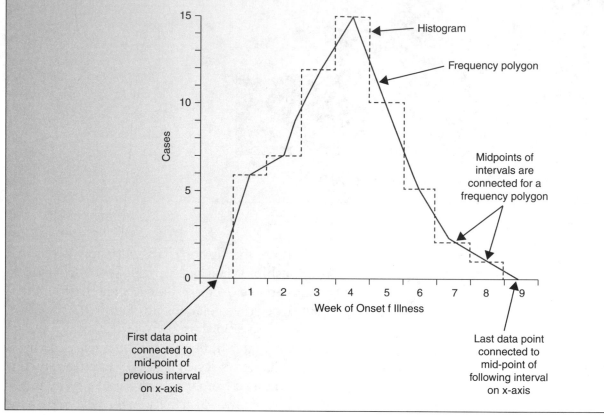

Source: CDC 2012.

Figure 13.12 Scatter chart showing a strong positive relationship between age and income

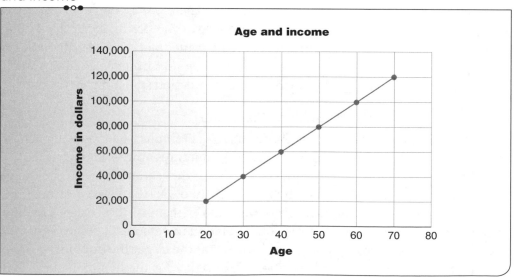

Figure 13.13 Scatter chart showing a strong negative relationship between age and physical ability

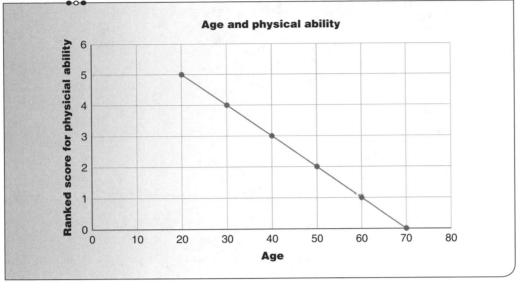

©AHIMA

the bubble, figure 13.14 shows that for those who made $20,000, their proportion of income to what they had to pay for hospital admission costs was the greatest, at 325 percent. The smallest bubble shows that for those who made $80,000, their proportion of income to what they had to pay for hospital admission costs was the lowest, at 63 percent.

Stem and Leaf Plots

In **stem and leaf plots**, data can be organized so that the shape of a frequency distribution is revealed. As an example, a stem and leaf plot is constructed on the number of discharges across cities in one particular state for Medicare severity diagnosis-related group (MS-DRG) 39, extracranial procedures without complication or comorbidity (CC) or major complication or comorbidity (MCC) (CMS 2014). The data are listed as follows and ranked from the smallest to largest number of discharges.

14, 14, 15, 18, 18, 21, 24, 25, 27, 27, 29, 31, 32, 33, 34, 43, 45, 51, 66, 67

Figure 13.14 Scatter chart showing no relationship between age and number of pets a person has in their household

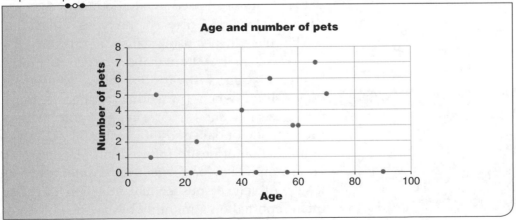

©AHIMA

Figure 13.15 Bubble chart showing a relationship of three variables

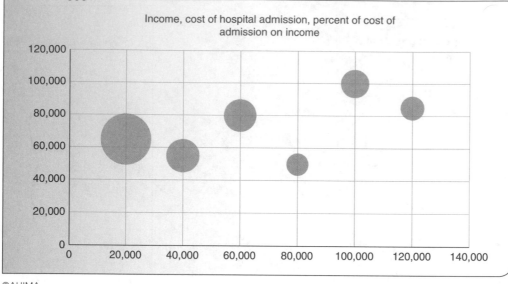

©AHIMA

To develop the stem and leaf plot, the numbers are separated into two parts. The first digit (in this example, the tens digit) is listed once as per occurrence in the stem column, and the last digit(s) (in this example, the ones digit) are placed in the leaf column. The first number, 14, is separated so that 1 goes in the stem column and 4 is the first listing in the leaf column. In the second 14, the first digit is already in the stem column (1) so the second (4) is placed in the leaf column as the second entry (44). Table 13.5 displays a continuation of the list of numbers in the given example.

The completed stem and leaf plot shows the distribution of the data set. It can immediately be seen that the lowest value in the distribution is 14 (created by using the digit in the first row in the first column [1] and the first digit in the first row

Table 13.5 Example of stem and leaf plot using discharges across a state for MS-DRG 39, extracranial procedures without CC or MCC

Stem	Leaf
1	44588
2	145779
3	1234
4	35
5	1
6	67

Source: CMS 2014.

of the second column [4]) and the highest is 67 (the digit in the last row in the first column [6] and the second digit in the last row of the second column [7]) and that there are six observations in the 20s group (created by adding the number of digits in the row that displays the tens digits for 2). With this type of display it is easy to see that the largest number of discharges is 67 (the digit in the last row in the first column and the second digit in the last row of the second column).

Statistical Packages and Presentation Software

There are many **statistical packages** that can be used to facilitate the data collection and analysis processes. These packages simplify the statistical analysis of data and are often used in addition to spreadsheet software. Table 13.6 displays the types of data that can be entered when using statistical software packages as well as the output that can be generated.

Presentation software is software used to build slides when presenting a specific topic, idea, research data, or any type of information. Presentation of data and information is an important function of health information management. For example, key performance indicators such as length of stay or nosocomial infection rates are often reported on a monthly basis. The HIM professional may be asked to present this information

Table 13.6   Common data configurations for statistical software

Data type	Description	Example
Data list or input	Data list or input includes the name of the variable, the type of the variable such as string, numeric, how long the variable is, and how many decimal places to keep in the number	Name of variable: codingtestscore, coderstatus Variable type (numeric or string): numeric Width of variable: 4 Number of decimals: 2
Value labels	Value labels assign a value to a specific variable and appears in the output for easy interpretation.	Coder Status 1 = advanced 2 = intermediate 3 = beginner
Missing values	Missing values are values that do not have a number or value assigned to the variable. Missing values can be displayed in output and can be recoded by the user if necessary. One may need to recode or add a number in case it was missed by the data entry.	**Statistics** |		Variable Name codingtestscore	Variable Name coderstatus
---	---	---	---
N	Valid	8	8
	Missing	2	2	 Key: N = population; n = sample Valid = all variables that have a value assigned to them Missing = variables that do not have a value assigned to them The numbers in the first column show the valid number of individuals that have a coding test score and the number of individuals that are missing a coding test score. The numbers in the second column show the valid number of individuals that have a coder status assigned (advanced, intermediate, beginner) and the number of individuals that are missing a coder status.
Output	Output includes statistics that can be generated from the data that is collected and entered into the software or spreadsheet. Statistics can be generated such as descriptive statistics (frequency tables, percentiles, graphs, measures of central tendency) as well as advanced statistics	**Report** codingtestscore | coderstatus	Mean	N	Standard Deviation
---	---	---	---
advanced	93.0000	3	5.00000
intermediate	89.5000	2	0.70711
beginner	73.3333	3	6.42910
Total	84.7500	8	10.51190	

in a way that clearly displays the information and also identifies trends that may need to be addressed. Different graphic designs, animations, and polls can also be added to slides to enhance and support the data presented. For example, an HIM professional would need to use presentation software when demonstrating how coding productivity changed after the implementation of ICD-10-CM/PCS and the slides would show an increase or decrease in coder productivity.

Check Your Understanding 13.1

Instructions: Answer the following questions.

1. True or false: Tables are excellent ways to organize and categorize data and can be useful to examine the detail of a specific concept, category, or response.

2. True or false: The easiest bar chart to build is the two-variable bar chart.

3. Which two graphs are best for displaying frequency distributions using continuous data?
   A. Histogram and frequency polygon
   B. Bar chart and line graph
   C. Scatter chart and stem and leaf plot
   D. Pie chart and frequency polygon

4. Which chart is best to compare data for three different variables?
   A. Bar chart
   B. Pie chart
   C. Bubble chart
   D. Scatter chart

5. Which of the following is an example of a value label variable?
   A. Coder status
   B. Coder test score
   C. Weight
   D. Height

Descriptive Statistics

Descriptive statistics include frequencies, percentiles, measures of central tendency (mean, median, and mode) and measures of variability (range, variance, and standard deviation). Descriptive statistics can be used in HIM, for example, to provide frequencies of the number of HIM professionals that believe they are leaders in information governance or how the age of a group of patients falls into the reimbursement amounts for a particular month in a healthcare facility vary. Measures of variability fall into the 25th, 50th, or 75th percentile; and how the mean, median, and mode of diagnosis-related group (DRG) can be used to further examine the spread of data and how outliers influence the distribution of the data.

Frequency and Percentile

Frequency is the number of times something occurs in a particular population or sample over a specific period of time. For example, if a researcher wanted to determine how often subjects considered themselves a leader in information governance (IG), they could ask the subjects whether they consider themselves a leader in IG and then count how many of the subjects said yes and how many said no.

They could then build a frequency table based on this question and its results. If there are 200 subjects in the study, the frequency table may look like table 13.7.

A **percentile** is a measure used in descriptive statistics that shows the value below which a given percentage of scores in a given group of scores fall. For example, the 40th percentile is the score below which 40 percent of the other scores in a given group of scores fall. Also, if a score is in the 95th percentile, it is higher than 95 percent of the other scores. A percentile can be broken up into quartiles. Quartiles are values that break up a list of numbers into quarters such as the 25th percentile or first quartile; 50th percentile or second quartile; and 75th percentile, or third quartile. For example, if a researcher wanted to determine how the age of their subjects were separated based on quartiles, they can collect age for each subject, create a spreadsheet, and use statistical software to provide percentiles of the data collected.

Table 13.7   Example of a frequency table

Do you consider yourself a leader in IG?	Frequency
Yes	150
No	45
No response	5
Total	200

Table 13.8 Example of percentiles

Statistics			
Age in years			
N	Valid		250
	Missing		0
Percentiles		25	36.00
		50	45.00
		75	53.25

N = Population

Table 13.8 demonstrates how the age of 250 individuals is categorized in 25th, 50th, and 75th percentiles. One can see that age 36 is at the 25th percentile, age 45 is at the 50th percentile, and age 53.25 is at the 75th percentile. This shows that age 36 is the age below which 25 percent of the other ages fall, 45 is the age below which 50 percent of the other ages fall, and 53.25 is the age below which 75 percent of the other ages fall within this particular group of subjects. This demonstrates that given the ages of the subjects, the majority of the not considered elderly, since elderly would include those equal to or over the age of 65.

Measures of Central Tendency

Measures of central tendency include the mean (average), the median (the middlemost point) and the mode (most frequent value).

Mean

The **mean** is the average of a group of values. The numerator in the formula is explained: You will need to add each observation (observations are indicated by the i) from the first observation ($i = 1$) up to and including the last observation. The denominator, or n, is the total number of observations.

For example, you are asked to calculate the mean length of stay for cardiac patients for the month of January. The lengths of stay for these six patients were 5, 8, 6, 4, 7, and 3. To calculate the mean of these lengths of stay you would add the days of stay together:

$$5 + 8 + 6 + 4 + 7 + 3 = 33 \text{ total days}$$

Then divide by 6, the total number of patients:

$$33/6 = 5.5 \text{ days}$$

The mean stay of days per patient is 5.5 days.

Median

When values are ranked, the **median** is the value in which there is the same amount of numbers above and below. It is the middlemost value when arranged in numerical order. For an odd number of observations, the median is the middle number in an ordered set of numbers; for an even number of observations it is the mean or average of the middle two numbers. For example, the systolic blood pressure of five patients is provided as follows.

$$140, 190, 120, 116, 109$$

The first step to compute the median will include ranking these values from lowest to highest:

$$109, 116, 120, 140, 190$$

The median is 120 since it is the middlemost value when counting from left to right and also from right to left. If there was one more systolic blood pressure value added to this data set, then the median would be determined by counting to the middle from left to right and right to left and then taking the average of the two values. For example, if 140 is added to the existing values then the new data set will include the following.

$$109, 116, 120, 140, 140, 190$$

The new median will be:

$$120 + 140 = 260/2 = 130$$

Mode

The **mode** is the value that occurs most frequently in a given set of observations or values. In the systolic blood pressure scores example, the mode is 140 because it occurs more than any of the other values. Sometimes data sets have two modes and are then called bimodal.

Modes are used mostly with nominal variables, medians are used mainly for ordinal or ranked variables, and the mean is used primarily with continuous or quantitative variables, such as interval or ratio.

Measures of Variability

Measures of variability examine the spread of different values around the measures of central tendency. The measures of variability include the range, variance, and standard deviation.

Range

The **range** is the simplest measure of variation to compute and is calculated by taking the difference between the highest and lowest values. It is quick and easy to do, but not that useful since it only considers extremes and not the entire sample of data values. The range in the systolic blood pressure data set is: 190 – 109 = 81.

Variance

The **variance** is the average of the squared deviations from the mean. Its symbol is σ^2 for populations and s^2 for samples.

Standard Deviation

The **standard deviation** is the measure of variability that is used most often and displays how data are related to the mean. The variance and standard deviation can be cumbersome to compute by hand but statistical applications make it easy to automatically generate results. Using the same array of data

Table 13.9 Example of range, variance, and standard deviation

Statistics		
Systolic blood pressure		
N	Valid	6
	Missing	0
Mean		135.8333
Standard Deviation		29.43750
Variance		866.567
Range		81.00

N = Number

for the systolic blood pressure, table 13.9 provides the mean, range, variance, and standard deviation. The interpretation of these measures is what is most important. In table 13.9, the variance and standard deviation are both fairly large values, which means there is great variability of the systolic blood pressure scores around the mean. This makes sense since the mean is 135.8 and the scores range from 109 to 190, which does demonstrate large amounts of variability.

Check Your Understanding 13.2

Instructions: **Answer the following questions.**

1. True or false: The mean is the best measure of central tendency to use with ordinal data. The median is the best measure to use with ordinal data since the mean should mainly be used with continuous data.

2. True or false: The 40th percentile is the score below which 40 percent of the other scores in a given group of scores fall.

3. Which of the following measures examine the spread of different values around the measures of central tendency?
   A. Measures of central tendency
   B. Measures of variability
   C. Measures of frequency
   D. Measures of percentile

4. Which of the following measures is simple to compute and calculated by taking the difference between the highest and lowest values?
   A. Mean
   B. Median
   C. Range
   D. Standard deviation

5. This is a measure used in descriptive statistics that shows the value below which a given percentage of scores in a given group of scores fall. It is called a:
   A. percentile
   B. frequency distribution
   C. standard deviation
   D. median

Normal Distribution

The **normal distribution** is where data follows a symmetrical curve. The normal distribution is actually a theoretical family of distributions that may have any mean or any standard deviation. In a normal distribution, the mean, median, and mode are equal. An example of a normal curve is shown in figure 13.16.

The properties of a standard normal distribution include:

- The appearance of a bell-shaped curve that is symmetrical about the mean and extends infinitely in both directions (positive and negative).
- The total area under the curve equals 1, so the area of one half of the curve is equal to .50 and the area of the other half is equal to .50. Also, the area under the curve between two points can be interpreted as the relative frequency of the values included between those points. One standard deviation from the mean = 68.26 percent of the area, two standard deviations = 95.45 percent of the area, and three standard deviations = 99.74 percent of the area under the curve.
- Being defined by two parameters: the mean, μ and the standard deviation, σ.

Figure 13.17 provides an example of a histogram with the normal curve superimposed. The center of the distribution, or mean, is 17. (The median and the mode also are 17.) The standard deviation is 2.595 or, with rounding, 2.6. This means that 68 percent of the observations in the frequency distribution fall within 1 standard deviation from the mean or 2.6 standard deviations from 17 (17 ± 2.6). Thus, approximately 68 percent of the observations fall between 14.4 and 19.6; 95 percent fall between 2 standard deviations from the mean or ($2.6 \times 2 = 5.2$) 5.2 standard deviations from 17 (17 ± 5.2) or between 11.8 and 22.2; and 99.7 percent fall between 3 standard deviations from the mean or ($2.6 \times 3 = 7.8$) 7.8 standard deviations from 17 (17 ± 7.8) or between 9.2 and 24.8.

Normal distribution plays a key role in statistics because many variables follow a normal distribution such as height, cholesterol, body temperature, and such. Determining if data follow a normal distribution is important because certain statistics can be computed on data that is normally distributed. One way to do this is by computing a Z-score. A Z-score is a standardized unit that provides the relative position of any observation in the distribution and is also the number of standard deviations that the observed value lies away from the mean, μ. Transforming the raw observations to Z values makes it possible to make comparisons between distributions. Using **inferential statistics**, researchers can then make inferences about certain types of data. Inferential statistics are techniques that can be used to make deductions based on the evidence of the data and reasoning.

$$Z\text{-score} = \frac{\text{Observation or x} - \text{Mean}(\mu)}{\text{Standard Deviation}(\sigma)}$$

Z-scores represent the number of standard deviations above or below the mean, so a Z-score of –2.5 represents a score that is 2.5 standard deviations below the mean.

For example, if a prospective employee scores a 95 percent on a billing exam, with an employee average of 80 percent and a standard deviation of 5, using the given formula, the Z-score will be:

$$\frac{95 - 80}{5} = 3$$

This means that the score of 95 percent is 3 standard deviations above the mean.

Figure 13.16 Example of a normal curve

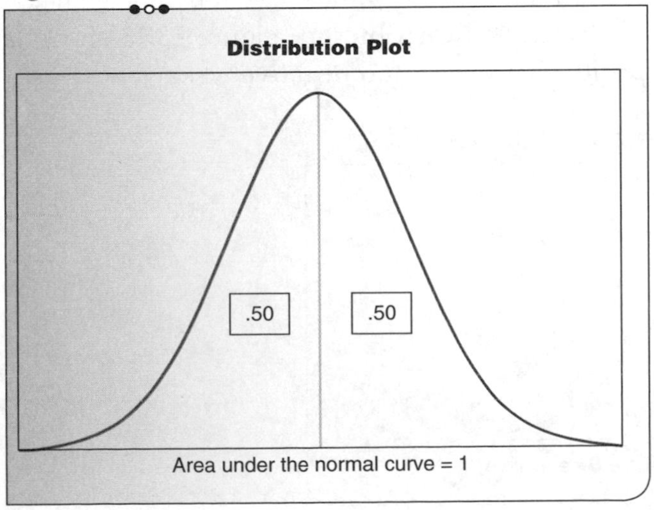

Distribution Plot

.50   .50

Area under the normal curve = 1

©AHIMA

Figure 13.17 Example of a histogram with a normal curve

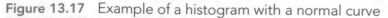

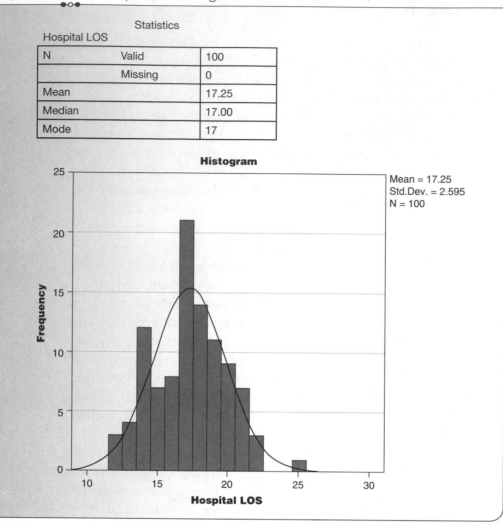

Statistics		
Hospital LOS		
N	Valid	100
	Missing	0
Mean		17.25
Median		17.00
Mode		17

Histogram

Mean = 17.25
Std.Dev. = 2.595
N = 100

©AHIMA

Sometimes data do not follow a normal distribution and are pulled toward the tails of the curve. When this occurs, it is referred to as having a skewed distribution. Because the mean is sensitive to extreme values or outliers, it gravitates in the direction of the extreme values thus making a long tail when a distribution is skewed. When the tail is pulled toward the right side, it is called a positively skewed distribution; when the tail is pulled toward the left side of the curve it is called a negatively skewed distribution. Figure 13.18 shows a positively skewed and negatively skewed curve.

Figures 13.18 Negatively skewed and positively skewed distribution

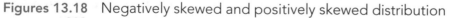

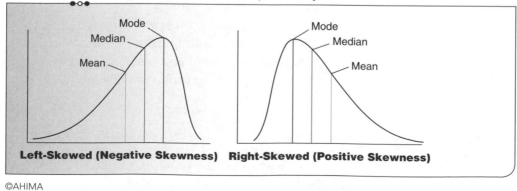

Left-Skewed (Negative Skewness) **Right-Skewed (Positive Skewness)**

©AHIMA

Check Your Understanding 13.3

Instructions: **Answer the following questions on a separate piece of paper.**

1. True or false: In a normal distribution, the mean, median, and mode are not equal.

2. True or false The total area under the curve of a normal distribution equals 1.

3. True or false: Z-scores represent the number of standard deviations above or below the mean, so a Z-score of −1.5 represents a score that is 1.5 standard deviations above the mean.

4. Determining if data follow a normal distribution is important because certain statistics can be computed on data that is normally distributed. Which of the following is one type of these statistics?
   A. Mean
   B. Median
   C. Z-score
   D. mode

5. Two standard deviations from the mean in a normal distribution equals what percent of the area?
   A. 68.26 percent
   B. 95.45 percent
   C. 99.74 percent
   D. 100 percent

6. A curve or distribution in which the tail is pulled to the right is called which of the following types of distribution?
   A. Negatively skewed
   B. Positively skewed
   C. Normal
   D. Bi-modal

7. If a student scores an 82 percent on an ICD-10-CM/PCS coding exam and the class average is 60 percent with a standard deviation of 4, what is the Z-score and what does this tell us about the student's coding exam score?
   A. Z = 5.5; the score of 82 percent is 5.5 standard deviations above the mean
   B. Z = 5.5; the score of 82 percent is 5.5 standard deviations below the mean
   C. Z = 5; the score of 82 percent is 5 standard deviations above the mean
   D. Z = 7.5; the score of 82 percent is 7.5 standard deviations above the mean

How to Analyze Information

Information can be analyzed in several ways in order to assess the quality, safety, and effectiveness of healthcare processes. There are several steps that should be taken in order to analyze information accurately. These steps include the following:

1. Know your objectives or purpose of the data analysis. What problem are you trying to solve? This includes obtaining the study objectives or specific aims for a quality, safety, or healthcare outcomes study. An example would be the comparison of nosocomial infection rates at a facility to establish CDC standards. If the rate is higher than the standard, there is an identified problem that needs corrective action to comply with accepted practice.

2. Know your audience.

3. Understand how the data was collected and for what purpose.

4. Recognize the different data types since this will dictate how to analyze the data.

5. Start with basic types of data analysis and work up to more sophisticated analysis, if appropriate.

6. Develop an interdisciplinary team of an HIM professional, a statistician and/or epidemiologist, information technologist, and administration to examine methods used to analyze the data early so that feedback on the approaches are incorporated from multiple potential users of the information. For example, if an HIM professional wanted to assess the feasibility of using natural language processing to extract quality measures from the EHR, these individuals would be an integral part of this team since the HIM professional knows the types of quality measures that are required as well as where these may be housed in the EHR and other data sources. Also, an interdisciplinary team of an epidemiologist and statistician working with the HIM professional to statistically examine manual versus automatic agreement levels would also be needed. The information technologist would determine how different types of electronic information may need to be connected through appropriate interfaces to obtain all of the correct data for extracting quality measures. Administration is always great to have on board—to make sure this work is supported at the top of the organization. Thus an interdisciplinary team is best for the project's success.

Quality, Safety, and Effectiveness of Healthcare

Using data to assess quality, safety, and healthcare outcomes such as the effectiveness of healthcare are prominent throughout healthcare organizations today. In fact, several federal government agencies, such as the Centers for Medicare and Medicaid Services (CMS) provide incentives for healthcare facilities that demonstrate high levels of quality, safety, and effectiveness of healthcare services. Quality measures developed by CMS are used in the pay-for-reporting programs for specific healthcare providers. The Joint Commission also uses data analysis to make decisions regarding patient safety and other measures of effectiveness of care. How is this data examined and how can HIM professionals assist? When the healthcare organization wants to measure variations within healthcare units—such as identifying variability across nursing units for the number or percentage of falls that occurred—a line graph would be an appropriate tool. Descriptive statistics in a table can also be used alongside the graph to provide more detail on the percentage of falls in total and also by nursing unit across the healthcare organization. Quality, safety, and effectiveness of healthcare are also assessed by many other organizations such as the National Commission for Quality Assurance (NCQA), which has developed Healthcare Effectiveness Data and Information Set (HEDIS) measures; Patient-Centered Outcomes Research Institute (PCORI), which focuses on the patient and engages the patient in the all phases of research related to healthcare outcomes; and the Agency for Healthcare Research and Quality (AHRQ), whose mission is to make healthcare safer, higher quality, more accessible, equitable, and affordable. The American Health Information Management Association (AHIMA) provides examples of publicly reported data by organizations such as the ones previously mentioned (AHIMA 2013). Much of the data collected is considered "big data" since it incorporates multiple sources from not only healthcare data but also financial, geographical, and human resource data. Analysis of big data does not necessarily mean that upper level statistics have to be used. One can start with descriptive levels of statistics and then move on to inferential statistics if the problem that needs to be solved needs this higher level of statistics.

Structure and Use of Health Information and Healthcare Outcomes

Data can be structured in many different ways. Healthcare facilities and organizations collect data that can fall into three different groups—individual, comparative, and aggregate.

Individual Data

Healthcare data that is housed within the EHR, or data collected from a case study, a focus group of individuals, or during an interview or survey are all considered individual data. This data can be helpful in providing direct care to patients, and for quality improvement studies or for larger descriptive studies. However, when using this type of data to make decisions related to a certain area of healthcare by evaluating it against other levels of data, then it becomes comparative data.

Comparative Data

When individual data is organized numerically and collated to evaluate against standards or benchmarks, it is described as being comparative data. For example, when a healthcare facility collects individual data on whether or not a patient acquired a healthcare-associated infection, such as ventilator-associated pneumonia (VAP), it is first documented in the individual patient's EHR. Queries throughout the entire EHR system will provide output on the number of cases of VAP that develops 48 hours or longer after mechanical ventilation is given by means of an endotracheal tube or tracheostomy, in order to designate it as a healthcare-associated infection. Once this data is gathered and collated, it can then be compared to other rates of VAP across the state, region, or nation.

Aggregate Data

Aggregate data is when individual, comparative, or other multiple sources of data are compiled and analyzed in order to draw conclusions about a specific topic or area. For example, in a focus group study, data, observation, and interview data were all compiled into an aggregate format so that none of the individuals in the multiple healthcare facilities that participated could be identified in any way. Varying methods and skills of leadership among HIM leaders and facilities were compared and contrasted in order to generate conclusions. However, since the focus group sample was small, not all of the conclusions could be generalized (Sheridan et al. 2016). In fact, any data compiled from samples of data have limitations since the sample of data may not accurately reflect the characteristics across that entire population. One way to reduce this is to compare the sample demographic characteristics to the population's demographics (if this information is available); if the characteristics prove similar, it increases the reliability of the sample data.

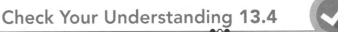

Check Your Understanding 13.4

Instructions: **Answer the following questions.**

1. True or false: The first step in analyzing data is to start with basic types of data analysis such as descriptive statistics.

2. True or false: Aggregate data is data that is individual in nature and not compiled for data analysis.

3. True or false: PCORI differs from other organizations that conduct evidence-based research because they focus on the patient and include patients in all steps of the research methodology.

4. True or false: Samples of data taken from populations have the same properties as the entire population.

5. True or false: When data is collected on the number of healthcare-associated infections, such as a catheter-associated urinary tract infection (CAUTI), in a healthcare facility and then compared to benchmark data across a region or the country, this is referred to as comparative data.

6. The focus group study previously mentioned is an example of using what type of data structure?
    A. Individual
    B. Comparative
    C. Aggregate
    D. Evaluative

7. Analysis of big data does not necessarily mean that upper level statistics have to be used. One can start with
_____ levels of statistics and then move on to _____ statistics if the problem that needs to be
solved requires this higher level of statistics.
   A. inferential; descriptive
   B. descriptive; inferential
   C. random; non-random
   D. social; scientific

Research Methodologies

There are several types of **research methodologies** that can be used to perform research on healthcare and HIM topics. Research studies can range from exploratory or descriptive studies that strive to generate new hypotheses based on data collected to experimental studies that provide interventions or treatments that can reduce the spread of an existing disease.

Quantitative Studies

When the data collected for the research studies are collated numerically with descriptive, inferential, or predictive statistics, it is normally referred to as a **quantitative study**—since it includes, if any, open-ended or qualitative-type responses by participants in the study. Descriptive studies contain research that is exploratory in nature and new hypotheses are generated from the data collected.

Correlational studies are similar to descriptive studies except that the correlational study determines if a relationship may exist between two variables. Retrospective studies (also called case-control studies) involve reviewing previous records or asking the subjects to recall past events in order to determine the presence or absence of the **independent variable** (an independent variable is one that is manipulated by the researcher) under study. A prospective study design is one in which a cohort of individuals are followed to determine if a particular characteristic or risk factor(s) may be causing the disease or outcome being studied. The experimental study design is the most powerful when trying to establish cause and effect and entails exposing participants to different interventions in order to compare the result of these interventions with the outcome. When study participants are arbitrarily chosen to be in the experimental, control, or comparison group using an indiscriminate method so each participant has an equal chance of being selected for one of the groups, it is called randomization. Ethical considerations need to be included in all of the study designs that are described in this section.

Descriptive Studies

Descriptive studies include research that is exploratory in nature and generate new hypotheses from the data collected. For example, a descriptive study approach was used to explore how the use of automated coding software (computer-assisted coding [CAC]) could be used to enhance anti-fraud activities. This study used a traditional descriptive study approach that consisted of the following steps.

1. Review of the literature on CAC software, anti-fraud software within CAC systems, and the extent of fraud and abuse related to CAC systems.

2. Interviews with federal agencies were conducted to gather information about instances of improper reimbursement or potential fraud involving the use of CAC software.

3. A description of products was developed based on a product information form completed by vendors.

4. Researchers then interviewed vendors and users about CAC and anti-fraud software to determine how they used these products.

5. Descriptive statistical results were reported through matrices, flowcharts, and tables to demonstrate the impact of automated coding tools on coding and billing accuracy. A model was designed that summarized features, processes, and staffing (Garvin et al. 2006).

Correlational Studies

Correlational studies are similar to descriptive studies except that the correlational study determines if a relationship may exist between two variables. This means that the researcher will try and determine if an increase or decrease in one variable corresponds to an increase or decrease in the other variable. The purpose of performing correlational studies is to determine which variables are connected in some way. However, correlation does not equal causation. For example, a researcher may be interested in patterns related to whether the use of electronic cigarettes or e-cigs affects school performance in teenagers. To determine a correlation, a researcher will interview teens to determine if and how often they smoke e-cigs and compare this to their grades in the past month. A correlation coefficient is then used to determine how strong the association is between two variables. The closer the correlation coefficient is to +1 or –1, the stronger the relationship between the variables. A strong positive relationship (closer to +1) means that as one variable increases the other also increases. A strong negative relationship (closer to –1) means that as one variable decreases the other variable increases. Hypothetically, if the research team collected data on the number of times a teen smoked an e-cig and on their SAT score, they may find that the correlation coefficient is a –0.845. The correlation coefficient of –0.845 is very close to –1. Therefore, this indicates a negative correlation and a negative correlation in this example means that as e-cig use increases, SAT scores decrease. There are two types of correlation coefficients: the Pearson Correlation coefficient and the Spearman Correlation coefficient. If continuous variables are collected by the researcher then the Pearson correlation coefficient should be used. If ordinal or ranked variables are collected then the Spearman correlation coefficient should be used.

Retrospective Studies

In epidemiology, **retrospective studies** (also called case-control studies) are conducted by reviewing records and asking the subjects to recall past events in order to determine the presence or absence of the independent variable under study. This is compared in samples of subjects with the disease under study (cases) and without the disease (controls). For example, if a researcher was interested in whether the use of estrogen replacement therapy (ERT) caused colon cancer in postmenopausal women, they would recruit a group of women with colon cancer (cases) and another group of women without colon cancer (controls) as subjects. Controls could be selected by recruiting subjects who also were treated by the same healthcare center as the cases or were friends or siblings of the cases. The more similar the controls are to the cases for everything except the disease under study (colon cancer), the better. The research team would then review their health records to determine if they ever used ERT. The research team may also want to validate the information found in the health record with interviews of the subjects asking them if they ever took ERT. This type of study is also called an analytic study because it tries to determine causation, or whether an independent variable (ERT) produced the dependent variable (colon cancer). Statistics used to determine causation include the odds ratio or the odds of getting the disease under study if you have the determinant variable or independent variable. Often the odds ratio is displayed in a two-by-two table, as shown in table 13.10.

To compute the odds ratio the formula is $AD/BC = (70 \times 80) / (20 \times 30) = 5,600/600 = 9.3$

The interpretation of this result for the odds ratio is that someone who takes ERT is approximately nine times more likely to get colon cancer than someone who does not take ERT.

Prospective Studies

A **prospective study** is one in which a cohort of individuals are followed to determine if a particular characteristic or risk factor(s) may be causing the disease or outcome under study. This type of study does something that the retrospective,

Table 13.10 Example of odds ratio for the retrospective (case-control) study

Independent variable ERT	Dependent variable (colon cancer)		
	Colon cancer	No colon cancer	Total
ERT use	70 (A)	30 (B)	100
No ERT use	20 (C)	80 (D)	100
Totals	90	110	200

Table 13.11 Example computing the incidence rates

	Disease	No Disease
Exposed	(A)	(B)
Not exposed	(C)	(D)
Totals		

Incidence rate of exposed = A / (A + B)
Incidence rate of unexposed = C / (C + D)
Relative risk: [A / (A + B)] / [C / (C + D)]

case-control design does not—it determines whether the characteristic(s) or risk factor(s) under study truly preceded the disease. The prospective study starts with subjects who have the risk factor (exposed group) but are free from the disease and compares them to individuals without the risk factor (unexposed group) who are also free of the disease. The two groups are then followed to determine if and when the subjects develop the disease. To begin, subjects are examined at a baseline to ensure they do not have the disease when the study commences. To do this, the researcher must collect data related to their occupation, medical history, and social habits. Physical exams and lab tests may also be necessary. It is important to collect other general characteristics such as age, sex, race, and such in addition to the characteristic of interest, in order to account for the influence of any factors that are known to be related to the disease. These are called confounding factors. Confounding factors are those characteristics other than the characteristic of interest that may also be related to the disease under study. If subjects cannot be correctly categorized into exposed and unexposed groups, the prospective design should not be used.

It is important to have correct classification of exposure because if participants' exposure to certain elements is not correctly classified it may lead to invalid study results. The most widely known example of a prospective study is the Framingham Heart Study, which began in 1948, is a project of the National Heart, Lung, and Blood Institute and Boston University, and is still in progress today (FHS 2015). Its original goal was to identify risk factors for cardiovascular disease (CVD) since the causes of heart disease and stroke were not known and the death rates were steadily

increasing. The researchers decided to study this over a long period of time using a large group of participants who had not yet developed CVD, or had a heart attack or stroke. The researchers recruited 5,209 men and women between the ages of 30 and 62 from Framingham, Massachusetts, and started physical exams and interviews to determine any type of CVD. The participants returned to the study every two years for follow-up physical exams, lab tests, and so forth, and in 1971 enrolled a second generation cohort of the participant's adult children and spouses. In 2002, a third generation of participants was recruited, which included the grandchildren of the original cohort. Based on its results, clinicians use many of its findings when treating CVD, since it identified major risk factors of CVD such as high blood pressure, high cholesterol, smoking, lack of physical activity, diabetes, and obesity. It was also instrumental in finding related factors that play a part in the development of CVD, such as triglyceride and HDL cholesterol levels, as well as psychosocial issues, age, and gender (FHS 2015). Prospective studies generate incidence—the number of new cases that occurred during a specific period of time in a population at risk for developing the disease—not the prevalence of a disease. The calculation for the incidence rate is given in table 13.11. **Incidence rates** can then be used to calculate the relative risk (table 13.12),

$$\frac{\text{Number of new cases over a time period} \times 1{,}000}{\text{Population at risk*}}$$

Those free of disease at the start of the study

An example of computing the incidence rates and relative risk is shown as follows.

Table 13.12 Example of computing relative risk

	CVD	No CVD
BMI > 27	50 (A)	20 (B)
BMI < 27	10 (C)	60(D)
Totals	60	80

Incidence rate of exposed = A / (A+B) = 50/ (50+20) = 0.71
Incidence rate of unexposed = C / (C + D) = 10 / (10 + 60) = 0.14
Relative risk: [A / (A + B)] / [C / (C + D)] = 0.71/0.14 = 5.1

Therefore, using this hypothetical data, one can say that the risk of developing CVD with a BMI of greater than 27 is approximately 5 times that of developing CVD with a BMI of less than 27. The difference between the odds ratio and the relative risk is that the odds ratio is an estimate of the risk since the study from which it was taken is based on retrospective data. The relative risk from a prospective study is considered "true risk" since it demonstrates that the risk factor under study actually came before the disease since participants were followed to collect the data and, therefore, determine the risk of disease.

Experimental Studies

The **experimental study** design is the most powerful when trying to establish cause and effect. It entails exposing participants to different interventions in order to compare the result of these interventions with the outcome. The intervention may include testing experimental drugs, new approaches to surgery, or other types of interventions such as smoking cessation treatments. Experimental studies can also be referred to as clinical trials. The National Institutes of Health (NIH) has a service that provides a registry and a database of results of clinical trials that have been conducted or are currently being conducted across the world (NIH 2015a). Pretests and posttests are used in observational experimental research. The pretest is performed to determine the baseline level of the independent variable under study and the posttest is determined to measure the same independent variable after the intervention. For example, blood pressure is taken before and after an experimental medication is used as the intervention in a sample of participants that were previously unable to control their blood pressure

with other medications. The independent variable is the experimental medication and the dependent variable is the blood pressure. In experimental research studies like clinical trials, researchers must pay attention to many things but three main areas are extremely important.

1. Eligibility of appropriate participants (inclusion and exclusion criteria)
2. Randomization
3. Ethical issues

Eligibility of appropriate participants includes the development of certain criteria so that the proper participants are recruited for the experimental study. For example, in a study entitled, "Evaluation of a Stepped Care Approach to Manage Depression in Diabetes" some of the inclusion criteria include:

- Age greater than or equal 18 and less than or equal to70
- Diabetes mellitus
- Elevated depressive symptoms

Some of the exclusion criteria include:

- Severe depressive episode
- Current psychotherapeutic or psychiatric treatment
- Current anti-depressive medication
- Severe physical illness (that is, cancer, multiple sclerosis, dementia)
- Terminal illness (NIH 2015b)

Randomization

When study participants are randomly chosen to be in the experimental, control, or comparison group using an indiscriminate method so each participant has an equal chance of being selected for one of the groups, it is called **randomization**. Randomization is important in effectively testing whether the specific intervention actually made a difference in the outcome of the disease. For example, if a researcher wanted to determine whether an experimental medication made a difference in a person's anxiety level, they would recruit participants who are diagnosed with anxiety and then randomly assign them to either a group that will take the experimental drug or a group that will take a placebo or pill that does not include the experimental drug. The researchers will also collect pretest data on the anxiety level of participants through interviews before they were randomized into the experimental or control group. They would then provide the medication over a period of time and collect data via interviews on the anxiety levels of participants in both the experimental and control groups. Anxiety level data should provide a score that can be compared pre- and post-intervention. Once this data is collected the difference in the average anxiety scores can be compared before and after the intervention in both the experimental and control groups. The *Paired t test* is a statistical test that can be used to determine if the differences seen pre- and post-intervention are significantly different statistically and not due to chance. If significant values are found more so in the experimental group than in the control group, then the researchers can conclude that the experimental drug was successful.

Ethics

Ethical considerations are vital when conducting research studies. These may include ensuring the research is accurate with minimal chance of error and that it can be valid to the public, providing credit in publications and other documents to those who are most involved in the research since it is a collaborative approach; protection of human subjects as well as protection and confidentiality of the data when collected from human subjects; and compliance with the law in all types of research conducted by organizations like the National Institutes of Health or the Food and Drug Administration. In most clinical trial research a control group or a group that will not receive any type of intervention (medicine or procedure) is used. However, there are times when it is not ethical to withhold a successful type of intervention to individuals who are suffering from a disease. When this occurs, the researcher can include a comparison group instead of a control group, and instead of providing a placebo (no medicine or intervention), another type of intervention can be provided to the comparison group. Other ethical considerations in experimental research include stopping the study when

researchers, upon collecting preliminary data, realize that the experimental intervention is highly successful. In this case, the researcher should stop the study and provide the intervention to both the experimental and control or comparison group, so that they can benefit from the intervention.

Quasi-Experimental Studies

The **quasi-experimental study** is similar to the experimental study except that randomization of participants is not included in a quasi-experimental study. Also, the independent variable may not be manipulated by the researcher and there may be no control or comparison group. Quasi-experimental studies can be performed over time and may not include individual participants but whole healthcare systems. For example, researchers performed a quasi-experimental study to examine the association between implementation of a certified outpatient EHR and control of diabetes in patients with the disease. They implemented the EHR system across 17 medical centers and then tested the difference in certain lab tests before and after implementation. They found the EHR improved drug treatment intensity, monitoring, and control for patients with diabetes (Reed et al. 2012).

Qualitative Research

Qualitative research designs involve collecting types of data that reflect a participant's perceptions, attitudes, feelings, or attitudes about a certain subject. The methods used to collect qualitative data can include observations, focus groups, case studies, informal conversational interviews, and in-depth interviews. An example of observation can be as simple as taking time to observe a physical object on your desk at home or at work. Look at the object in relation to its shape, size, color, material composition, and its purpose and write these observations down. This also can be performed in an HIM department, where the researcher will observe how coders react to their first exposure to the use of a clinical documentation improvement software system. The researcher could observe them as they are trained on the system or as they use the system and then document their observations. Qualitative research is chosen because it can provide robust data on a new topic or it can provide background for larger studies on the same topic. Grounded theory and ethnography are explained in more detail as follows since HIM professionals may find themselves conducting research in these areas.

Grounded Theory

Grounded theory is a research method that enables the researcher to develop a theory that is substantiated or confirmed by the data. It is a systematic method that can use multiple methods (both quantitative and qualitative findings) and pull it all together to develop a theory. Because it includes types of data like conversing with subjects on a specific topic it is usually categorized under qualitative research, but it can also include quantitative information (Grounded Theory Institute 2014). First, the researcher should identify the topic area such as information governance. The study will then consult all the previous research and possibly the researchers that have defined and discussed information governance. Data collection may include several types of data—qualitative, quantitative, or a mixture of both—in the particular topic area. Data can be from sources such as articles, news reports, pictures, photographs, videos, recordings, and the like. It can also include conversing with individuals or groups. For example, in order to learn more about information governance, the researcher may choose leaders in the field of IG and create focus groups of individuals with a background in IG and ask them questions about the topic. In grounded theory, the researcher codes the data as it is collected and makes memos and observations simultaneously so that at the end of this refining process, the research is used to develop a theory. It is also important that the researcher be familiar with literature on the topic so that his or her theory coincides with what is currently published and accepted. The researcher's theory is then published or presented in a model that can be used by others to conduct further research in that area.

Ethnography

Ethnography is a methodology where the researcher delves into a particular culture or organization in great detail in order to learn everything there is to know about them and to develop new hypotheses. Ethnography is not objective and includes opinions of the researcher. No two ethnographers will examine a specific culture or organization the same way. Ethnography's focus is on people, culture, and life. The researcher takes notes while out in the field observing the people and their experiences in a particular culture so the researcher can create a more thorough and specific description of all interactions, experiences, perceptions, and opinions. In one particular example of an ethnographic study, a researcher examined the social relationship between a physician and patient as the patient is diagnosed with clinical illness. The specific aims of the research were to identify and describe the most important social practices between urologists and patients as they are diagnosed with cancer. The researcher worked in urology offices and hospitals primarily using participant observation to collect his data, which is one of the primary tools of ethnographic research. He found that a healing relationship between the patient and clinician emerged as the diagnosis unfolded (Meza 2013).

Mixed-Methods Approach

A mixed-methodology approach includes using both quantitative and qualitative data in a research study design. According to the NIH Office of Behavioral and Social Science Research, mixed-methods research includes the following aspects:

- Research questions that focus on real life, multilevel perspectives, across many cultures
- Using multiple methods (for example, intervention trials and in-depth interviews)
- Integrating these multiple methods or combining them to extract the strengths of each
- Focusing the research within philosophical and theoretical positions (Creswell et al. 2011)

According to NIH, mixed-methods research is more than collecting qualitative data from interviews or observations, or gathering multiple types of quantitative evidence through surveys and diagnostic tests. It involves the intentional collection of both quantitative and qualitative data in order to combine the strengths of both to answer the research questions. Mixed-methods research designs are usually performed when qualitative or quantitative data alone are not sufficient to answer the research question. For example, if an HIM professional wanted to explore the underutilization of the cancer registry at one healthcare facility, he or she could first collect quantitative data on the number of requests the cancer registry received. However, more qualitative informal interviews with physicians and other potential users may also be needed. Therefore, a mixed-methods approach would be the best research design in this case.

Check Your Understanding 13.5

Instructions: **Answer the following questions by matching the corresponding research study design with its appropriate description.**

1. _____ Uses a combination of quantitative and qualitative data

2. _____ Exploratory, generates new hypotheses

3. _____ Determines if a relationship exists between two variables

4. _____ Case-control study

5. _____ Framingham Heart Study

6. _____ Randomization

7. _____ Kaiser Permanente study to examine the impact of implementation of EHR on outcomes of diabetes patients

8. _____ Studies a particular culture in great detail

9. _____ Uses multiple methods to determine a new theory

10. _____ Collect robust types of data

   A. Qualitative research
   B. Quasi-experimental study
   C. Retrospective study
   D. Prospective study
   E. Mixed-methods approach
   F. Ethnography
   G. Experimental study
   H. Grounded theory
   I. Descriptive study
   J. Correlational study

Institutional Review Board

The Department of Health and Human Services (HHS), describes the role of the **Institutional Review Board (IRB)**, as one that protects human subjects as they are involved in research activities. The IRB determines whether research conducted on human subjects is appropriate and protects the participant's rights. The major focus of the IRB is not whether the research is appropriate for the organization or researcher to conduct, but that it contains all the appropriate protections for human subjects involved in the research (45 CFR 46). There are three major categories for IRB review and approval and they include exempt, expedited, and full board approval. Exempt research activities that are the most closely related to HIM fall into three main categories:

- Research conducted in an educational setting involving normal education practices such as testing different teaching methods
- Research conducted that includes using tests, interviews, or observations, unless identifiable and pose risks
- Collection or study of existing data or specimens, if publicly available or deidentified (45 CFR 46)

Expedited research include those studies that pose only minimal risk to human subjects; examples include those studies that collect information on human subjects that is identifiable and may include sensitive information such as identifiable health information on subjects that are HIV positive.

Full board approval is required for those studies that do not fall under exempt or expedited. Most of the studies performed by HIM professionals are categorized as exempt or expedited. It is best to meet with a member of the IRB at the healthcare organization to determine under which category the research study would fall. Once the review category is determined the researcher must then submit their research protocol to the IRB for review and approval. This takes about two weeks and if a decision is made that the research falls under the exempt category then the researcher does not have to renew the study annually, as they must do under expedited and full board reviews. Also, informed consent is normally not required under exempt research as it is for expedited and full board study reviews (45 CFR 46).

Researchers should always remember that whenever any human subjects are used in research, the IRB should be consulted and the research protocol should be submitted to the organization's IRB for review and approval. Even if research is conducted on individuals that are not patients—such as interviewing employees, students, or even collecting data on human subjects from existing records—IRB approval should still be obtained.

Check Your Understanding 13.6

Instructions: **Answer the following questions.**

1. True or false: The IRB determines whether research conducted on human subjects is appropriate and protects the participant's rights.

2. True or false: Once the review category is determined, the researcher must then submit their research protocol to the IRB for their review and approval.

3. True or false: Informed consent is only required for exempt research studies.

4. Which type of IRB review category most closely relates to HIM research activities?
   A. Exempt
   B. Expedited
   C. Full board approval
   D. HIM does not do IRB research

5. Which type of research include those studies that pose only minimal risk to human subjects?
   A. Exempt
   B. Expedited
   C. Full board approval
   D. Clinical trial research

Healthcare Research Organizations

There are many different types of **healthcare research organizations** that conduct, promote, or support research across healthcare organizations. The Centers for Disease Control and Prevention (CDC), the World Health Organization (WHO) and the Agency for Healthcare Research and Quality (AHRQ) are discussed in the following sections.

Centers for Disease Control and Prevention (CDC)

The **Centers for Disease Control and Prevention (CDC)** is a US government organization whose mission is to collaborate with the public to create the expertise, information, and tools people and communities need to protect their health, through health promotion, prevention of disease, injury and disability, and preparedness for new health threats. The CDC does this by confronting global diseases such as helping to combat the recent Ebola virus outbreak, tracking diseases (like influenza or foodborne outbreaks) to find out what is causing individuals to become ill, and helping healthcare organizations and cultivating public health. The CDC employs researchers to meet many of these goals, but they also provide funding and support to other researchers who can then submit grants in order to conduct research to meet their objectives. Also, the CDC and the National Center for Health Statistics provides mounds of data, statistical reports, and surveys that can be used to conduct research as well (CDC 2015).

World Health Organization

The **World Health Organization (WHO)** works to direct and coordinate authority on international health through the United Nations' Its health-related focus areas include:

- Health systems
- Noncommunicable diseases such as heart disease, cancer, stroke, diabetes, chronic lung disease, and mental health conditions

- Promoting health throughout the course of life to include environment and social determinants of health as well as gender, equity, and human rights
- Communicable diseases such as HIV, tuberculosis, and malaria
- Preparedness, surveillance, and response through emergencies that occur worldwide
- Corporate services that includes all of WHO's tools, functions, and resources

WHO provides data, publications, and funding support to researchers across the world (WHO, 2015).

Agency for Healthcare Research and Quality (AHRQ)

The **Agency for Healthcare Research and Quality (AHRQ)** is a federal agency within the US Department of Health and Human Services (HHS) whose mission is to make healthcare safer, higher quality, more accessible, equitable, and affordable, and to work within HHS and with other partners to make sure that the evidence is understood and used. Its priority areas of focus include:

- Improving healthcare quality by accelerating implementation of patient-centered outcomes research (PCOR). This priority is being met through the Patient-Centered Outcomes Research Institute (PCORI), which provides funding to researchers to perform research that is patient centered and patient engaged. Every research study funded by PCORI must include patients within all aspects of the research methodology process.
- Making healthcare safer by preventing healthcare-associated infections (HAI), accelerating patient safety in healthcare facilities, reducing harm associated with obstetrical care, improving safety and reducing medical liability, and accelerating patient safety in nursing homes.
- Increasing accessibility to healthcare.

- Improving healthcare affordability, efficiency, and cost transparency through improved data measures and public reporting strategies.

Similar to the CDC and WHO, AHRQ also provides multiple sources of data, information, funding, and support to researchers in the healthcare sector (AHRQ 2015).

Check Your Understanding 13.7

Instructions: **Answer the following questions.**

1. True or false: Although the CDC provides a great deal of data and reports, it does not provide funding for researchers to conduct their research.

2. True or false: The major difference between WHO and the CDC and AHRQ is that WHO focuses its efforts across the world whereas the CDC and AHRQ focus on the United States.

3. True or false: PCORI provides funding to researchers to perform research that is patient centered and patient engaged.

4. Which organization focuses one of its main priorities on patient-centered outcomes research?
   A. CDC
   B. AHRQ
   C. WHO
   D. HHS

5. Which organization's primary focus is improving healthcare across the world?
   A. CDC
   B. WHO
   C. AHRQ
   D. Joint Commission

6. Patients must be involved in the design of the research study if the researcher is to receive funding from which of the following organizations?
   A. PCORI
   B. CDC
   C. WHO
   D. AHA

Real-World Case 13.1

Researchers were interested in assessing the relationship between obesity and breast cancer recurrence and fatality in postmenopausal African-American and Caucasian women with primary breast cancer. Data was collected on women with primary breast cancer and included the following variables:

- Age
- Age at diagnosis of breast cancer

- Weight
- Height
- Data of diagnosis of breast cancer
- Menopausal status
- Diagnosis and coding of tumor (histopathology and topography)
- Stage of tumor

- Size of tumor
- Number of positive lymph nodes
- Estrogen receptor analysis
- Progesterone receptor analysis
- Site of distant metastasis
- First course of treatment (surgery, radiation, chemotherapy)
- Additional treatment
- Five-year recurrence and survival rates

Recurrence and survival status were determined by reviewing the cancer registry follow-up data and medical record information across the multiple healthcare sites involved in this study. The cancer registries were accredited by the American College of Surgeons and used active follow-up on all cancer patients. Postmenopausal status was determined as subjects older than 55 years. In those subjects younger than age 55, determination was made by consulting the cancer registry data, the medical record, and physician's office records. Premenopausal patients and patients whose menopausal status could not be determined from the data were excluded from the study. Body mass index (BMI) was based on height and weight collected from the medical record or cancer registry at the date of diagnosis only. Values greater than 27 were considered to indicate obesity. The effect of weight changes during the follow-up period was not evaluated.

 Real-World Case 13.2

A descriptive research study was performed to investigate the completeness of the ICD-10-CM coding system in capturing public health diseases when compared to ICD-9-CM. In order to do this, the infectious and reportable public health conditions—such as avian flu, smallpox, anthrax, and such—were examined first by reviewing each state department of health's website to determine which diseases are required to be reported. Once this list was developed, it was supplemented with the CDC national reportable disease listing. The final list of public health reportable infectious diseases included all the reportable infectious diseases by state as well as those required by CDC. This list was supplemented with two other areas that are very pertinent to public health—the top 10 causes of mortality:

- Accidents
- Alzheimer's disease
- Cerebrovascular disease
- Diabetes mellitus
- Influenza
- Lower respiratory disease
- Nephritis
- Septicemia
- Heart disease
- The top five malignant neoplasms

And the classification of death and injury resulting from terrorism list, including 10 major categories as follows:

- Terrorism involving explosion of marine weapons
- Destruction of aircraft
- Other explosions and fragments
- Fires
- Firearms
- Nuclear weapons
- Biological weapons
- Chemical weapons
- Terrorism other specified
- Sequelae of terrorism

A total of 248 public health disease categories were developed. When coding the diseases, several more codes and descriptions were listed so that the number of codes far exceeded the 248 disease categories. A website was then developed so that all of the public health diseases and descriptions could be easily accessed by the researchers and the focus group members. For example, when organizing the reportable disease list on the website, every disease was categorized alphabetically. When the specific reportable disease was accessed, a spreadsheet with each of the ICD-9-CM and ICD-10-CM codes could be easily viewed. This was extremely useful for reviewing the codes, rankings, explanations for using a specific ranking, and so forth. Although the list of 248 disease categories is not exhaustive of all public health diseases, it was believed to provide an adequate number to make comparisons between the two coding systems. The 248 public health diseases were then coded using both ICD-9-CM and ICD-10-CM so that comparisons between the two coding systems could be made. The research coder for this study has a master's of science degree in information science and is a registered health information administrator (RHIA) and has taught coding for more than 20 years. She was also trained and educated on the ICD-10-CM coding system through AHIMA's online ICD-10-CM coding seminars. The research assistant, who performed data entry and assisted in some of the ICD-10-CM coding, has a master's of science degree in health information systems and was also trained and educated on the ICD-10-CM coding system. All final codes were approved by a research coder. Quality checks for final codes were performed by a secondary investigator, who has a doctorate in public health and is an RHIA and certified coding specialist (CCS); and also by the principal investigator, who has a doctorate in epidemiology and is an RHIA.

Comparison tables that describe the specificity of the coding for ICD-9-CM and ICD-10-CM for each of the public health diseases were developed. A ranked score was assigned to each public health disease for both the ICD-10-CM and ICD-9-CM coding systems. The ranking was determined by comparing the number of codes, level of specificity, and ability of the code description to fully capture the diagnostic term. The ranked or ordinal scale consisted of the following:

5 = Diagnosis is fully captured by the code(s) (all codes, specificity, description is found)

4 = Diagnosis is almost fully captured by the code(s) (minor detail is missing)
3 = Diagnosis is partially captured by the code(s) (moderate detail is missing)
2 = Diagnosis is less than partially captured by the code(s) (major detail is missing)
1 = Diagnosis is not captured by the code(s) (codes, specificity, description is not found)

The ranking scale was developed by the research team and reviewed and approved by the focus group members. All assigned rankings were also reviewed and approved by the research team and by all focus group members. Researchers do acknowledge that there was some subjectivity involved in the assignment of the rankings.

Once all rankings were assigned, a focus group that included seven experts in ICD-9-CM, ICD-10-CM, and public health convened. Two of the focus group members have medical degrees, two are working on their doctorates in public health and have extensive education and training in coding, and three have coding credentials and have worked in the coding field for more than 10 years. The purpose of the focus group was to review and examine the information accumulated from the study and provide feedback and recommendations regarding where changes need to be made in the ICD-10-CM system. Therefore, the focus group examined the rankings and made changes. The researchers reviewed and discussed all comments from the focus group, clarifying any questions, and then made the appropriate changes to the rankings and code descriptions. In the analysis of all the public health diseases, such as reportable diseases ($p < 0.001$), top 10 causes of death ($p < 0.001$), and those related to terrorism ($p < 0.001$), it was found that the overall rankings for disease capture for ICD-10-CM were significantly higher than the rankings for ICD-9-CM. In this example the p value is a statistic that demonstrates statistical significance. It is computed by running statistical tests to determine if the differences between ICD-9-CM and ICD-10-CM rankings were real or due to chance. If the p value is less than 0.05, the differences seen are not due to chance and it demonstrates that what was found in this study is real. (Watzlaf et al. 2007).

References

Agency for Healthcare Research and Quality. 2015. http://www.ahrq.gov/.

American Health Information Management Association. 2013 (September). Understanding publicly available healthcare data. *Journal of AHIMA.* 84(9):expanded web version. http://library.ahima.org/doc?oid=300183#.VxE-MvkrK9I.

Brewer N.T., M.B. Gilkey, S.E. Lillie, B.W. Hesse, and S.L. Sheridan. 2012. Tables or bar graphs? Presenting test results in electronic medical records. *Medical Decision Making.* 32(4):545–553.

Centers for Disease Control and Prevention. 2015. http://www.cdc.gov/about/organization/mission.htm.

Centers for Disease Control and Prevention. 2012. *Principles of Epidemiology in Public Health Practice,* 3rd ed. http://www.cdc.gov/ophss/csels/dsepd/ss1978/ss1978.pdf.

Centers for Disease Control and Prevention. 2004. Prevalence of overweight and obesity among adults with diagnosed diabetes–United States, 1988–1994 and 1999–2002. *MMWR Morb Mortal Wkly Rep.* 53:1066–1068.

Centers for Medicare and Medicaid Services. 2016. National Health Expenditure Data. https://www.cms.gov/Research-Statistics-Data-and-Systems/Statistics-Trends-and-Reports/NationalHealthExpendData/index.html.

Centers for Medicare and Medicaid Services. 2014. Inpatient Prospective Payment System (IPPS) Provider Summary. https://data.cms.gov/Medicare/Inpatient-Prospective-Payment-System-IPPS-Provider/97k6-zzx3.

Creswell, J.W., A.C. Klassen, V.L. Plano Clark, and K.C. Smith for the Office of Behavioral and Social Sciences Research. 2011 (August). *Best Practices for Mixed-Methods Research in the Health Sciences.* https://www2.jabsom.hawaii.edu/native/docs/tsudocs/Best_Practices_for_Mixed_Methods_Research_Aug2011.pdf.

Framingham Heart Study (FHS). 2015. A Project of the National Heart, Lung and Blood Institute and Boston University. https://www.framinghamheartstudy.org/.

Garvin, J.H., V. Watzlaf, and S. Moeini. 2006. Development and Use of Automated Coding Software to Enhance Anti-fraud Activities. *Perspectives in Health Information Management*, CAC Proceedings.

Grounded Theory Institute. 2014. http://www.groundedtheory.com/what-is-gt.aspx.

Meza, J.P. 2013. *The Diagnosis Narratives and the Healing Ritual* [dissertation]. Paper 848. Detroit, MI: Wayne State University.

National Archives and Record Administration. 2015 (September 8). Proposed Rules. *Federal Register.* 80(173). https://www.gpo.gov/fdsys/pkg/FR-2015-09-08/pdf/2015-21756.pdf.

National Institutes of Health. 2015a. ClinicalTrials.gov. https://clinicaltrials.gov/ct2/home.

National Institutes of Health. 2015b. Evaluation of a Stepped Care Approach to Manage Depression in Diabetes, https://clinicaltrials.gov/ct2/show/NCT01812291.

Productivity-Quality Systems. 2015. Pareto Diagram. http://www.pqsystems.com/qualityadvisor/DataAnalysisTools/pareto_diagram.php.

Reed, M., J. Huang, I. Graetz, R. Brand, J. Hsu, B. Fireman, and M. Jaffe. 2012. Outpatient electronic health records and the clinical care and outcomes of patients with diabetes mellitus. *Annals of Internal Medicine.* 157(7):482–489.

Sheridan, P., V. Watzlaf, and L. Fox. 2016. HIM Leaders and the Practice of Leadership through the Lens of Bowen Theory. *Perspectives in Health Information Management.* Spring.

Watzlaf, V., Z. Alakrawi, S. Meyers, and P. Sheridan. 2015. Physicians' outlook on ICD-10-CM/PCS and its effect on their practice. *Perspectives in Health Information Management.* Winter:1–23.

Watzlaf V.J.M., J.H. Garvin, S. Moeini, and P. Anania-Firouzan. 2007. The effectiveness of ICD-10-CM in capturing public health diseases. *Perspectives in Health Information Management.* 4(6).World Health Organization. 2015. http://www.who.int/en/.

45 CFR 46: Basic HHS policy for protection of human research subjects. 2009.

14

Healthcare Statistics

Loretta A. Horton, MEd, RHIA, FAHIMA

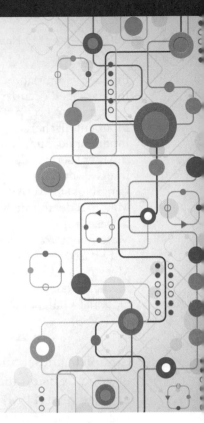

Learning Objectives

- Define measurement
- Differentiate among nominal-level, ordinal-level, interval-level, and ratio-level data
- Identify various ways in which statistics are used in healthcare
- Define hospital-related statistical terms
- Calculate hospital-related inpatient and outpatient statistics
- Define community-based morbidity and mortality rates

- Calculate community-based morbidity and mortality rates
- Calculate the case-mix index
- Calculate population-based statistics
- Differentiate between incidence and prevalence and calculate their rates
- Identify the use of the National Notifiable Diseases Surveillance System

Key Terms

Ambulatory care
Ambulatory surgery center (ASC)
Average daily census
Average length of stay (ALOS)
Bed count
Bed count day
Bed turnover rate
Case fatality rate
Case mix
Case-mix index (CMI)
Cause-specific mortality rate
Census
Clinic outpatient

Consultation rate
Continuous data
Coroner
Crude birth rate
Crude death/mortality rate
Daily inpatient census
Descriptive statistics
Discrete data
Emergency patient
Encounter
Fetal autopsy rate
Fetal death (stillborn)
Fetal death rate

Gross autopsy rate
Gross death rate
Hospital-acquired (nosocomial) infection rate
Hospital autopsy
Hospital autopsy rate
Hospital death rate
Hospital inpatient
Hospital inpatient autopsy
Hospital newborn inpatient
Hospital outpatient
Incidence rate
Infant mortality rate

379

Inpatient admission
Inpatient bed occupancy rate (per-
    centage of occupancy)
Inpatient discharge
Inpatient hospitalization
Inpatient service day (IPSD)
Interval-level data
Length of stay (LOS)
Maternal death rate (hospital
    based)
Maternal mortality rate (communi-
    ty-based)
Measurement
Medical examiner
National Vital Statistics System
    (NVSS)

Neonatal mortality rate
Net autopsy rate
Net death rate
Newborn (NB)
Newborn autopsy rate
Newborn death rate
Nominal-level data
Nosocomial (hospital-acquired)
    infection
Notifiable disease
Occasion of service
Ordinal-level data
Outpatient
Outpatient visit
Population-based statistics
Postneonatal mortality rate

Postoperative infection rate
Prevalence rate
Proportion
Proportionate mortality
    rate (PMR)
Rate
Ratio
Ratio-level data
Referred outpatient
Scales of measurement
Surgical operation
Surgical procedure
Total length of stay
    (discharge days)
Vital statistics

Complete and accurate information is at the heart of good decision making. The health information management (HIM) professional is responsible for ensuring that data collected are accurate and organized into information that is useful to healthcare decision makers.

The primary source of clinical data in a healthcare facility is the health record. To be useful in decision making, data taken from the health record must be as complete and accurate as possible. Data are compiled in various ways to help make decisions about patient care, the facility's financial status, and facility planning.

This chapter discusses common statistical measures and types of data used by organizations in different healthcare settings. A discussion of normal distribution and descriptive statistics is given.

Before discussing statistical measures used in healthcare, it is important to define measurement and how the data collected are classified. **Measurement** refers to the systematic process of data collection, repeated over time or at a single point in time. The process of collecting the data must be consistent in order to ensure the results are the same no matter who is collecting the data. If there is consistency in the data collection, comparisons can be made within and across facilities.

Data collected falls on one of four **scales of measurement**: nominal, ordinal, interval, or ratio. Furthermore, the data collected is described as either continuous or discrete. **Continuous data** are those that represent measurable quantities but are not restricted to certain specified values while

discrete data are data that represent separate and distinct values or observations. These characteristics influence the type of graphic technique used to display the data and the types of statistical analyses that can be performed.

Nominal-level data fall into groups or categories. This is a scale that measures data by name only. The groups or categories are mutually exclusive; that is, a data element cannot be classified to more than one group. Some examples of nominal data collected in healthcare are related to patient demographics such as third-party payer, race, and gender. There is no order to the data collected within these categories.

Data that fall on the ordinal scale have some inherent order, and higher numbers are usually associated with higher values. In **ordinal-level data**, the order of the numbers is meaningful, not the number itself. Staging of Parkinson's disease is an example of a variable that has order. Parkinson's disease is often classified in five stages—with stage I showing mild symptoms, to stage V that takes over a patient's physical movements. In this example, the higher number is associated with the most severe type of symptoms; however, we cannot measure the difference between the levels in exact numerical terms. A Likert scale is often used in this level of measurement. A Likert, or rating scale, is one that is commonly used in questionnaires to gather data. It primarily has five potential choices (strongly agree, agree, neutral, disagree, strongly disagree) but will sometimes include 10 or more (BusinessDictionary.com 2016).

The most important characteristic of **interval-level data** is that the intervals between successive values are equal. On the Fahrenheit scale, for example, the interval between 20°F and 21°F is the same as between 21°F and 22°F. But because there is no true zero on this scale, it is not appropriate to say that 40°F is twice as warm as 20°F.

In **ratio-level data** there is a defined unit of measure, a real zero point, and the intervals between successive values are equal. A real zero point means there is an absolute zero. Only when a zero on a scale truly means the total absence of a property being assessed can that scale be described as ratio-level. For example, consider the variable length of stay. **Length of stay (LOS)** has a defined unit of measurement, day, and a real zero point—0 days. Because there is a real zero point, we can state that an LOS of six days is twice as long as a LOS of three days. Multiplication on the ratio scale by a constant does not change its ratio character, but addition of a constant to a ratio measure does. For example, if two days is

Table 14.1 Scales of measurement

Scale of measurement	Examples
Nominal	Name, gender, race
Ordinal	Likert scale (a rating scale), anything that is ordered
Interval	Temperature
Ratio	Age, height, length of stay

added to each LOS so that the stays are eight and five days respectively, the ratio of their stays is no longer 2:1. However, if the respective lengths of stay is multiplied by two (for example, 6 × 2 and 3 × 2), the ratio between the two lengths of stay remains 2:1.

This four-fold structure is a useful classification for data and the four levels are hierarchically arranged so that higher levels include the key properties of the levels so that ratio-level data include the three key properties found in nominal-, ordinal-, and interval-level data. Table 14.1 lists the scales of measurement and examples.

Discrete versus Continuous Data

Another way to classify data involves categorizing them as either being discrete or continuous. Data that are nominal or ordinal are also considered discrete. Discrete data are finite numbers; that is, they can have only specified values. The number of children in a family is an example of discrete data. A family can have two or three children but cannot have 2.25 or 3.5 children. The numbers represent actual measurable quantities rather than labels.

Other examples of discrete data include the number of motor vehicle accidents in a particular community, the number of times a woman has given birth, the number of new cases of cancer in a state within the past five years, and the number of beds available in a hospital.

In discrete data, a natural order exists among the possible data values. In the example of the number of times a woman has given birth, a larger number indicates that she has had more children; the difference between one and two births is the

same as the difference between four and five; and the number of births is restricted to whole numbers (a woman cannot give birth 2.3 times). For the most part, measurements on the nominal and ordinal scales are discrete (Horton 2012).

Continuous variables are either interval or ratio-level, but some ratio-level variables are discrete. Continuous data represent measurable quantities but are not restricted to certain specified values. A variable that is continuous can take on a fractional value. For example, a patient's temperature may be 102.6°F. Another example is height. One could say that someone is approximately 6 feet tall, refine it to 5 feet 10 inches, and refine it still further to 5 feet 10.5 inches. Age is yet another example. A person may have been 20 years old on his or her last birthday, but now the person would be 20 plus some part of another year. Arithmetic operations—addition, subtraction, multiplication, and division—may be performed on continuous variables (Horton 2012).

Check Your Understanding 14.1

Instructions: Identify the scale of measurement for each of the following variables and indicate whether each variable is discrete (D) or continuous (C).

1. _____ Zip code

2. _____ Blood pressure

3. _____ Heart failure classification I, II, III, IV

4. _____ Age

5. _____ Ethnicity

6. _____ Marital status

7. _____ Length of stay

8. _____ Discharge disposition (home, SNF, and such)

9. _____ Weight

10. _____ Level of education

11. _____ Race

12. _____ Temperature in degrees Fahrenheit

13. _____ Types of third-party payers

14. _____ Gender

15. _____ Height

Common Statistical Measures Used in Healthcare

Healthcare data are collected to describe the health status of groups or populations. The data reported about healthcare facilities and communities describe the occurrence of illnesses, births, and deaths for specific periods of time. Data that are collected may be either facility based or population based. The sources of facility-based statistics are acute-care facilities, long-term care facilities, and other types of healthcare organizations. The population-based statistics are gathered from cities, counties, states, or specific groups within the population, such as individuals affected by diabetes.

Reporting statistics for a healthcare facility is similar to reporting statistics for a community. Rates for healthcare facilities are reported as per 100 cases or percent; a community rate is reported as per 1,000, 10,000, or 100,000 people. For example, if a hospital experienced 4 deaths in a given month and 100 patients were discharged in the same month, the death rate would be 4 percent ([4 × 100]/100). If there were 400 deaths in a community of 80,000 for a given period of time, the death rate would be reported as 50 deaths per 10,000 population ([400 × 10,000]/80,000) for the same period of time. The following terms are common for the HIM professional to use in determining statistics.

Ratios, Proportions, and Rates: Three Common Examples of Ratio-Level Data

Many healthcare statistics are reported in the form of a ratio, proportion, or rate (discussed in the following sections). A **ratio** is a calculation that compares two quantities found by dividing one quantity by another. A **proportion** is the relation of one part to another or to the whole with respect to magnitude, quantity, or degree. A **rate** is a measure used to compare an event over time.

These measures are used to report morbidity (illness), mortality (death), and natality (birth) at the local, state, and national levels. These measures indicate the number of times something happened relative to the number of times it could have happened. All three measures are based on formula 14.1. In this formula, x and y are the quantities being compared and x is divided by y. Further, 10^n is 10 to the nth power. The size of 10^n may equal 10, 100, 1,000, 10,000, and so on, depending on the value of n:

$$10^0 = 1$$
$$10^1 = 10$$
$$10^2 = 10 \times 10 = 100$$
$$10^3 = 10 \times 10 \times 10 = 1,000$$

Formula 14.1. General formula for calculating rates, proportions, and ratios

$$\text{Ratio, proportion, rate} = x/y \times 10^n$$

Ratios

In a ratio, the two quantities are compared, such as patient discharge status (x = alive, y = dead), may be expressed so that x and y are completely independent of each other, or x may be included in y. For example, the outcome of patients discharged from Community Hospital could be compared in one of two ways:

Alive/dead, or x/y
Alive/(alive + dead), or $x/(x + y)$

In the first example, x is completely independent of y. The ratio represents the number of patients discharged alive compared to the number of patients who died. In the second example, x is part of the whole ($x + y$). The ratio represents the number of patients discharged alive compared to all patients discharged. Both expressions are considered ratios.

Proportions

A proportion is a particular type of ratio in which x is a portion of the whole ($x + y$). In a proportion, the numerator is always included in the denominator. Figure 14.1 describes the procedure for calculating ratios and figure 14.2 describes the procedures for calculating proportions.

Figure 14.1 Calculation of a ratio; discharge status of patients discharged in a month

1. Define x and y:
   x = number of patients discharged alive
   y = number of patients who died
2. Identify x and y:
   $x = 250$
   $y = 20$
3. Set up the ratio x/y:
   250/20
4. Reduce the fraction so that either x or y equals 1:
   12.5/1

There were 12.5 live discharges for every patient who died.

©AHIMA

Rates

Rates are often used to measure events over a period of time. Sometimes they also are used in performance improvement studies. Like ratios and proportions, rates may be reported daily, weekly, monthly, or yearly. This allows for trend analysis and comparisons over time. The basic formula for calculating a rate is shown in formula 14.1.

Healthcare facilities calculate many types of morbidity and mortality rates. For example, the C-section rate is a measure of the proportion, or percentage, of C-sections performed during a given period of time. C-section rates are closely monitored because they present more risk to the mother and baby and because they are more expensive than vaginal deliveries. In calculating the C-section rate, the number of C-sections performed during the specified period of time is counted and this value is placed in the numerator. The number of cases, or the population at risk, is the number of women who delivered during the same time period. This number is placed in the denominator. By convention, inpatient hospital rates are reported as the rate per 100 cases ($10^n = 10^2 = 10 \times 10 = 100$) and are expressed as percentages. The formula for calculating the risk of contracting a disease is shown in formula 14.2.

Formula 14.2. Calculating risk for contracting a disease

$$\text{Risk rate} = \frac{\text{Number of cases occurring during a given time period}}{\text{Total number of cases or population at risk during the same time period}}$$

Figure 14.2 Calculation of a proportion; discharge status of patients discharged in a month

1. Define x and y:
   x = number of patients discharged alive
   y = number of patients who died
2. Identify x and y:
   $x = 250$
   $y = 20$
3. Set up the ratio $x/(x + y)$:
   $250/(250 + 20) = 250/270$
4. Reduce the fraction so that either x or y equals 1:
   $0.93/1$

The proportion of patients discharged alive was 0.93.

©AHIMA

Figure 14.3 Calculation of a rate; C-section rate for June 20XX

During June, 705 women delivered; of these, 45 deliveries were by C-section. What is the C-section rate for June at University Hospital?

1. Define the numerator (number of times an event occurred) and the denominator (number of times an event could have occurred):
   Numerator = total number of C-sections performed during the time period
   Denominator = total number of deliveries, including C-sections, in the same time period
2. Identify the numerator and the denominator:
   Numerator = 45
   Denominator = 705
3. Set up the rate:
   45/705
4. Multiply the numerator by 100 and then divide by the denominator:
   $([45 \times 100]/705) = 6.38\%$

The C-section rate for June is 6.438 percent.

©AHIMA

Figure 14.3 shows the procedure for calculating a rate. In the example, 45 of the 705 deliveries at University Hospital during the month of June were C-sections. In the formula, the numerator is the number of C-sections performed in June (the given period of time) and the denominator is the total number of deliveries including C-sections (the population at risk) performed within the same time frame. In calculating the rate, the numerator is always included in the denominator. Also, when calculating a facility-based rate, the numerator is first multiplied by 100, and then divided by the denominator.

Because hospital rates rarely result in a whole number, they are usually rounded. The hospital should set a policy on whether rates are to be reported to one or two decimal places. The division should be carried out to at least one more decimal place than desired.

When rounding, if the last number is five or greater, the preceding number should be increased one digit. In contrast, if the last number is less than five, the preceding number remains the same. For example, in the example given in figure 14.3, when rounding 6.38 percent to one decimal place, the rate becomes 6.4 percent because the last number is greater than five. When rounding, for example, 2.563 percent to two places, the rate becomes 2.56 percent because the last digit is less than five. Rates of less than 1 percent are usually carried out to three decimal places and rounded to two. For rates less than 1 percent, a zero should precede the decimal to emphasize that the rate is less than 1 percent, for example, 0.56 percent.

Check Your Understanding **14.2**

Instructions: **Identify the following statements as a rate, a ratio, or a proportion.**

1. Medicare admissions outnumber commercial insurance admissions three to two.

2. At the annual state HIM meeting, 85 of the registrants were female and 35 were male. Therefore 0.71 percent of the registrants were female.

3. Of the 250 patients admitted in the last 6 months, 36 percent had Type II diabetes mellitus.

4. In a study of acute myocardial infarction, there were seven males to nine females.

5. In many healthcare insurance policies the insurance company covers 0.80 of the amount.

Acute-Care Statistical Data

In the daily operations of any organization, whether in business, industry, or healthcare, data are collected for decision making. To be effective, the decision makers must have confidence in the data collected. Confidence requires the data collected be accurate, reliable, and timely. The types of data collected in the acute-care setting are discussed in the following sections.

Administrative Statistical Data

Hospitals collect data on both inpatients and outpatients on a daily basis. Hospitals use these statistics to monitor the volume of patients treated daily, weekly, monthly, annually, or within some other specified time frame. The statistics give healthcare decision makers the information needed to plan facilities and services and to monitor inpatient and outpatient revenue streams. For these reasons, the HIM professional must be well versed in data collection, reporting, and analysis methods.

Standard definitions have been developed to ensure that all healthcare providers collect and report data in a consistent manner. The *Pocket Glossary of Health Information Management and Technology* (the most recent edition was published in 2014), developed by the American Health Information Management Association (AHIMA), is a resource commonly used to describe the types of healthcare events for which data are collected. It includes definitions of terms related to healthcare organizations, health maintenance organizations (HMOs), and other health-related programs and facilities and emerging HIM and HIT topics. The following terms and definitions will be used in this chapter:

- **Hospital inpatient:** A patient who is provided with room, board, and continuous general nursing service in an area of an acute-care facility where patients generally stay at least overnight

- **Hospital newborn inpatient:** A patient born in the hospital at the beginning of the current inpatient hospitalization
  - Newborns are usually counted separately because their care is so different from that of other inpatients
  - Infants born on the way to the hospital or at home and later admitted to a hospital are considered hospital inpatients, not hospital newborn inpatients

- **Inpatient hospitalization:** The period during an individual's life when he or she is a patient in a single hospital without interruption except by possible intervening leaves of absence. A leave of absence is the authorized absence of an inpatient from a hospital or other facility for a specified period of time occurring after admission and prior to discharge.

- **Inpatient admission:** An acute-care facility's formal acceptance of a patient who is to be provided with room, board, and continuous nursing service in an area of the facility where patients generally stay at least overnight

- **Inpatient discharge:** The termination of hospitalization through the formal release of an inpatient by the hospital
  - The term includes patients who are discharged alive (by physician's order), who are discharged against medical advice (AMA), or who died while hospitalized
  - Unless otherwise directed by your healthcare facility's administration inpatient discharges include deaths

- **Hospital outpatient:** A hospital patient who receives services in one or more of the hospital's facilities when he or she is not currently an inpatient or home care patient
  - An outpatient may be classified as either an emergency patient or a clinic outpatient

- An emergency patient is admitted to the emergency services department of a hospital for the diagnosis and treatment of a condition that requires immediate medical, dental, or allied health services in order to sustain life or to prevent critical consequences
- A clinic outpatient is a patient who is admitted to a clinical service of a clinic or hospital for diagnosis and treatment on an ambulatory basis (AHIMA 2014)

Inpatient Census Data

It is an ongoing responsibility of the HIM professional to verify the **census** data that are collected daily. The census reports patient activity for a 24-hour reporting period. Included in the census report is the number of inpatients admitted and discharged for the previous 24-hour period as well as the number of intra-hospital transfers. An intra-hospital transfer is a patient who is moved from one patient care unit to another (for example, a patient may be transferred from the intensive care unit [ICU] to the medicine unit). The usual 24-hour reporting period begins at 12:01 a.m. and ends at 12:00 midnight. In the census count, adults and children (A&C) are reported separately from newborns.

Before compiling census data, however, it is important to understand related terminology. The census is the number of hospital inpatients present in a hospital at any given time. For example, the census in a 300-bed hospital may be 250 patients at 2:00 p.m. on June 1, but 245 patients an hour later. Because the census may change throughout the day as admissions and discharges occur, hospitals designate an official census-taking time. In most facilities, the official count takes place at midnight. The census-reporting time can be any other time, but it must be consistent throughout the healthcare facility and occur at the same time each day.

The result of the official count taken at midnight is called the **daily inpatient census**. This is the number of inpatients present at the census-taking time each day plus any patients who were admitted and discharged that same day. For example, if a patient was admitted to the intensive care unit (ICU) at 1:00 p.m. on June 1 and died at 4.00 p.m. on the same day, he would be counted as a patient who was both admitted and discharged the same day. Most facilities have a census-taking policy that outlines the process for census reporting and tracking.

Because patients admitted and discharged the same day may not be present at the census-taking time, hospitals must account for them separately. If it did not, credit for the services provided these patients would be lost. The daily inpatient census reflects the total number of patients treated during the 24-hour period. Figure 14.4 displays a sample daily inpatient census report.

A unit of measure that reflects the services received by one inpatient during a 24-hour period is called an **inpatient service day (IPSD)**. The number of IPSDs for a 24-hour period is equal to the daily inpatient census, that is, one service day for each patient treated. In figure 14.4, the total number of inpatient service days for June 2 is 260.

IPSDs are compiled daily, weekly, monthly, and annually. They reflect the volume of services

Figure 14.4 Daily inpatient census report—A&C

June 2	
Number of patients in hospital at midnight, June 1	250
+ Number of patients admitted June 2	+40
– Number of patients discharged, including deaths, June 2	–35
Number of patients in hospital at midnight, June 2	255
+ Number of patients both admitted and discharged, including deaths	+5
Daily inpatient census at midnight, June 2	260
Total inpatient service days, June 2	260

©AHIMA

Table 14.2 Number of IPSDs

Day	Census	Same day admissions and discharges	Inpatient service days
Day 1	250	0	250
Day 2	255	0	255
Day 3	240	2	242
Total			**747**

Formula 14.4. Calculating the average daily census for adults and children

$$\text{Average daily census for A\&C} = \frac{\text{Total number of inpatient service days for A\&C for a given period}}{\text{Total number of days in the same period}}$$

provided by the healthcare facility—the greater the volume of services, the greater the revenues to the facility. Daily reporting of the number of IPSDs is an indicator of the healthcare facility's financial condition.

As mentioned, the daily inpatient census is equal to the number of IPSDs provided for that day as shown in table 14.2.

The total number of IPSDs for a week, a month, and so on can be divided by the total number of days in the period of interest to obtain the **average daily census.** In the previous example, 747 IPSDs is divided by three days to obtain an average daily census of 249. The average daily census is the average number of inpatients treated during a given period of time. The general formula for calculating the average daily census is shown in formula 14.3.

In calculating the average daily census, A&C and **newborns (NB)** are reported separately. This is because the intensity of services provided to adults and children is greater than it is for newborns. To calculate the A&C average daily census, the general formula is modified as shown in formula 14.4. Many facilities use a whole number when reporting the census.

The formula for calculating the average daily census for newborns is shown in formula 14.5. For example, the total number of IPSDs provided to adults and children for the week of June 1 is 1,825, and the total for newborns is 125. Using the formulas, the average daily census for adults and children is 261 (1,825/7) and for newborns it is 18 (125/7). Notice that the answer to the newborn average daily census was 17.9, but using the standard practice of reporting census information as a whole number, the figure reported would be 18. The average daily census for all hospital inpatients for the week of June 1 is 278.6 or 279 ([1,825 + 125]/7). Table 14.3 compares the various formulas for calculating the average daily census.

Formula 14.5. Calculating the average daily census for newborns

$$\text{Average daily census for NBs} = \frac{\text{Total number of inpatient service days for NBs for a given period}}{\text{Total number of days in the same period}}$$

Table 14.3 Calculation of census statistics

Indicator	Numerator	Denominator
Average daily inpatient census	Total number of inpatient service days for a given period	Total number of days for the same period
Average daily inpatient census for adults and children (A&C)	Total number of inpatient service days for A&C for a given period	Total number of days for the same period
Average daily inpatient census for newborns (NBs)	Total number of inpatient service days for NBs for a given period	Total number of days for the same period

Formula 14.3. Calculating the average daily census

$$\text{Average daily census} = \frac{\text{Total number of inpatient service days for a given period}}{\text{Total number of days in the same period}}$$

Check Your Understanding **14.3**

Instructions: **Answer the following questions.**

1. Community Hospital reported the following statistics for adults and children at 12:01 a.m. April 1: Census 160; Admissions 20; Discharges 15; 1 patient admitted and died the same day; 1 patient admitted and discharged alive the same day. Calculate the following for April 2:
   A. Inpatient census
   B. Daily inpatient census
   C. Inpatient service days

2. Community Hospital reported the following statistics for their newborn unit at 12:01 a.m. June 1: Census 10; Births 5; Discharges 3; 1 Newborn born and transferred to University Hospital. Calculate the following for June 2:
   A. Inpatient census
   B. Daily inpatient census

3. Community Hospital reported the following statistics for their intensive care unit at 12:01 a.m. June 1: Census 12; 1 patient admitted directly from the Emergency Services Department (ESD); 1 patient transferred from surgery unit; 1 patient transferred from the medicine unit; 1 patient transferred to the medicine unit; 1 patient admitted and died the same day. Calculate the following for June 2:
   A. Inpatient census
   B. Daily inpatient census

Inpatient Bed Occupancy Rate

Another indicator of the hospital's financial position is the **inpatient bed occupancy rate**, also called the percentage of occupancy. The inpatient bed occupancy rate is the percentage of official beds occupied by hospital inpatients for a given period of time. In general, the greater the occupancy rate, the greater the revenues for the hospital. For a bed to be included in the official count, it must be set up, staffed, equipped, and available for patient care. The total number of inpatient service days is used in the numerator because it is equal to the daily inpatient census or the number of patients treated daily. The occupancy rate compares the number of patients treated over a given period of time to the total number of beds available for the same period of time.

For example, if 250 patients occupied 300 beds on June 2, the inpatient bed occupancy rate would be 83.3 percent ([250/{300 × 1}] × 100). If the rate were for more than one day, the number of beds would be multiplied by the number of days within that particular time frame. For example, if 1,830 IPSDs were provided during the week of June 1 in the same hospital, the inpatient bed occupancy rate for that week would be 87.1 percent ([1,830/{300 × 7}] × 100).

The denominator in this formula is actually the total possible number of inpatient service days. That is, if every available bed in the hospital were occupied every single day, this would be the maximum number of IPSDs that could be provided. This is an important concept, especially if the official **bed count** changes for a given reporting period. For example, if the bed count changed from 300 beds to 310, the bed occupancy rate would reflect the change. The total number of inpatient beds times the total number of days in the period is called the total number of **bed count days**. The general formula for the inpatient bed occupancy rate is shown in formula 14.6.

Formula 14.6. Calculating the inpatient bed occupancy rate

$$\text{Inpatient bed occupancy rate} = \frac{\text{Total number of inpatient service days for a given period}}{\text{Total number of inpatient bed count days for the same period}} \times 100$$

What happens when the bed count changes? For example, the bed count changed on June 20 from 300 beds to 310 beds and the total number of inpatient service days provided was 8,327. To calculate the inpatient bed occupancy rate for

June, the total number of bed count days must be determined. There are 30 days in June; therefore, the total number of bed count days is calculated as:

Number of beds, June 1-June 19 = 300 × 19 days

= 5,700 bed count days

Number of beds, June 20-June 30 = 310 × 11 days

= 3,410 bed count days

5,700 + 3,410 = 9,110 bed count days

The inpatient bed occupancy rate for the month of June is 91.4 percent ([8,327/9,110] × 100).

As with the average daily census, the inpatient bed occupancy rate for adults and children is reported separately from that of newborns. To calculate the total number of bed count days for newborns, the official count for newborn bassinets is used. Table 14.4 reviews the formulas for calculating inpatient bed occupancy rates.

It is possible for the inpatient bed occupancy rate to be greater than 100 percent. This occurs when the hospital faces an epidemic or disaster. In this type of situation, hospitals set up temporary beds that usually are not included in the official bed count. As an example, Community Hospital experienced an excessive number of admissions in December because of an outbreak of pneumonia. In December, the official bed count was 125 beds. On December 5, the daily inpatient census was 135. Therefore, the inpatient bed occupancy rate for December 5 was 108 percent ([135/125] × 100).

Table 14.4   Calculation of inpatient bed occupancy rates

Rate	Numerator	Denominator
Inpatient bed occupancy rate	Total number of inpatient service days for a given period × 100	Total number of inpatient bed count days for the same period
Inpatient bed occupancy rate for adults and children (A&C)	Total number of inpatient service days for A&C for a given period × 100	Total number of inpatient bed count days for A&C for the same period
Newborn (NB) bed occupancy rate	Total number of NB inpatient service days for a given period × 100	Total number of bassinet bed count days for the same period

Bed Turnover Rate

The **bed turnover rate** is a measure of hospital utilization. It includes the number of times each hospital bed changed occupants. The formula for the bed turnover rate is shown in formula 14.7. For example, Community Hospital had 2,120 discharges and deaths for the month of October. Its bed count for October averaged 700. The bed turnover rate is 3.1 (2,120/700). This simply means that on average, each hospital bed had three occupants during October.

Formula 14.7. Calculating the bed turnover rate

$$\text{Bed turnover rate} = \frac{\text{Total number of discharges, including deaths, for a given period}}{\text{Average bed count for the same time period}}$$

Check Your Understanding 14.4

Instructions: **Answer the following questions.**

1. Fill in table 14.5 with the inpatient bed occupancy rate for each of the following patient care units at Community Hospital for the month of September. (Calculate to one decimal point.)

Table 14.5   Community Hospital occupancy rate for September

Inpatient unit	Service days	Bed count	Occupancy rate
Medicine	680	38	
Surgery	790	37	
Pediatric	235	20	
Psychiatry	927	40	
Obstetrics	252	12	
Newborn	252	16	

2. Use the preceding information to determine the inpatient bed occupancy rate for Community Hospital—all A&C (exclude newborns). Calculate to one decimal point.

3. On July 1, Community Hospital expanded the number of patient beds from 165 to 200. Use the following information in table 14.6 to determine the inpatient bed occupancy rate for January to June; July to December; and the total for the year (non-leap year).

Table 14.6 Community Hospital number of service days and bed count

Months	Service days	Bed count
January–June	25,720	165
July–December	27,852	200

Length of Stay Data

LOS data is calculated for each patient after he or she is discharged from the hospital. It is the number of calendar days from the day of patient admission to the day of patient discharge. When the patient is admitted and discharged in the same month, the LOS is determined by subtracting the date of admission from the date of discharge. For example, the LOS for a patient admitted on June 12 and discharged on June 17 is five days (17 − 12 = 5)

When the patient is admitted in one month and discharged in another, the calculations must be adjusted. One way to calculate the LOS in this case is to subtract the date of admission from the total number of days in the month the patient was admitted and then add the total number of hospitalized days for the month in which the patient was discharged. For example, the LOS for a patient admitted on June 28 and discharged on July 6 is eight days ([June 30–June 28 = 2 days] and [July 1–July 6 = 6 days]; LOS = 8 days).

When a patient is admitted and discharged on the same day, the LOS is one day. A partial day's stay is never reported as a fraction of a day. The LOS for a patient discharged the day after admission also is one day. Thus, the LOS for a patient who was admitted to the ICU on June 10 at 9:00 a.m. and died at 3:00 p.m. on the same day is one day. Likewise, the LOS for a patient admitted on June 12 and discharged on June 13 is one day.

When the LOS for all patients discharged for a given period of time is summed, the result is the **total length of stay (discharge days)**. As an example, five patients were discharged from the pediatric unit on June 9. The LOS for each patient was as follows in table 14.7.

In the preceding example, the total LOS is 32 days (3 + 7 + 2 + 1 + 19). The total LOS is also referred to as the number of days of care provided to patients who were discharged or died (discharge days) during a given period of time.

The **average length of stay (ALOS)** is calculated from the total LOS. The total LOS divided by the number of patients discharged is the ALOS. Using the data in the preceding example, the ALOS for the five patients discharged from the pediatric unit on June 9 is 6.4 days (32/5)

The general formula for calculating ALOS is shown in formula 14.8. As with the measures already discussed, the ALOS for adults and children is reported separately from the ALOS for newborns. Table 14.8 reviews the formulas for ALOS. Table 14.9 displays an example of a hospital statistical summary prepared by the HIM department using census and discharge data.

Formula 14.8. Calculating the average length of stay

$$\text{Average length of stay} = \frac{\text{Total length of stay for a given period}}{\text{Total number of discharges, including deaths, for the same period}}$$

Table 14.7 Length of stay for five patients discharged June 9

Patient	LOS
1	3
2	7
3	2
4	1
5	19
Total	**32**

Table **14.8** Calculation of LOS statistics

Indicator	Numerator	Denominator
Average LOS	Total length of stay (discharge days) for a given period	Total number of discharges, including deaths, for the same period
Average LOS for adults and children (A&C)	Total length of stay for A&C (discharge days) for a given period	Total number of discharges, including deaths, for A&C for the same period
Average LOS for newborns (NB)	Total length of stay for all NB (discharge days) for a given period	Total number of NB discharges, including deaths, for the same period

Table **14.9** Statistical summary, Community Hospital, for the period ending July 20XX

	July 20XX		Year-to-Date 20XX	
Admissions	Actual	Budget	Actual	Budget
Medicine	728	769	5,075	5,082
Surgery	578	583	3,964	3,964
OB/GYN	402	440	2,839	3,027
Psychiatry	113	99	818	711
Physical medicine and rehab	48	57	380	384
Other adult	191	178	1,209	1,212
Total adult	2,060	2,126	14,285	14,380
Newborn	294	312	2,143	2,195
Total admissions	**2,354**	**2,438**	**16,428**	**16,575**
Average length of stay	Actual	Budget	Actual	Budget
Medical	6.1	6.4	6.0	6.1
Surgical	7.0	7.2	7.7	7.7
OB/GYN	2.9	3.2	3.5	3.1
Psychiatry	10.8	11.6	10.4	11.6
Physical medicine and rehab	27.5	23.0	28.1	24.3
Other adult	3.6	3.9	4.0	4.1
Total adult	6.3	6.4	6.7	6.5
Newborn	5.6	5.0	5.6	5.0
Total ALOS	**6.2**	**6.3**	**6.5**	**6.3**
Patient Days	Actual	Budget	Actual	Budget
Medical	4,436	4,915	30,654	30,762
Surgical	4,036	4,215	30,381	30,331
OB/GYN	1,170	1,417	10,051	9,442
Psychiatry	1,223	1,144	8,524	8,242
Physical medicine and rehab	1,318	1,310	10,672	9,338
Other adult	688	699	4,858	4,921
Total adult	12,871	13,700	95,140	93,036
Newborn	1,633	1,552	12,015	10,963
Total patient days	**14,504**	**15,252**	**107,155**	**103,999**
Other key statistics	Actual	Budget	Actual	Budget
Average daily census	485	482	498	486
Average beds available	677	660	677	660
Clinic visits	21,621	18,975	144,271	136,513
Emergency visits	3,822	3,688	26,262	25,604
Inpatient surgery patients	657	583	4,546	4,093
Outpatient surgery patients	603	554	4,457	3,987

Check Your Understanding 14.5

Instructions: Using the data provided for patient discharges in table 14.10, answer the following questions. Calculate to two decimal points.

Table 14.10   Patient discharges

Day	Number of patients discharged	Discharge days
September 1	10	82
September 2	12	75
September 3	17	68
September 4	8	153
September 5	9	43
September 6	11	101
September 7	18	77
September 8	12	93
September 9	13	42
September 10	15	97

1. Total length of stay.

2. Number of patients discharged.

3. Average length of stay.

4. What is the ALOS for September 10th?

5. What is the ALOS for September 1st to (and including) September 5th?

Patient Care and Clinical Statistical Data

Thus far, this chapter discussed statistical measures that are indicators of volume of services and utilization of services. The collection of data related to morbidity and mortality is also an important aspect of evaluating the quality of hospital services. Morbidity and mortality rates are reported for all patient discharges within a certain time frame. They also may be reported by service or by physician or other variable of interest in order to identify trends, issues, or opportunities for improvement that may require corrective action. The most frequently collected morbidity and mortality rates are presented in this section.

Hospital Death (Mortality) Rates

The **hospital death rate** is based on the number of patients discharged, alive and dead, from the hospital. Deaths are considered discharges because they are the end point of a period of hospitalization. In contrast to the rates discussed in the preceding section, newborns are not counted separately from adults and children. The following sections will discuss the different statistics for death including gross, net, newborn, fetal, maternal death rates.

Gross Death Rate

The **gross death rate** is the proportion of all hospital discharges that ended in death. It is the basic indicator of mortality in a healthcare facility. The gross death rate is calculated by dividing the total number of deaths occurring in a given time period by the total number of discharges, including deaths, for the same time period. The formula for calculating the gross death rate is shown in formula 14.9.

Formula 14.9. Calculating the gross death rate

$$\text{Gross death rate} = \frac{\text{Total number of inpatient deaths, including NBs, for a given period}}{\text{Total number of discharges, including A\&C and NB deaths, for the same period}}$$

As an example, Community Hospital experienced 15 deaths (A&C and NBs) during the month of June. There were 278 total discharges, including deaths. The gross death rate is 5.4 percent ([15/278] × 100).

Net Death Rate

The net death rate is an adjusted death rate. It is calculated with the assumption that certain deaths should not count against the hospital. The net death rate is an adjusted rate because it does not include patients who die within 48 hours of admission. The reason for excluding these deaths is that historically it has been believed that 48 hours is not enough time to positively affect patient outcome. In other words, the patient was not admitted to the hospital in a manner timely enough for treatment to have an effect on his or her outcome. The formula for calculating the net death rate is shown in formula 14.10.

Formula 14.10. Calculating the net death rate

$$\text{Net death rate} = \frac{\text{Total number of inpatient deaths, including NBs, minus deaths} <48 \text{ hours for a given period}}{\text{Total number of discharges, including A\&C and NB deaths, minus deaths} <48 \text{ hours for the same period}} \times 100$$

Continuing with the preceding example of the 15 patients who died at Community Hospital in June, three died within 48 hours of admission. Therefore, the net death rate is 4.4 percent ([{15 − 3}/{278 − 3}] × 100). The fact that the net death rate is less than the gross death rate is favorable to Community Hospital because lower death rates may be an indicator of better care.

Newborn Death Rate

Even though newborn deaths are included in the hospital's gross and net death rates, the newborn death rate is often calculated separately. Newborns include only infants born alive in the hospital. The newborn death rate is the number of newborns who died in comparison to the total number of newborns discharged, alive and dead. To qualify as a newborn death, the newborn must have been delivered alive. A stillborn infant is not included in either the newborn death rate or the gross or net death rate. The formula for calculating the newborn death rate is shown in formula 14.11.

Formula 14.11. Calculating the newborn death rate

$$\text{Newborn death rate} = \frac{\text{Total number of NB deaths deaths for a given period}}{\text{Total number of NB discharges, including deaths, for the same period}} \times 100$$

For example, Community Hospital experienced three newborn deaths during the month of June. There were 47 newborn discharges (including these three deaths). The newborn death rate is 6.4 percent ([3/47] × 100)

Fetal Death Rate

In healthcare terminology, the death of a stillborn baby is called a fetal death. A fetal death is the death of a product of human conception before its complete expulsion or extraction from the mother in a hospital facility, regardless of the duration of the pregnancy. Thus, fetal deaths are neither admitted nor discharged from the hospital. A fetal death occurs when the fetus fails to breathe or show any other evidence of life, such as a heartbeat, a

Table 14.11 Classifications of fetal death

Classification	Length of gestation	Weight
Early fetal death	Less than 20 weeks	500 g or less
Intermediate fetal death	20 weeks completed, but less than 28 weeks	501 to 1,000 g
Late fetal death	28 weeks completed	Over 1,000 g

pulsation of the umbilical cord, or a movement of the voluntary muscles.

Fetal deaths also are classified into categories based on length of gestation or weight. (See table 14.11.) To calculate the **fetal death rate**, divide the total number of intermediate and late fetal deaths for the period by the total number of live births and intermediate and late fetal deaths for the same period. The formula for calculating the fetal death rate is shown in formula 14.12. For example, during the month of June, Community Hospital experienced 97 live births and 3 intermediate and 2 late fetal deaths. The fetal death rate is 4.9 percent ([{3 + 2}/{97 + 3 + 2}] × 100).

Formula 14.12. Calculating the fetal death rate

$$\text{Fetal death rate} = \frac{\text{Total number of intermediate and late fetal deaths for a given period}}{\text{Total number of live births plus total number of intermediate and late fetal deaths for the same period}} \times 100$$

Maternal Death Rate

Hospitals are also interested in calculating their **maternal death rates** (hospital based). A maternal death is the death of any woman from any cause related to, or aggravated by, pregnancy or its management, regardless of the duration or site of the pregnancy. Maternal deaths that result from accidental or incidental causes are not included in the maternal death rate.

Maternal deaths are classified as either direct or indirect. A direct maternal death is the death of a woman resulting from obstetrical (OB) complications of the pregnancy, labor, or puerperium (the period including the six weeks after delivery). Direct maternal deaths are included in the maternal death rate. An indirect maternal death is the death

of a woman from a previously existing disease or a disease that developed during pregnancy, labor, or the puerperium that was not due to obstetric causes, although the physiological effects of pregnancy were partially responsible.

The maternal death rate may be an indicator of the availability of prenatal care in a community. The hospital also may use it to help identify conditions that could lead to a maternal death. The formula for calculating the maternal death rate is shown in formula 14.13. For example, during the month of June, Community Hospital experienced 150 maternal discharges. Two of these patients died. The maternal death rate for May is 1.33 percent ([2/150] × 100). Table 14.12 summarizes hospital-based mortality rates.

Formula 14.13. Calculating the maternal death rate

$$\text{Maternal death rate} = \frac{\text{Total number of direct maternal deaths for a given period}}{\text{Total number of maternal (OB) discharges, including deaths, for the same period}} \times 100$$

Table 14.12 Calculation of hospital-based mortality rates

Rate	Numerator (x)	Denominator (y)
Gross death rate	Total number of inpatient deaths, including NBs, for a given period × 100	Total number of discharges, including A&C and NB deaths, for the same period
Net death rate (institutional death rate)	Total number of inpatient deaths, including NBs, minus deaths <48 hours for a given period × 100	Total number of discharges, including A&C and NB deaths, minus deaths <48 hours for the same period
Newborn death rate	Total number of NB deaths for a given period × 100	Total number of NB discharges, including deaths, for the same period
Fetal death rate	Total number of intermediate and late fetal deaths for a given period × 100	Total number of live births plus total number of intermediate and late fetal deaths for the same period
Maternal death rate	Total number of direct maternal deaths for a given period × 100	Total number of maternal (obstetric) discharges, including deaths, for the same period
Infant death rate	Number of deaths under one year of age during a given time period	Number of live births during the same time period

Check Your Understanding 14.6

Instructions: Using the data provided on deaths and discharges at Community Hospital for the past calendar year in table 14.13, answer the following questions. Calculate to two decimal points.

Table 14.13   Community Hospital death and discharge data

Type of death or discharge	Total
Total discharges, including deaths (A&C)	2,703
Total deaths (A&C)	43
Deaths less than 48 hours after admission (A&C)	2
Fetal deaths (intermediate and late)	5
Live births	175
Newborn deaths	1
Newborn discharges, including deaths	175
Maternal deaths (direct)	1
OB discharges, including deaths	175

1. _____ What is the gross death rate for adults and children?

2. _____ What is the net death rate for adults and children?

3. _____ What is the newborn death rate?

4. _____ What is the fetal death rate?

5. _____ What is the gross death rate for adults and children and newborns combined?

6. _____ What is the maternal death rate (direct)?

7. _____ What is the net death rate for adults and children and newborns combined?

Autopsy Rates

An autopsy is the postmortem (after death) examination of the organs and tissues of a body to determine the cause of death or pathological conditions; also known as a postmortem examination or necropsy examination. Autopsies are a powerful tool in medical education and research. In addition, the autopsy can alert family members to conditions or diseases for which they may be at risk.

Two categories of hospital autopsies are conducted in acute-care facilities: hospital inpatient autopsies and hospital autopsies. A **hospital inpatient autopsy** is an examination performed on the body of a patient who died during an inpatient hospitalization by a hospital pathologist or a physician of the medical staff who has been delegated the responsibility.

A **hospital autopsy** is a postmortem examination on the body of a person who at some time in the past had been a hospital patient but was not a hospital inpatient at the time of death. A pathologist or some other physician on the medical staff performs this type of autopsy as well. The following sections describe the different types of autopsy rates calculated by acute-care hospitals.

Gross Autopsy Rates

A **gross autopsy rate** is the proportion or percentage of deaths that are followed by the performance of autopsy (see formula 14.14). For example, during the month of June, Community Hospital experienced 19 deaths. Autopsies were performed on three of these patients. The gross autopsy rate is 15.8 percent ($[3/19] \times 100$).

Formula 14.14. Calculating the gross autopsy rate

$$\text{Gross autopsy rate} = \frac{\text{Total inpatient autopsies for a given period}}{\text{Total number of inpatient deaths for the same period}} \times 100$$

Net Autopsy Rates

The bodies of patients who have died are not always available for autopsy. For example, a coroner or medical examiner may claim a body for an autopsy for legal reasons. A **coroner** is the official (elected or appointed, physician or nonphysician) who is responsible for determining the cause, time, and manner of death in unattended, violent, or unexplained deaths, or a case where a law may have been broken. Coroners may also have other duties depending on their state.

In some areas of the country, the coroner has been replaced with a **medical examiner (ME)**. The medical examiner is usually an appointed official who is a physician, commonly holding a specialty in pathology or forensic medicine. Large metropolitan areas usually have a forensic pathologist who acts as the coroner and performs the postmortem examination. In smaller areas, the coroner may be a physician practicing in the community who is not trained as a pathologist. It may also be a mortician or sheriff who is also serving as the coroner (Horton 2012).

The hospital calculates a **net autopsy rate**. In calculating the net autopsy rate, bodies that have been removed by the coroner or medical examiner are excluded from the denominator because they were not available for an autopsy. The formula for calculating the net autopsy rate is shown in formula 14.15. Continuing with the example in the preceding section, the medical examiner claimed three of the patients for autopsy. The numerator remains the same because three autopsies were performed by the hospital pathologist. However, because three of the deaths were identified as medical examiner's cases and removed from the

hospital, 3 is subtracted from 19. The net autopsy rate is 18.8 percent ($[3/\{19-3\}] \times 100$).

Formula 14.15. Calculating the net autopsy rate

$$\text{Net autopsy rate} = \frac{\text{Total inpatient autopsies on inpatient deaths for a given period}}{\text{Total number of inpatient deaths minus unautopsied coroners' or medical examiners' cases for the same period}} \times 100$$

Hospital Autopsy Rates

A third type of autopsy rate is called the **hospital autopsy rate**. This is an adjusted rate that includes autopsies on anyone who may have at one time been a hospital patient. The formula for calculating the hospital autopsy rate is shown in formula 14.16. The hospital autopsy rate includes autopsies performed on any of the following:

- Bodies of inpatients, except those removed by the coroner or medical examiner. When the hospital pathologist or other designated physician acts as an agent in the performance of an autopsy on an inpatient, the death and the autopsy are included in the percentage.
- Bodies of other hospital patients, including ambulatory care patients, hospital home care patients, and former hospital patients who died elsewhere, but whose bodies have been made available for autopsy to be performed by the hospital pathologist or other designated physician. These autopsies and deaths are included in computations of the percentage.

Formula 14.16. Calculating the hospital autopsy rate

$$\text{Hospital autopsy rate} = \frac{\text{Total number of hospital autopsies for the period}}{\text{Total number of deaths of hospital patients with bodies available for hospital autopsy for the period}} \times 100$$

Generally, it is difficult to determine the number of bodies of former hospital patients who may have died in a given time period. In the formula, the phrase available for hospital autopsy involves several conditions, including:

- The autopsy must be performed by the hospital pathologist or a physician who treated the patient at some time at the hospital.
- The report of the autopsy must be filed in the patient's health record and in the hospital laboratory or pathology department.
- The tissue specimens must be maintained in the hospital laboratory.

Figure 14.5 explains how to calculate the hospital autopsy rate.

Newborn Autopsy Rates

Autopsy rates usually include autopsies performed on newborn infants unless a separate rate is requested. The formula for calculating the **newborn autopsy rate** is shown in formula 14.17.

For example, three newborn deaths occurred at Community Hospital in June, one of the deaths was autopsied. This represents 33.3 percent ($[1/3] \times 100$).

Formula 14.17. Calculating the newborn autopsy rate

$$\text{Newborn autopsy rate} = \frac{\text{Total number of autopsies on NB deaths for a given period of time}}{\text{Total number of NB deaths for the same period}} \times 100$$

Figure 14.5 Calculation of hospital autopsy rate

In June, 19 inpatient deaths occurred at Community Hospital. Three of these were medical examiner's cases. Two of the bodies were removed from the hospital and so were not available for hospital autopsy. One of the medical examiner's cases was autopsied by the hospital pathologist. Three other autopsies were performed on hospital inpatients that died during the month of June. In addition, autopsies were performed in the hospital on:

- A child with congenital heart disease who died in the emergency department
- A former hospital inpatient who died in an extended care facility and whose body was brought to the hospital for autopsy
- A former hospital inpatient who died at home and whose body was brought to the hospital for autopsy
- A hospital outpatient who died while receiving chemotherapy for cancer
- A hospital home care patient whose body was brought to the hospital for autopsy
- A former hospital inpatient who died in an emergency vehicle on the way to the hospital

Calculation of total hospital autopsies:

```
 1 autopsy on medical examiner's case
+3 autopsies on hospital inpatients
+6 autopsies on hospital patients whose bodies were available for autopsy
10 autopsies performed by the hospital pathologist
```

Calculation of number of deaths of hospital patients whose bodies were available for autopsy:

```
19 inpatient deaths
−2 medical examiner's cases
+6 deaths of hospital patients
23 bodies available for autopsy
```

Calculation of hospital autopsy rate:

$$\text{Hospital autopsy rate} = \frac{\text{Total number of hospital autopsies for the period}}{\text{Total number of deaths of hospital patients with bodies available for hospital autopsy for the period}} \times 100$$

$(10 \times 100)/23 = 43.5\%$

Table 14.14   Calculation of hospital autopsy rates

Rate	Numerator	Denominator
Gross autopsy rate	Total number of autopsies on inpatient deaths for a given period × 100	Total number of inpatient deaths for the same period
Net autopsy rate	Total number of autopsies on inpatient deaths for a given period × 100	Total number of inpatient deaths minus unautopsied coroner or medical examiner cases for the same period
Hospital autopsy rate	Total number of hospital autopsies for a given period × 100	Total number of deaths of hospital patients whose bodies are available for hospital autopsy for the same period
Newborn (NB) autopsy rate	Total number of autopsies on NB deaths for a given period × 100	Total number of NB deaths for the same period
Fetal autopsy rate	Total number of autopsies on intermediate and late fetal deaths for a given period × 100	Total number of intermediate and late fetal deaths for the same period

Fetal Autopsy Rates

Hospitals sometimes also calculate the **fetal autopsy rate**. Fetal autopsies are important for the clinician to determine the cause of the fetal loss and to the parents to determine if they need genetic counseling or other types of prenatal care in the future. Fetal autopsies are performed on stillborn infants who have been classified as either intermediate or late fetal deaths (see table 14.11). This is the proportion or percentage of autopsies performed on intermediate or late fetal deaths out of the total number of intermediate or late fetal deaths. The formula for calculating the fetal autopsy rate is shown in formula 14.18.

Formula 14.18. Calculating the fetal autopsy rate

$$\text{Fetal autopsy rate} = \frac{\text{Total number of autopsies on intermediate and late fetal deaths for a given period of time}}{\text{Total number of intermediate and late fetal deaths for the same period}} \times 100$$

In a previous example there were five intermediate and late fetal deaths at Community Hospital during a year. Three of those deaths were autopsied. The fetal autopsy rate is 60.0 percent ([3/5] × 100).

Table 14.14 summarizes the different hospital autopsy rates.

✓ Check Your Understanding 14.7

Instructions: Read the following scenario and use the table below to answer the questions. Calculate to one decimal point.

Community Hospital January through June	Total
Number of inpatient deaths (all deaths)	35
Hospital inpatient autopsies (all autopsies)	9
Coroner's cases	2
Former patient brought to hospital for autopsy	1
Newborn deaths	5
Newborn autopsies	1
Fetal deaths (intermediate and late)	12
Fetal autopsies	1

1. What is the gross autopsy rate for this month?
2. What is the net autopsy rate for this month?
3. What is the hospital autopsy rate?
4. What is the newborn autopsy rate?
5. What is the fetal autopsy rate?

Healthcare-Associated Infection Rates

The most common morbidity rates calculated for hospitals are related to hospital-acquired infections, called **nosocomial (hospital-acquired) infections**. Morbidity refers to the state of being ill. The hospital must continuously monitor the number of infections that occur in its various patient care units because infection can adversely affect the course of a patient's treatment and possibly result in death. The Joint Commission requires hospitals to follow written guidelines for reporting all types of infections. Examples of the different types of infections are respiratory, gastrointestinal, surgical wound, skin, urinary tract, septicemias, and infections related to intravascular catheters.

Healthcare-Associated Infection Rates

Hospital-acquired (nosocomial) infection rates, now referred to as healthcare-associated infections or HAIs by the CDC, may be calculated for the entire hospital or for a specific unit in the hospital. They also may be calculated for the specific types of infections. Ideally, the hospital should strive for an infection rate of zero. The formula for calculating the hospital-acquired or nosocomial infection rate is shown in formula 14.19. For example, Community Hospital discharged 226 patients during the month of June. Thirteen of these patients experienced hospital-acquired infections. The hospital-acquired infection rate is 5.8 percent ([13/226] × 100). If, of those 13 patients who had infections, there were eight who had a catheter-associated urinary tract infections (CAUTI) the rate would be 61.5 percent ([8/13] × 100). This information would be extremely important to the Infection Control Committee because if they could control CAUTIs, then more than half of their infections would be eliminated.

> **Formula 14.19. Calculating the nosocomial infection rate**
>
> $$\text{Hospital-acquired infection rate} = \frac{\text{Total number of hospital-acquired infections for a given period of time}}{\text{Total number of discharges, including deaths, for the same period}} \times 100$$

Many healthcare facilities report their infection rates to the CDC. The CDC is primarily interested in central line-associated bloodstream infection (CLABSI), catheter-associated urinary tract infection (CAUTI), surgical site infection (SSI), and ventilator-associated pneumonia. These rates are reported as indicators of unsafe practices such as failure to wash hands and other means to reduce infections.

Postoperative Infection Rates

Hospitals often track their **postoperative infection rate**. The postoperative infection rate is the proportion or percentage of infections in clean surgical cases out of the total number of surgical operations performed. A clean surgical case is one in which no infection existed prior to surgery. The postoperative infection rate may be an indicator of a problem in the hospital environment or of some type of surgical contamination.

Two terms must be considered here—*surgical procedure* and *surgical operation*. A **surgical procedure** is any single, separate, systematic process upon or within the body that can be complete in itself. It is normally performed by a physician, dentist, or some other licensed practitioner with or without instruments, to:

- Restore disunited or deficient parts
- Remove diseased or injured tissues
- Extract foreign matter
- Assist in obstetrical delivery
- Aid in diagnosis

A **surgical operation** involves one or more surgical procedures that are performed at one time for one patient by way of a common approach or for a common purpose. An example of a surgical operation is the resection of a portion of both the intestine and the liver in a cancer patient. This involves two procedures, removal of a portion of the liver and removal of a portion of the colon; but it is considered only one operation because there is only one operative approach or incision. In contrast, an esophagogastroduodenoscopy (EGD) and a colonoscopy performed at the same time are two procedures with two different approaches. In the former, the approach is the upper gastrointestinal tract; in the latter, the approach is the lower gastrointestinal tract. In this case, the two procedures do not have a common approach or purpose. The formula for calculating the postoperative infection rate is shown in formula 14.20. For example, Community Hospital reported that 258 surgical operations were performed during the month of June. There were two postoperative infections in clean surgical cases. The postoperative infection rate is 0.78 percent ([2/258] x 100).

Formula 14.20. Calculating the postoperative infection rate

$$\text{Postoperative infection rate} = \frac{\begin{array}{c}\text{Number of infections}\\\text{in clean surgical cases}\\\text{for a given period}\\\text{of time}\end{array}}{\begin{array}{c}\text{Total number of}\\\text{surgical operations for}\\\text{the same period}\end{array}} \times 100$$

Consultation Rates

A consultation is the response by one healthcare professional to another healthcare professional's request to provide recommendations or opinions regarding the care of a particular patient or resident. The attending physician requests the consultation and explains his or her reason for doing so. The consultant then examines the patient and the patient's health record and makes recommendations in a written report. Higher consultant rates for a given specialty indicates the need to acquire the services of such a physician in the community or at the hospital. The formula for calculating the consultation rate is shown in formula 14.21.

During June, Community Hospital had 226 discharges and deaths. Fifty-seven patients received consultations. The consultation rate for June is 25.2 percent ([57/226] × 100).

Formula 14.21. Calculating the consultation rate

$$\text{Consultation rate} = \frac{\begin{array}{c}\text{Total number of patients}\\\text{receiving consultations for}\\\text{a given period of time}\end{array}}{\begin{array}{c}\text{Total number of}\\\text{discharges and deaths}\\\text{for the same period}\end{array}} \times 100$$

Check Your Understanding 14.8

Instructions: **Answer the following questions. Calculate all answers to one decimal point.**

1. During the month of September, Community Hospital discharged 278 patients. Twelve of those patients were seen by a consultant. Six patients had an infection acquired in the hospital.
   A. What is the consultation rate?
   B. What is the healthcare-associated infection rate?

2. Using the following information, answer the following questions.

Community Hospital surgery service
Number of surgical discharges: 203
Number of clean surgical operations: 205
Number of patients operated: 203
Number of postoperative infections: 15
Number of consultations in the surgery service: 3

   A. What is the postoperative infection rate?
   B. What is the consultation rate?

Case-Mix Statistical Data

Case mix is a description of a patient population based on any number of specific characteristics including age, gender, type of insurance, diagnosis, risk factors, treatment received, and resources used. It is generally used as a distribution of patients into categories reflecting differences in severity of illness or resource consumption. Medicare severity diagnosis-related groups (MS-DRGs) are often used to determine case mix in hospitals. MS-DRGs is the US government's revision of the DRG system. MS-DRGs were developed to allow the CMS to provide greater reimbursement to hospitals who serve severely ill patients. MS-DRGs are covered in chapter 15.

When calculating case mix using MS-DRGs, the case-mix index (CMI) is the average relative weight of all cases treated at a given facility or by a given physician, which reflects the resource intensity or clinical severity of a specific group in relation to the other groups in the classification system. More information on case mix can be found in chapter 15.

The CMI is a measure of the resources used in treating the patients in each hospital or group of hospitals. A sample of a case mix report by payer (table 14.15), by physician (table 14.16), or by top 10 MS-DRGs (table 14.17) is given for Community Hospital. The CMI is calculated by multiplying the number of cases for each MS-DRG by the relative weight of the MS-DRG,

summing the result (696.2095) and dividing by the total number of cases (484). By convention, the CMI is calculated to five decimal points and rounded to four.

The CMI can be used to indicate the average reimbursement for the hospital. From table 14.15, the reimbursement is approximately 1.4798 multiplied by the hospital's base rate. It also is a measure of the severity of illness of Medicare patients. In table 14.15, you can see that Medicare patients, as expected, have the highest CMI at 2.0059.

Other data analyzed by MS-DRG include LOS and mortality rates. LOS and mortality data are benchmarked against a particular hospital and national data. The process of benchmarking involves comparing the hospital's performance against an external standard or benchmark. An excellent source of information for benchmarking purposes is the Healthcare Cost Utilization Project database

Table 14.16 Case mix of physicians, 20XX

Physician	CMI	N
A	1.0235	71
B	1.6397	71
C	1.1114	86
Average case mix by physician	**1.2582**	**228**

Table 14.15 Case-mix index by payer, Community Hospital, 20XX

Payer	CMI	N
Commercial	1.8830	283
Government managed care	0.9880	470
Managed care	1.4703	2,326
Medicaid	1.3400	962
Medicare	2.0059	1,776
Other	1.3251	148
Self-pay	1.3462	528
Average case mix by payer	**1.4798**	**6,493**

Table 14.17 Calculation of case-mix index for the top 10 MS-DRGs, Community Hospital, 20XX

MS-DRG	Number (N)	MS-DRG weight	N X MS-DRG weight
286	84	2.1240	178.4160
293	62	0.6762	41.9244
982	61	2.8150	171.7150
986	51	1.0453	53.3103
434	45	0.6229	28.0305
391	43	1.1976	51.4968
378	41	1.0021	41.0861
287	40	1.1290	45.1600
871	31	1.8072	56.0232
689	26	1.1172	29.0472
Total	**484**		**696.2095**
CMI			**1.4384**

(HCUPnet). HCUPnet is an online query system that provides access to statistics from the Healthcare Cost and Utilization Project (HCUP). Data for conditions, procedures, MS-DRGs, and Major Diagnostic Categories (MDCs) are available by patient characteristics such as age, sex, payer, and hospital characteristics such as bed size, location, and ownership; information is provided by each state.

Table 14.16 shows the case mix by physician and table 14.17 shows the case mix for the top 10 MS-DRGs. A comparison of hospital and national data for MS-DRG 293 appears in table 14.18.

Gross analysis of the data indicates that Community Hospital's mortality rate and ALOS are slightly better than the national average. But, at the same time, the hospital's average charges are higher than the national average.

Table 14.18 Benchmark data, Community Hospital versus national average for MS-DRG 293, Heart failure and shock without complication/comorbidity/major complication/comorbidity (CC/MCC)

	ALOS	Mortality rate	Average charges
Community Hospital	2.5	0.9%	$22,375
National average	2.6	1.1%	$18,192

Check Your Understanding 14.9

Instructions: **Answer the following questions. Calculate to four decimal points.**

Table 14.19 Community Hospital number of patients Dr. Green discharged by MS-DRG, August, 20XX

MS-DRG	MS-DRG title	Relative weight	Number of patients	Total weight
179	Respiratory infections and inflammations w/o CC/MCC	0.9693	5	
187	Pleural effusion w/ CC	1.0691	2	
189	Pulmonary edema and respiratory failure	1.2136	3	
194	Simple pneumonia and pleurisy w/ CC	0.9688	1	
208	Respiratory system diagnosis w/ ventilator support < 96 hours	2.2969	1	
280	Acute myocardial infarction, discharged alive w/ MCC	1.7289	3	
299	Peripheral vascular disorders w/ MCC	1.4094	2	
313	Chest pain	0.6138	4	
377	G.I. hemorrhage w/ MCC	1.7775	1	
391	Esophagitis, gastroenteritis. and miscellaneous digestive disorders w/ MCC	1.1976	1	
547	Connective tissue disorders w/o CC/MCC	0.7985	1	
552	Medical back problems w/o MCC	0.8698	1	
684	Renal failure w/o CC/MCC	0.6085	1	
812	Red blood cell disorders w/o MCC	0.8182	2	
872	Septicemia w/o MV 96+ hours w/o MCC	1.0528	1	
918	Poisoning and toxic effects of drugs w/o MCC	0.6412	1	
Total				
Case-mix index =				

1. Last month, Community Hospital had 68 discharges from its medicine unit. Six patients developed a catheter-associated urinary tract infection while in the hospital. Calculate the CAUTI rate for the last month.
2. During June, Community Hospital had 127 patients discharged. Fifty-seven patients had consultations from specialty physicians. What was the consultation rate for June?
3. Dr. Green discharged patients from medicine service during the month of August. Table 14.19 presents the number of patients discharged by Dr. Green by MS-DRG. Determine the total number of patients, calculate the total weight for each MS-DRG, and the CMI for Dr. Green.
4. A name given to describe an infection acquired in a healthcare facility is _____.
5. The CDC's term for hospital-acquired infections is _____.

Ambulatory Care Statistical Data

Ambulatory care includes healthcare services provided to patients who are not hospitalized (that is, who are not considered inpatients or residents and do not stay in the healthcare facility overnight). Such patients are referred to as outpatients. Most ambulatory care services today are provided in freestanding physicians' offices, emergency care centers, and ambulatory surgery centers that are not owned or operated by acute-care organizations. Hospitals do, however, provide many hospital-based healthcare services to outpatients. Hospital outpatients may receive services in one or more areas within the hospital, including clinics, same-day surgery departments, diagnostic departments, and emergency departments.

Outpatient statistics include records of the number of patient visits and the types of services provided. Many different terms are used to describe outpatients and ambulatory care services, including:

- **Ambulatory care**: Preventive or corrective healthcare services provided on a nonresident basis in a provider's office clinic setting, or hospital emergency setting

- **Outpatient**: A patient who receives ambulatory care services in a hospital-based clinic or department

- **Hospital outpatient**: A hospital patient who receives services in one or more of a hospital's facilities when he or she is not currently an inpatient or a home care patient

- **Emergency patient**: A patient who is admitted to the emergency services department of a hospital for diagnosis and treatment of a condition that requires immediate medical, dental, or allied health services in order to sustain life or to prevent critical consequences

- **Clinic outpatient**: A patient who is admitted to a clinical service of a clinic or hospital for diagnosis or treatment on an ambulatory basis

- **Referred outpatient**: An outpatient who is provided special diagnostic or therapeutic services by a hospital on an ambulatory basis but whose medical care remains the responsibility of the referring physician

- **Outpatient visit**: A patient's visit to one or more units or facilities located in the ambulatory services area (clinic or physician's office) of an acute-care hospital in which an overnight stay does not occur

- **Encounter**: The face-to-face contact between a patient and a provider who has primary responsibility for assessing and treating the condition of the patient at a given contact and exercises independent judgment in the care of the patient

- **Occasion of service**: A specified, identifiable service involved in the care of a patient that is not an encounter (for example, a lab test ordered during an encounter)

- **Ambulatory surgery center or ambulatory surgical center (ASC)**: Under Medicare, an outpatient surgical facility that has its own national identifier; is a separate entity with respect to its licensure, accreditation, governance, professional supervision, administrative functions, clinical services, recordkeeping, and financial and accounting systems; has as its sole purpose the provision of services in connection with surgical procedures that do not require inpatient hospitalization; and meets the conditions and requirements set forth in the Medicare Conditions of Participation
  - May be referred to as short-stay surgery, one-day surgery, same-day surgery, or come-and-go surgery services (Horton 2012).

Because outpatient care represents a large part of a healthcare organization's activity, statistics are collected and calculated on this group of patients. Many of the statistics covered in this chapter apply to ambulatory care.

✓ Check Your Understanding 14.10

Instructions: **Match the term to the definition.**

1. _____ A patient's visit to one or more units or facilities located in the ambulatory services area (clinic or physician's office) of an acute-care hospital in which an overnight stay does not occur

2. _____ A specified, identifiable service involved in the care of a patient that is not an encounter (for example, a lab test ordered during an encounter)

3. _____ Preventive or corrective healthcare services provided on a nonresident basis in a provider's office, clinic setting, or hospital emergency setting

4. _____ A patient who receives ambulatory care services in a hospital-based clinic or department

5. _____ An outpatient who is provided special diagnostic or therapeutic services by a hospital on an ambulatory basis but whose medical care remains the responsibility of the referring physician

6. _____ The face-to-face contact between a patient and a provider who has primary responsibility for assessing and treating the condition of the patient at a given contact and exercise

7. _____ A patient who is admitted to a clinical service of a clinic or hospital for diagnosis or treatment on an ambulatory basis

8. _____ A hospital patient who receives services in one or more of a hospital's facilities when he or she is not currently an inpatient or a home care patient

9. _____ A patient who is admitted to the emergency services department of a hospital for diagnosis and treatment of a condition that requires immediate medical, dental, or allied health services in order to sustain life or to prevent critical consequences

10. _____ An outpatient surgical facility that has its own national identifier; is a separate entity with respect to its licensure, accreditation, governance, professional supervision, administrative functions, clinical services, recordkeeping, and financial and accounting systems

11. _____ An ambulatory surgery center that is owned and operated by a hospital but is a separate entity with respect to its licensure, accreditation, governance, professional supervision, administrative functions, clinical services, recordkeeping, and financial and accounting systems.

    A. Ambulatory surgery center
    B. Outpatient visit
    C. Encounter
    D. Occasion of service
    E. Referred outpatient
    F. Clinic outpatient
    G. Emergency outpatient
    H. Hospital outpatient
    I. Hospital ambulatory care
    J. Outpatient
    K. Hospital-affiliated ambulatory surgery center

Public Health Statistics and Epidemiological Information

Just as statistics are collected in the healthcare organizational setting, they also are collected on a community, regional, and national basis. Vital statistics are an example of data collected and reported at these levels. The term *vital statistics* refers to the collection and analysis of data related to the crucial events in life: birth, death, marriage, divorce, fetal death, and induced terminations of pregnancy. These statistics are used to identify trends. For example, a higher-than-expected death rate among newborns may be an indication of the lack of prenatal services in a community. A number of deaths in a region due to the same cause may indicate an environmental problem. For example, the World Health Organization (WHO) has found that poor outdoor air quality is a cause of lung cancer deaths.

These types of data are used as part of the effort to preserve and improve the health of a defined population—the public health. The study of factors that influence the health status of a population is called epidemiology. The following sections will cover national vital statistics and population-based statistics.

National Vital Statistics System

The National Vital Statistics System (NVSS) is the oldest and most successful example of intergovernmental data sharing in public health, and the shared relationships, standards, and procedures that form the mechanism by which the National Center for Health Statistics (NCHS) of the Centers for Disease Control and Prevention (CDC) collects and disseminates the nation's official vital statistics. These data are provided through contracts between NCHS and vital registration systems operated in the various jurisdictions and legally responsible for the registration of vital events—births, deaths, marriages, divorces, and fetal deaths.

To facilitate consistent data collection, the National Vital Statistics System uses standard forms and procedures for the uniform registration of events are developed and they recommend each state use the same forms. The standard certificates represent the minimum basic data set necessary for the collection and publication of comparable national, state, and local vital statistics data. The standard forms are revised about every 10 years, with the last revision completed in 2003. To effectively implement these new certificates, the NCHS collaborates with its state partners to improve the timeliness, quality, and sustainability of the vital statistics system, along with collection of the revised and new content of the 2003 certificates (CDC 2016).

The certificate of live birth is used for registration purposes and is composed of two parts. The first part contains the information related to the child and the parents. The second part is used to collect data about the mother's pregnancy. This information is used for the collection of aggregate data only. No identification information appears on this portion of the certificate nor does it ever appear on the official certificate of birth. Pregnancy-related information includes complications of pregnancy, concurrent illnesses or conditions affecting pregnancy, and abnormal conditions or congenital anomalies of the newborn. Lifestyle factors such as use of alcohol and tobacco also are collected. Thus, the birth certificate is the major source of maternal and natality statistics. A listing of pregnancy-related information appears in figure 14.6.

Data collected from death certificates are used to compile causes of death in the United States. The certificate of death contains decedent information, place of death information, medical certification, and disposition information. Data on causes of death are classified and coded using the International Classification of Diseases (ICD). Beginning in 1999, the United States implemented ICD-10 for the coding of causes of death. Examples of the content of death certificates appear in figure 14.7.

Figure 14.6 Content of US certificate of live birth, 2003

Child's information	Pregnancy history
Child's name	Date of first prenatal care visit
Time of birth	Date of last prenatal care visit
Sex	Total number of prenatal visits for this pregnancy
Date of birth	Mother's height
Facility (hospital) name (if not an institution, give street address)	Mother's prepregnancy weight
City, town, or location of birth	Mother's weight at delivery
County of birth	Did mother get Women Infant Child (WIC) food for herself during this pregnancy?
Mother's Information	Number of previous live births
Current legal name	Number now living
Date of birth	Number now dead
Mother's name prior to first marriage	Date of last live birth
Birthplace	Number of other pregnancy outcomes
Residence (state)	Other outcomes
County	Date of last other pregnancy outcomes
City, town, or location	Cigarette smoking before and during pregnancy
Street number	Principal source of payment for this delivery
Apartment number	Date last normal menses began
Zip code	Mother's medical record number
Inside city limits?	Risk factors in this pregnancy
Mother's mailing address	Infections present and treated during this pregnancy
Mother married?	Obstetric procedures
If no, has paternity acknowledgment been signed in the hospital?	Onset of labor
Social Security number (SSN) requested for child?	Characteristics of labor and delivery
Mother's SSN	Method of delivery
Education	Maternal mortality
Hispanic origin?	Newborn Information
Race	Newborn medical record number
Place where birth occurred	Birth weight
Attendant's name, title, and National Provider Identifier	Obstetric estimate of gestation
Mother transferred for maternal, medical, or fetal indications for delivery?	Apgar score (1 and 5 minutes)
Father's Information	Plurality
Current legal name	If not born first (born first, second, third)
Date of birth	Abnormal conditions of newborn
Birthplace	Congenital anomalies of the newborn
Education	Was infant transferred within 24 hours of delivery?
Hispanic origin?	Is infant living at time of report?
Race	Is infant being breastfed at discharge?
Father's SSN	

Source: CDC 2016.

Figure 14.7   Content of US certificate of death, 2003

Decedent information

Name
Sex
Social Security number
Age
   Under 1 year—month; days
   Under 1 day—hours; minutes
Date of birth
Birthplace
Residence (state)
County
City or town
Street and number
Apartment number
Zip code
Inside city limits?
Ever in US armed forces?
Marital status at time of death
Surviving spouse's name (if wife, give name prior to first marriage)
Father's name
Mother's name (prior to first marriage)
Informant's name
Relationship to decedent
Mailing address
Decedent's education
Hispanic origin?
Race

Disposition information

Method of disposition
Place of disposition (cemetery, crematory, other)
Location—city, town, and state
Name and complete address of funeral facility
Signature of funeral service licensee or other agent
License number

Place of death information

Place of death
If hospital, indicate inpatient, emergency room or outpatient, dead on arrival
If somewhere other than hospital, indicate hospice, nursing home or long-term care facility, decedent's home, other
Facility name
City or town, state, zip code
County

Medical certification

Date pronounced dead
Time pronounced dead
Signature of person pronouncing death
Date signed
Actual or presumed date of death
Actual or presumed time of death
Was medical examiner contacted?
Immediate cause of death
Due to _____
Due to _____
Due to _____
Other significant conditions contributing to death
Was an autopsy performed?
Were autopsy findings available to complete the cause of death?
Did tobacco use contribute to death?
If female, indicate pregnancy status
Manner of death
For deaths due to injury:
Date of injury
Time of injury
Place of injury
Injury at work?
Location of injury
Describe how injury occurred
If transportation injury, specify if driver or operator, passenger, pedestrian, other

Certifier information

Certifier
Name, address, and zip code of person completing cause of death
Title of certifier
License number
Date certified

Source: CDC 2016.

A report of fetal death is completed when a pregnancy results in a stillbirth. This report contains information on the parents, the history of the pregnancy, and the cause of the fetal death. Information collected on the pregnancy is the same as that recorded on the birth certificate. To assess the effects of environmental exposures on the fetus, the parents' occupational data are collected. A listing of the content of the fetal death certificate appears in figure 14.8.

Figure 14.8 Content of US standard report of fetal death, 2003

Mother's information

Name of fetus (optional—at the discretion of the parents)
Time of delivery
Sex
Date of delivery
City, town, or location of delivery
Zip code of delivery
County of delivery
Place where delivery occurred
Facility name
Facility ID
Mother's current legal name
Date of birth
Mother's name prior to first marriage
Birthplace
Residence of mother (state)
County
City, town, or location
Street number
Apartment number
Zip code
Inside city limits?
Education
Hispanic origin?
Race
Mother married at delivery, conception, or any time between?
Date of first prenatal care visit
Date of last prenatal care visit
Total number of prenatal visits for this pregnancy
Mother's height
Mother's pre-pregnancy weight
Mother's weight at delivery
Did mother get WIC food for herself during this pregnancy?
Number of previous live births
    Number now living
    Number now dead
    Date of last live birth

Number of other pregnancy outcomes
Other outcomes
Date of last other pregnancy outcomes
Cigarette smoking before and during pregnancy
Date last normal menses began
Plurality
If not born first (born second, third)
Mother transferred for maternal, medical, or fetal indications
    for delivery?

Medical and health information
Risk factors in this pregnancy
Infections present and treated during this pregnancy
Method of delivery
Maternal mortality
Congenital anomalies of the newborn

Father's information
Current legal name
Date of birth
Birthplace

Disposition
Method of disposition

Attendant and registrant information
Attendant's name, title, and National Provider Identifier
Name of person completing report
Date report completed
Date received by registrar

Cause of fetal death
Initiating cause or condition
Other significant causes or conditions
Weight of fetus
Obstetric estimate of gestation at delivery
Estimated time of fetal death
Was an autopsy performed?
Was a histological placental examination performed?
Were autopsy or histological placental examination results
    used in determining the cause of fetal death?

Source: CDC 2016.

The report of induced termination of pregnancy records information on the place of the induced termination of pregnancy, type of termination procedure, and patient. (See figure 14.9.)

A tool for monitoring and exploring the interrelationships between infant death and risk factors at birth is the linked birth and infant death data set. This is a service provided by the NCHS. In this data set, the information from the death certificate (such as age and underlying or multiple causes of death) is linked to the information in the birth certificate (such as age, race, birth weight, prenatal care, maternal education, and so on) for each infant who dies in the United States, Puerto Rico, the Virgin Islands, and Guam. The purpose of the data set is to use the many additional variables available from the birth certificate to conduct a detailed analysis of infant mortality patterns.

Birth, death, fetal death, and termination of pregnancy certificates provide vital information for use in medical research, epidemiological studies, and other public health programs. In addition, they are the source of data for compiling morbidity, birth, and mortality rates that describe the health

Figure 14.9 Content of US standard report of induced termination of pregnancy, 1997

Place of induced termination

Facility name
City, town, or location of pregnancy termination
County of pregnancy termination

Patient information

Patient identification
Age at last birthday
Marital status
Date or pregnancy termination
Residence (state)
County
City, town, or location
Inside city limits?
Zip code

Hispanic origin?
Race
Education
   Elementary/secondary
   College
Date last normal menses began
Clinical estimate of gestation
Previous pregnancies
   Live births
   Other terminations
      Type of termination procedure

Other information
Name of attending physician
Name of person completing report

Source: CDC 2010.

of a given population at the local, state, or national level. Because of their many uses, the data on these certificates must be complete and accurate.

Population-Based Statistics

Population-based statistics are based on the mortality and morbidity rates from which the health of a population can be inferred. The entire defined population is used in the collection and reporting of these statistics. The size of the defined population serves as the denominator in the calculation of these rates, which are discussed in the following sections.

Birth Rates and Measures of Infant Mortality

Two community-based rates that are commonly used to describe a community's health are the crude birth rate and measures of infant mortality. WHO's definition of a live birth is "the complete expulsion or extraction from its mother of a product of conception, irrespective of the duration of the pregnancy, which after such separation, breathes or shows other evidence of life such as beating of the heart, pulsation of the umbilical cord, or definite movement of voluntary muscles, whether or not the umbilical cord has been cut or the placenta is attached" (WHO 2016).

Rates that describe infant mortality are based on age. Therefore, the definitions for the various age groups must be strictly followed. Table 14.20 summarizes the calculations for community-based birth and infant mortality rates. These mortality or death rates are broken down as follows.

Crude birth rate is the number of live births divided by the population at risk, meaning the population affected (as shown in table 14.20). Community rates are calculated using the multiplier 1,000, 10,000, or 100,000. The purpose is to bring the rate to a whole number, as discussed earlier in the chapter. The result of the formula would be stated as the number of live births per 1,000 population. Formula 14.22 for calculating the crude birth rate is as follows.

Formula 14.22. Calculating the crude birth rate

$$\text{Crude birth rate} = \frac{\substack{\text{Number of live births} \\ \text{for a given community} \\ \text{for a specified period of time}}}{\substack{\text{Estimated population} \\ \text{for the same community} \\ \text{and the same time period}}} \times 1,000$$

Table 14.20 Calculation of community-based birth and infant death (mortality) rates

Measure	Numerator (x)	Denominator (y)	10^n
Crude birth rate	Number of live births for a given community for a specified time period	Estimated population for the same community and the same time period	1,000
Neonatal mortality rate	Number of deaths of infants from birth up to, but not including, 28 days of age during a given time period	Number of live births during the same time period	1,000
Postneonatal mortality rate	Number of deaths of infants from 28 days of age up to, but not including, one year of age during a given time period	Number of live births minus neonatal deaths during the same time period	1,000
Infant mortality rate	Number of deaths of infants under one year of age during a given time period	Number of live births during the same time period	1,000

For example, if there were 5,392 live births in a community of 500,000 in 20XX, the crude birth rate for that year would be 11 per 1,000 population ($[5,392/500,000] \times 1,000$).

The **neonatal mortality rate** can be used as a measure of the quality of prenatal care and the mother's prenatal behavior (for example, alcohol, drug, or tobacco use). The neonatal period is the period of an infant's life from the hour of birth through the first 27 days, 23 hours, and 59 minutes of life. In the formula for calculating the neonatal mortality rate, the numerator is the number of deaths of infants in the neonatal period during a given time period and the denominator is the total number of live births during the same time period. See formula 14.23 to calculate the neonatal mortality rate.

Formula 14.23. Calculating the neonatal mortality rate

$$\text{Neonatal mortality rate} = \frac{\text{Number of deaths of infants from birth up to, but not including, 28 days of age during a given time period}}{\text{Number of live births during the same time period}} \times 1,000$$

For example, in your community there were 5,392 live births in 20XX and 12 infants who died within the neonatal period in that year. The neonatal mortality rate is 2 per 1,000 live births for the period ($[12/5,392] \times 1,000$).

The **postneonatal mortality rate** is often used as an indicator of the quality of the home or community environment of infants. The postneonatal period is from 28 days of age up to, but not including, one year of age. In the formula for calculating the postneonatal mortality rate, the numerator is the number of deaths among infants from 28 days of age up to, but not including, one year of age during a given time period and the denominator is the total number of live births minus the number of neonatal deaths during the same time period. The formula for calculating the postneonatal mortality rate is shown in formula 14.24.

Formula 14.24. Calculating the postneonatal mortality rate

$$\text{Postneonatal mortality rate} = \frac{\text{Number of deaths of infants from 28 days of age up to, but not including, one year of age during a given time period}}{\text{Number of live births minus neonatal deaths during the same time period}} \times 1,000$$

For example, in your community there were 5,392 live births, 12 neonatal deaths, and 9 postneonatal deaths during 20XX. The postneonatal mortality rate is 2 per 1,000 live births minus neonatal deaths for the period ($[9/\{5,392-12\}] \times 1,000$).

The **infant mortality rate** is the summary of the neonatal and postneonatal mortality rates. In the formula for calculating the infant mortality rate, the numerator is the number of deaths among infants under one year of age (364 days, 23 hours, and 59 minutes from the moment of birth) and the denominator is the number of live births during the same period. The infant mortality rate is the most commonly used measure for comparing health status among nations. All the rates are expressed in terms of the number of deaths per 1,000 live births. The formula for calculating the infant mortality rate is found in formula 14.25.

Formula 14.25. Calculating the infant mortality rate

$$\text{Infant mortality rate} = \frac{\text{Number of deaths of infants under one year of age during a given period of time}}{\text{Number of live births during the same period}} \times 1,000$$

For example, in your community there were 12 neonatal deaths, 9 postneonatal deaths, and 5,392 live births in 20XX. The infant mortality rate is 4 per 1,000 live births in that year ([{12 + 9}/5,392] × 1,000).

Other Death (Mortality) Rates

Other measures of mortality with which the HIM professional should be familiar include the following.

Crude death/mortality rate is a measure of the actual or observed mortality in a given population. Crude death rates apply to a population without regard to characteristics such as age, race, and sex. They measure the proportion of the population that has died during a given period of time (usually one year) or the number of deaths in a community per 1,000 for a given period of time. In the formula, the numerator is the total number of deaths in a population for a specified time period and the denominator is the estimated population for the same time period. The formula

for calculating the crude death/mortality rate is found in formula 14.26.

Formula 14.26. Calculating the crude death/mortality rate

$$\text{Crude death / mortality rate} = \frac{\text{Total number of deaths for a population during a specified period of time}}{\text{Estimated population for the same time period}} \times 1,000$$

For instance, in our previous examples we used a community population of 500,000. There were 1,327 deaths in 20XX. Dividing 1,327 by 500,000 equals 0.002654. Using a multiplier of 1,000 gives a crude death rate of 2.7 deaths per 1,000 population for 20XX ([1,327/500,000] × 1,000).

As its name indicates, the **cause-specific mortality rate** is the rate of death due to a specified cause. It may be calculated for an entire population or for any age, sex, or race. In the formula, the numerator is the number of deaths due to a specified cause for a given time period and the denominator is the estimated population for the same time period. Table 14.21 displays cause-specific mortality rates for men and women due to influenza and pneumonia for the year 2013. The cause-specific death rates for each age group are consistently higher for men than for women, but the overall rate is higher for women. This information could lead to an investigation of why this occurs. The formula for calculating the cause-specific mortality rate can be found in formula 14.27.

Formula 14.27. Calculating the cause-specific mortality rate

$$\text{Cause-specific mortality rate} = \frac{\text{Total number of deaths due to a specific cause during a specified period of time}}{\text{Estimated population for the same time period}} \times 100,000$$

Table 14.21   Cause-specific mortality rates, by sex, due to influenza and pneumonia (ICD-10 codes J10–J18.9), age 45+, in the United States, 2013

Age group	Women			Men		
	Population	Deaths	Rate/100,000	Population	Deaths	Rate/100,000
45–54	22,198,448	956	4.3	21,569,084	1,277	5.9
55–64	20,359,676	2,034	10.0	18,956,755	2,745	114.5
65–74	13,419,124	3,310	24.7	11,797,642	4,131	35.0
75–84	7,686,002	6,852	89.1	5,760,517	7,097	123.2
85+	3,999,007	16,152	403.9	2,041,782	10,489	513.7
Total	**67,662,257**	**29,304**	**43.3**	**60,125,780**	**25,739**	**43.1**

Source: CDC 2015a.

The **case fatality rate** measures the total number of deaths among the diagnosed cases of a specific disease, most often acute illness. In the formula for calculating the case fatality rate, the numerator is the number of deaths due to a specific disease that occurred during a specific time period and the denominator is the number of diagnosed cases during the same time period. The higher the case fatality rate, the more virulent the infection. The formula for calculating the case fatality rate is found in formula 14.28.

Formula 14.28. Calculating the case fatality rate

$$\text{Case fatality rate} = \frac{\text{Total number of deaths due to a specific disease during a specified period of time}}{\text{Total number of cases due to a specific disease during the same time period}} \times 100$$

For example, in our community there were seven cases of meningitis resulting in two deaths. The case fatality rate of meningitis is 28.6 percent ([2/7] × 100).

The **proportionate mortality rate (PMR)** is a measure of mortality due to a specific cause for a specific time period. In the formula for calculating the PMR, the numerator is the number of deaths due to a specific disease for a specific time period and the denominator is the

number of deaths from all causes for the same time period. Table 14.22 displays the PMRs for influenza and pneumonia in the United States in 2013 by age groups. The formula for calculating the proportionate mortality rate is found in formula 14.29.

Formula 14.29. Calculating the proportionate mortality rate

$$\text{Proportionate mortality rate} = \frac{\text{Total number of deaths due to a specific cause during a specified period of time}}{\text{Total number of deaths from all causes during the same time period}} \times 100$$

The **maternal mortality rate (community based)** measures the deaths associated with pregnancy for a specific community for a specific period of time. It is calculated only for deaths that are directly related to pregnancy. In the formula for calculating the maternal mortality rate, the numerator is the number of deaths attributed to causes related to pregnancy during a specific time period for a given community and the denominator is the number of live births reported during the same time period for the same community. The maternal mortality rate is expressed as the number of deaths per 100,000 live births. The formula for calculating the maternal mortality rate (community based) is found in formula 14.30.

Table 14.22 Proportionate mortality rates for influenza and pneumonia (ICD-10 codes J10–J18.9), all ages, in the United States, 2013

Age group	Influenza and pneumonia deaths	Total deaths	PMR/100
< 1 year	159	23,629	0.67
0–4	93	4,218	2.20
5–14	85	5,200	1.63
15–24	147	29,182	0.50
25–34	356	44,591	0.80
35–44	685	69,162	0.99
45–54	1,825	179,463	1.02
55–64	3,929	329,606	1.19
65–74	6,269	432,346	1.45
75–84	13,040	620,428	2.10
85+	24,046	805,307	2.99

Source: CDC 2013.

Formula 14.30. Calculating the maternal mortality rate

$$\text{Maternal mortality rate} = \frac{\text{Total number of deaths due to pregnancy-related conditions during a specified period of time}}{\text{Total number of live births during the same time period}} \times 100,000$$

For example, according to the CDC in the United States in 2013 there were 3,932,181 live births and 1,111 maternal deaths. This is a maternal mortality rate of 29 maternal deaths per 100,000 live births ($[1,111/3,932,181] \times 100,000$). Table 14.23 shows how to calculate community-based mortality rates.

Measures of Morbidity

Two measures are commonly used to describe the presence of disease in a community or specific location (for example, a nursing home)—incidence and prevalence rates. *Disease* is any illness, injury, or disability. Incidence and prevalence measures can be broken down by race, sex, age, or other characteristics of a population.

An **incidence rate** is used to compare the frequency of new cases of disease in populations. Populations are compared using rates instead of raw numbers because rates adjust for differences in population size. The incidence rate is the probability or risk of illness in a population over a period of time. The denominator represents the population from which the case in the numerator arose, such as a nursing home, school, or organization. For 10^n, a value is selected so that the smallest rate calculated results in a whole number. In a small population such as a nursing home you might select 100, in studying a larger population you might select 1,000. For example, in a local nursing home of 174 patients, 8 new cases of H1N1 (a strain of influenza A virus) occurred during January. Using

Table 14.23 Calculation of community-based mortality rates

Measure	Numerator (x)	Denominator (y)	10^n
Crude death/mortality rate	Total number of deaths for a population during a specified time period	Estimated population for the same time period	1,000 or 10,000 or 100,000
Cause-specific mortality rate	Total number of deaths due to a specific cause during a specified time period	Estimated population for the same time period	100,000
Case fatality rate	Total number of deaths due to a specific disease during a specified time period	Total number of cases due to a specific disease during the same time period	100
Proportionate mortality rate	Total number of deaths due to a specific cause during a specified time period	Total number of deaths from all causes during the same time period	N/A
Maternal mortality rate	Total number of deaths due to pregnancy-related conditions during a specified time period	Total number of live births during the same time period	100,000

✓ Check Your Understanding 14.11

Instructions: **Answer the following questions.**

1. Review the mortality data in table 14.24 and then answer the questions that follow.

Table 14.24   Mortality Rates, United States, 2013

Age group	Female Population	Female Deaths	Male Population	Male Deaths
Less than 1 year	1,925,056	10,321	2,016,727	13,119
1–4 years	7,790,614	1,745	8,135,691	2,323
5–14	20,159,538	2,263	21,061,497	3,077
15–24	21,429,247	7,622	22,525,155	20,864
25–34	21,203,096	14,001	21,641,491	31,462
35–44	20,307,429	26,501	20,145,261	43,072
45–54	22,198,448	69,727	21,569,084	107,997
55–64	20,359,676	131,802	18,956,755	206,325
65–74	13,419,124	196,531	11,797,642	257,898
75–84	7,686,002	309,673	5,760,517	315,340
85+	3,999,007	520,736	2,041,782	304,462
Total				

Source: CDC 2015a.

   A. What is the crude death rate per 10,000 for men all ages?
   B. What is the crude death rate per 10,000 for women all ages?
   C. What is the crude death rate per 10,000 for the entire group?
   D. What is the crude death rate per 10,000 for men ages 15 to 24?
   E. What is the crude death rate per 10,000 for women ages 15 to 24?

2. In a community of 750,000 there were reported 4,899 live births. What is the crude birth rate?

3. In this same community there were eight infants who died in the neonatal period. What is the neonatal mortality rate?

4. In this same community there were 14 children who died in the neonatal period. What is the postneonatal mortality rate?

5. What is the infant mortality rate in this community?

6. In this same community there were 4,225 deaths. What is the crude death rate?

7. In this same community, 125 people died of lung cancer. What is cause-specific mortality rate?

8. In this same community, 37 people reported a *Clostridium difficile (C. diff)* infection; of these, four people died. What is the case fatality rate?

9. What is the proportionate mortality rate for *Clostridium difficile (C. diff)* in this community?

10. In this same community there were 4,012 live births. Two mothers died of causes associated with their pregnancies. What is the maternal mortality rate?

this formula, the incidence rate is 5.5 percent ($[8/147] \times 100$). The formula for calculating the incidence rate is found in formula 14.31.

Formula 14.31. Calculating the incidence rate

$$\text{Incidence rate} = \frac{\begin{array}{c}\text{Total number of new} \\ \text{cases of a specified} \\ \text{disease during a} \\ \text{given period of time}\end{array}}{\begin{array}{c}\text{Total population at} \\ \text{risk during the} \\ \text{same time period}\end{array}} \times 10^n$$

The **prevalence rate** is the proportion of persons in a population who have a particular disease at a specific point in time or over a specified period of time. The prevalence rate describes the magnitude of an epidemic and can be an indicator of the medical resources needed in a community for the duration of the epidemic. For example, in a community of 750,000 individuals, there were 1,875 individuals identified as having AIDS and an additional 93 cases identified in 20XX. The prevalence rate is 2.62 cases per 1,000 population ($[\{1,875 + 93\}/750,000] \times 1,000$). The formula for calculating the prevalence rate is found in formula 14.32.

Formula 14.32. Calculating the prevalence rate

$$\text{Prevalence rate} = \frac{\begin{array}{c}\text{All new and preexisting} \\ \text{cases of a specific} \\ \text{disease during a given} \\ \text{period of time}\end{array}}{\begin{array}{c}\text{Total population during} \\ \text{the same time period}\end{array}} \times 10^n$$

It is easy to confuse incidence and prevalence rates. The distinction is in the numerators of their formulas. The numerator in the formula for the incidence rate is the number of new cases occurring in a given time period. The numerator in the formula for the prevalence rate is all cases present during a given time period. In addition, the incidence rate includes only patients whose illness began during a specified time period whereas the prevalence rate includes all patients from a specified cause regardless of when the illness began. Moreover, the prevalence rate includes a patient until he or she recovers.

National Notifiable Diseases Surveillance System

In 1878, US Congress authorized the US Marine Hospital Service, the precursor to the Public Health Service, to collect morbidity reports on cholera, smallpox, plague, and yellow fever from US consuls overseas. This information was used to implement quarantine measures to prevent the spread of these diseases to the United States. To provide for more uniformity in data collection, Congress enacted a law in 1902 that directed the surgeon general to provide standard forms for the collection, compilation, and publication of reports at the national level. In 1912, the states and US territories recommended that infectious disease be immediately reported by telegraph. By 1928, all states, the District of Columbia, Hawaii, and Puerto Rico were participating in the national reporting of 29 specified diseases. In 1961, the CDC assumed responsibility for the collection and publication of data concerning nationally notifiable diseases.

A **notifiable disease** is one that must be reported to a government agency so that regular, frequent, and timely information on individual cases can be used to prevent and control future cases of the disease. The list of notifiable diseases varies over time and by state. The Council of State and Territorial Epidemiologists (CSTE) collaborates with the CDC to determine which diseases should be reported. State reporting to the CDC is voluntary. However, all states generally report the internationally quarantinable diseases in accordance with WHO's International Health Regulations. Completeness of reporting varies by state and type of disease and may be influenced by a number of factors, for example type of illness and resources for reporting.

Information that is reported includes date, county, age, sex, race and ethnicity, and disease-specific epidemiologic information; personal identifiers are not included. A strict CSTE Data Release Policy regulates dissemination of the data. A list of nationally notifiable infectious diseases appears in figure 14.10. The list is updated annually; the list in figure 14.10 is not an exhaustive list.

Selected national morbidity data are reported weekly by the 50 states, New York City, the District of Columbia, and the US territories. Then they are collated and then published by the CDC in the Morbidity and Mortality Weekly Report. Public health managers and providers use the reports to rapidly identify disease epidemics and to understand patterns of disease occurrence. Case-specific information is included in the reports. Changes in age, sex, race and ethnicity, and geographic distributions can be monitored and investigated as necessary (CDC 2015b).

Figure 14.10 Nationally notifiable infectious diseases in the United States, 2015

Anthrax	Measles (Rubeola)
Arboviral neuroinvasive and non-neuroinvasive diseases	Meningococcal disease
Babesiosis	Mumps
Botulism, *C.botulinum*	Novel influenza A virus infections
Brucellosis	Pertussis (Whooping cough)
Campylobacteriosis	Pesticide-related illness and injury, acute
Cancer	Plague
Carbon monoxide poisoning	Poliomyelitis, paralytic
Chancroid	Poliovirus infection, nonparalytic
Chlamydia trachomatis, infection	Psittacosis (Ornithosis)
Cholera	Q fever
Coccidioidomycosis/Valley fever	Rabies, animal
Congenital syphilis	Rabies, human
Cryptosporidiosis	Rubella (German measles)
Cyclosporiasis	Rubella, congenital syndrome (CRS)
Dengue virus infections	Salmonellosis
Diphtheria	Severe acute respiratory syndrome–associated coronavirus (SARS) disease
Ehrlichiosis and anaplasmosis	
Food-borne disease outbreak	Shiga toxin-producing *Escherichia coli* (STEC)
Giardiasis	Shigellosis
Gonorrhea	Silicosis
Haemophilus influenzae, invasive disease	Smallpox (Variola)
Hansen disease and leprosy	Spotted fever rickettsiosis
Hantavirus infection, non-Hantavirus pulmonary syndrome	Streptococcal toxic-shock syndrome (STSS)
Hantavirus pulmonary syndrome (HPS)	Syphilis
Hemolytic uremic syndrome, post-diarrheal (HUS)	Tetanus, *c. tetani*
Hepatitis A, B, and C, acute; Hepatitis B chronic and perinatal infection	Toxic-shock syndrome (other than streptococcal) (TSS)
	Trichinellosis (Trichinosis)
HIV infection (AIDS has been reclassified as HIV stage III) (AIDS/HIV)	Tuberculosis (TB)
	Tularemia
Influenza-associated pediatric mortality	Typhoid fever
Invasive pneumococcal disease (IPD), *Streptococcus pneumoniae,* invasive disease	Vancomycin-intermediate *Staphylococcus aureus* and vancomycin-resistant *Staphylococcus aureus* (VISA/VRSA)
Lead, elevated blood levels	Varicella (Chickenpox)
Legionellosis (Legionnaire's disease) or Pontiac fever	Varicella deaths
Leptospirosis	Vibriosis
Listeriosis	Viral hemorrhagic fevers (VHF)
Lyme disease	Waterborne disease outbreak
Malaria	Yellow fever

Source: CDC 2015c.

Check Your Understanding 14.12

Instructions: **Answer the following questions.**

1. Define *incidence rate* and *prevalence rate*.

2. What is a notifiable disease?

3. Calculate the incidence rate, per 100,000, for the following hypothetical data: In 20XX, 189,000 new cases of coronary artery disease were reported in the United States. The estimated population for 20XX was 301,623,157.

4. In a community of 50,000, there were four cases of hantavirus pulmonary syndrome during the first half of 20XX. What is the incidence rate?

5. In the same community, three more cases of hantavirus pulmonary syndrome were reported for the remaining months of the year. What is the prevalence rate?

Real-World Case 14.1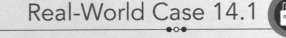

The performance improvement committee of Community Regional Medical Center wanted to study MS-DRG 689 kidney and urinary tract infections with MCC (Major Complication or Comorbidity) because of wide variations in LOS and total charges (refer to chapter 15 for a more information on MS-DRGs and MCCs). The committee asked the HIM director to prepare a profile of patients discharged from MS-DRG 689. A summary of the patients discharged from MS-DRG 689 at Community Hospital was prepared using information found in the hospital's online database.

Real World Case 14.2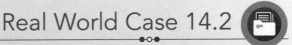

A facility is looking into the possibility of adding or deleting procedures to their surgery product line in the cardiothoracic area. The following table lists the types of procedures they are reviewing.

MS-DRG	Description	Relative weight	National LOS
2	Heart Transplant or Implant of Health Assist System w/o MCC	15.6820	15.7
216	Cardiac Valve and Other Maj Cardiothoracic Proc w Card Cath w/ MCC	9.2380	13.0
232	Coronary Artery Bypass w PTCA w/o MCC	5.5976	7.9
237	Major Cardiovas proc w/ MCC	5.0843	6.7

References

American Health Information Management Association. 2014. *Pocket Glossary of Health Information Management and Technology,* 3rd ed. Chicago: AHIMA.

BusinessDictionary.com. 2016. Likert Scale. http://www.businessdictionary.com/definition/Likert-scale.html.

Centers for Disease Control and Prevention. 2016. "2003 Revisions of the U.S. Standard Certificates of Live Birth and Death and the Fetal Death Report." 1 Jan. 2016.

Centers for Disease Control and Prevention. 2015a. CDC Wonder. http://wonder.cdc.gov.

Centers for Disease Control and Prevention. 2015b. Morbidity and Mortality Weekly Reports. http://www.cdc.gov/mmwr/publications/index.html.

Centers for Disease Control and Prevention. 2015c. National Notifiable Conditions. http://wwwn.cdc.gov/nndss/conditions/notifiable/2015/.

Centers for Disease Control and Prevention. 2013. Mortality Multiple Cause Micro-data Files. Deaths: Final Data for 2013. http://www.cdc.gov/nchs/data/nvsr/nvsr64/nvsr64_02.pdf.

Centers for Disease Control and Prevention. 2010 (updated). State Definitions and Reporting Requirements for Live Births, Fetal Deaths and Induced Termination of Pregnancy. http://www.cdc.gov/nchs/products/other/miscpub/statereq.htm.

Horton, L. 2012. *Calculating and Reporting Healthcare Statistics.* Chicago: AHIMA.

World Health Organization. 2016. Health Statistics and Information Systems. http://www.who.int/healthinfo/statistics/indmaternalmortality/en/.

Part V
Revenue Management and Compliance

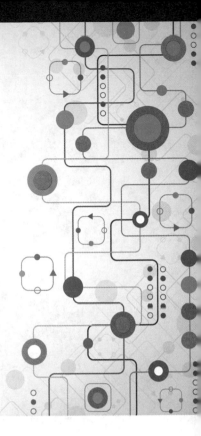

15

Revenue Management and Reimbursement

Leslie L. Gordon, MS, RHIA, FAHIMA
Morley L. Gordon, RHIT

Learning Objectives

- Describe the reimbursement process, forms, and support practice for healthcare reimbursement
- Differentiate commercial, private, and employer-based healthcare insurance
- Describe the purpose and benefits of government-sponsored health programs
- Describe managed care

- Identify different fee-for-service reimbursement methods
- Understand the purpose and use of fee schedules, chargemaster, and auditing procedures that support the reimbursement process
- Outline the revenue cycle process

Key Terms

Accept assignment
Adjudication
Affordable Care Act
Ambulatory payment classification
Ambulatory surgery center (ASC) payment rate
Balanced billing
Beneficiaries
Capitation
Case management
Case-mix index
Centers for Medicare and Medicaid Services (CMS)
Charge description master
Chargemaster

Children's Health Insurance Program
Civilian Health and Medical Program of the Department of Veterans Affairs
Claims
Clinical data
Coinsurance
Concurrent review
Consumer-directed health plans (CDHP)
Coordination of benefits
Cost sharing
Copayment
Deductible

Demographic data
Diagnosis-related group
Disproportionate share hospital
Dual eligible
Eligibility
Episode of care reimbursement
Exclusive provider organizations (EPO)
Explanation of benefits
Federal poverty level
Fee-for-service reimbursement
Fee schedule
Global payment
Health insurance marketplace or exchange

Health maintenance organization
Healthcare insurance
Home health prospective
    payment system
Hospital-acquired condition
Indian Health Service
Inpatient prospective payment
    system
Managed care
Managed care organization
    (MCO)
Mandatory eligibility groups
Medicaid
Medical necessity
Medicare
Medicare administrative
    contractors
Medicare Advantage Plan
Medicare Part A
Medicare Part B

Medicare Part D
Medicare severity diagnosis-related
    groups (MS-DRGs)
National Committee for Quality
    Assurance (NCQA)
Out of pocket
Outpatient Prospective Payment
    System
Pay for performance
Point of service plans
Policy
Policyholder
Precertification
Preferred provider organization
Premium
Preventive services
Prior approval
Private healthcare insurance
Professional component
Prospective payment system

Prospective review
Reimbursement
Remittance advice
Resource-based relative value
    scale
Retrospective review
Revenue cycle
Skilled nursing facility prospective
    payment system
Technical component
Third-party administrator
Third-party payer
Traditional fee-for-service
    reimbursement
TRICARE
Usual, customary, and reasonable
    charges
Utilization management
Veterans Health Administration
Workers' compensation

Payment for healthcare services, called **reimbursement**, is complex in the United States. Reimbursement begins before a patient enters a healthcare facility, with the collection of demographic and patient-specific data and insurance coverage information, and ends with the final **adjudication** of all medical charges. *Adjudication* is a term used by the insurance industry and refers to the process of paying, denying, and adjusting claims based on the patient's healthcare insurance coverage benefits. Information about a patient is collected during the course of receiving healthcare services. This includes **demographic data**, used to identify an individual, and **clinical data**, which is the patient's medical condition or treatment. This information is used to bill for healthcare services. Reimbursement for services is what keeps healthcare providers and

facilities in business. Healthcare providers submit **claims**, which represent the services and supplies provided to a patient during his or her encounter with the facility or provider, for reimbursement to insurance companies on behalf of patients. Health information management (HIM) professionals play a vital role in the submission of accurate claims by ensuring the documentation supports the services billed, assigning proper diagnostic and procedure codes, and ensuring accurate information is captured throughout the patient's encounter with the healthcare organization.

This chapter discusses healthcare insurance, revenue cycle management, reimbursement systems (including private and government plans), managed care, healthcare reimbursement methodologies, and utilization and case management.

Healthcare Insurance

Americans without healthcare insurance must pay for healthcare expenses **out-of-pocket**, meaning they pay for the services provided with their own funds. Those without the ability to pay for healthcare either do not receive care or are not able pay for the care they receive (Hazelwood

and Venable 2012). **Healthcare insurance** protects a person from paying the full cost of healthcare by prepaying for a healthcare coverage plan. Before the early 1900s, Americans paid for all of their healthcare out-of-pocket. The cost of healthcare was not a significant part of the American family's budget and the need for health insurance was not a consideration because in 1900 the average yearly amount spent on healthcare was $5 (equivalent to $100 today) (Blumberg and Davidson 2009). During this time hospitals were places for injured soldiers, those who were very sick, the poor, and those who had contagious diseases. Hospitals were known as a last resort—a place where people went to die (Ferenc 2014). By the late 1920s, with modern medicine and the discovery of antibiotics, hospitals started marketing themselves as places with positive health outcomes. Hospitals wanted to fill beds and wanted people who were not deathly ill to come in and fill these empty beds because more patients filling the beds means revenue for the hospital (Blumberg and Davidson 2009). In 1929, in Dallas, Texas, Baylor Hospital started a prepaid hospital insurance program with a local teachers union. The teachers paid 50 cents a month to cover the care they received at Baylor and the teachers would not be billed for care. This plan created what is thought to be the nation's first example of modern healthcare insurance. The Baylor program was popular across America, initiating a system where employers paid for health insurance for employees (Blumberg and Davidson 2009).

Health insurance coverage for all Americans began to be a political hot topic as early as 1912. While campaigning for the US presidency, Theodore Roosevelt called for a national healthcare insurance program. He did not win the presidency and, therefore, national healthcare insurance was not implemented at that time (CMS 2015a). Many politicians and presidents throughout the years championed for universal health coverage and almost 100 years after Theodore Roosevelt campaigned for national health coverage, the **Affordable Care Act (ACA)** was signed into law in 2010 providing health coverage for all Americans. The ACA mandated many changes in reimbursement methodologies, which are discussed in this chapter. More information on the ACA is found in chapter 2.

To understand the process of healthcare reimbursement as defined in this chapter, it is important to understand basic terms. When a person has healthcare insurance they receive a **policy**, or contract, in which they pay a **premium**—a set amount per month or year—to help cover the cost of medical expenses. The **policyholder** is the person covered by the policy. The purchaser of a healthcare insurance policy can be an individual, group, or employer.

Revenue Cycle Management

The **revenue cycle** is the process of patient financial and health information moving into, through, and out of the healthcare facility, culminating with the facility receiving reimbursement for services provided. HIM professionals are vital to the management of the revenue cycle. The revenue cycle begins with patient registration, known as the front-end of the cycle. The documentation of the encounter in the health record, charge capture, coding, and charge entry comprise the middle section of the cycle. The back-end of the revenue cycle includes claims transmission and accounts receivable management (Fahrenholz 2010). Financial viability of the healthcare organization rests with

the revenue cycle and every aspect of it having accurate and complete information and data capture. Management of the revenue cycle is the process of supervising the entire claims process from determining patient eligibility for insurance, collecting money owed on copayments (co-pays) and deductibles, and ensuring correct and timely capture of all charges. Monitoring, or working, the revenue cycle from the patient's first contact with the organization to the final account balance of zero includes numerous steps and professionals (Fahrenholz 2010). This entire process will be discussed in further detail as follows.

Patient Registration

Patient registration is a vital first step to ensure the claims submitted to a payer will receive proper reimbursement. Responsibilities include preregistration, registration, insurance verification, and prior approval (authorization) for some services.

The patient registration department of a hospital is frequently called Patient Access and is responsible for capturing demographic information for each patient. This is a critical first step in ensuring insurance information for the patient is correct. The capture of demographic information on a patient begins before the patient encounter with preregistration involving collection of data including name, date of birth, insurance coverage, and address. If a patient is not covered by an insurance plan he or she is considered a self-pay patient and are responsible for all charges incurred during his or her encounter. The term **third-party payer** is used to identify an insurance company that pays for the medical care of covered individuals. The terms *first party*, the patient, and *second party*, the healthcare provider, are not used as frequently.

If a patient is covered by more than one insurance, **coordination of benefits (COB)**—determining which insurance coverage is the primary, secondary, and tertiary payer—takes place. For example, a patient is covered under the group plan A offered at her place of work and is also covered under the group plan B, offered at her spouse's place of work. Her own insurance A is primary and her spouse's insurance B is billed after her plan A has made its payment. The birthday rule is used to determine which coverage is billed first when a child is covered by both parents' plan. The parent whose birthday falls first in the calendar year (not who is oldest, or who has insurance for the longest amount of time) is primary; for example, if the mother's birthday is May 15 and the father's birthday is October 10, the mother's insurance plan is primary.

Registration staff monitor the organization's appointments and schedules and are responsible for contacting the health insurance carriers for procedures that require prior approval. **Prior approval** (authorization) for services involves obtaining approval from the insurance company before receiving services. For example, a patient with a strong family history of breast cancer may require a breast ultrasound yearly. If this service does not receive prior approval, the claim may be denied by the insurance company for payment.

Documentation, Coding, and Charge Capture

Healthcare services should be documented in the health record and captured either through an electronic system or manually entered into the patient's financial account as they are provided. The charge capture process involves entering codes for all procedures and supplies provided during patient care. The codes include diagnoses, procedure, and supply codes.

A **charge description master (CDM)**, sometimes called **chargemaster**, is a financial management list that contains information about the organization's charges for healthcare services it provides to patients. The CDM is a listing of every service and supply the facility provides. As the patient is seen at the facility the charges are captured either electronically or manually for services such as the following:

- Accommodations (room and board)
- Room use (for example, emergency room, recovery room, operating room)
- Supplies used during the course of stay (bandages, splints, venipuncture tray)
- Ancillary services (such as radiology, laboratory, pharmacy)
- Clinical services (such as anesthesia, cardiology, physician rounds)

Hospitals charge facility fees—the technical component of healthcare services, for laboratory and radiology tests. It covers the cost and overhead for providing the service. The portion of work performed by a physician or other healthcare professional is the professional component of the charge capture. More information on the professional and technical component of healthcare charges is found in the global payment section of this chapter. The charge capture process flow for a paper-based physician practice is outlined in figure 15.1. Starting with the front office and patient check-in where a new charge slip is generated, payment

Figure 15.1 Paper-based charge capture process for a physician practice

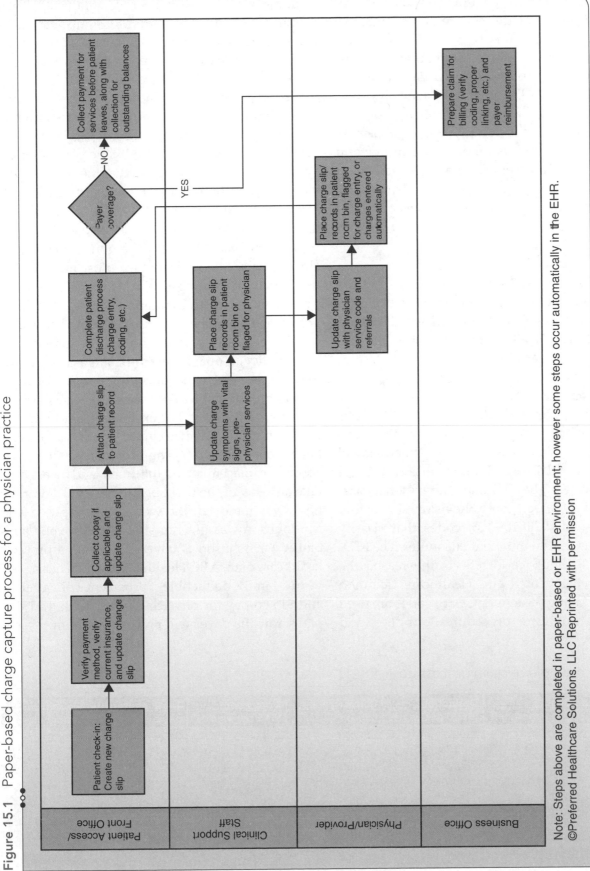

Note: Steps above are completed in paper-based or EHR environment; however some steps occur automatically in the EHR.
©Preferred Healthcare Solutions. LLC Reprinted with permission

Source: Fahrenholz 2010.

method and insurance coverage is verified, co-pay is collected, and the charge slip is attached to the patient record for the visit. The next two steps involve clinical support staff and physicians or providers who update the charge slip as services are rendered. The next step again involves the front office staff where the discharge process is completed. The final step involves the business office, where the claim is prepared for billing and the insurance plan is sent the claim. If the patient does not have insurance coverage the front office staff collects the payment for services rendered (Farenholz 2010).

Healthcare Claims Processing

After all the charges for an episode of care are captured the healthcare facility creates a claim for reimbursement based on the CDM fees listed for each service. The Health Insurance Portability and Accountability Act (HIPAA) mandated the use of electronic transaction for healthcare claims using the *HIPAA X12 837 Healthcare Claim: Professional* for the professional charges and *HIPAA X12 837 Healthcare Claim: Institutional* for the facility and technical component claims. Claim forms include International Classification of Disease, Tenth Revision, Clinical Modification (ICD-10-CM) and International Classification of Disease, Tenth Revision, Procedure Coding System (ICD-10-PCS) codes that classify the diagnosis for the inpatient encounter. The ICD-10-CM, ICD-10-PCS code reflects the reason the patient is being treated and Healthcare Common Procedure Coding System (HCPCS) codes are used to identify healthcare procedures, supplies, and equipmentforoutpatientencountersandhaveadollar value associated with them. More information on ICD-10 and HCPCS codes is found in chapter 5.

The third-party payer receives the claim for reimbursement, determines the eligibility of the patient for coverage, and the medical necessity of the services. **Eligibility** is verification the patient is currently covered by the plan on the date of service and the services provided are covered by the plan. **Medical necessity** is the determination that the services provided will benefit the patient and are needed.

The insurance policy determines the amount the patient pays for deductible, coinsurance, and copayment. **Deductible** is the amount of cost, usually annually, the policyholder must incur before the plan will assume liability for the remaining covered expenses. **Coinsurance** is a pre-established percentage of eligible expenses after the deductible is met (such as 20 percent, though the amount varies by policy). **Copayment (co-pay)** is a cost-sharing measure in which the policyholder pays a fixed dollar amount (flat fee) per service, such as $15 per physician office visit. For example, David Johnson is seen in the urgent care clinic for removal of a fish hook from his thumb. The provider was not sure about the placement of the hook and needed to take an x-ray of the hand before removal. After the hook was removed, the wound was cleaned and Mr. Johnson was given a shot of cefitraxone antibiotic. Mr. Johnson is covered by his employer's healthcare plan, ABC HealthCare, which has a $500 yearly family deductible, 20 percent coinsurance, and $15 co-pay for physician visits. Table 15.1 displays how the payer will process the claim.

Table 15.1 Example of claim processing

Service	Cost (fee schedule)	Deductible ($500 per year)	Coinsurance (20%)	Copayment ($15 per visit)	Total insurance pays	Patient responsibility
Physician visit	$100.00	$50.00	$10.00	$15.00	$25.00	$75.00
Comment		Patient has already paid $450 this year, he has now met his deductible	20% of cost of visit after the deductible is paid. $100 – $50 = $50 and 20% of $50 = $10	Patient pays $15 out of pocket for each visit		
X-ray	$250.00	$0.00	$50.00	$0.00	$200.00	$50.00
Antibiotic	$50.00	$0.00	$10.00	$0.00	$40.00	$10.00
Total	$400.00	$50.00	$70.00	$15.00	$265.00	$135.00

A provider may choose to **accept assignment**, meaning payment is based on a **fee schedule**—a list of services and the amount that the healthcare insurance plan will pay for healthcare claims. The provider will accept the amount paid as payment in full for the service, as opposed to **balance billing** where the provider charges the patient for the remainder of the costs not paid by the insurance plan. Therefore there may be different payment of services within the same facility for the same service depending on the contracted price for that service with each third-party payer. Using the previous example with Mr. Johnson, if the provider accepts assignment from ABC HealthCare the physician agrees to accept $75.00 for the doctor visit instead of his normal $100.00 fee.

Healthcare insurance payers have a variety of reimbursement plans and contract with individual providers and employers for payment such that the same type of service to two different patients may be paid differently depending on each patient's contract or insurance. After a claim is processed, the third-party payer will send notification to the patient in the form of an **explanation of benefits (EOB)**, detailing how the payer processed the claim for payment. The third-party payer will also send a **remittance advice (RA)** to the healthcare provider explaining the process used for the claim and how much they are paying the healthcare provider.

Working the Accounts Receivable

Billing department employees (billers) are responsible for maintaining and working the organization's accounts receivable (AR). AR is a record of the payments owed to the organization by outside entities such as third-party payers and patients. Billers work the AR by monitoring charges payments, adjustments, and write-offs. If a claim has not been paid billers will resubmit the claim to insurance carriers or determine why the claim has not been paid. When a healthcare organization has a contract with a third party payer for services, the difference between what is charged by the healthcare provider and what is paid by the payer is the contractual adjustment (Fahrenholz 2010). The billing department has a detailed list of adjustment codes to monitor all adjustments made to AR.

If a claim was accepted by the payer but payment was denied for any reason, it is important for the billers to explore the reason for the denial and correct any errors in the claim or submit additional documentation requirements requested by the payer. This process is called denial management.

Check Your Understanding 15.1

Instructions: **Answer the following questions by matching the terms with their definitions.**

1. _____ Pre-established percentage of eligible expenses after the deductible is met, such as 20 percent

2. _____ Cost sharing measure in which the policyholder pays a fixed dollar amount per service

3. _____ Process of how patient financial and health information moves into, through, and out of the healthcare facility

4. _____ Policy or contract in which the purchaser (insured) pays a set amount to help cover the cost of medical expenses

5. _____ Paying for services provided with own funds

6. _____ Insurance company

7. _____ Fixed amount paid by policyholder per month

8. _____ Amount of cost (usually annually) the policyholder must incur before the plan will assume liability for the remaining covered expenses
   A. Revenue cycle
   B. Premium
   C. Copayment
   D. Third-party payer
   E. Deductible
   F. Coinsurance
   G. Out-of-pocket
   H. Healthcare insurance

Healthcare Insurers

Healthcare reimbursement systems in the United States are complex and include commercial, managed care, and government-sponsored plans. Each insurer or payer has their own set of reimbursement guidelines, defined by payer contracts with providers, or they may follow federal regulations for reimbursement methodologies. Each insurer or payer may use different reimbursement methodologies for claims from providers (reimbursement methodologies will be discussed in detail later in this chapter).

Commercial Insurance

Many Americans are covered by commercial insurance plans through their employer, purchased individually, or through a group, such as a professional association. These healthcare plans are private, employer-based self-insurance, not-for-profit, and for-profit.

Private Healthcare Insurance

Individuals, self-employed business people, and groups of people (such as associations and religious organizations) are able to purchase commercial insurance, called **private healthcare insurance**, for themselves and their dependents. Typically these plans have high deductibles or limited covered services. A premium for coverage is paid each month to the third-party payer and those funds are used to help pay for healthcare services. Private healthcare insurance plans use the premiums collected from policyholders to pay for healthcare incurred by all the members of the plan who are covered during a particular month.

Employer-Based Coverage

Employer-based coverage is obtained when employees and employers share the cost of premium payment—the employer contributes a portion of the premium amount and the employee also contributes, usually with a direct deduction from his or her paycheck. Employees are usually able to pay an additional premium amount to cover dependents. For example, employees of a company called Cydney's Safe Shelter for Women employs 17 people and the company pays to enroll the employees and their dependents in a Blue Cross Blue Shield plan. Blue Cross and Blue Shield offered the first healthcare plans in the United States in 1929 and remains an insurer to this day.

Employer-Based Self-Insurance Plans

In the 1970s, large companies started to self-insure employees instead of paying into private plans. Companies set aside the cost they would have paid for premiums for health coverage and used those funds to pay the healthcare claims. Employer-based self-insurance is a self-funding arrangement in which an employer funds medical expenses for the covered beneficiaries and contracts with a **third-party administrator (TPA)** to provide the administrative oversight to process the medical claims payments for the employer. A third-party administrator is responsible for payment of healthcare claims on behalf of the company. For example, Community Hospital has 4,000 employees and offers healthcare insurance coverage for those employees. Community Hospital is self-insured and contracts with ABC Insurance Provider to administer the insurance plan for the hospital. Community Hospital sets aside the amount of money they would pay for premiums for healthcare coverage. When an employee healthcare claim is sent to ABC Insurance Provider the claim is paid from these funds Community Hospital has allocated. Many factors affect an employer's decision to self-fund, particularly the ability to assume the risk involved when a claim for high-cost services is experienced. For example, one case of cancer in an employee may cost the employer a large amount of money in a short period of time causing the employer to not be able to assume the risk for future high-cost medical cases.

Not-for-Profit and For-Profit Healthcare Plans

Commercial healthcare insurance plans are either not-for-profit or for-profit plans. Not-for-profit third-party payers do not focus on making money; the premiums collected pay for the administrative costs of running the company and the company receives tax breaks that the for-profit plan does not. As part of the ACA, Consumer Operated and Oriented Plans or CO-OPs were created. Low-interest loans are available to eligible nonprofit groups to provide insurance coverage to the nonprofit organization (CMS 2015b).

A for-profit plan exists to make money from the premiums collected. The ACA requires healthcare insurance companies to report the amount of premium revenue it collects that is spent on clinical services and quality improvement; this is known as the medical loss ratio (MLR). The MLR requires companies spend at least 80 percent of premium money on medical care. The ACA also requires the company to issue rebates to enrollees if the percentage falls below these standards (CMS 2015c).

Managed Care

Managed care is a healthcare delivery system, or network, organized to manage cost, utilization, and quality. Managed care plans contract with healthcare providers and medical facilities to provide care for members of the plan at reduced costs. Plans restricting choices usually cost less while a flexible plan will cost more. There are three types of managed care plans addressed:

- Health maintenance organizations (HMO)
- Preferred provider organizations (PPO)
- Point of service (POS) (MedlinePlus 2016)

A managed care organization (MCO) is a type of healthcare organization that delivers medical care and handles all aspects of the care and payment for care by limiting providers of care, discounting payment to providers of care, or limiting access to care. For example, a provider may agree to see enrollees of an MCO for a set payment per member per month, also referred to as capitation, which is discussed in full later in the chapter. Members of an MCO are called enrollees and have access to services including physician, inpatient, preventive, prenatal, emergency, and home healthcare (Casto 2015). The National Committee for Quality Assurance (NCQA) is a private, not-for-profit organization whose mission is to improve healthcare quality by accrediting, assessing, and reporting the quality of managed care plans. Enrollees can find information regarding the quality of care, access, and cost, and compare managed care plans, because the Centers for Medicare and Medicaid Services (CMS) collects data via the Healthcare Effectiveness Data and Information Set (HEDIS) (NCQA 2016).

Health Maintenance Organization

A health maintenance organization (HMO) is an entity that combines the provision of healthcare insurance and the delivery of healthcare services. It is characterized by an organized healthcare delivery system to a specific geographic area. The HMO has a set of basic and supplemental health maintenance and treatment services that are provided to voluntarily enrolled members. The members pay a predetermined fixed amount per month or year as prepayments for coverage. HMOs provide for care within their network, where patients are seen by providers and within facilities the HMO controls and owns. A wide range of healthcare services are offered through HMOs such as family health, gynecology, well-child visits, radiology, surgical, obstetrics, inpatient, or therapies. Typically HMOs offer a broader range of preventative healthcare services than other managed care plans (CMS 2011).

HMOs started as a way to provide healthcare at reduced cost to the consumer. The Health Maintenance Organization Act of 1973 established federal rules defining the operation of HMOs. The Act made it easier for HMOs to grow and attract clients and required all employers that offered traditional healthcare to their employees to sign up for an HMO if they had more than 25 employees. Under all types of HMOs, every employer pays the same monthly premium for services. Each employee is assigned a primary care physician—a doctor who bears the ultimate responsibility for ensuring the employee receives the medical care he or she needs. If an employee has a medical condition, he or she first visits the primary care physician. If the condition is beyond the physician's expertise or scope, the physician refers the employee to another doctor within the HMO. If emergency treatment is needed, the employee is referred to hospitals within the HMO; likewise, the employee obtains medication from pharmacies within the HMO network. Most HMOs are extensive enough to offer a wide variety of providers, described as follows.

- *Group model HMOs:* In this model the HMO contracts with more than one physician; for example, a medical group that includes physicians in multiple fields of expertise. The members of the medical group provide the care to the HMO enrollees on a fee-for-service basis (Casto 2015).
- *Open-panel model or independent practice associations:* This model is created when the HMO contracts with a physician who has his or her own practice and the physician agrees

to see the patients who belong to the HMO in addition to their regular patients (Casto 2015).

- *Network model HMOs:* In this model the HMO contracts with a network of providers who provide multispecialty group practices. Reimbursement for healthcare is either on a fee-for-service or capitation basis.
- *Staff model HMOs:* In this model HMO the physicians are employed by the HMO. Physicians see only members of the HMO and are paid a salary by the HMO. The premiums paid by enrollees to the HMO are used to cover the cost of services and facilities.

Preferred Provider Organization

A **preferred provider organizations (PPO)** is a managed care contract-coordinated care plan with the following elements:

- Contains a network of providers who have agreed to a contractually specified reimbursement for covered benefits with the organization offering the plan
- Provides for reimbursement for all covered benefits regardless of whether the benefits are provided with the network of providers
- Offered by an organization that is not licensed or organized under state law as an HMO (CMS 2011)

A PPO is a form of managed care closest to a fee-for-service where providers agree to accept lower fees from the insurer for services to be part of the network, with the patient paying a set copayment. If a patient sees a provider outside the network, the patient will pay a higher fee (CMS 2011).

Point-of-Service Plans

A **point-of-service plan (POS)** allows enrollees to choose between an HMO or PPO each time he or she is in need of care. Payment for services outside of the network is covered by the plan with the patient paying a percentage of the bill. If the primary care provider refers a patient outside of the network of providers, the plan pays all or most of the bill. If the patient sees a provider outside the network and the service is covered by the plan, the patient will have to pay a percentage of the bill as coinsurance, or if the service is not covered by the plan the patient will pay out of pocket for the entire bill

Exclusive Provider Organizations

Exclusive provider organizations (EPO) are hybrid MCOs in that they provide benefits to subscribers only when healthcare services are performed by network providers. Self-insured (self-funded) employers or associations use this model that has characteristics of both HMOs and PPOs.

Government-Sponsored Healthcare Plans

The US government is the largest payer of healthcare insurance. According to CMS, 100 million people are covered through Medicare, Medicaid, the Children's Health Insurance Program, and the Health Insurance Marketplace (CMS 2015d). Medicare Part A, Part B, and Part D; the Medicare Advantage Plan; and the Conditions of Participation will be described in the sections that follow, as well as Medicaid eligibility criteria, services, the Medicare–Medicaid relationship, State Children's Health Insurance plans, TRICARE, the Veterans Administration, CHAMPVA, Indian Health Services, and workers' compensation.

Medicare

Medicare was enacted as Title XVIII amendment to the Social Security Act of 1935. Implemented in 1965, Medicare extended health coverage to most Americans age 65 or older or those receiving retirement benefits from Social Security or the Railroad Retirement Board (CMS 2015e). Medicare is financed through payroll taxes paid by workers. CMS is responsible for management of the Medicare program. To be eligible for Medicare coverage, enrollees—called **beneficiaries**—must fall into one of six benefit categories: be age 65 or older, be a retired federal employees who is enrolled in the civil service retirement system, have end-stage renal disease, be a disabled adult, have become disabled before the age of 18, or be

a spouse of an entitled individual. Medicare contracts with **Medicare Administrative Contractors (MAC)**, which are private insurance companies that serve as Medicare's agent in the administration of the Medicare program, including payment of claims (CMS 2015e).

The next section will define Medicare Parts A and B, Medicare Advantage Plan, and Medicare Part D. The Medicare Conditions of Participation are also discussed.

Medicare Part A Hospital Insurance

Medicare Part A hospital insurance assists in covering inpatient care in hospitals, including critical access hospitals and skilled nursing facilities (not custodial or long-term care). It also assists in covering hospice care and some home healthcare. Beneficiaries must meet certain conditions to receive these benefits such as having paid enough Medicare taxes while they were working, being age 65 or older, or being disabled before the age of 65 (CMS 2015f). Most people do not have to pay for Part A coverage because they or a spouse paid Medicare and payroll taxes while working that funds their part A coverage. Individuals may be able to buy coverage if they are not entitled to Medicare if they did not pay enough Medicare taxes while working. Some states may help pay for Part A for people with limited income and resources (CMS 2015f).

Medicare Part B Medical Insurance

Medicare Part B medical insurance is an optional and supplemental portion of Medicare for which beneficiaries pay a monthly premium. Part B assists with coverage for physicians' services and outpatient care. It also insures other medical services not covered under Part A, such as some physical and occupational therapists' services, and some home healthcare. Part B pays for these covered services and supplies when they are medically necessary (CMS 2015b). To be **medically necessary**, the services or supplies required to diagnose or treat a medical condition meet accepted standards of medical practice. Services covered may include physicians' services, outpatient care, home health, durable medical equipment, ambulance, and preventive services. Preventive services include healthcare services to prevent illness (for example, vaccinations to prevent diseases like polio) or early detection tests and diagnostic tools, when treatment is most likely to be effective (CMS 2015g).

Medicare Part C: Medicare Advantage Plan

Medicare Advantage (MA) Plans were created as part of the Balanced Budget Act (BBA) of 1997. They are sometimes called Part C or MA Plans, and are insurance plans offered by private companies approved by Medicare. For example, United Healthcare insurance plan contracts with Medicare to cover beneficiaries who choose this plan. MA Plans cover all Medicare services, but may also offer extra coverage, such as dental, vision, and acupuncture. Beneficiaries who join an MA Plan have Medicare Part A and B coverage through the MA Plan and not from original Medicare Part A (CMS 2015h).

Medicare pays a fixed amount for the beneficiary's care each month to the companies offering MA Plans. Each MA Plan can charge different out-of-pocket costs and have different guidelines for how services are received; for example, requiring a referral before seeing a specialist (CMS 2015h).

Medicare Part D, Prescription Drug Coverage

Medicare Part D provides various plan options for beneficiaries to obtain prescription drug coverage. Medicare Part D was created by the Medicare Prescription Drug Improvement and Modernization Act (MMA) in 2003. Medicare contracts with private insurance companies to provide drug coverage to beneficiaries. Enrollment is voluntary and only available to people who are covered under Parts A and B. Benefits and cost vary by the plan in which the beneficiary is enrolled and can be as low as $15 per month, with an annual deductible and co-pay required (CMS 2015c).

Out-of-Pocket Expenses and Medigap Insurance

Medicare does not pay 100 percent of medical claims. Medicare beneficiaries pay out-of-pocket for the deductible, co-pay, and noncovered services portions of healthcare claims. Beneficiaries may purchase supplemental insurance—known as Medigap—to help cover those expenses.

Medicaid

Medicaid helps with medical costs for millions of Americans with low incomes and limited resources including the mandatory eligibility groups of children, pregnant women, elderly adults, people with disabilities, and low-income adults. The program is funded jointly by the US federal government and state governments (CMS 2015i). Each state administers its own Medicaid program and determines the type, amount, duration, and scope of services above and beyond the basic broad federal guidelines. This means that Medicaid programs can vary widely between states. The federal government establishes a set of mandatory benefits and states can choose to provide additional optional benefits beyond the required benefits.

States can apply to CMS for a waiver of federal law to expand health coverage beyond the mandatory eligibility groups. Many states have opted to expand Medicaid coverage, especially for children, above the federal minimums because they feel that the federal minimums do not provide enough coverage. Medicaid eligibility criteria, services, the Medicaid–Medicare relationship, and the state Children's Health Insurance Plan are defined as follows.

Medicaid Eligibility Criteria

Medicaid eligibility is based on the annual income of a person or his or her family and is calculated in relation to a percentage of the federal poverty level (FPL), which is the minimum amount of gross income that a family receives in a year to be able to be eligible for Medicaid coverage. The FPL is determined by the Department of Health and Human Services (HHS) and is updated annually on the Medicaid website (CMS 2015j). The ACA set the national Medicaid minimum eligibility level at 133 percent of the FPL, for nearly all Americans under the age of 65. This means if the FPL for a family of one is $11,770 per year the 133 percent FPL would be $15,651 ($11,770 \times 133\% = 15,651$).

Non-financial eligibility criteria include proof of federal and state residency, immigration status, and documentation of US citizenship.

Medicaid Services

States establish and administer Medicaid programs and determine the type, amount, duration, and scope of services within broad federal guidelines. Common mandatory benefit services include coverage of the following care and services.

- Inpatient hospital
- Outpatient hospital
- Nursing facility
- Physician
- Home healthcare
- Rural health clinic
- Laboratory and x-ray
- Family planning
- Tobacco cessation

Common optional benefits include coverage of the following care and services.

- Prescription drugs
- Physical, occupational, speech, hearing, and language therapy
- Optometry
- Dental
- Chiropractic
- Hospice

The Medicare–Medicaid Relationship

The Federal Coordinated Healthcare Office (Medicare–Medicaid Coordination Office) serves people who are enrolled in both Medicare and Medicaid and are known as **dual eligible**, meaning they are covered under both Medicare and Medicaid. The goal is for enrollees who are dual eligible to have full access to seamless, high quality healthcare and to make the system as cost-effective as possible (CMS 2015k). The Medicare–Medicaid Coordination Office, established by the ACA, works across federal and state agencies to align coordination of benefits (COB) between the programs. COB determines the financial responsibility for payment of medical claims when one or more payers are involved. The goals of the office are to:

- Provide access to people who are covered by both Medicare and Medicaid
- Make the process easier for dual eligible people

- Provide quality healthcare
- Help with understanding the programs
- Eliminate regulatory conflicts
- Prevent shifting costs from one program to the other
- Improve the transitions of care
- Improve the quality of service and suppliers (CMS 2015l)

State Children's Health Insurance Plan

The **Children's Health Insurance Program (CHIP)** provides healthcare coverage to eligible children through both Medicaid and individual state CHIP programs. Eligibility is based on a percentage of the family's annual income based on the FPL for the current year. Like all Medicaid programs, CHIP is administered by states according to federal requirements and is funded jointly by states and the federal government. States are able to choose to impose limited enrollment fees, premiums, deductibles, coinsurance, and copayments for children and pregnant women, usually five percent of a family's annual income. **Cost sharing** is prohibited for some services. Cost sharing is the amount that a patient pays for a medical service out of pocket; for example, a healthcare provider who performs a well-baby check must accept the amount Medicaid pays as payment in full.

TRICARE

The US Department of Defense operates **TRICARE**, which is a major part of the Military Health System and is the healthcare program for uniformed service members (active, Guard or Reserve, and retired) and their families. TRICARE is managed by the Defense Health Agency under leadership of the Assistant Secretary of Defense for Health Affairs and is a regionally managed healthcare program with an expansive provider network that combines the resources of military hospitals and clinics with civilian healthcare networks (DHA 2015). Several healthcare plan options are available for members, depending on their circumstances, and include emergency care, urgent care, preventative services, hospitalization, dental, and pharmacy coverage. Table 15.2 displays some of the plan options.

Table 15.2 TRICARE options

Option	Definition	Annual fee	Annual deductible	Co-pay amount
TRICARE Prime and Prime Remote	Managed care option offering the most affordable and comprehensive coverage Prime remote covers remote US stations Overseas options for active duty families living overseas	No annual fee	No deductible	No co-pay
TRICARE Standard and Extra	A fee-for-service plan available to all nonactive duty beneficiaries Most freedom to choose providers	No annual fee	$50/Individual $100/Family	15% of negotiated fee
TRICARE Reserve Select and Retired Reserve	A premium-based healthcare plan that qualified National Guard and Reserve members may purchase	Monthly premiums apply	$50/Individual $100/Family	No co-pay
TRICARE For Life	Offers secondary coverage to people who have Medicare Parts A and B	No annual fee but must have Medicare	No deductible	No co-pay
TRICARE Young Adult Options	A premium-based, worldwide healthcare plan that qualified adult children of eligible sponsors may purchase	Monthly premiums apply	No deductible	$12 per visit outpatient $11 per day inpatient
US Family Health Plan	Available through networks of community-based, not-for-profit healthcare systems in six areas of the United States	Enrollment is required with one year commitment to receive care from the plan	No deductible	No co-pay

Source: Adapted from TRICARE 2015.

Veterans Health Administration

The US Department of Veterans Affairs operates the nation's largest integrated healthcare system, **Veterans Health Administration (VA)**, with more than 1,700 hospitals, clinics, community living centers, domiciliaries, readjustment counseling centers, and other facilities. The VA offers a variety of healthcare services from basic primary care to nursing home care for eligible veterans. The number of veterans who can be enrolled in the healthcare program is determined by the amount of money Congress gives the VA each year.

Civilian Health and Medical Program of the Department of Veterans Affairs

The **Civilian Health and Medical Program of the Department of Veterans Affairs (CHAMPVA)** is a comprehensive healthcare program in which the VA shares the cost of covered healthcare services and supplies with eligible beneficiaries.

The program is administered by the Chief Business Office Purchased Care (CBOPC). CHAMPVA covers most healthcare services medically and psychologically necessary. To be eligible for CHAMPVA, you cannot be eligible for TRICARE, and you must be in one of these categories:

- The spouse or child of an eligible veteran
- The spouse or child of a veteran who died as a result of service injury
- The spouse or child of a veteran who was totally disabled at the times of their death.
- The spouse or child of a military member who died while serving in the military (DVA 2015)

Indian Health Services

The **Indian Health Service (IHS)** is an HHS agency responsible for providing healthcare to American Indians and Alaska Natives within the

United States. The provision of health services to members of federally recognized Native tribes grew out of a special government-to-government relationship between the federal government and Indian tribes. The Indian Self-Determination Act of 1975 turned control of healthcare facilities and programs over to Native and Indian tribes within the United States (IHS 2015). Each tribal government is responsible for the healthcare of its tribal members. The IHS is divided into 12 physical areas of the United States, Alaska, Albuquerque, Bemidji, Billings, California, Great Plains, Headquarters, Nashville, Navajo, Oklahoma, Phoenix, Portland, and Tucson. Each area works collaboratively to provide healthcare services to all American Indians and Alaska Natives who live within its areas (IHS 2015). For example, a Native Alaskan living in California can receive care at an IHS facility in California. If an IHS facility is not available for a patient the tribe may use contract funds to pay for coverage at another facility. This relationship, established in 1787, is based on Article I, Section 8 of the Constitution. Numerous treaties, laws, Supreme Court decisions, and executive orders are responsible for what the agency is today. The IHS is the principal federal healthcare provider and health advocate for American Indian and Native people, and its goal is to raise their health status to the highest possible level (IHS 2015). Every IHS facility in the United States sets its own standard of coverage and services. For example, in Alaska there are 10 service areas, some with hospitals, clinics, or small rural health centers.

Workers' Compensation

Most employers in the United States are required to carry **workers' compensation** insurance for employees who are injured on the job. Workers' compensation laws are regulated by state and federal government and vary by state. A notice of injury report is completed by the employee and provider for claim payment to be processed. The notice of injury report details what happened and how the injury occurred, the provider then adds details to the report indicating the diagnosis and anticipated healthcare services that will be required. When a claim is sent to the workers' compensation insurance carrier the notice of injury report must be submitted with each claim for payment.

Federal Workers' Compensation Funds

Federal employees are covered under the Federal Employees' Compensation Act (FECA) of 1916. The Department of Labors' Office of Workers' Compensation Programs (OWCP) administers four major disability compensation programs for federal employees or their dependents if the employee is injured at work. The four programs include:

- Divisions of Federal Employees' Compensation (DFEC)
- Division of Energy Employees Occupational Illness Compensation (DEEOIC)
- Division of Longshore and Harbor Workers' Compensation (DLHWC)
- Division of Coal Mine Workers' Compensation (DCMWC)

The benefits include disability, wage replacement, medical treatment, and vocational rehabilitation for workers injured on the job (DOL 2015).

State Workers' Compensation Funds

Before state workers' compensation laws were introduced, companies were reluctant to provide insurance coverage for employees because of the high costs for workers injured on the job. Most states addressed the concern by introducing state workers' compensation insurance funds as a source of coverage for claims occurring because of workplace injury. State workers' compensation funds are maintained by each state from employer-paid premiums. Benefits may include compensation for burial, life insurance coverage for dependents upon death, compensation for lost income, and health coverage for medical care (Casto 2015).

Check Your Understanding 15.2

Instructions: **Answer the following questions.**

1. Which insurance provides coverage to most Americans age 65 or older?
   A. TRICARE
   B. IHS
   C. Medicare
   D. Medicaid

2. The number of veterans who can be enrolled in the healthcare program is determined by the amount of money Congress allocates to whom each year?
   A. VA
   B. TRICARE
   C. CHAMPVA
   D. Workers' compensation

3. Mandatory eligibility groups fall under which insurance?
   A. CHAMPVA
   B. CHIP
   C. IHS
   D. Medicaid

4. The spouse or child of a veteran who has been rated permanently and totally disabled for a service-connected disability would qualify for which program?
   A. TRICARE
   B. CHAMPVA
   C. VA
   D. CHIP

5. If a hospital employee lifts a box filled with medical records off of a shelf and subsequently pulls a shoulder muscle, for which type of insurance would he or she be eligible?
   A. Workers' compensation
   B. Medicaid
   C. IHS
   D. TRICARE

6. Which government health program was introduced out of a special government-to-government relationship?
   A. Medicare
   B. Tricare
   C. IHS
   D. Workers' compensation

7. A patient visits a primary care physician and the medical issue is beyond the physician's expertise or scope, so the patient is referred to another doctor within which of the following?
   A. HMO
   B. PPO
   C. POS
   D. High-deductible plan

New Trends

Revenue management and reimbursement professionals must stay current with changes in laws and regulations that affect the revenue cycle and billing guidelines. New trends in recent years include the healthcare insurance marketplace, consumer-directed healthcare plans, hospital-acquired conditions, and present on admission indicator reporting.

Health Insurance Marketplace or Exchange

The Patient Protection and Affordable Care Act (ACA) was signed into law in 2010. The ACA established a health insurance marketplace or exchange where uninsured, eligible Americans are able to purchase federally regulated and subsidized healthcare insurance. People who are not covered by insurance through a job, Medicare, Medicaid, CHIP, or another source are able to purchase insurance through a marketplace exchange. The exchange offers healthcare insurance to members based on their income. Most people who apply qualify for premium tax credits, which lowers the cost of coverage. All plans cover essential health benefits, pre-existing conditions, and preventive care (HealthCare.gov 2015).

Consumer-Directed Health Plans

Consumer-directed health plans (CDHP), also known as high-deductible plans (HDPs) because the deductible is at least $1,200 per year, are managed care organizations characterized by influencing patients and clients to select cost-efficient healthcare through the provision of information about health benefit packages and through financial incentives. Employers shift payment responsibility to plan members causing employees to opt for the HDP option to save money on premiums. The ACA mandates that HDPs purchased after March 2010 provide free preventive services even if the deductible has not been met.

Hospital-Acquired Conditions and Present on Admission Indicator Reporting

The ACA established the hospital-acquired conditions (HAC) reduction program to encourage hospitals to reduce HACs. An HAC is a reasonably preventable condition that a patient did not have upon admission to a hospital, but that developed during the hospital stay. Examples of HACs include foreign object retained after surgery, blood incompatibility, falls, and infections.

Hospital performance under the HAC reduction program is determined based on a hospital's total HAC score, which can range from 1 to 10. The higher a hospital's total HAC score, the worse the hospital performed under the HAC reduction program. Hospitals are given an opportunity to review their data and request a recalculation of their scores if they believe an error in the score calculation has occurred. The law requires the Secretary of the Department of Health and Human Services to reduce payments to hospitals that rank in the quartile of hospitals with the highest total HAC scores by one percent (CMS 2015l). Present on admission (POA) indicates that a condition was present at the time the patient was admitted to the hospital. When submitting claims to Medicare for MS-DRG reimbursement the POA indicator includes:

Y: Diagnosis was present at the time of admission

N: Diagnosis was not present

U: Documentation is insufficient to determine if condition was present

W: It is clinically undermined if the condition was present (CMS 2015m)

Patient Protection and the Affordable Care Act

The ACA includes a number of provisions designed to encourage improvements in the quality of care and includes comprehensive healthcare insurance reforms. For example, Medicare's hospital readmissions reduction program requires a reduction in payment to a hospital if the hospital has what is considered excessive readmission rates. A readmission includes hospital admission within 30 days of a subsequent hospitalization (CMS 2015l). Another outcome of the ACA is the creation of accountable care organizations (ACO). The ACO agrees "to be held accountable for improving the health and experience of care for individuals and improving the health of populations while reducing the rate of growth in healthcare spending" (CMS 2015l).

Utilization Management

Utilization management (UM) is the evaluation of the medical necessity, appropriateness, and efficiency of the use of healthcare services, procedures, and facilities under the provisions of the applicable health benefits plan, sometimes called utilization review. **Prospective review** refers to the review that takes place prior to elective procedures and admissions. This is achieved through a precertification process for elective admissions, certain diagnostic procedures, and outpatient surgeries. Utilization management professionals, who may be clinical nurses, physicians or mid-level providers, use clinical screening processes to apply consistent standards when determining if the service is medically necessary. One tool is preauthorization, which reviews proposed surgeries and other inpatient and outpatient healthcare services before the patient is admitted. **Concurrent review** involves screening for medical necessity and the appropriateness and timeliness of the delivery of medical care from the time of admission until discharge. **Retrospective review** includes review and analysis of actual utilization data after the patient has been discharged. The retrospective review may be conducted by a committee of the organization or an outside quality improvement organization (QIO), which is an organization that performs medical peer review of coding information for completeness, adequacy, and quality of care, as well as the appropriateness of payments. An outside review may find errors in daily operations performance that are missed by the organization. UM professionals monitor inpatient utilization daily by reviewing a list of all patients, their diagnosis, the requested length of stay versus the actual length of stay, and other information that help to continually manage inpatient activity to determine medical necessity as well as reimbursement for the inpatient stay.

Case Management

Case management is collaboration between healthcare and service providers to aid in the process of assessment, planning, facilitation, care coordination, evaluation, and advocacy to meet the comprehensive health needs of an individual or family. This is accomplished through communication and coordination of available resources to promote quality and cost-effective outcomes. The primary reason for case management is the facilitation of care across the continuum of care for the patient. For example, a patient newly diagnosed with cancer may require surgery, laboratory services, chemotherapy, radiation, and counseling services. Case management helps navigate all the services and providers for the patient.

The ultimate goal of case management is for the individual to reach the optimum level of wellness and functional capability. A case manager is usually a nurse, physician, or social worker who arranges all services that are needed by a patient and his or her family, for example, continued care or social services. They accomplish this by identifying the continued needs of the patient and determine the resources that are available to the patient.

Case managers use a multi-disciplinary approach to optimize the outcome. This approach brings together many services from medical, social service, therapies, and such (CMSA 2015).

Healthcare Reimbursement Methodologies

Healthcare services can be reimbursed in a number of ways depending on the type of insurance coverage and the type of service provided. This section discusses fee-for-service, episode of care, capitation, global payment, resource-based relative value scale, skilled nursing payment, and prospective payments.

Fee-for-Service Reimbursement

Fee-for-service reimbursement is a reimbursement method through which providers retrospectively receive payment based on either billed charges for services provided or annually updated fee schedules. A provider submits a claim form to a healthcare plan with all charges itemized. In fee-for-service reimbursement, the itemized charges are individually assessed and paid.

Pay for Performance

Pay for performance is a type of incentive to improve clinical performance using the electronic health record resulting in additional reimbursement or eligibility for grants or other subsidies to support further health information technology efforts. The goal is to improve the quality, efficiency, and overall value of healthcare. The ACA expands the use of pay for performance in Medicare with the idea that paying providers to achieve better outcomes should improve those outcomes (CMS 2013).

The typical pay-for-performance program provides a bonus to healthcare providers if they meet or exceed agreed-upon quality or performance measures; for example, reductions in hemoglobin

A1c in diabetic patients. The programs may also reward improvement in performance over time, such as year-to-year decreases in the rate of avoidable hospital readmissions (CMS 2013).

Traditional Fee-for-Service Reimbursement

In **traditional fee-for-service (FFS) reimbursement** systems, third-party payers or patients issue payments to healthcare providers after healthcare services have been received (for example, after the patient has been discharged from the hospital). Payments are based on the specific services delivered.

After services are rendered an itemized claim for all service charges is submitted to a healthcare plan for payment. Payment is based on the billed charges taking into account discounted charges, negotiated rates, and usual or customary charges for a geographic area. **Usual, customary, and reasonable (UCR) charges** is a type of fee-for-service payment method in which the third-party payer remunerates fees that are usual for the provider's practice, customary for the community, and reasonable for the situation.

The traditional FFS reimbursement methodology is used by many commercial insurance companies for visits to physician's offices.

Managed Fee-for-Service Reimbursement

Managed FFS reimbursement involves utilization controls for reimbursement under traditional fee-for service insurance plans, in that managed care plans control costs by handling their members' use of healthcare services. Managed care plans negotiate with providers to develop discounted fee schedules.

Controlling utilization of services includes both prospective and retrospective reviews of planned healthcare services. A type of prospective review involves precertification, or obtaining approval from a healthcare insurance company before a healthcare service is rendered. For example, a patient with a strong family history of colon cancer needs prior approval to receive a screening colonoscopy before the age approved by a healthcare plan.

Retrospective utilization review process involves evaluation of utilization information after the patient has been discharged or the care has been completed. Utilization review also includes discharge planning—coordinating the activities related to the release of a patient when inpatient hospital care is no longer needed. The managed care plan controls cost by providing a less intensive, and therefore less expensive, care setting as soon as possible.

Episode-of-Care Reimbursement Methodologies

An episode-of-care (EOC) reimbursement is given for a relatively continuous medical treatment provided by the healthcare professional in relation to a particular clinical problem or situation. For example, an obstetrician who charges a patient a flat fee for the entire episode of pregnancy and delivery; or a patient receiving follow-up care for the first 60 days after a stroke. In home health services, all services and supplies provided to a patient for a 60-day period are paid by EOC reimbursement.

Capitation

Capitation is a specified amount of money paid to a healthcare plan or doctor to cover the cost of a healthcare plan member's services for a certain length of time (CMS 2016a). The healthcare plan negotiates with an employer or agency for a pre-established amount of money to care for the health services of members. The MCO agrees to provide health services for a period of time, usually one year. Capitated premiums are calculated on the projected cost of providing covered services per patient per month or per member per month.

Global Payment

Global payment methodology involves payment that combines the professional and technical components of a procedure and disperses payments as a lump sum to be split between the physician and the healthcare facility. The professional component of a service is considered the part of the service supplied by physicians (for example, the radiologist), the technical component (for example, supplies, equipment, and support services) is supplied by a hospital or freestanding surgical center. For example:

> A patient receives a chest x-ray.
>
> *Professional component:* Services of the radiologist
>
> *Technical component:* Radiology department use, x-ray equipment
>
> *Global payment:* The facility received a lump-sum payment for the radiologist reading the x-ray and the facility fees to take the x-ray

Prospective Payment

A prospective payment system (PPS) is a method of reimbursement in which Medicare payment is made based on a predetermined, fixed amount. The payment amount for a particular service is derived based on the classification system of that service. CMS uses separate PPSs for reimbursement of the following:

- Acute inpatient hospitals
- Home health agencies
- Hospice
- Hospital outpatient
- Inpatient psychiatric facilities
- Inpatient rehabilitation facilities
- Long-term care hospitals
- Skilled nursing facilities (CMS 2014a)

Medicare Acute Inpatient Prospective Payment System (IPPS)

The inpatient prospective payment system (IPPS) under Medicare Part A is a payment methodology in which payment is based on the diagnosis of the patient. An inpatient stay is categorized into a diagnosis-related group (DRG). A DRG is a unit of case-mix classification in a prospective payment system where diseases are placed into groups because related diseases and treatments tend to consume similar amounts of healthcare resources and incur similar amounts of cost to the hospital. A patient's hospitalization may fall into one of more than 500 diagnostic classifications in which cases demonstrate similar resource consumption and length of stay patterns. Hospitals are paid a set fee for treating patients in a single DRG category, regardless of the actual cost of care. A hospital may receive an adjustment of additional reimbursement of payment if it is a **disproportionate share hospital (DSH)**, which occurs when the DSH treats a high percentage of low income patients (CMS 2015l).

Medicare Severity Diagnosis-Related Groups

The DRG system was updated to **Medicare severity diagnosis-related groups (MS-DRG)** to better account for severity of illness and resource use for inpatient services. The three levels of severity in the MS-DRG system include:

- Major complication/comorbidity (MCC): The patient has a medical condition that arises during an inpatient stay, like a wound infection (complication) or a medical condition that coexists with the primary reason for admission and affects the patient's treatment or length of stay (comorbidity)

- Complication/comorbidity (CC): The patient has a medical condition that is not considered major

- Non-CC: All severity levels are based on the secondary diagnosis; this level of severity indicates the patient does not have a CC (CMS 2013a)

A hospital's **case-mix index (CMI)** represents the average DRG relative weight for a particular hospital. It is calculated by adding the DRG weights for all Medicare discharges for a defined period of time (month, quarter, year) and dividing by the number of discharges within that period of time. The CMI allows administration to measure the

hospital's performance based on MS-DRG cases. CMIs are calculated using both transfer-adjusted cases and unadjusted cases, meaning a patient who is transferred from facility A to facility B to receive a higher level of care and is only at facility A for one day will not receive the entire DRG payment for the patient's diagnosis because the patient was transferred out of the first facility. The payment rate is based on the type of case and resources required to treat the patient. By analyzing the CMI of a facility a manager is able to compare the CMI against other similar facilities in the area, or the year-to-year changes of the facility in its CMI. This analysis allows coding managers to correct coding errors resulting in improper DRG payments in a timely manner and allows administrators to understand the type of patient in the facility to allow and plan for future clinical allocations.

Resource-Based Relative Value Scale System

A **resource-based relative value scale system (RBRVS)** is a payment methodology in which physician payments are determined by the resource costs needed to provide care. The RBRVS scale contains national uniform relative values for all physicians' services. The relative value of each service must be the sum of relative value units representing the physicians' work, practice expenses including the cost of medical malpractice insurance, and the cost of professional liability insurance (AMA 2015). The calculation for payment is based on the three components listed. There may also be an adjustment based on geographical resource costs (CMS 2016b).

Skilled Nursing Facility Prospective Payment System

The BBA of 1997 modified how facilities are paid for skilled nursing facility (SNF) services. SNFs are paid a comprehensive per diem under a PPS, meaning they receive a set amount for each day of service instead of being paid for itemized charges or services. Payment includes all reasonable costs incurred by the facility to provide care in the SNF. The **skilled nursing facility prospective payment** system issues case-mix adjusted payments based on resource utilization group (RUG) classifications, from data collected in the patient assessment.

Adjustments to federal rates are made yearly to reflect geographic differences in wage rates, the hospital wage index, and patient case mix (the relative resource intensity that would typically be associated with each patient's clinical condition) (CMS 2014b).

Outpatient Prospective Payment System

As part of the BBA, CMS started using the **outpatient prospective payment system (OPPS)**—the Medicare prospective payment system used for hospital-based outpatient services and procedures that is predicated on the assignment of **ambulatory payment classifications (APC)**. A single payment is made for all outpatient services that fall within an APC, which is a group consisting of diagnoses and procedures that are similar in terms of resources used, complexity of illness, and conditions represented. A single payment for the outpatient services provided is made. A single visit can result in multiple APC groups. APC groups consist of five types of services: significant procedures, surgical services, medical visits, ancillary services, and partial hospitalization. The OPPS reimburses some hospital outpatient services and certain Medicare Part B services furnished to hospital inpatients when Part A payment cannot be made; for example, implantable devices used in diagnostic testing (CMS 2014a)

Ambulatory Surgery Center Prospective Payment System

For Medicare purposes, an **ambulatory surgery center (ASC)** is a distinct entity that operates exclusively for the purpose of furnishing surgical services to patients who do not require hospitalization and when the expected duration of services does not exceed 24 hours following admission. This definition applies to the ASC no matter who the payer is for the ASC's services (CMS 2015b). Medicare makes a single payment to ASCs for covered surgical procedures, including ASC facility services furnished in connection with the covered

procedure; this is known as the **ambulatory surgery center (ASC) payment rate**. Examples of ASC-covered services include nursing, surgical dressing, administrative costs for the facility, and ancillary services (CMS 2014c).

Home Health Prospective Payment System

The **home health prospective payment system (HH PPS)** was mandated by the BBA. CMS implemented a series payment methodology where visits can be billed in a series of 6, 14, or 20 visits at a time and are paid as a series instead of billing each visit separately. Payment for services provided by home health require that the patient have a current plan of care (POC) from a healthcare provider that defines the services to be provided to the patient. Payment includes all services and supplies provided to the patient during care, except some medication and durable medical equipment provided to the patient. The HH PPS model includes different resource costs for early home health episodes versus later home health episodes and is variable for certain wound and skin conditions (CMS 2014d).

Ambulance Fee Schedule

The BBA mandated the implementation of a national ambulance fee schedule for Medicare Part B. Ambulance transport includes both vehicular and air travel. Medicare will determine the medical necessity for the transportation of a patient by ambulance and if the facility to which the patient is taken is appropriate. For example, a patient living on an island with only a small clinic healthcare facility is in a car accident and receives a broken femur. The clinic calls an air ambulance service to transport the patient to a larger trauma center on the mainland. Payment for ambulance services includes a base rate payment plus a mileage payment to the nearest facility. So, if the base rate for air ambulance for the patient with the broken femur is $3,000 and the mileage was 100 miles at $45 per mile, the total payment would be $3,000 (base rate) + $4,500 ($45 per mile) for a total of $7,500. Rates vary based on geographic area across the United States (CMS 2014e).

Check Your Understanding 15.3

Instructions: **Answer the following questions.**

1. What lump-sum payment is distributed among physicians who perform a procedure or interpret its results and the healthcare facility that provided the equipment, supplies, and technical support required?
   A. OPPS
   B. PPS
   C. Global payment
   D. Case-mix index

Instructions: **Match the terms to the descriptions.**

   A. Resource-based relative value scale
   B. Prospective review
   C. Utilization management
   D. Hospital-acquired conditions
   E. Case management

2. _____ The evaluation of the medical necessity, appropriateness, and efficiency of the use of healthcare services, procedures, and facilities under the provisions of the applicable health benefits plan

3. _____ A group of reasonably preventable conditions that patients do not have upon admission to a hospital, but which develop during the hospital stay

4. _____ Collaboration between healthcare and service providers to aid in the process of assessment, planning, facilitation, care coordination, evaluation, and advocacy to meet the comprehensive health needs of an individual or family

5. _____ Payments for services are determined by the resource costs needed to provide them

6. _____ The review that takes place prior to requested procedures and admissions

Real-World Case 15.1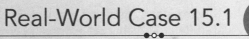

A student from an accredited HIM program was given the project of mapping the revenue cycle for a simple outpatient visit to the Community Health Clinic where she was doing her internship. She started with the registration department and determined the clerks were not obtaining copies of insurance cards but were taking the information orally from patients. She then determined that the coding department was using CPT (current procedural terminology) codes that were from the prior year. Finally, in reviewing the remittance advice notice from the insurance carriers she noticed that the patients were never balance billed for the claim amount for which they were responsible.

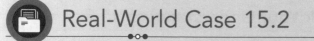 Real-World Case 15.2

Emily Kelley was taken to Sitlan Community Hospital for pain in her side. She was admitted and taken into surgery, where her appendix was removed. In recovery her temperature spiked, and after looking at Emily's labs it was determined she had developed an infection from the surgery. This was not the first surgery where an infection subsequently developed, and the current total HAC score for this hospital was 8. As a result of the high HAC score, the reimbursement to the hospital for Emily's surgery was less than it should have been based on APC grouping. The billers started noticing a decrease in reimbursement, and brought it up to the manager.

References

American Medical Association. 2015. Overview of the RBRVS. http://www.ama-assn.org/ama/pub/physician-resources/solutions-managing-your-practice/coding-billing-insurance/medicare/the-resource-based-relative-value-scale/overview-of-rbrvs.page.

Blumberg, A. and A. Davidson. 2009 (October 22). Accidents of History Created US Health System. National Public Radio. http://www.npr.org/templates/story/story.php?storyId=114045132.

Case Management Society of America (CMSA). 2015. http://www.cmsa.org/.

Casto, A.B. 2015. *Principles of Healthcare Reimbursement*. Chicago: AHIMA.

Centers for Medicare and Medicaid Services. 2016a. Capitation. https://www.cms.gov/apps/glossary/search.asp?Term=capitation&Language=English&SubmitTermSrch=Search.

Centers for Medicare and Medicaid Services. 2016b. Resource-Based Relative Value Scale. https://www.cms.gov/apps/glossary/search.asp?Term=resource-based+relative+value&Language=English&SubmitTermSrch=Search.

Centers for Medicare and Medicaid Services. 2015a. Tracing the History of CMS Programs: From President Theodore Roosevelt to President George W. Bush. https://www.cms.gov/About-CMS/Agency-Information/History/Downloads/PresidentCMSMilestones.pdf.

Centers for Medicare and Medicaid Services. 2015b. Loan Program Helps Support Customer-Driven Non-Profit Health Insurers. https://www.cms.gov/CCIIO/Resources/Grants/new-loan-program.html.

Centers for Medicare and Medicaid Services. 2015c. Medical Loss Ratio. https://www.cms.gov/CCIIO/Programs-and-Initiatives/Health-Insurance-Market-Reforms/Medical-Loss-Ratio.html.

Centers for Medicare and Medicaid Services. 2015d. Medicare. https://www.cms.gov/Medicare/Medicare.html.

Centers for Medicare and Medicaid Services. 2015e. History: CMS' Program History. https://www.cms.gov/About-CMS/Agency-Information/History/index.html?redirect=/History/.

Centers for Medicare and Medicaid Services. 2015f. Medicare Part A. https://www.cms.gov/Medicare/Medicare-General-Information/MedicareGenInfo/Part-A.html.

Centers for Medicare and Medicaid Services. 2015g. Medicare Part B. https://www.cms.gov/Medicare/Medicare-General-Information/MedicareGenInfo/Part-B.html.

Centers for Medicare and Medicaid Services. 2015h. Health Plans—General Information. https://www.cms.gov/Medicare/Health-Plans/HealthPlansGenInfo/.

Centers for Medicare and Medicaid Services. 2015i. Medicaid and CHIP Eligibility Levels. http://www.medicaid.gov/medicaid-chip-program-information/program-information/medicaid-and-chip-eligibility-levels/medicaid-chip-eligibility-levels.html.

Centers for Medicare and Medicaid Services. 2015j. Federal Policy Guidance. http://www.medicaid.gov/federal-policy-guidance/federal-policy-guidance.html.

Centers for Medicare and Medicaid Services. 2015k. About the Medicare-Medicaid Coordination Office. Advance Care for People with Medicaid and Medicare. https://www.cms.gov/Medicare-Medicaid-Coordination/Medicare-and-Medicaid-Coordination/Medicare-Medicaid-Coordination-Office.

Centers for Medicare and Medicaid Services. 2015l. Readmissions Reduction Program. https://www.cms.gov/medicare/medicare-fee-for-service-payment/acuteinpatientpps/readmissions-reduction-program.html.

Centers for Medicare and Medicaid Services. 2015m. Hospital-Acquired Conditions. https://www.cms.gov/Medicare/Medicare-Fee-for-Service-Payment/HospitalAcqCond/Hospital-Acquired_Conditions.html.

Centers for Medicare and Medicaid Services. 2014a. Hospital Outpatient Prospective Payment System. http://www.cms.gov/Outreach-and-Education/Medicare-Learning-Network-MLN/MLNProducts/downloads/HospitalOutpaysysfctsht.pdf.

Centers for Medicare and Medicaid Services. 2014b. Skilled Nursing Facility Prospective Payment System. http://www.cms.gov/Outreach-and-Education/Medicare-Learning-Network-MLN/MLNProducts/downloads/snfprospaymtfctsht.pdf.

Centers for Medicare and Medicaid Services. 2014c. Ambulatory Surgical Center Fee Schedule. https://www.cms.gov/Outreach-and-Education/Medicare-Learning-Network-MLN/MLNProducts/downloads/AmbSurgCtrFeepymtfctsht508-09.pdf.

Centers for Medicare and Medicaid Services. 2014d. Home Health Prospective Payment System. http://www.cms.gov/Outreach-and-Education/Medicare-Learning-Network-MLN/MLNProducts/Downloads/Home-Health-Prospective-Payment-System-Text-Only.pdf.

Centers for Medicare and Medicaid Services. 2014e. Ambulance Fee Schedule. http://www.cms.gov/Medicare/Medicare-Fee-for-Service-Payment/AmbulanceFeeSchedule/.

Centers for Medicare and Medicaid Services. 2013. Acute Care Hospital Inpatient Prospective Payment System. https://www.cms.gov/Outreach-and-Education/Medicare-Learning-Network-MLN/MLNProducts/downloads/AcutePaymtSysfctsht.pdf.

Centers for Medicare and Medicaid Services. 2011. Medicare Managed Care Manual: Chapter 1—General Provisions. https://www.cms.gov/Regulations-and-Guidance/Guidance/Manuals/downloads/mc86c01.pdf.

Defense Health Agency (DHA). 2015. TRICARE. http://www.tricare.mil.

Fahrenholz, C.G. 2010 (September). Show Me the Money… A Look at the Revenue Cycle from the Billing Perspective. 2010 AHIMA Convention Proceedings.

Ferenc, D. 2014. *Understanding Hospital Billing and Coding*, 3rd ed. St. Louis, MO: Elsevier.

Hazelwood, A. and C. Venable. 2012. Reimbursement Methodologies. Chapter 6 in *Health Information Management Technology: An Applied Approach*, 4th ed. Edited by N.B. Sayles. Chicago: AHIMA.

HealthCare.gov. 2015. A Quick Guide to the Health Insurance Marketplace: 4 Tips about the Health Insurance Marketplace. https://www.healthcare.gov/quick-guide/one-page-guide-to-the-marketplace/.

Indian Health Service. 2015. https://www.ihs.gov/.

MedlinePlus. 2016. Managed Care Summary. US National Library of Medicine. https://www.nlm.nih.gov/medlineplus/managedcare.html.

National Committee for Quality Assurance. 2016. About NCQA Overview. http://www.ncqa.org/AboutNCQA.aspx.

TRICARE. 2015. Compare Plans. http://www.tricare.mil/Plans/ComparePlans.aspx.

US Department of Labor (DOL). 2015. Office of Workers' Compensation Programs (OWCP). http://www.dol.gov/owcp/.

US Department of Veterans Affairs (DVA). 2015 CHAMPVA Family Members Insurance. http://www.va.gov/hac/forbeneficiaries/champva/handbook.asp.

16

Fraud and Abuse Compliance

Darline A. Foltz, RHIA
Karen M. Lankisch, PhD, RHIA
Nanette B. Sayles, EdD, RHIA, CCS, CHPS, CHDA, CPHIMS, FAHIMA

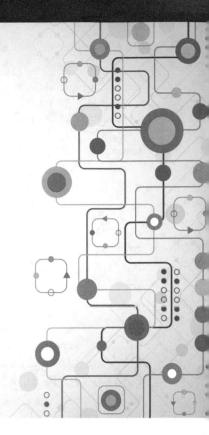

Learning Objectives

- Differentiate among fraud, abuse, and waste
- Identify the elements of a compliance program
- Examine the legal and regulatory requirements related to the management of a compliance program
- Justify the need for the involvement of health information management (HIM) professionals in clinical documentation improvement

- Justify the need for audits
- Assist in the monitoring of compliance metrics
- Identify the standards required to meet the terms of the compliance plan

Key Terms

Abuse
All patient refined diagnosis-related groups (APR-DRGs)
Anti-Kickback Statute
Audit
Automated reviews
Balanced Budget Act of 1997
Benchmarking
Certified EHR technology
Clinical documentation improvement
Coding compliance plan

Compliance
Compliance program
Comorbidity
Complex review
Complication
Computer-assisted coding (CAC)
Eligible professional
False Claims Act
Fraud
Health Care Fraud Prevention and Enforcement Action Team (HEAT)

Health Insurance Portability and Accountability Act (HIPAA)
Hospital-acquired conditions (HAC)
Key indicator
Meaningful Use
Medicare Fraud Strike Force
Natural language processing (NLP)
Noncovered services
Office of Inspector General (OIG)
Overpayment

Present on admission (POA)	Reasonable cause	Severity of illness (SOI)
Quality improvement organization (QIO)	Reasonable diligence	Unbundling
	Recovery audit contractor (RAC)	Upcoding
	Risk of mortality (ROM)	Waste
Qui tam	Semi-automated reviews	Willful neglect

Payers of healthcare services, including federal and state governments, private insurance companies, and patients trust that physicians and all healthcare professionals render high quality medical care to their patients and submit accurate claims for payment while upholding the highest ethical standards. While most healthcare professionals strive to meet these expectations, there are some dishonest healthcare professionals who exploit the healthcare system illegally for personal gain. In addition to dishonest healthcare professionals, there are healthcare organizations that have poor billing policies and procedures in place resulting in unintentional billing errors. These instances have created the need for laws to combat fraud and abuse to ensure appropriate quality medical care.

While the terms *fraud* and *abuse* are often used together, there is a distinct difference between them. Fraud is "when someone intentionally executes or attempts to execute a scheme to obtain money or property of any healthcare benefit program" (CMS 2014a, 4). The key word in this definition is *intentionally*. An example of fraud is billing for services not provided to the patient. Abuse occurs "when healthcare providers or suppliers perform actions that directly or indirectly result in unnecessary costs to any healthcare benefit program" (CMS 2014a, 4). An example of abuse is a pattern of coding errors. In the case of abuse, the healthcare provider is entitled to payment but requests more reimbursement than he or she deserves. Mistakes happen in the course of doing business, so one or two errors will not usually result in accusations of abuse. It is only when a consistent pattern is evident that abuse allegations occur. Another related term is waste, the overutilization or inappropriate utilization of services and misuse of resources, and typically is not a criminal or intentional act. Examples of waste include having too many supplies on hand and being required to destroy them when the expiration date passes, or ordering more

ancillary tests than may be required to treat the patient (NAMD 2012).

Any inappropriate payment made to a healthcare organization for any reason is considered an improper or inappropriate payment. Improper payments are discussed later in the chapter. Mistakes will occur in the process of billing for healthcare services and may result in an incorrect payment to a healthcare organization. A mistake is considered the most innocent of improper payments since there is no intent to falsely receive an incorrect payment from a healthcare plan. The next level in the spectrum of improper payment is inefficiencies. This is a more serious type of error that occurs when billing insurance companies since ongoing inefficiencies may demonstrate a lack of an effort to bill correctly, resulting in improper payments and waste of insurance plan staff and resources. Bending the rules is the next level of improper payments, and meets the definition of abuse, since it demonstrates that a healthcare provider consistently chooses to bill in the provider's favor when billing rules allow for some interpretation. Intentional deception is clearly the most serious and highest level of improper payments since this reflects a healthcare provider's purposeful incorrect billing to result in improper payments, falling under the definition of fraud. This progression is shown in figure 16.1.

The risk for fraud and abuse exists in all organizations so compliance measures must be taken. Compliance is the process of establishing an organizational culture that promotes the prevention, detection, and resolution of instances of conduct that do not conform to federal, state, or private payer healthcare program requirements or the healthcare organization's ethical and business policies. In other words, compliance actively prevents fraud and abuse. This chapter will cover the regulations and initiatives, organizations involved and tools used in fighting fraud, coding fraud and abuse, and clinical documentation improvement.

Figure 16.1 Progression, types, and causes of inappropriate payments

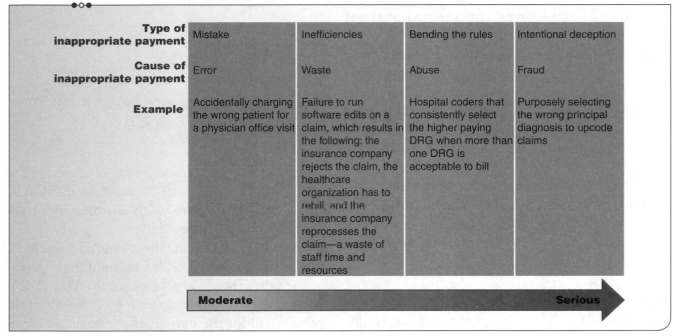

Type of inappropriate payment	Mistake	Inefficiencies	Bending the rules	Intentional deception
Cause of inappropriate payment	Error	Waste	Abuse	Fraud
Example	Accidentally charging the wrong patient for a physician office visit	Failure to run software edits on a claim, which results in the following: the insurance company rejects the claim, the healthcare organization has to rebill, and the insurance company reprocesses the claim—a waste of staff time and resources	Hospital coders that consistently select the higher paying DRG when more than one DRG is acceptable to bill	Purposely selecting the wrong principal diagnosis to upcode claims

Moderate → **Serious**

Source: CMS 2014b.

Federal Regulations and Initiatives

There are a number of federal regulations and initiatives used to combat fraud and abuse. These include the False Claims Act, Anti-Kickback Statute, Stark Law, Balanced Budget Act of 1997, Health Insurance Portability and Accountability Act (HIPAA), Health Care Fraud Prevention and Enforcement Action Team, Office of the Inspector General, recovery audit contractor, quality improvement organizations, Recovery Audit Contractor, Quality Improvement Organizations, and Meaningful Use.

False Claims Act

Fraud is not a new concept, as the **False Claims Act** was passed during the Civil War. The law allows penalties to be awarded to those who knowingly submit fraudulent claims to the US government for payment. "Knowing" includes "deliberate ignorance or reckless disregard of the truth or falsity of the information related to the claim" (CMS 2014c, 2). The law has been the foundation upon which fraud and abuse efforts have been based, with revisions and other legislation added to it over the years. One of the key components of the False Claims Act is qui tam. **Qui tam** is the whistleblower provisions of the False Claims Act—private persons, known as relators, may enforce the Act by filing a complaint, under seal, alleging fraud committed against the government. For example, if a coder is told to assign codes in violation of coding rules, then he or she can report the facility for fraud. The individual who submits the allegations can receive 15 to 30 percent of the penalties collected by the federal government.

Anti-Kickback Statute

The **Anti-Kickback Statute** dictates that physicians cannot receive money or other benefits for referring patients to a healthcare facility (CMS 2015a). For example, a hospital cannot give a physician $100 for every patient referred to the hospital for care.

The Stark Law

The Physician Self-Referral Law, otherwise known as the Stark Law, builds on the Anti-Kickback Statute and prohibits a physician from referring patients to a business in which he or she or a member of the physician's immediate family has financial interests. For example, if the physician owns a dialysis center, he or she cannot refer a patient for dialysis at that location. If he or she does refer a patient to the facility, then the physician cannot receive Medicare or Medicaid funding (CMS 2014c). There are exceptions to the Stark Law; for example, healthcare facilities can help physicians with limited costs of implementation of an electronic health record (EHR).

Balanced Budget Act of 1997

The **Balanced Budget Act of 1997 (BBA)** excludes healthcare organizations that are convicted of healthcare-related crimes from participating in Medicare programs. The exclusion includes 10 years for the first offense and permanent exclusion for the second. The BBA also permits Medicare to refuse to allow convicted felons into the Medicare program (BBA 1997). The BBA also educates Medicare beneficiaries on how they can assist in preventing fraud as well as how to report fraud when they when they identify it. It also gives the Medicare beneficiaries the right to receive a copy of their detailed bill from the healthcare provider. A healthcare fraud registry was created to keep track of all confirmed fraud (Casto and Forrestal 2015).

Health Insurance Portability and Accountability Act (HIPAA)

The **Health Insurance Portability and Accountability Act (HIPAA)** of 1996 addresses many topics such as privacy and security of health information as well as fraud and abuse. HIPAA created a joint venture between the Department of Health and Human Services (HHS) and the Department of Justice (HHS 2009). It also increased the civil monetary penalty for fraud and abuse convictions. The penalty was increased from $2,000 per incident to $10,000 per incident plus three times the total amount of the fraudulent claims

Figure 16.2 Example of civil monetary penalties

Community Hospital submitted 150 claims where they unbundled laboratory charges. They were overpaid $100 on each claim.

150 claims × $100 overpayment = $15,000

3 × total amount of overpayment = $15,000 × 3 = $45,000

Community Hospital would be fined $45,000.

©AHIMA

(OIG 1998). For additional information on HIPAA, refer to chapter 8. Figure 16.2 is an example of how civil monetary penalties work.

Under HIPAA, organizations, entities, and individuals can be penalized for unbundling, upcoding, or other fraudulent practices (McWay 2016). **Unbundling** is the practice of using multiple codes to bill for the various individual steps in a single procedure rather than using a single code that includes all of the steps of the comprehensive procedure code. For example, a code for a complete blood count should be used rather than a code for a red blood count, a white blood count, a hematocrit and all of the other tests that make up a complete blood count. Unbundling can result in the facility receiving an overpayment and is considered abuse as it violates coding guidelines.

Upcoding is the practice of assigning diagnostic or procedural codes that represent higher payment rates than the codes that actually reflect the services provided to patients. For example, billing with the procedure code for an open procedure when the procedure was actually laparoscopic. This difference in surgical approach would provide the healthcare provider with an **overpayment**—a higher reimbursement than deserved. Overpayments occur in the following scenarios.

- Two or more claims are submitted for the same service
- Payment is billed for medically unnecessary services
- Payment is billed for noncovered services
- Payment is made to the wrong provider
- Payment is made for services performed after the patient's death (Green and Rowell 2015)

Noncovered services are healthcare services that are not reimbursable under a healthcare plan. These services vary by medical plan but typically include plastic surgery, procedures that are not medically necessary, infertility treatments, and dental cleaning.

Healthcare providers must make a concerted effort to comply with best practices regarding reimbursement and monitoring for fraud and abuse. Best practices include monitoring and auditing (covered later in this chapter). When HHS determines the civil monetary penalties for the instance of fraud or abuse, the level of efforts put into fraud and abuse prevention is considered. These efforts can be grouped into the following three categories.

- **Reasonable cause:** It would be unreasonable to expect the healthcare provider to comply with the requirements of HIPAA.

- **Reasonable diligence:** The healthcare provider has taken reasonable actions to comply with the legislative requirements.

- **Willful neglect:** Intentionally failing to comply with or being indifferent to the HIPAA provisions. (45 CFR 160.401)

Health Care Fraud Prevention and Enforcement Action Team

The HHS, along with the Department of Justice created the **Health Care Fraud Prevention and Enforcement Action Team (HEAT)** in 2009. Their mission is to:

- Prevent waste, fraud, and abuse
- Identify those who participate in fraud and abuse
- Reduce healthcare costs
- Improve the quality of care provided to Medicare and Medicaid patients
- Provide best practices in combating fraud and abuse
- Expand partnership between HHS and the Department of Justice (STOP Medicare Fraud 2016)

The result of this partnership was the creation of the **Medicare Fraud Strike Force** who use data analytics to look for evidence of fraud and abuse. The individual teams are known as a strike forces (STOP Medicare Fraud 2016).

Office of the Inspector General

The **Office of Inspector General (OIG)** is an office in the federal government working to combat fraud, waste, and abuse and to improve the efficiency of HHS programs (OIG 2016a). The mission of the OIG is to protect the integrity of the HHS programs as well as the health and welfare of individuals enrolled in federal programs such as Medicare and Medicaid. The OIG is responsible for monitoring Medicare and Medicaid, which provide health insurance to one in three Americans at the cost of hundreds of billions of taxpayer dollars. The sheer size of Medicare and Medicaid make these programs vulnerable to criminals. One of the vital roles of the OIG is to keep these programs less prone to waste, fraud, and abuse. The OIG has the federal government's largest team of auditors and is the premier healthcare law enforcement agency. Every year the OIG investigates, prosecutes, and convicts hundreds of individuals who misuse or steal taxpayer dollars. This results in the recovery of billions of dollars for the federal government (OIG 2016a).

The majority of the OIG's resources go to the oversight of Medicare and Medicaid, but also extend to programs under other HHS institutions, including the Centers for Disease Control and Prevention (CDC), the, National Institutes of Health (NIH), and the Food and Drug Administration (FDA) (OIG 2016a).

The OIG is organized into five divisions, categorized as follows and illustrated in figure 16.3.

- *Office of Audit Services:* The Office of Audit Services is responsible for auditing HHS programs to ensure that the agencies and their contractors are meeting their responsibilities. Their findings can be used in criminal and other investigations.

- *Office of Evaluation and Inspections:* This division evaluates the HHS programs in order to make them more effective and to prevent fraud, abuse, or waste within HHS.

Figure 16.3 OIG organizational structure

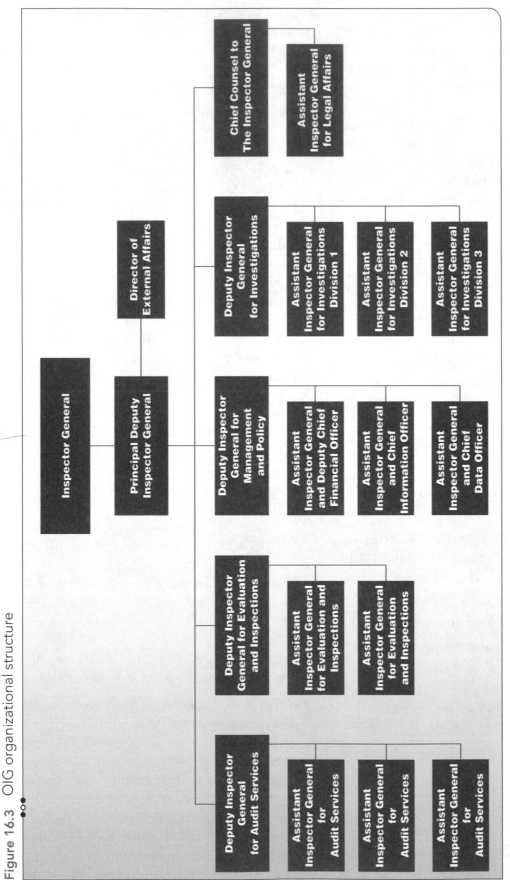

Source: OIG 2016b.

- *Office of Management and Policy:* This division ensures that the OIG has the resources that they need in order to fulfill their responsibilities.

- *Office of Investigations:* This is the OIG division responsible for monitoring and enforcing fraud and abuse regulations in HHS programs, operations, and beneficiaries. These efforts include operating the fraud hotline where individuals can call and report fraudulent activities, working with the Department of Justice to coordinate fraud investigations, protecting the Secretary of HHS and participating in public safety and security management activities, and working to enforce and update the fraud and abuse efforts of the OIG to continue to improve programs.

- *Office of Counsel to the Inspector General:* The Office of Counsel to the Inspector General provides legal advice to the OIG (OIG 2016a).

Recovery Audit Contractor

Recovery Audit Contractor (RAC) is a governmental program whose goal is to identify improper payments made on claims of healthcare services provided to Medicare beneficiaries. Improper payments may be overpayments or underpayments. RAC was established as a demonstration project to test the Medicare program on payments made to healthcare providers. The program was found to be effective by identifying over one billion dollars in overpayments and so it was implemented across the country as per the Tax Relief and Health Care Act of 2006. Medicare contracted with several organizations to conduct the audits required by the program (OIG 2013). The RAC program has significantly impacted the workload of HIM departments primarily in the functions of release of information, coding, and auditing.

A request for additional documentation from a healthcare provider to support the submitted claim is an additional documentation request (ADR). ADRs for the RAC program increased the number of record requests for all healthcare providers providing services to Medicare patients as the Centers for Medicare and Medicaid Services (CMS) is permitted to present a large number of ADRs to a provider based primarily on the percentage of Medicare claims of the healthcare organization. There are minimum and maximum limits of the ADRs that may be presented to an organization within each 45-day timeframe (CMS 2013). Most affected are HIM departments that handle the record requests for the entire healthcare enterprise. An enterprise is a term that describes all of the healthcare provider organizations within one company. For example, an enterprise may consist of a hospital, multiple physician offices, ambulatory surgical centers, outpatient therapy sites, a rehab facility, and a long term care facility that are all owned by one company. An HIM department that handles all HIM functions for an enterprise would experience a significant increase in workload since they would be handling record requests for all of the healthcare providers in the enterprise. HIM departments of healthcare providers that have a higher Medicare payment denial rate also experience a higher number of requests for copies of health records as CMS associates a high payment denial rate with potential coding and billing errors and therefore increases the number of RAC audits for these facilities to ensure compliance.

HIM departments have increased coding audits prior to billing claims in the areas that RAC audits are targeting with the goal of avoiding coding and billing errors. These coding audits are good professional practice as they not only potentially improve the accuracy of claims processing but also provide data for health information managers regarding areas of education needed for coders. In addition to including coding audits prior to billing claims, healthcare organizations have also increased coding audits related to the focus or target areas of the RAC program and also in the top issues found by RAC auditors that are published quarterly. These coding audits are also examples of good HIM professional practice as potential coding errors may be identified and corrected or provide content for coder education.

RAC utilizes three different types of audits. Automated reviews are performed electronically rather than by humans. A software program ana-lyzes claims data to identify improper payments. In a **complex review**, humans analyze health records for accuracy (Casto and Forrestal 2015). A complex review can be used for situations where no coding or other guidelines exist (AHIMA 2009). **Semi-automated reviews** start with an automated review but also incorporate health record docu-ments analyzed by humans. When required, the RAC requests a health record in question from the healthcare provider. If the review of the health record identifies an improper payment, the health-care provider receives a RAC demand letter with instructions to refund the improper payment and the reason for the request for funds. The health-care facility has the right to appeal the request for the refund and needs to make a decision whether or not to appeal the RAC findings. Table 16.1 pro-vides some potential reasons for appealing or not appealing the RAC findings.

There are five levels in the appeal process described below and displayed in figure 16.4.

1. *Redetermination:* The appeal is submitted to the Medicare Administrative Contractor (MAC) for redetermination. "A Medicare Administrative Contractor (MAC) is a private health care insurer that has been awarded a geographic jurisdiction to process Medicare Part A and Part B (A/B) medical claims or Durable Medical Equipment (DME) claims for Medicare Fee-For-Service (FFS) beneficiaries" (CMS 2016b). Reviewing appeals for redetermination is one task of a MAC. MACs are also responsible for the initial processing of Medicare fee for service (FFS) claims, making and accounting for the

Medicare FFS payments, enrolling providers in the Medicare FFS program and responding to provider inquiries, educating providers, reviewing health records, and several other tasks related to the FFS process (CMS 2016b).

2. *Reconsideration:* If the redetermination does not rule in their favor, the facility has the right to appeal to the qualified independent contractor, an outside organization contracted by Medicare to audit the reconsideration.

3. *Administrative law judge:* The third level is a review by an administrative law judge. Attorneys may be involved in this level (and beyond) of appeal to facilitate the process.

4. *Appeals council review:* The fourth level is to send the appeal to the appeals council, a department of HHS responsible for Medicare appeals.

5. *Final judicial review:* This last level sends the appeal to federal district court for a final ruling (HFMA n.d.)

Quality Improvement Organizations

Quality Improvement Organizations (QIO) per-form medical peer review of Medicare and Medicaid claims, including review of validity of hospital diagnosis and procedure coding data completeness, adequacy, and quality of care; and appropriateness of prospective payments for outlier cases and nonemergent use of the emer-gency room. While the focus of the RAC audits is payment-related, the QIO audits are patient care-focused. Many of the audits conducted by the QIOs result in findings that may assist healthcare organizations in the improvement of quality of

Table 16.1 Appealing RAC findings

Reasons to appeal after review of the RAC findings by the coding manager or physician reviewer	Reasons not to appeal after review of the RAC findings by the coding manager or physician reviewer
When the healthcare provider's review of the health record ref-erenced in the demand letter does not match the findings of the RAC audit.	When the healthcare provider's review of the health record referenced in the demand letter matches the findings of the RAC audit; there would not be any point to an appeal and would be a waste of the organization's time and money.
When the amount of repayment specified in the demand letter is of a significant amount that the staff time involved in an appeal merits time well spent.	When the amount of repayment specified in the demand letter is such a low amount that it would not be worth the organization's time and money to file an appeal as appeals can be very labor intensive in terms of staff reviewing the record.

Figure 16.4   Five levels in the RAC appeal process

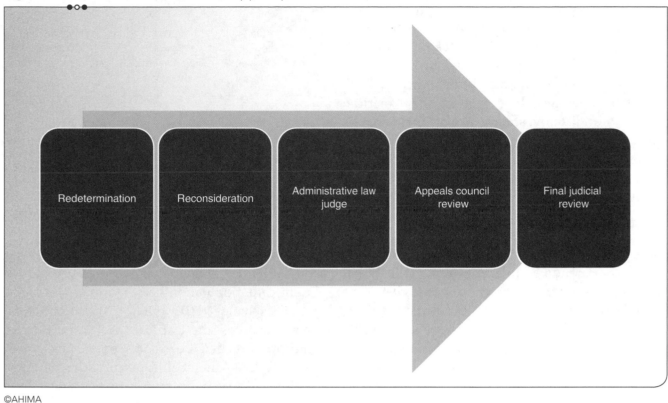

| Redetermination | Reconsideration | Administrative law judge | Appeals council review | Final judicial review |

©AHIMA

care such as reduction of pressure ulcers or fewer avoidable hospital admissions. QIOs frequently conduct audits to determine if healthcare services have been provided in the appropriate setting. The following are a few examples.

- Establishing if the emergency room of a major hospital is clogged with patients with nonemergent conditions that could be taken care of at an outpatient clinic.

- Determining if patients are staying too long in an acute care environment when they could be treated at a long term acute care hospital or nursing home.

- Identifying patients with chronic conditions, such as CHF, being cared for at home with hospice to avoid unnecessary hospital admissions.

These are the types of utilization audits that are conducted by QIOs. QIOs are contracted by Medicare to review health records for quality of care provided, the appropriateness of the reimbursement requested, treatment at the appropriate level of care (such as inpatient vs. ambulatory) and the billing of noncovered services (OIG 2007). Because of their role in monitoring coding quality, QIOs are an important part of Medicare's fraud and abuse efforts. QIOs are required to report any evidence of fraud that they identify. Obviously, the QIOs must review health records to be able to carry out the duties listed above. The QIOs request copies of the health records from the HIM department. Healthcare organizations should analyze the QIO requests for patterns related to specific DRGs, diagnoses, procedures, and physicians to identify opportunities for education and improvement.

Meaningful Use

Meaningful Use (MU) is an incentive program issued by CMS for eligible professionals, hospitals, and critical access hospitals participating in Medicare and Medicaid programs that adopt and successfully demonstrate meaningful use of certified electronic health record (EHR) technology

(ONC 2016). **Certified EHR technology** are EHRs that have been approved for use in the MU program by organizations hired by CMS to evaluate EHRs (Sayles 2014). The MU program was put into effect as part of the Health Information Technology for Economic and Clinical Health (HITECH) Act, which is part of the American Recovery and Reinvestment Act of 2009 (ARRA). **Eligible professionals (EP)** include physicians, dentists, ophthalmologists, and others who can participate in the MU program.

MU is a three-stage program with specific requirements for the use of certified EHR technology for each stage. Each stage becomes gradually more sophisticated in the demands of the EHR. EPs are not mandated to implement certified EHR technology but those who chose not to forfeit the incentive payments and will see reduced Medicare payments at the end of the program. Access to electronic information is a key tool in monitoring fraud and abuse as more electronic data will be available for analysis by the OIG, Medicare Fraud Strike Force, and others involved in fighting fraud and abuse. Figure 16.5 shows the emphasis of each

Figure 16.5 Stages of Meaningful Use

2011–2012	2014	2016
Stage 1	Stage 2	Stage 3
Data capture and sharing	Advance clinical processes	Improved outcome

Source: OIG 2016b.

stage in the MU program. The first stage focuses on the implementation of the EHR to be used in capturing patient data and then sharing the data with the patients. The rigor of the requirements increases in stage 2 to require the use of the EHR in quality improvement activities (CMS 2016a). For additional information on quality improvement, see chapter 18. Stage 3 focuses on outcomes of patient care, population health, and health information exchange (HIE) (ONC 2013). Population health includes the capture and reporting of healthcare data that are used for public health purposes. It allows the healthcare provider to report infectious diseases, immunizations, cancer, and other reportable conditions to public health officials. For information on HIE, refer to chapter 12.

 ## Check Your Understanding 16.1

Instructions: **Answer the following questions.**

1. Which of the following is an example of abuse?
   A. Billing for healthcare services
   B. Knowingly charging an inappropriate amount for healthcare services or supplies
   C. Unbundling codes
   D. Consistently upcoding to receive higher payments

2. Which of the following is an example of fraud?
   A. Accidentally overbilling for healthcare services
   B. Charging an inappropriate amount for healthcare services or supplies
   C. Knowingly submitting bills for healthcare services not provided
   D. Unbundling codes

3. Which of the federal fraud and abuse laws prohibits a physician's referral of designated health services for Medicare and Medicaid patients if the physician has a financial relationship with the entity?
   A. False Claims Act
   B. Anti-Kickback Statute
   C. Stark Law
   D. HIPAA

4. Which of the following organizations is responsible for coordinating the Medicare fraud programs?
    A. Quality improvement organizations
    B. Recovery audit contractor
    C. Office of Inspector General
    D. The Joint Commission

5. Meaningful Use is which of the following?
    A. A state monitored program
    B. An incentive program
    C. An accreditation program
    D. A fraud investigation program

Compliance Program

Each healthcare facility should have a compliance program. A **compliance program** in a healthcare organization is a set of internal policies and procedures that a healthcare entity puts into place to comply with applicable state and federal laws. An effective compliance program can enhance a healthcare organization's operations and improve quality of care and reduce overall costs as well as reduce the liability with regards to fraud and abuse. The compliance program can help the healthcare organization identify problems and correct them before they become systemic and costly.

There are seven basic elements that should be included in an effective compliance program:

- *Policies, procedures, and standards of conduct:* A healthcare organization should put, in writing, all policies, procedures, and standards of conduct related to their compliance program. These are discussed later in this chapter.

- *Identifying a compliance officer and committee:* The chief compliance officer and compliance committee are responsible for the overall compliance program for the organization. Besides the chief compliance officer, the compliance committee should consist of representatives from the healthcare organization's departments that have the most responsibility for monitoring compliance within the organization. These departments would likely include HIM, revenue cycle management, patient billing, medical staff, and patient accounting. The privacy officer, general counsel, and risk management should also be represented on the committee. An organization may also want to include members from Administration such as the chief executive officer or chief operations officers as well as a member of the governing board since the compliance committee typically reports directly to the governing board. The governing board has ultimate responsibility of compliance for the organization. The compliance committee will also review the OIG work plan and then determine what items they want to include in their compliance activities and review for the upcoming year. This plan will change from year to year as the OIG focus and the needs of the facility change.

- *Educating staff:* It is imperative that all staff be trained in compliance policies, procedures, and standards of conduct as it applies to their position in the organization. This training should occur, at a minimum, in their initial orientation training and on an annual basis. This is discussed later in this chapter.

- *Establish communication channels:* There should be methods in place for employees to report fraud and abuse; this can be a confidential hotline or comment box where employees can report fraud and abuse without fear of reprisal.

- *Perform internal monitoring:* Organizations must be diligent to ensure compliance with policies and procedures such as through the use of audits and data analysis.

- *Penalties for noncompliance with standards:* There should be appropriate consequences for employees who do not comply with policies and procedures and who participate in fraud and abuse activities. These consequences might include some form of disciplinary action or termination, depending on the severity of the employee's action.

- *Taking immediate corrective action when a problem is identified:* Healthcare facilities must take action when fraud and abuse is identified; failure to do so could increase their risk of fraud and abuse accusations (OIG n.d.).

Elements of an effective compliance program are discussed in the following sections. These elements include fraud and abuse prevention strategies and audits.

Fraud and Abuse Prevention Strategies

A number of fraud and abuse prevention strategies can be used by the healthcare provider to protect themselves from fraud and abuse allegations. These strategies include:

- *Policies and procedures:* Policies and procedures are a critical part of a compliance program and tell the "who" and "what" should be done to combat fraud and abuse. Policies should include internal coding procedures, how and when to write physician queries, billing practices, and audits.

- *Education of employees and medical staff of the healthcare organization:* Laws and regulations change from time to time. A healthcare organization's employees and medical staff must be kept up to date on these changes. They must also understand their role in preventing fraud and abuse and what to do if they are requested to act in a fraudulent manner. Coders also must stay informed of changes in coding practices. A component

of compliance training is typically a part of a healthcare organization's orientation programs for newly hired employees and newly appointed medical staff members. In addition, annual compliance training for rules and regulations at a minimum is usually carried out for all employees of a healthcare organization. More detailed and complex compliance training should be conducted for employees whose positions in the healthcare organization require a more in-depth knowledge and understanding of the rules and regulations surrounding healthcare compliance. For example, employees involved in the revenue cycle should receive education regarding the False Claims Act.

- *Routine review of coding and billing reports:* There are billing and coding reports that organizations use on a routine basis to gauge the status of the billing and coding processes. A routine review of these coding and billing reports can be useful in the identification of significant changes in coding and billing practices. Identified coding changes may or may not be justified. For example, there may have been a change in coding rules that would justify the use of different codes. A consultant may have given the facility improper information regarding coding, billing, or other reimbursement practices that resulted in changes that should not have occurred. The data that can be reviewed are discussed later in this chapter.

- *Documentation strategies:* A strong clinical documentation improvement (CDI) program is important to fighting fraud and abuse. CDI is discussed later in this chapter. An example documentation issue is the use of the copy and paste functionality in an EHR. This practice presents opportunities for clinicians to duplicate previous documentation and insert it into current notes, which presents an opportunity for incorrect data to be carried forward and may result in the appearance of fraud or abuse (AHIMA 2014). Refer to chapter 3 for more information regarding EHR documentation strategies.

Audits

Audits are a function that allows retrospective reconstruction of events, including who executed the events in question, why, and what changes were made as a result. Internal audits are conducted routinely by employees of healthcare organizations. The audit can be performed on an ongoing basis, monthly, annually, or by some other schedule. The audits allow the facility to confirm that the policies and procedures of the organization are being met and to identify problems that need to be addressed and corrected.

Audits serve a number of purposes including:

- Reducing improper reimbursement
- Improving the accuracy of healthcare claims
- Improving patient care
- Showing commitment to complying with laws and regulations (CMS 2015b)

Many of the audits conducted by healthcare organizations are performed internally meaning that they are performed by healthcare facility employees, such as the coding manager. The following section will address preparing for and conducting internal and external audits.

Preparing for and Conducting Audits

Before an audit can be conducted, the organization must first identify the objective of the audit. For example, an objectives may be to monitor billing practices or coding quality. Once the objective is established, the audit method can be determined. Audit methods include analyzing electronic data, reviewing documents, collecting data, adding and inputting it into a database, or assembling data using a manual data collection tool. The method will control the resources needed such as the health record, bills, queries, and so forth. The number of cases needed and how the cases will be identified must be established. For example, the organization may choose to review 20 percent of the queries written every month. A number of statistical methods can be used to select the specific queries such as:

- *Simple random sampling:* This model gives every bill, patient, and so forth so that each has the same chance of being chosen.
- *Systematic random sampling:* In this model, there is a pattern used to select patients such as every 10th patient admitted.
- *Convenience sampling:* In this model, the bills, for example, are chosen based on which ones are available to the auditor (Horton 2012).

While audits vary based on what is being audited, there is a basic process—identify areas of risk that need to be monitored, conduct audits on these areas of risk, document the findings of the audit, analyze the data, and correct any problems identified. To conduct the audit, the auditors will need access to the necessary resources being audited. The areas of risk can be HHS focus areas, problems that have previously been identified at the facility, or areas where problems are suspected. There should be a database, spreadsheet, or other tool where the audit is recorded. The data elements collected during the audit vary based on the audit objective. For example, auditing a claim for healthcare services in the emergency department might consider the following areas:

- Procedures are reported at the appropriate level
- Claims are not submitted more than once
- Coding guidelines are followed such as not unbundling
- Documentation supports services reported on the claim
- Copayments and deductibles are collected from the patient (CMS 2015b)

The general rule for documentation in the health record is "if it is not documented, it was not done". That is true in compliance as well. The documentation of audits is a significant part of this proof. The documentation should include where the data was obtained, why it was gathered, what was done with the data, what the facility learned and what the audit tells the facility (CMS 2015b). Figure 16.6 is an example of an audit data collection tool.

Figure 16.6 Sample audit data collection tool

Query Audit

Patient name _____   Encounter number _____

Physician name _____   Query author _____

What impact on reimbursement did the query have?   ___Increased

                                                      ___Decreased

                                                      ___No change

Justification for query: ___Contradictory information

                           ___Incomplete information

                           ___Present on admission status unclear

                           ___Ambiguous information

                           ___Other: _____

Queries contain the following information: ___Patient name

                                               ___Date of service

                                               ___Health record number

                                               ___Date of query

                                               ___Name and contact information of coder

Appropriate physician queried? ___Yes   ___No

Query appropriately written based on policy?   ___Yes   ___No

Auditor: _____   Date of audit: _____

Comments:

©AHIMA

The health information management (HIM) professional is the keeper of the health record and therefore must control the release of data needed for the audit. In preparation for an audit, the HIM professional must review the audit request documents to validate the auditor's right to review the health record. The HIM professional must also ensure that the audit will take place in an atmosphere that maintains the security of protected health information (PHI) during audit activities. The healthcare organization will be best served if the audit processes in place are proactive rather than reactive. A proactive approach enables an organization to identify areas of concern, opportunities for documentation improvement, and educational needs, and to address and correct these issues prior to any audit request from an external organization.

The HIM professional should plan audit activities, keeping in mind that both internal and external audit requests can arrive at any time. Audit planning should include the following:

- Identification of the audit requestor
- Information requested
- Information is needed
- Identification of individuals from the healthcare organization that need to be involved in the audit, keeping in mind these individuals may be from other departments such as patient accounting, revenue management, charge description

master control, clinical services, clinical documentation improvement (CDI), or utilization review (UR)

- Timeline of audit activities

- Designation of individual responsible for the management of the audit activities

- Determination of when audit results will be reviewed and who will review them

The traditional role of the HIM professional in the audit process typically includes providing the health records to be audited or auditing health records. The audit may have particular requirements, specifications, and criteria regarding the health records to be included. Then the HIM professional will apply privacy regulations and organizational policies and procedures to ensure that the audit is lawful and that the health record may be used or released.

External Audits

External audits are performed routinely, such as once a year, to confirm that the facility's internal audits are effective. The external auditors are hired by the healthcare facility to conduct the reviews. The external audits help ensure that the organization's policies and procedures are in compliance with laws, regulations, and their own policies and procedures. External audits may be conducted at the request of the healthcare provider such as a coding consulting company hired to validate coding accuracy. It may also be accreditation, insurance companies, or other organizations monitoring the healthcare provider for compliance with their standards or regulations. Regardless of who performs the external audits, they are conducted by with the same goal of determining the healthcare organization's level of compliance. For example, an insurance company may conduct a billing audit to determine if the items charged on a patient's bill are supported by documentation in the health record, or, the Joint Commission may conduct an audit to determine compliance with the Joint Commission standards regarding patients' rights.

Coding and Fraud and Abuse

Codes are used to determine reimbursement, therefore code assignment is critical. Assigning the incorrect codes with the intent of receiving more money is fraudulent. The following questions should be asked when monitoring and auditing the coding process at a healthcare organization:

- Is the diagnosis-related group correct?
- Is there any unbundling?
- Are the codes assigned for the appropriate level of service?
- Are codes changed so that a noncovered service is billed as a covered service?
- Is there a discrepancy between the codes provided by the physician and the hospital? (Prophet 1997)

The following section addresses coding compliance and computer-assisted coding.

Coding Compliance

Healthcare organizations should have a **coding compliance plan** in addition to the organization's compliance plan. It should contain the same components as the facility's compliance plan with a primary focus on coding practices. Benefits of the coding compliance plan include the following.

- Improved documentation in the health record
- Retention of a high standard of coding
- Reduction in denials of healthcare services reimbursement based on coding errors
- Correction of coding-related risks (Schraffenberger and Kuehn 2011)

The coding compliance plan should include expectations for coding quality (such as 98 percent accuracy in code assignment), use of office coding guidelines and official resources such as the American Health Association's Coding Clinic for ICD-10-CM and ICD-10-PCS and CPT Assistant.

The following are strategies that can be used to combat fraud and abuse in coding.

- Provide ongoing training to all coding staff
- Implement comprehensive policies and procedures
- Examine the quality of coding through the use of audits
- Ensure that coding practices follow official coding guidelines
- Ensure that for each procedure code there is a corresponding or supporting diagnosis code
- Support codes with health record documentation
- Support evaluation and management code assignment with the documentation
- Educate physicians on how to improve their documentation
- Use best practices to write a query to clarify documentation
- Disseminate memorandums on changes in regulations and insurers' policies
- Verify the advice of consultants prior to implementation of their recommendations
- Monitor changes in regulations
- Compare facility metrics with national data
- Monitor claims denials and coding changes
- Review data to identify any significant changes in the facility's case-mix index or coding practices

- Ensure the person maintaining the chargemaster is knowledgeable in coding, billing, and documentation
- Report any possible fraud to the facility's compliance officer or attorney (Prophet 1997)

Other issues that must be addressed in the coding compliance plan include upcoding and unbundling, discussed earlier in this chapter.

Computer-Assisted Coding

Computer-assisted coding (CAC) is the process of extracting and translating dictated and then transcribed free-text data (or dictated and then computer-generated discrete data) into International Classification of Diseases, Tenth Revision, Clinical Modification (ICD-10-CM) and Current Procedural Terminology (CPT) evaluation and management codes for billing and coding purposes. CAC uses **natural language processing (NLP)** to review the documentation in the EHR and assign a code number. NLP is a technology that converts human language into data that can be translated then manipulated by computer systems and is a branch of artificial intelligence. In 2013, the AHIMA Foundation conducted a research study to determine whether coding timeliness and accuracy is effected by the use of CAC. The study determined that the best scenario for coding accuracy is for a credentialed coder to code in conjunction with the use of a CAC. Study results demonstrated that credentialed coders that used a CAC were able to reduce the amount of time it took to code a record by 22 percent. A coder that did not use a CAC, or the use of a CAC alone without a credentialed coder, resulted in lower coding accuracy. (AHIMA 2013).

CAC does not eliminate the need for coders, but the roles of the coder changes as he or she will validate the codes assigned by the computer rather than assign the code. The CAC can help prevent fraudulent coding and ensure consistent, complete coding. Figure 16.7 is an example of how the EHR documentation is used to assign codes via computer-assisted coding.

Figure 16.7   ICD-10-CM CAC example

In this example, the CAC software assigned the code T15.91xA based on documentation in the emergency department record that states the patient had a "foreign body in the right eye." The coder is presented with the decision to accept the code or reject it based on further analysis.

Review of the documentation revealed that the foreign body was located on the edge of the cornea, which changes the fourth character in ICD-10-CM from 9 to 0. The coding professional replaces the T15.91xA with T15.01xA, Foreign body in cornea, right eye.

Emergency Department Record

A patient is brought to the emergency department with a foreign body in the right eye. He was working with metal, and a piece flew in his eye. He reports slight irritation to the right eye but no blurred vision. A slit lamp shows a foreign body approximately 2 to 3 o'clock on the edge of the cornea. The foreign body appears to be metallic. The iris is intact.

Procedure:

   Two drops of Alcaine were used in the right eye. Foreign body is removed from the right eye.

Computer-Generated Codes:

   T15.91xA, Foreign body, external eye, right

Final Coding Decision:

   Coding professional selects the more specific code for foreign body of cornea, T15.01xA

Source: Smith and Bronnert 2010.

Check Your Understanding 16.2

Instructions: **Answer the following questions.**

1. The coder assigned separate codes for individual tests when a combination code exists. This is an example of which of the following?
   A. Upcoding
   B. Complex coding
   C. Query
   D. Unbundling

2. Benefits of a compliance plan include which of the following?
   A. Reduction in denials
   B. Elimination of denials
   C. Maintenance of the status quo
   D. Documentation audits

3. True or false: Compliance plans are a reconstruction of events that include who executed the events in question, why, and what changes were made as a result.

4. True or false: In systematic random sampling there is a pattern used to select patients such as every 10th patient admitted.

5. True or false: Internal monitoring should be part of a compliance plan.

Clinical Documentation Improvement

Clinical documentation improvement (CDI) is the process an organization undertakes that will improve clinical specificity and documentation that will allow coders to assign more concise classification codes. For example, ensuring that the organism for pneumonia is documented and coded. The CDI process can be performed either concurrently or retrospectively to the patient encounter. Concurrent CDI is performed while the patient is admitted and still in the hospital and can enhance the quality of care as the improved documentation is available for all care providers. Retrospective CDI is performed after the patient is discharged. The review is frequently performed during the coding process. The CDI review of the health record looks for "conflicting, incomplete, or nonspecific provider documentation" (AHIMA 2014, 2). The improved documentation helps ensure that the documentation supports code assignment. For example, the documentation should indicate whether the fractured arm is the left or right one so that the proper code can be chosen.

An important tool in CDI is the physician query process in which questions are posed to a provider to obtain additional, clarifying documentation to improve the specificity and completeness of the data used to assign diagnosis and procedure codes in the patient's health record and computer-assisted coding programs that help guide coders to the correct codes. This chapter focuses on CDI as it relates to fraud and abuse; for additional information on CDI, refer to chapter 6. Information systems and CDI metrics are other tools used in this process and are discussed further.

Information Systems and CDI

CDI computer systems can evaluate documentation in an EHR and make improvement suggestions. Queries can also be documented through a computer system. These systems allow the CDI specialists to query the physician, the physician to view the EHR, and the physician to document his or her response both in the query and in the EHR. These systems are used by the CDI specialists or coders depending on the organization. The role of HIM professionals in CDI is discussed later in this chapter.

Clinical Documentation Improvement Metrics

CDI metrics are key indicators used to monitor the effectiveness of CDI programs. A key indicator is a quantifiable measure used over time to determine whether some structure, process, or outcome in the provision of care to a patient supports high-quality performance measured against best practice criteria. These measures are reported to the appropriate administrator or committee routinely.

One of the most widely used key indicators for a CDI program to use to monitor is the case-mix index (CMI). CMI is the average relative weight of all cases treated at a given facility or by a given physician, which reflects the resource intensity or clinical severity of a specific group in relation to the other groups in the classification system. The CMI is calculated by dividing the sum of the weights of diagnosis-related groups (DRGs) for patients discharged during a given period by the total number of patients discharged. The CMI is a strong indicator of the healthcare facility's financial state. A significant unexplained increase in the CMI should be investigated as it may be an indication of improper coding or fraud and abuse. Sometimes changes in CMI are expected in situations; for example, with the addition or termination of healthcare services such as the performance cardiac surgery or kidney transplants, which are extremely high-weighted DRGs that would have a large impact in the CMI. It may also result from the addition of a new specialist, such as a cardiologist, to the medical staff. A strong CDI program will strengthen the CMI because the quality and specificity of the documentation help the coders to choose the appropriate codes (Schraffenberger and Kuehn 2011).

Many DRGs are impacted by the presence of a complication or comorbidity or a major complication or comorbidity. These paired DRGs, DRGs with and without complications and comorbidities, are another important key indicator for a CDI program to monitor. A **complication** is a medical condition that arises during an inpatient hospitalization (for example, a postoperative wound infection). A **comorbidity** is a medical condition that coexists with the primary cause for hospitalization and affects the patient's treatment and length of stay (for example, a chronic condition like diabetes mellitus). Major complications and major comorbidities are identified by CMS as more serious conditions and therefore have greater impact on the reimbursement. Incorrect documentation of these conditions can increase reimbursement by thousands of dollars. DRGs that are impacted by complications, comorbidities, major complications, and major comorbidities should be reviewed to ensure that the documentation supports correct coding of the conditions.

The distribution of the cases between these levels of DRGs can be benchmarked with other facilities (AHIMA 2015a). **Benchmarking** is the systematic comparison of the products, services, and outcomes of one organization with those of a similar organization; or the systematic comparison of one organization's outcomes with regional or national standards. Benchmarking allows the facilities to determine if their distribution of DRGs is within normal expectations and therefore, can also be a key indicator. Though benchmarking is typically considered an external comparison against regional or national standards, it can be performed internally as well. Internal benchmarking compares the facility to its own statistics from a year ago, five years ago, or for some other denoted period (Casto and Forrestal 2015). This is important as it allows the facility to identify changes that may indicate fraud or abuse. More information on benchmarking can be found in chapter 18.

Another key indicator is comparing the codes assigned by the CDI specialist to the final codes assigned by the coders. Differences between the two sets of codes may indicate that improved documentation caused the changes in codes and possibly reimbursement or fraud and abuse. The codes assigned by the coders are submitted on the healthcare claims.

Clinical Outcomes Measures and Monitoring

Healthcare organizations are interested in monitoring the clinical outcomes of patients who received care at their facility to determine if the patients are receiving quality care by providers and if providers are following proper procedures and standards of care. HIM professionals are involved in the monitoring process for quality improvement of documentation and data capture within the health record and EHR systems. Documentation in the health record is used to provide the information necessary to report **present on admission (POA)** and **hospital-acquired conditions (HAC)**. For each diagnosis code on inpatient claims, the coder must determine and record whether or not the condition was POA to the hospital as an inpatient based on the documentation in the health record. HACs are diagnoses and complications that CMS indicates should not occur while the patient is a hospital inpatient. Medicare will no longer pay healthcare facilities to treat HACs that occur after admission (Wiedemann 2013). Examples of HACs are foreign bodies left in a patient during surgery, fractures from a fall at the facility, or a catheter-associated urinary tract infection. More information on POA and HACs is found in chapter 15. A healthcare organization that is monitoring clinical outcomes as part of an ongoing quality assurance program will be able to determine that a HAC is the responsibility of the organization and could have been prevented with proper clinical processes and healthcare providers following the standard of care.

Part of clinical outcomes measuring allows for systems to be in place to determine a patient's severity of illness and risk of mortality. **Severity of illness (SOI)** is a type of supportive documentation reflecting objective clinical indicators of a patient illness (meaning the patient is sick enough to be at an identified level of care) and referring to the extent of physiological decompensation or organ system loss of function. **Risk of mortality (ROM)** is the likelihood of an inpatient death for a patient. One of these systems is the **all-patient refined diagnosis-related groups system (APR-DRG)**. The APR-DRG not only assigns a DRG, but it also assigns an SOI and ROI subclass. The subclasses assigned in

APR-DRGs are 1-minor, 2-moderate, 3-major, and 4-extreme (Schraffenberger and Kuehn 2011). Like DRGs, the SOI and ROM are based on the codes assigned so the stronger the documentation, the more accurate the SOI and ROM.

Roles in CDI

CDI cannot be adequately performed by one group or individual. It takes a team with specified skills in order to be successful.

Physicians play an important role in the CDI process as it is their documentation that is used to code health record. Education programs for physicians should be conducted by HIM professionals and other physicians in order to train physicians on best documentation practices. The training should be focused on the physician's specialty. For example, for a pregnant patient who enters a facility with pneumonia, a pulmonologist would be trained on the importance of documenting the organism causing the pneumonia—not documenting the patient's gestational age since a pulmonologist generally would not treat obstetric

patients. A physician advisor is a physician who is an employee of the hospital and acts as a liaison between the healthcare facility and the physicians. He or she generally works a few hours a week as a champion for the CDI program and to help the physician understand the importance of the program.

While some healthcare facilities hire nurses as CDI specialists, HIM professionals are uniquely qualified for this role because of the combination of skills they possess. These skills include clinical understanding, documentation knowledge, and coding expertise. They also have knowledge of reimbursement systems. Other skills of CDI specialists include strong interpersonal and communication skills, leadership abilities, and solid organizational skills (AHIMA 2014). Combining these skills with effective communication will help the CDI specialists to work with healthcare providers in ensuring health record documentation contains the information needed to support reimbursement, quality initiatives, and patient care (AHIMA 2015b).

 Check Your Understanding 16.3

Instructions: **Answer the following questions.**

1. According to CMS, diagnoses and complications that should not occur while the patient is a hospital inpatient are known as which of the following?
   A. Queries
   B. Hospital-acquired conditions
   C. Present on admission indicators
   D. Complications

2. Which of the following is the average relative weight of all cases treated at a given facility or by a given physician?
   A. Case-mix index
   B. Sampling
   C. Hospital-acquired condition
   D. Present on admission indicator

3. True or false: HIM professionals make excellent CDI specialists because of their clinical, documentation, and coding skills.

4. True or false: CDI specialists should have strong communication skills.

5. True or false: Changes in the CMI are always evidence of fraud.

Real-World Case 16.1

On June 18, 2015, the Medicare Fraud Strike Force charged 243 healthcare professionals with Medicare fraud resulting in $712 million in false billings. This was the largest one day arrest ever conducted by the Medicare Fraud Strike Force. These individuals are accused of conspiracy to commit fraud, kickbacks, and identity theft. The defendants are physicians, pharmacy owners, and home health providers. Specific alleged fraudulent behavior includes billing for durable medical equipment and services that were not provided, as well as healthcare services that were not medically necessary (DOJ 2015). Inspector General Levinson stated:

> This record-setting takedown sends a message to would-be perpetrators that healthcare fraud is a risky way to line your pockets. Our agents and our law enforcement partners stand ready to protect these vital programs and ensure that those who would steal from federal healthcare programs ultimately pay for their crimes (DOJ 2015).

Real-World Case 16.2

The University of New Mexico Hospitals created a CDI program. They identified physician advisors to educate physicians on the importance of clinical documentation in the health record. In the first five months of 2015, the University of New Mexico Hospitals realized an increase of more than $1.8 million as a result of improved documentation. In the first 16 months of the program, the hospitals' CMI improved by 18.6 percent. The facilities have also seen improvement in the quality of care they provide based on SOI and ROM measures (Precyse n.d.).

References

American Health Information Management Association. 2015a. Best practices in the art and science of clinical documentation improvement. *Journal of AHIMA*. 86(7):46–50. http://bok.ahima.org/doc?oid=107704#.Vsxwe_krK9I.

American Health Information Management Association. 2015b. HIM Role. http://www.ahima.org/topics/cdi.

American Health Information Management Association. 2014. Clinical Documentation Improvement Toolkit. http://library.ahima.org/doc?oid=300359.

American Health Information Management Association. 2013. Study Reveals Hard Facts on CAC http://bok.ahima.org/doc?oid=106668#.Vu9SIebx2b8.

American Health Information Management Association. 2009. Recovery Audit Contractor (RAC) Toolkit. http://library.ahima.org/PdfView?oid=98673.

Balanced Budget Act of 1997. Public Law 105-32.

Casto, A.B. and E. Forrestal. 2015. *Principles of Healthcare Reimbursement*, 5th ed. Chicago: AHIMA.

Centers for Medicare and Medicaid Services. 2016a. Electronic Health Records (EHR) Incentive Programs. https://www.cms.gov/Regulations-and-Guidance/Legislation/EHRIncentivePrograms/index.html?redirect=/EHRIncentivePrograms/01_Overview.asp#BOOKMARK4.

Centers for Medicare and Medicaid Services. 2016b. What Is a MAC and What Do They Do? https://www.cms.gov/Medicare/Medicare-Contracting/Medicare-Administrative-Contractors/What-is-a-MAC.html.

Centers for Medicare and Medicaid Services. 2015a. Physician Self Referral. https://www.cms.gov/Medicare/Fraud-and-Abuse/PhysicianSelfReferral/index.html?redirect=/physicianselfreferral/.

Centers for Medicare and Medicaid Services. 2015b. Self-Audit Toolkit. https://www.cms.gov/Medicare-Medicaid-Coordination/Fraud-Prevention/Medicaid-Integrity-Education/Downloads/audit-selfaudit-booklet[April-2015].pdf.

Centers for Medicare and Medicaid Services. 2014a. 2014 National Training Program Module: 10 Medicare and Medicaid Fraud and Abuse Prevention Workbook. https://www.cms.gov/Outreach-and-Education/Training/CMSNationalTrainingProgram/Downloads/2014-Medicare-and-Medicaid-Fraud-and-Abuse-Prevention-Workbook.pdf.

Centers for Medicare and Medicaid Services. 2014b. Medicare Fraud and Abuse. https://www.cms.gov/Outreach-and-Education/Medicare-Learning-Network-MLN/MLNProducts/downloads/fraud_and_abuse.pdf.

Centers for Medicare and Medicaid Services. 2014c. Avoiding Medicare and Medicaid Fraud and Abuse: A Roadmap for Physicians. https://www.cms.gov/Outreach-and-Education/Medicare-Learning-Network-MLN/MLNProducts/Downloads/Avoiding_Medicare_FandA_Physicians_FactSheet_905645.pdf.

Centers for Medicare and Medicaid Services. 2013. Medicare Fee-for-Service Recovery Audit Program Additional Documentation Limits for Medicare providers (Except suppliers and physicians). https://www.cms.gov/Research-Statistics-Data-and-Systems/Monitoring-Programs/Recovery-Audit-Program/Downloads/April-2013-Provider-ADR-Limit-Update.pdf.

Healthcare Financial Management Association. n.d. Tool: RAC Timeframes and Deadlines. http://www.hfma.org/WorkArea/DownloadAsset.aspx?id=12770.

Green, M.A. and J.C. Rowell. 2015. *Understanding Health Insurance: A Guide to Billing and Reimbursement*. Stamford, CT: Cengage Learning.

Horton, L.A. 2012. *Calculating and Reporting Healthcare Statistics*. Chicago: AHIMA.

McWay, D.C. 2016. *Legal and Ethical Aspects of Health Information Management*, 4th ed. Clifton Park, NY: Cengage Learning.

National Association of Medicaid Directors (NAMD). 2012. Rethinking Medicaid Program Integrity: Eliminating Duplication and Investing in Effective, High-Value Tools. http://medicaiddirectors.org/wp-content/uploads/2015/08/namd_medicaid_pi_position_paper_final_120319.pdf.

Office of Inspector General. n.d. Health Care Compliance Program Tips. http://oig.hhs.gov/compliance/provider-compliance-training/files/Compliance101tips508.pdf.

Office of Inspector General. 2016a. About Us. http://oig.hhs.gov/about-oig/about-us/.

Office of Inspector General. 2016b. Organizational Chart. http://oig.hhs.gov/about-oig/organization-chart/index.asp.

Office of Inspector General. 2013. Medicare Recovery Audit Contractors and CMS's Actions to Address Improper Payments, Referrals of Potential Fraud, and Performance. http://oig.hhs.gov/oei/reports/oei-04-11-00680.pdf.

Office of Inspector General. 2007. Quality Concerns Identified Through Quality Improvement Organization Medical Record Reviews. http://oig.hhs.gov/oei/reports/oei-01-06-00170.pdf.

Office of Inspector General. 1998. 42 CFR Parts 1003, 1005 and 1006. Health care programs: Fraud and abuse; revised OIG civil money penalties resulting from the Health Insurance Portability and Accountability Act of 1996. *Federal Register*. http://oig.hhs.gov/authorities/docs/hipaacmp.pdf.

Office of the National Coordinator for Health Information Technology (ONC). 2016. Electronic Health Records (EHR) Incentive Programs. https://www.cms.gov/Regulations-and-Guidance/Legislation/EHRIncentivePrograms/index.html?redirect=/EHRIncentivePrograms/.

Office of the National Coordinator for Health Information Technology (ONC). 2013. How to Obtain Meaningful Use. https://www.healthit.gov/providers-professionals/meaningful-use-definition-objectives.

Precyse. n.d. UNM Hospitals Turns the Tide on Clinical Documentation. https://www.precyse.com/resources/Precyse%20UNMH%20CDI%20Success%20Story%20Web%20Version.pdf.

Prophet, S. 1997. Fraud and abuse implications for the HIM professional. *Journal of AHIMA*. 68(4):52–56.

Sayles, N.B. 2014. *Introduction to Computer Systems for Health Information Technology*, 2nd ed. Chicago: AHIMA.

Schraffenberger, L.A. and L. Kuehn. 2011. *Effective Management of Coding Services*, 4th ed. Chicago: AHIMA.

Smith, G. and J. Bronnert. 2010. Transitioning to CAC: The skills and tools required to work with computer-assisted coding. *Journal of AHIMA.* 81(7):60–61. http://library.ahima.org/doc?oid=101090#.VxUObfkrLDc.

STOP Medicare Fraud. 2016. HEAT Task Force. https://www.stopmedicarefraud.gov/aboutfraud/heattaskforce/.

US Department of Health and Human Services (HHS). 2009. Testimony. http://www.hhs.gov/asl/testify/2009/10/t20091028a.html.

US Department of Justice. 2015. National Medicare Fraud Takedown Results in Charges Against 243 Individuals for Approximately $712 Million in False Billing. http://www.justice.gov/opa/pr/national-medicare-fraud-takedown-results-charges-against-243-individuals-approximately-712.

Wiedemann, L.A. 2013. Using CDI to Meet Federal Quality Measures. http://bok.ahima.org/doc?oid=105918#.VsZtb-Y2DAk.

45 CFR 160.401: Definitions. 2009.

Part VI
Leadership

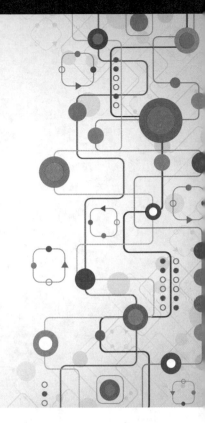

17

Leadership

Donald W. Kellogg, PhD, CPEHR, RHIA, FAHIMA

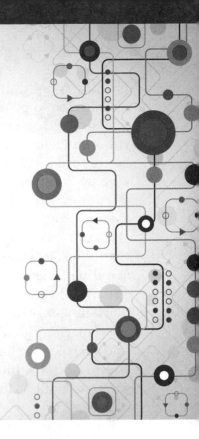

Learning Objectives

- Critique the different leadership theories
- Differentiate among leadership styles
- Summarize the impact of change management on processes, people, and systems
- Execute the fundamentals of team leadership
- Execute and facilitate meetings
- Summarize health information-related leadership roles

Key Terms

Active listening
Authoritarian leadership
Behavior theory
Benevolent autocracy
Bureaucracy
Business-related partnerships
Change management
Chief executive officer (CEO)
Chief financial officer (CFO)
Chief information officer (CIO)
Coercive power
Conflict management
Consultative leadership
Consensus building
Consensus-oriented decision-making model

Contingency theory
Critical thinking
Democratic leadership
Distal attributes
Expert power
Exploitive autocracy
Great Person theory
Laissez-faire leadership
Leader–member relations
Leadership criteria
Leadership grid
Leading
Leading by example
Legitimate power
Participative leadership
Power and influence theory

Proximal attributes
Referent power
Reward power
Team building
Team charter
Team leader
Team member
Team norms
Theory X and Y
Timekeeper
Trait theory
Transactional leadership
Transformational leadership
Transitional model

Leading is one of the four management functions (in addition to planning, organizing, and controlling) in which people are directed and inspired toward achieving specific goals. Leaders should not be confused with managers. "Leaders are people who do the right thing; managers are people who do things right" (Manktelow 2015). Yet, while leaders provide direction, they must also use the skills of a manager to guide their followers to successful results in an effective and efficient way. By inspiring others, creating a vision, and mapping out what needs to be done, a leader can ensure that everyone in the group or team is successful.

Former President Dwight D. Eisenhower once said that "leadership is the art of getting someone else to do something you want done because he wants to do it." How a person perceives himself or herself as a leader may be different than an employee's view of that person as a leader. There are numerous definitions for leadership with multiple approaches to identify and explain the multifaceted factors that shape leadership and how it is accomplished. These theories evaluate the relationship of the leader to others and examine styles of leadership, adding to the general knowledge of leader behavior and effectiveness.

Though created over 50 years ago, Robert Blake and Jan Mouton's **leadership grid** is still one of the most used tools to determine leadership style and presents five different personal leadership styles that depend on a person's concern for people (plotted on the y-axis) versus his or her concern for production (plotted on the x-axis) (see figure 17.1). The first style is *impoverished management* (IM) where a leader has a low concern for people and

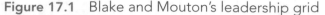

Figure 17.1 Blake and Mouton's leadership grid

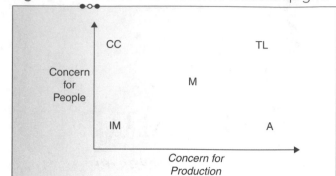

©AHIMA

a low concern for production (near the zero point on a graph). The *country club* (CC) style shows that a leader has a high concern for people and yet still has a low concern for production. The *authoritarian* (A) leadership style reflects a very low concern for people and a very high concern for production. The *team leader* (TL) style has a very high concern for people and also a very high concern for production. Finally, the *middle of the road* (MR) leadership style produces medium results with a medium concern for both people and production (Blake and Mouton 1964).

This chapter will discuss the various leadership theories, styles, patterns of leadership, and transformational leadership, as well as characteristics of leaders who create, motivate a group of people, and deliver an inspiring vision of the future. Also discussed are change management, critical thinking, and identifying the executive level of management, the chapter concludes with discussions of teams including team leadership and business-related partnership and holding meetings.

Leadership Theories

How does someone become a leader? Is it inherent in the way a person is perceived or can an individual learn the necessary skills to become a leader? There are four major theories on how one becomes a leader:

- *Trait theory*: Leadership is an inherited set of traits and not learned

- *Behavior theory*: Leadership can be learned
- *Contingency theory*: Leadership is based on the situation and context
- *Power and influence theory*: Leadership can be based on position and title

Each of the four theories is discussed in the following sections.

Trait Theory

Trait theory is one of the earliest leadership theories, sometimes referred to as the "**Great Person Theory**." which states that some people have innate leadership skills that are not due to training and exercises but, rather, to one's natural ability. Leadership is considered a unique property of extraordinary people that cannot be learned (Galton 1869).

Traits can be divided into three divisions: distal attributes, proximal attributes, and leadership criteria. **Distal attributes**—such as personality, cognitive abilities, motives, and values—are traits that surround the leader as a person. **Proximal attributes**—such as problem-solving skills, social appraisal skills, and expertise and tacit knowledge—are derived from the distal attributes and are part of a leader's operating environment. From these proximal attributes, a leader possesses **leadership criteria**—leader emergence, leader effectiveness, as well as advancement and promotion. Criticisms of this model is that it is too simplistic–perceptions of leaders by their followers does not necessarily reflect the effectiveness of the leader, in the context of the leader's position is not considered, and this model focuses too much on personality traits and not on social skills and problem solving ability.

Table 17.1 illustrates how leadership traits are organized into three categories: demographic, task competence, and interpersonal attributes (DeRue et al. 2011). Gender differences have been the main focus of research for the demographics category, though most scholars have found both genders are equally effective as leaders. Task competence

Table 17.1   Division of leadership traits

Demographic	Task competence	Interpersonal attributes
Gender	Execution of tasks	Approaches social interactions
	Performance of tasks	Extraversion
	Intelligence	Agreeableness
	Conscientiousness	
	Openness to experience	
	Emotional stability	

Source: DeRue et al. 2011.

relates to how individuals approach the execution and performance of individual tasks (Bass and Bass 2008). Intelligence, conscientiousness, openness to experience, and emotional stability fit into this category (Hoffman et al. 2011). Finally, interpersonal attributes are related to how a leader approaches social interactions. Extraversion and agreeableness are grouped into this category (Hoffman et al. 2011).

More recently, researchers determined that there are six leadership traits including:

1. *Physiological*: Appearance, height, and weight
2. *Demographic*: Age, education, and socioeconomic background
3. *Personality*: Self-confidence and aggressiveness
4. *Intellective*: Intelligence, decisiveness, judgment, and knowledge
5. *Task-related*: Achievement drive, initiative, and persistence
6. *Social characteristics*: Sociability and cooperativeness (Management Study Guide 2015)

Behavior Theory

In response to the trait theory advocates, a group of researchers proposed the behavior-based theory to better define what makes a leader. Whereas the proponents of the trait theory believe leaders are born with these characteristics, the behaviorists determined leaders can be made and that successful leadership is based on definable, learnable behavior.

The **behavior theory** opened the door to leadership development rather than looking for those individuals who were born into a leadership role. Using different techniques, researchers at The Ohio State University and the University of Michigan developed two broad categories of behavioral characteristics—task-oriented (initiating structure) and people-oriented (consideration) behaviors. Task-oriented behaviors include setting goals, defining roles, organizing work, assigning tasks, establishing standards, and emphasizing meeting deadlines. People-oriented behaviors include sensitivity toward subordinates, establishing mutual trust, exhibiting concern for workers, showing appreciation, and being fair and just (Thye 2010).

Contingency Theory

Contingency theory states leadership exists between persons in social situations; and persons who are leaders in one situation may not necessarily be leaders in other situations (Stogdill 1948). The first contingency approach to leadership stated that leadership effectiveness (in terms of team performance) depends on the interaction of the leader's task motivations and certain aspects of the situation. This model postulates that the leader's task motivations are dependent on whether he or she can control and predict the team's outcomes. Whether those outcomes are in alignment with the situation (context) depends on three calculations: (1) whether the leader perceives supportive relations with team members (leader–member relations); (2) whether the task is highly structured with standardized procedures and measures of performance (task structure); and (3) whether the leader's position of authority is harsh or satisfying to the team members (position power) (Fielder 1964).

Many contingency theories have defined leadership effectiveness in terms of team performance or satisfaction. However, a decision model created by Victor Vroom and Arthur Jago emphasized that situational factors are more important than leadership behaviors (Vroom and Jago 1995). The model relies on decision making to determine leadership style. A set of five different decision-making strategies that range on a continuum from directive to participative decision making are outlined. These strategies include two types of autocratic styles, in which one person has complete control and decision making authority (type A1: the leader decides alone, and type A2: leader collects information from followers and then decides alone), two types of consultative styles (type C1: the leader consults followers individually and then decides alone, and type C2: leader consults followers as a group and then decides alone), and a group decision-making option (group consensus). Figure 17.2 illustrates the relationships between the leader and followers.

Power and Influence Theory

The **power and influence theory** of leadership takes a different approach in that there are various ways leaders use authority, control, and their influence on others to get things done. Perhaps the best-known of these theories is the model that social psychologists John R. P French Jr. and Bertram Raven's proposed listing five forms of power (French and Raven 1960). This model identifies three types of positional power and two sources of personal power.

Figure 17.2 Vroom and Jago's decision-making strategies

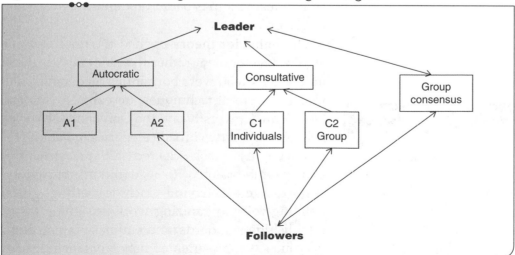

Adapted from: Vroom and Jago 1995.

Positional power is divided into legitimate power, reward power, and coercive power. **Legitimate power** is afforded by a persons' position or status within the organization. The team leader expects the team members to follow their orders and their status allows the leader to act as a liaison between the team and upper management. Use caution when relying too much on legitimate power as it is only effective in situations in which the team believes the team leader has the right or power to influence them.

Reward power is based on the leader's ability to give rewards to team members for outstanding work such as letters of recommendation, additional training or responsibilities, and additional compensation for working on the team. Reward power and legitimate power go hand in hand as the leader can only provide rewards if he or she is in a position of power.

Finally, **coercive power**, considered the opposite of reward power, occurs when the team leader uses threats and punishments to get his or her way. Extensive use of coercive power should be avoided as many leaders abuse this power and use it inappropriately (French and Raven 1960).

Personal power is divided into referent power and expert power. **Referent power** (also known as charismatic power) is the ability of the team members to identify with leaders who have desirable resources or personal traits. This may come from the leader's energy, endurance, empathy, toughness, humor, or charm. **Expert power** refers to leaders who are experts in their field or have knowledge or skills that are in short supply. Team members have a tendency to listen to those who demonstrate expertise. A person does not have to be in a position of power to have expert power. A team leader can take maximum advantage of expert power by using their knowledge to offer guidance and support to the team to motivate them. A leader should not be a know-it-all and must listen to the concerns of the team members to create credibility and respect. The team leader does not have to have all the knowledge and expertise in the group and should acknowledge the expertise of other team members (French and Raven 1960).

Two additional power and influence theories are transactional leadership and leading by example. **Transactional leadership** assumes that the team members will accept and complete their responsibilities for no other reason than to receive rewards. Therefore, leaders need to design a task and reward system to ensure that the team's work progresses at a satisfactory pace. **Leading by example** places the leader in a role model position. If the team members see the leader assume responsibilities and complete them on time then the team members are likely to do the same (French and Raven 1960).

Leadership Styles

After all leadership styles are evaluated they can be divided into three basic groups: authoritarian, democratic, and laissez-faire. As expected from the name, the **authoritarian leadership** style is domineering; and decisions are made from a distance and far away from the workers that they affect. Rulemaking, task assignments, and problem solving are done solely by the leader and enforced through punishment, threats, demands, orders, and regulations (Lewin et al. 1939).

The **democratic leadership** style is participative and supports collective decision making by offering others in the group choices and then empowering its members by facilitating group deliberations and encouraging and rewarding active member involvement. The leader gains authority by taking personal responsibility for the group's outcomes and accepts accountability for the results. The pluses for this type of leadership style are that it builds consensus of the group members, encourages creativity, builds commitment, and creates a shared vision. One negative of the democratic style is that it is not particularly effective when decisions have to be made quickly and the group feels the leader is not leading but, rather, depending too heavily on the group. This style is difficult to use when there is little communication and the group is comprised of inexperienced people. A type of leadership style included in the democratic method is value-based leadership—an approach that emphasizes values, ethics, and stewardship as central to effective leadership (Lewin et al. 1939).

The third leadership style is **laissez-faire** (also known as delegative leadership). This style reflects a leader who holds a title and responsibility but is strictly hands-off and has everyone else perform the work. This style is commonly associated with negative outcomes though it can be highly effective if the group members are already highly accomplished and motivated. Some of the negatives associated with laissez-faire include the need for some group members to have direction and guidance, some of the members might be inexperienced and likely to struggle with the task at hand, and the leaders give the appearance of being uninterested. A type of leadership style associated with laissez-faire is path–goal leadership, which emphasizes the role of the leader in removing barriers to goal achievement but otherwise having a hands-off attitude after the group is established (Lewin et al. 1939).

Patterns of Leadership

Leadership reveals itself in a continuum of five distinct styles (see figure 17.3). On one side of the continuum is **exploitive autocracy**—the harshest form of leadership, as the leader wields absolute power and uses the team to serve his or her own personal interests. This is followed by **benevolent autocracy** where the leader also wields absolute power but is generally kind and sincere in the use of the team for the good of the organization.

Subsequently, in a **bureaucracy** the leader relies primarily on rules and regulations but sometimes those rules and regulations become more important than the team's purpose. Next is **consultative leadership** where the leader remains open to input from members of the team but still retains full decision-making authority. And at the most lenient end of the continuum is **participative leadership** where plans and decisions are made by the team and the leader is there to provide advice and assistance (McConnell 2015).

Perhaps the single most important factor that defines a true leader is the acceptance (and not just obedience) by his or her followers; that is, a leader's real effectiveness is related to the amount of influence that individual has on the team performance, satisfaction of team members, and overall team effectiveness (DeRue et al. 2011). **Leader–member relations**—the acceptance of and confidence in the leader by the team members, as well as the loyalty and commitment they show toward the leader—is vital for any leadership style.

Douglas McGregor investigated that leadership styles may be related to a leader's philosophy about the members in a group or team; and his investigations resulted in **Theory X and Y**. Theory X is pure authoritative leadership, in which the team leader believes team members perform best under supervision that involves close control, centralized authority, authoritarian practice, and minimal participation of the group members in the decision-making process. The leader feels that the team is lazy, has no motivation, and will do nothing productive if not overseen closely. In theory X, leaders are pessimistic about the team members and the quality of their work; and assume the average person dislikes work and must be forced to accomplish the group's goals. This theory may be self-fulfilling because if the leader believes the

Figure 17.3 The continuum of leadership styles

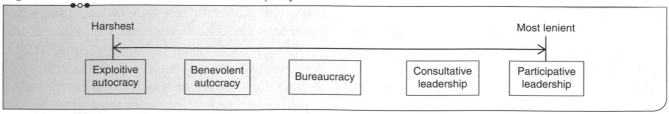

team members are lazy, they may, indeed, become lazy (McGregor 1960).

Theory Y relates to participative leadership where the team leader believes team members are eager to do well, have the motivation to perform their best, and are capable of doing so. In theory Y, leaders are optimistic about the team members and expects great results from their work. The Theory Y leader assumes that work is not avoided, self-motivation and inherent satisfaction will work toward the benefit of the group, and each group member seeks responsibility. Leaders will delegate tasks and responsibilities as much as possible and open communication is encouraged (McGregor 1960).

While the reality is that neither of these theories is used exclusively by leaders, there are elements of each that reflect how one anticipates working with others. As an example of Theory X, some people may dread being placed on a particular team feeling they will have to do all the work because other members of the team will not carry their weight. However, there are some groups for which people volunteer either because they know other people in the group or believe the work is worthwhile. In this Theory Y example, leaders rarely have to threaten, punish, or look over the shoulders of the team members because the members enjoy being a part of that group.

Transformational Leadership

The theory of **transformational leadership** is exemplified by leaders who inspire and motivate a group of people, and create a vision of the future. The leader becomes a role model who coaches and builds a team of committed members. The leader identifies a needed change, creates the vision of how to accomplish this change, and aligns the group members with tasks that will not only achieve the goals and objectives of the vision but also enhance the performances of group members.

There are four common components of transformational leaders. First, leaders serve as a role model to the group, referred to as idealized influence (II). Second, leaders have the ability to inspire and motivate their followers, also known as inspirational motivation (IM). Third, leaders demonstrate individualized consideration (IC), or a genuine concern for the needs and feelings of their followers. Finally, leaders challenge their followers to be innovative and creative, referred to as intellectual stimulation (IS).

Transformational leaders recognize many of today's problems cannot be solved with the same solutions of the past. New problems require new answers. Therefore, transformational leaders need to think outside of the box for new and innovative solutions and inspire their group members to do the same.

Check Your Understanding 17.1

Instructions: **Answer the following questions.**

1. Which of the following leadership theories state leaders are made not born?
   A. Trait
   B. Behavior
   C. Contingency
   D. Power and influence

2. The leadership trait of "appearance" is which of the following?
   A. Demographic
   B. Intellective
   C. Physiological
   D. Social

3. Creating a vision to guide a change through inspiration is characteristic of which of the following?
   A. Transformational leadership
   B. Exploitive autocracy
   C. Bureaucracy
   D. Path–goal leadership

4. A person may be a leader in one situation but not in another is the basis of what leadership theory?
   A. Trait
   B. Behavioral
   C. Contingency
   D. Power and influence

5. In which of the following theories would a leader feel that he or she cannot trust group members and has to micromanage?
   A. Theory X
   B. Theory Y
   C. Transformational leadership theory
   D. Participative leadership theory

6. Which of the following is the most lenient pattern of leadership?
   A. Bureaucracy
   B. Consultative leadership
   C. Exploitive autocracy
   D. Participative leadership

7. In Blake and Mouton's leadership grid, which leadership style reflects a high concern for people but a low concern for productivity?
   A. Country club
   B. Middle of the road
   C. Team leader
   D. Authoritarian

8. True or false: The Great Person Theory is closely associated with the contingency leadership theory.

9. True or false: Intellectual stimulation is a common component of transformational leadership.

10. True or false: Laissez-faire leadership is also known as delegative leadership.

Change Management

Change in healthcare is constant and may be impacted by internal and external forces outside of one's control. Within an organization, change generally occurs when someone perceives a need for a process or procedural improvement. It is the role of the leader to influence and guide others through the change so the group feels the change was worthwhile and they are not threatened by the finished result—whether by loss of employment, change in work responsibilities, or reduced income.

Methods of Change Management

Change management is a controlled method to ensure change can be managed smoothly. The underlying tenet is all human beings prefer doing things that have the most meaning for themselves. When people believe change is going to be harmful to themselves or their career they are resistant to change. To overcome this resistance, leaders need to patiently sell the idea of change by educating their team and carefully disseminating information.

The following sections explain various methods of change management: Kotter's eight step method to leading change, Lewin's change management model, and Bridge's Transitional Model of Change.

Kotter's Eight-Step Method to Leading Change

While a professor at Harvard's Business School, John Kotter developed an eight-step method of leading change within the organization. The eight steps to creating a climate of change in the organization include the following. Creating a climate of change starts with establishing a sense of urgency, building a team to guide change, and developing an informed vision and strategy to deal with the change. To engage and enable change in the entire organization includes generating short-term wins, empowering broad-based action, and communicating the change vision to all employees. To implement and sustain change involves consolidating gains and anchoring the new approaches within the culture of the organization (see table 17.2) (Kotter 1995). An example of this method of change management in HIM is the implementation of new healthcare regulations mandated by a new federal legislative Act. For example, a new law may change the way an HIM department processes healthcare disclosures. The manager of the HIM department could follow Kotter's eight step method to alleviate the anxiety caused by the required change.

Lewin's Change Management Model

Kurt Lewin, one of the first researchers in social psychology, proposed an alternative model of change management by advocating that organizations must first *unfreeze* or disrupt current processes, meaning the organization's existing mindset is interrupted. Often organizations continue using the same work processes believing the "if it ain't broke, don't fix it" adage. However, the organization's recognition that change must occur is the unfreezing of current work processes. This stage can lead to employees and management having feelings of denial and anxiety that must be overcome before the organization can move on to the second stage.

The second stage—*create the change*—occurs when people resolve their uncertainty and look for new ways to do things. This is typically a period of confusion and even anger and fear as they realize change must occur. There is usually resistance as the change is not clearly defined yet; however, the organization is beginning to move in a positive direction.

The final stage is *refreezing* the environment so the change is integrated into the processes and procedures within the organization. The change now becomes the status quo and produces a positive impact in the organization (Lewin 1947). Using the example of implementation of a new coding system in the United States, unfreezing would involve preparing for the implementation date. Transition and the refreezing would involve getting all staff and teams comfortable with the change and then getting productivity back up to where it was prior to unfreezing.

It is not the change itself that leads to so much misunderstanding as it is the manner in which a change is introduced. Leaders should introduce the change well in advance of the change's implementation so the employees can adapt to the idea, consider the implications, and ask questions for more clarification. Involving employees change management will reduce their uncertainty and potentially increase their acceptance rather than feeling the change was thrust upon them without their input.

Table 17.2 Kotter's eight-step method of leading change

Create a climate of change	Engage and enable change in the whole organization	Implement and sustain change
1. Establish a sense of urgency	4. Generate short-term wins	7. Consolidate gains
2. Build a team to guide change	5. Empower a broad-based action	8. Anchor changes in organizational culture
3. Develop vision and strategy	6. Communicate vision to all employees	

Source: Kotter 1995.

When providing the information and directives of how the change will occur, a leader must consider the types of employees impacted by the change, the work situation where the change will occur, and how supervisors will work with their staff—including their attitudes toward their staff members. Care must be given to how the directive for change is presented to the staff. For example, directives should be reasonable, intelligible, worded appropriately, compatible with the desired end result of the change, and indicate that the change can occur within a reasonable time frame.

Presenting the directive for change takes a great deal of forethought and is not to be rushed into without considering how the staff will react. Employees will be better able to acknowledge the directive if they understand the purpose behind the change. A better informed employee is more likely to accept the change. However, do not provide too much information as this may result in the leader spending excessive time clarifying the minute details rather than focusing employees on the bigger picture.

Bridge's Transitional Model of Change

William Bridges, a management consultant, focused his research on transitional process rather than change implementation. He created a **transitional model** that defines three stages: (1) ending, losing, and letting go; (2) a neutral zone; and (3) new beginnings. Each stage identifies the different emotions employees have as their daily work is either changed or replaced. The emotions associated with stage 1 are fear, denial, anger, sadness, disorientation, frustration, uncertainty, and a sense of loss. In stage 2 people may experience resentment toward the change initiative; low morale and productivity; anxiety about their role, status, or identity; and skepticism about the change initiative. Finally, in stage 3 employees may experience high energy, openness to learning, and renewed commitment to the group or their role in the organization (table 17.3). Understanding what a member of a group is feeling during the change process will help a leader anticipate potential issues and allow the leader to better guide the employees to a successful resolution.

Table 17.3 Bridges's list of feelings for a transitional model

Stage 1	Stage 2	Stage 3
Fear	Resentment	High energy
Denial	Low morale and productivity	Openness to learning
Anger	Anxiety about role, status, or identity	Renewed commitment
Sadness	Skepticism	
Disorientation		
Frustration		
Uncertainty		
Sense of loss		

Source: Bridges 2009.

Mergers

Mergers are a joining of two or more companies into one; this is a major source of change as hospitals and other healthcare entities are combined. During and after the merging of two healthcare entities, employees will wonder if there will be duplication or replacement of positions. Will the new entity need two HIM directors or can one position handle both departments? Perhaps the healthcare entity will create a corporate HIM position and only have supervisors at each location. The employee might wonder if his or her pathway to advancement has been lost as a result of a change in the organizational culture. One entity may have an organizational culture that encourages promotion from within while another entity may see the benefit of bringing in professionals from outside the organization. Which entity will dominate and thus offer an advantage to that company's employees? Will one entity's staff be given preference over the other? Mergers can create unsettling times but by being prepared for a leadership role an individual can provide extra security as either an asset in the new entity or by moving to another healthcare entity that can better appreciate his or her leadership abilities.

New Systems

Another major source of change is the development and implementation of the electronic health record (EHR) in a healthcare entity. Traditionally, HIM has been very labor intensive with people whose sole job is to move paper; from patient care sites, to analysis and assembly, to incomplete files, to coding, and then to permanent files—not to mention moving paper for release of information and off-site storage. However, with the creation of the EHR most document movement is handled electronically, thus reducing staffing levels previously necessary in HIM departments (see chapter 3 for more information about change within the EHR environment. This change is significant and affects all employees as the physical size of the department may be reduced since there is less paper to be stored and used for patient care. It is a leader's duty to explain the benefits of the change to staff and set a vision of where the department needs to transform; and clarify that while some jobs may be eliminated (file clerks) new jobs may be created (scanning). A leader must feel comfortable with his or her own role and convey that sense of job security to the other employees in the department.

Critical Thinking Skills

HIM leaders are confronted with a changing profession, whether it is in reimbursement, technology, or release of information. One of the most useful tools an HIM leader can possess is to think critically. **Critical thinking** is a disciplined process of actively and skillfully conceptualizing, analyzing, synthesizing, applying, and evaluating information. The information can be gathered from or generated by observation, experience, reflection, reasoning, or communication, and used as a guide to belief and action (Critical Thinking Community 2015). It involves the examination of the purpose, problem, or question-at-hand; any assumptions; concepts; reasoning leading to conclusions; implications and consequences; objections from alternative viewpoints; and a frame of reference. Critical thinking has two components—belief generating and processing skills, or the habit of using those skills to guide behavior (Critical Thinking Community 2015).

Critical thinking varies according to underlying motivation of one's self. When used for selfish purposes, it is often revealed as the skillful handling of ideas for the personal interest of an individual or group. When used in good faith, it is seen as ethical and perhaps idealistic, especially by those with other agendas. Critical thinking of any kind is never universal—everyone is subject to episodes of undisciplined or irrational thought. The quality of critical thinking is a matter of degree and dependent on, among other things, the quality and depth of experience in a given domain of thinking or with respect to a particular class of questions. The development of critical thinking skills is a lifelong endeavor as no one thinks critically in all situations (Critical Thinking Community 2015).

The list of core critical thinking skills includes observation, interpretation, analysis, inference, evaluation, explanation, and metacognition (Critical Thinking Community 2015). There are tools that can be used to help with critical thinking in a group. These include brainstorming, nominal group technique, and Ishikawa diagrams. Brainstorming is the aggregation of ideas from a group, where no response is considered bad and the goal is to generate quantity not necessarily quality. Using the nominal group technique, the group writes down their suggestions anonymously and then votes on which ideas are the most appropriate for the context of the discussion. This technique focuses on finding a communally acceptable solution. An Ishikawa diagram (also referred to as a root-cause diagram) is used to determine the root causes of a problem by constantly asking the question "Why?"

The following is a list of specific abilities that critical thinking requires.

- Recognize problems and find workable means for approaching those problems
- Understand the importance of prioritization and order of precedence in problem solving
- Gather and organize pertinent (relevant) information

- Recognize unstated assumptions and values
- Comprehend and use language with accuracy, clarity, and discernment
- Interpret data to appraise evidence and evaluate arguments
- Recognize the existence (or nonexistence) of logical relationships between propositions
- Draw warranted conclusions and generalizations
- Test these conclusions and generalizations
- Reconstruct one's patterns of beliefs on the basis of wider experience
- Render accurate judgments about qualities in everyday life (Reynolds 2011)

C-Suite

The HIM department does not stand alone, but reports to administrators in the C-suite (also referred to as the C-level). The C-suite is a slang term for the uppermost management level in an organization and refers to the executive titles that start with the letter C, referring to the word *chief* as in chief executive officer (CEO), chief information officer (CIO), and chief financial officer (CFO). It is important to note these executives report to the board of directors and the decisions they make affect the subordinate levels in an organization. At this level of management, technical and functional expertise matters less than leadership skills and a strong grasp of business fundamentals. The knowledge and skills that may have propelled an employee to this level of management might not be sufficient once he or she arrives at this level (Groysberg et al. 2011).

Chief Executive Officer (CEO)

The **chief executive officer (CEO)** is generally accountable solely to the board of directors (see chapter 2 for more information about the board of directors). The major responsibilities of the CEO are to develop and implement high-level strategies; set a vision; make major organizational decisions; manage the overall operations and resources of a company; build culture; set the budget to be presented to the board of directors for approval; and act as the main point of communication between the board of directors, the corporate operations, and public (SHRM 2015). The CEO position requires strong communication skills,

collaboration with others in upper management, and trust building between the CEO and upper management as well as subordinates (Groysberg et al. 2011).

Chief Information Officer

The **chief information officer (CIO)** is responsible for leading, planning, budgeting, resourcing, and training the information technology (IT) staff. The CIO needs to know how to create business models and make rigorous decisions based on the analysis of the return on investment. It is important the CIO understands new technologies and their potential impact (both good and bad) on the organization and its employees and how these technologies can create a competitive advantage as applied to the overall business strategy (Groysberg et al. 2011).

Chief Financial Officer

The **chief financial officer (CFO)** typically reports to the CEO or board of directors and is the chief financial spokesperson for the organization. Most CFOs have a master's in business administration (MBA) or are even a certified public accountant (CPA). This position oversees the financial unit and while they are good stewards of the organization's financial resources they are also focused on finding new opportunities for investments and assessing their strategic and financial merits and risks as well as developing risk management strategies (Groysberg et al. 2011).

Check Your Understanding 17.2

Instructions: **Answer the following questions.**

1. Which of the following is a problem-solving technique that focuses on working with individuals to find a mutually acceptable solution?
   A. Nominal group technique
   B. Change management
   C. Brainstorming
   D. New beginnings

2. Which of the following is a tool designed to find the root cause of a problem?
   A. Brainstorming
   B. Ishikawa diagram
   C. Nominal group technique
   D. Transitional modeling

3. When should a leader introduce the topic of upcoming changes to a group?
   A. As soon as the leader knows of the change
   B. Right before the change is to begin
   C. At the time of change
   D. Four to six months prior to the change

4. The C in C-level stands for which of the following?
   A. Clinical
   B. Chief
   C. Core
   D. Critical

5. Which of the following is not a specific ability used in critical thinking?
   A. Interpret data
   B. Recognize a problem
   C. Render accurate judgments
   D. Disorganize priorities

6. Which of the following statements is true about the C-suite?
   A. Every member of the C-suite reports to the board of directors.
   B. Only the CEO reports to the board of directors.
   C. The CEO may have a position on the board of directors.
   D. The CFO is only concerned with the operating budget.

7. Bridge's model of managing change indicates that there will be a negative impact on the organization in all but one of the change phases. Which phase shows a positive impact through the entire stage?
   A. Change phase
   B. Disruption phase
   C. Exploration phase
   D. Rebuilding phase

8. True or false: Critical thinking implies that human beings prefer to do things that have the most meaning for them.

9. True or false: Change is the same as transition.

10. True or false: The CFO's primary role is to develop and implement high-level strategies.

Team Leadership

HIM professionals work with other healthcare professionals (such as nurses, information technologists, informaticists, therapists) throughout the organization. As such, they are often placed in teams, an important part of any organization. By assembling a diverse group of people with technology knowledge as well as users and stakeholders, teams provide a valuable asset to the future of any healthcare entity. It should be noted teams and committees are not the same, as teams have a relatively short life span, whereas committees are part of the formal organizational structure. The **team leader** is someone who provides leadership, instruction, and direction to a team for the purpose of achieving a set goal or objective. It is the team leader who is responsible for the team's outcomes and ensuring everyone on the team contributes in a meaningful way.

There are certain leadership traits and qualities he or she must project to the team members to ensure the team's objectives are met. These include the following:

- *Communication:* An essential function to ensure all members of the team are aware of their role and responsibilities

- *Organization:* The composition and set of responsibilities of the team members is essential for any successful outcome

- *Confidence:* Through his or her actions, the team leader must show the team that the goals are important and each member has his or her own worth

- *Respectful:* All members of the team have to be shown respect for their input and who they represent on the team

- *Fair:* All members of the team must be treated fairly and no favoritism shown because of title or relationship to the team leader

- *Integrity:* The team's leader must not appear to change or waiver when difficulties occur but rather keep a constant viewpoint and direction

- *Influential:* The team leader must be able to bring the team to a consensus when differences of opinion occur to achieve a common outcome

- *Delegation:* The team leader cannot do it all; therefore, various tasks and objectives should be delegated to different team members

- *Facilitator:* When disagreements occur among the team members, it is the team leader's responsibility to keep everyone on task and focused on the projected outcomes

- *Negotiator:* When a stalemate occurs on the team's decision regarding the final deliverable, it is the team leader's responsibility to work toward a common agreement (Scott 2015)

Factors that contribute to team success are a team leader and members who have effective and excellent communication skills and member roles and responsibilities are clearly defined. When there is disagreement among members, it needs to be productive disagreement instead of accusations; and when decisions are made all parties agree to support those decisions. Next, the team needs to have strong external relationships with not only executive management but the other stakeholders who have an interest in the team's goals and objectives. Finally, the team needs to perform a routine self-assessment to determine what worked and what the bottlenecks were to finding the end result.

Teams that fail often have unclear goals or changing objectives so the team is constantly trying to achieve a moving target. Leadership is ineffective when there is no clear decision maker in the group so the lack of leadership results in conflicts between team members as they struggle to understand and take ownership of the process.

As with all new initiatives, support from the upper levels of management is essential for a team to accomplish its targeted goals. The support is often in the form of a team charter, providing a team purpose, help with team member selection, and creation of team norms. Without executive support, the team loses its champion to defend the team before the other top executives and the board. Executive support also ensures the team will have the resources (time, personnel, and money) needed to complete the team's objectives successfully.

Team Charter

The **team charter**, provided by upper management, is the document that describes the concerns the team was created to address, the team's goal or vision, and lists the initial members of the team and their respective departments. A team's success or failure at collaborating will depend on executives participating in supporting social relationships, demonstrating collaborative behavior, and creating a culture where the interaction among colleagues is viewed as valuable (Gratton and Erickson 2007).

Team Purpose

The main purpose for creating teams is to provide a formal framework so its members can participate in planning, problem solving, and decision making to better serve the organization. Therefore, the team purpose needs to be well defined by the team charter. When everyone knows the team's objectives then the team will not waste time with unnecessary or unproductive communication.

Team Selection

Once management determines a team should be formed to accomplish a set of specific goals and objectives and a person has been delegated as the team leader, it is time to appoint the **team members**. Every team should have the input and expertise of people from different parts of the organization who have direct relationships to the outcomes associated with the goals and objectives of the team. Membership should include people with technical expertise, knowledge of the process under consideration, employees who actually work with the process after the changes have been integrated, as well as other people who may affect or be affected by the outcomes of the team. By having members with diverse backgrounds, more insight and a variance of opinions and perspectives are

offered, rather than just a homogeneous approach (Gratton and Erickson 2007).

The size of the team depends on the scope of the outcomes required. For example, in a large organization strategic planning may have as many as 100 members who are then placed on teams and subcommittees to work on specific objectives. On the other hand, deciding what documents need to be scanned in an HIM department may only need five or six members to accomplish the task. A general rule of thumb is a team should be no greater than 20 members to run efficiently and achieve the stated goals and objectives in a reasonable time frame (Gratton and Erickson 2007).

Team and Member Participation

Comprising a team of diverse members is a risky venture that can prolong the desired outcomes of the team. This is especially true if the team members do not know each other, each member's area of expertise, or the task ahead. It can also occur when multiple managers are placed on one team as each might try to take control from the team leader. Ideally, the team leader should lead the team in **team building** exercises at the beginning of the process so the members can learn to work better as a group rather than individually. An example of a team building exercise is dividing the group into a group of 3 to 5 members and having them design a system to prevent an egg from cracking when the egg is dropped from a height of 10 feet.

Diversity of team members is needed for varying viewpoints; however, that same diversity can cause problems as people work better with others who they view as equals in terms of similar viewpoints and perspectives. This also may result in the lack of sharing of knowledge and less collaborative efforts (Gratton and Erickson 2007).

Each team goes through group dynamics that often take the form proposed by Bruce Tuckman (a professor at The Ohio State University). Referred to as Tuckman's model of forming-storming-norming-performing this four-stage model is a simple way to determine where a team dynamic is at any given point. *Forming* is the process of putting the team together. This is the first exposure of the team members to each other and making first impressions that are either on target or off base from reality. These first impressions will color a person's viewpoint of other team members throughout most of the team's existence. *Storming* is the phase when personalities clash as each team members are trying to find what their role is on the team and attempting to establish their relative position in the team dynamics. During this time the leader may have to institute **conflict management**, which focuses on working with individuals to find a mutually acceptable solution (Tuckman 1965). For more information of conflict management see chapter 20. *Norming* is the phase where conflicts are reduced, everyone knows their positions and responsibilities, and actual work to achieve the goals and objectives can begin. Finally, *performing* is the phase where actual results are obtained as the team is productive and reaches its final outcomes and deliverables.

Each of these phases can exist for different times depending on the composition of the team and people's personalities. For example, if a team is comprised of members who have worked before on other teams then the storming phase can be shortened. However, if the team is comprised of members that have never met or are representing different departments that have not traditionally worked well together than the storming phase can take up a lot of time that could otherwise have been productive (Tuckman 1965).

Eventually team members must work together to reach the common goals and objectives of the team. Each member must take the responsibility to communicate not only with the team leader but with each other, do not blame others but support group members' ideas, leave the egos at the door and do not brag, use **active listening** (a communication method that requires the listener to provide feedback to the speaker), and finally get involved by being a participant not a bystander. The four rules for active listening are: (1) seek to understand before you seek to be understood; (2) be nonjudgmental; (3) give your undivided attention to the speaker; and (4) use silence effectively (US Department of State 2015).

Team Norms

Team norms help determine what is both acceptable and unacceptable behavior for a team. Team norms may be *explicit* as in rules and regulations or *unwritten behavior* that is formed over time or through peer pressure. Most newly created teams start out with a preliminary set of norms that will be reviewed and modified frequently as conflicts or disagreements among team members occur. Some teams review norms at the beginning or end of each meeting and discuss which are working effectively and which need to be retooled. The establishment and adherence to team norms help build team discipline, trust between team members, and supports a safe environment.

Some norms that are common to most teams are as follows.

- Meetings will start on time
- Designated secretary will take notes
- An agenda is published in advance of the meeting
- Decision making is by consensus
- Silence means consent
- Teams members are held accountable for their work, or lack thereof, on the team
- Team members treat each other with respect and refrain from accusations or personal attacks.
- Everyone is regarded as equal (Establishing Group Norms 2015)

Team Meetings

Once the team is formed, a leader has been selected, team members establish their roles on the team, and a charter is presented by upper management, it is then the team leader's responsibility to set an agenda, schedule meetings, conduct the meeting, build consensus, and handle any follow-up tasks required to ensure the next meeting runs smoothly. The frequency of meetings is determined by the time constraints given in the team charter. Some teams may meet once a month while others need to meet weekly to reach a goal within the time frame given. For example, moving the HIM department to an off-site location may require teams meeting more infrequently when compared to implementing computer-assisted coding.

Scheduling of Meetings

One of the most difficult parts of organizing and running a team is the scheduling of meetings. The greater the number of team members, the more difficult it is to arrange a meeting. Be sure team members are informed in advance of the meeting to reduce scheduling conflicts.

Conducting Effective Meetings

Everyone on the team must be ready to participate and be an active member on the team. This means members coming prepared for the meeting by reading any material issued beforehand, being ready to discuss the material, and understanding what will be covered in the meeting. Often team members represent a division or unit within the organization, so the team member should collaborate with other people in his or her department and bring their collective views to the meeting. This will provide a richer discussion as a single person might not have considered all of the nuances that someone else from the department might have observed and shared with the team member representing the unit.

Prior to the meeting, the team leader should send requests to team members for input on meeting agenda items. This is not to say everything suggested will be included, but it is a starting point and indicative of what members feel are important issues that need discussion. The team leader controls the amount of information and discussion presented in the meeting to a reasonable amount so the meeting does not exceed its allotted time. The agenda and any other materials to be read should be sent to the members well in advance (4 to 5 days) of the meeting so they have enough time to review and prepare for the meeting.

The team leader must start the meeting on time to be cognizant and respectful of the members' schedules. The meeting should begin with a review of the agenda and ask for any additional comments before continuing. A team member delegated to be secretary will take notes (minutes) during the meeting. It is also helpful to have a member be a **timekeeper** to ensure the meeting stays on track without too many digressions. When confronted with numerous tasks to complete in a limited amount of time, the team leader must delegate several tasks and responsibilities to the team members, which allows everyone to share in the decision-making process.

At the end of the meeting, the leader should conduct a review of what was discussed and remind everyone who is responsible for individual tasks for future meetings. Be sure to end the meeting on time or even a little early; the team members will appreciate the thoughtfulness behind an efficient meeting. Finally, once the secretary has completed his or her notes, they should be distributed to the team members for review and clarification, if needed.

Consensus Building

When a group of people converge from diverse backgrounds to search for a solution to a problem, conflicts and differences of opinion often occur. It is the responsibility of the team leader to use **consensus building**—a decision-making method that seeks consent of all participants to resolve those differences so an acceptable result can be found. Note that a successful result does not mean it is favored by all, but only that it is acceptable to the members of the team.

The **consensus-oriented decision-making model (CODM)** presents a seven-step progression that allows groups the flexibility to come to a consensus by approaching important topics with open discussion rather than presenting a preformulated proposal; gathering a list of all the needs and concerns expressed by the group to form a list of conditions for possible proposals to address; taking turns in a unified attempt to shape each idea into the best possible proposal before choosing among them; and using empathy in the closure stage to address any unresolved feelings from the process.

The following are the seven CODM steps.

1. Framing the topic
2. Open discussion
3. Identifying underlying concerns
4. Collaborative proposal building
5. Choosing a direction
6. Synthesizing a final proposal
7. Closure (Hartnett 2011)

Consensus building is needed so the team is inclusive and not limited in their perspective. The team members represent diverse backgrounds and everyone should be encouraged to participate and all voices heard. Team members need to collaborate for further development of ideas into final results. Consensus building seeks to have everyone reach a common agreement so that implementation of the team's deliverables will be acceptable to all parts of the organization. It also results in more informed, collaborative, decisions and outcomes as everyone on the team has an ownership of the results and can relay them to their counterparts in their respective organizational units (Hartnett 2015).

Communication

Communication is vital for an effective leader. Direct communication with team members is important so they understand everything that concerns their work on the team. Communication can take different forms, whether through the use of meetings, minutes, reports (a summary of the data collection, conclusions, and recommendations of the team at a specific period of time), and storytelling (whose purpose is to summarize an entire project using words, pictures, or graphs in a fashion that permits listeners to grasp the team's accomplishments and to understand its specific application).

Most forms of communication use the same process, as shown in figure 17.4. The first step is to determine the concept of the message (ideation), which is the most difficult part of the process as the message must be clearly and concisely Formulated prior to sending the message to the receiver. The second step is to designate the sender. Usually is the team leader who communicates to those people outside of the team and also ensures the message is sent to each team member. The third stage is encoding, where the message is put into a clear and understandable format for everyone. For example, when communicating with a person who is not an HIM professional, it would be wise not to use jargon that HIM professionals use such as ROI, DRG, and MPI. The fourth stage is selecting the medium in which the message should be sent—via e-mail, letter, text, conversation, or posting on the organization's intranet. Each type of medium has a specific intimacy for the receiver that may

Figure 17.4 Stages of communication

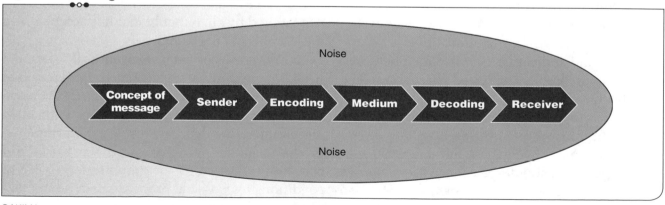

or may not be appropriate depending on the circumstances. The fifth stage is decoding, where the receiver acquires the message and has to internalize the message accurately so the meaning is not lost. The last step in the communication process is the establishing the receiver. This will impact not only the concept of the message but also the encoding, medium, and decoding. Surrounding the entire message is the background noise, those things that are distracting to the receiver when interpreting the correct perspective of the message being received, for example the tone of voice and mannerisms of the person attempting to communicate.

It is also important to know while much of the communication a team leader oversees is verbal, there is a great amount of nonverbal communication that adds significant importance to the message. Nonverbal communication is both written (text and graphs) and visual (behavior, body language, clothing, and intentional and unintentional signals). For a team leader to be a successful communicator he or she needs to adapt to the intended receivers' learning styles. Those learning styles include sensory (people who learn by doing), personality (some people prefer to work at night and sleep during the day), information processing (reading and writing out notes), social interaction (forming study groups), and instructional and environmental preference (some people prefer to learn in a classroom rather than online).

Lastly, there are barriers to effective communication. The first is *selective perception*, which means an individual will tune out information if it does not meet his or her preconceived ideas or conclusions. The next is *information overload*. Healthcare professionals are constantly being presented with a plethora of information and data, often much more than they need to accomplish their jobs. Having too much information slows down the communication process by not being able to distinguish what is of value and what is not. *Emotions* often interfere with the coding and decoding of a message. *Attitude* will determine if the receiver is receptive to a message presented by the team leader. In the United States today, *language* can play an important role as a barrier to effective communication. Many hospitals in western states are now looking for bilingual employees to speak with not only employees but also patients whose primary language is Spanish. *Silence* can be used effectively as a communication tool (namely, waiting until someone responds to a message) or as a barrier (indicating the receiver is either ignoring or in disagreement with the message). Some people have *communication apprehension* and do not like to speak in front of a group or present ideas that conflict with the group's opinion. Sometimes *differences in gender* can result in a single message having multiple interpretations based on the gender of the receiver. Another barrier to communication is *political correctness* where the intent of the message may be skewed so as to not offend the receiver. In this case, the message may be completely different than the original intent, that the true intent of the message cannot be received. Finally, the actual *presentation of the information* may create a barrier. Many times a clearer message can be received visually rather than through a narrative format. For example, this paragraph is over 300 words long. Many people would grasp this information better in the form of bullets, shown as follows.

- Selective perception
- Information overload
- Emotions
- Attitudes
- Language
- Silence
- Communication apprehension
- Differences in gender
- Political correctness
- Presentation of information

Check Your Understanding 17.3

Instructions: **Answer the following questions.**

1. Who has the responsibility for setting the meeting agenda?
   A. Team leader
   B. Executive sponsor
   C. Team recorder
   D. Team timekeeper

2. Accountability of team members is an example of which of the following?
   A. Team charter
   B. Group dynamic
   C. Group think
   D. Team norm

3. Group members trying to find their role within the team is part of which stage of Tuckman's model?
   A. Forming
   B. Storming
   C. Conforming
   D. Performing

4. Posture is an example of what type of communication?
   A. Verbal
   B. Nonverbal
   C. Explicit
   D. Tacit

5. When should a meeting's minutes be distributed to the team for clarification?
   A. As soon as the meeting is over
   B. Just before the next meeting starts
   C. At the beginning of the next meeting
   D. Five to six days prior to the next meeting

6. What is the rule of thumb for the size of a team?
   A. No more than 5
   B. No more than 10
   C. No more than 20
   D. No more than 100

7. CODM stands for which of the following?
   A. Computer-oriented decision making
   B. Consensus-oriented decision making
   C. Competency-oriented decision making
   D. Communication-oriented decision making

8. True or false: Teams and committees are not essentially the same.

9. True or false: While meetings should start on time it is acceptable for a meeting to go beyond the time allotted as a certain amount of material must be covered at each meeting.

10. True or false: Active listening allows a group member to listen and participate in the proceedings.

Business-Related Partnerships

Often it is beneficial for people in leadership positions to make **business-related partnerships**. A business-related partnership, which can be internal or external to the healthcare entity, is an agreement between two parties to cooperate for the advancement of their mutual interests and the entity's strategic goals. To create a successful partnership, each party must agree on a shared vision and mission and ensure each partner's needs and expectations will be met. It is important to identify the strengths and weaknesses of each partner so the tasks and accountability can be assigned to each partner appropriately.

Internal Business Partnerships

Within a healthcare entity, business partnerships can exist between individual managers or across entire departments. This is necessitated by the need to share resources, whether it is project funding, capital equipment, knowledge, expertise, or personnel. The main advantage of developing a partnership within an organization is that two heads are often better than one—sometimes great ideas can be generated with input from and the perspective of two people. Also, high-caliber employees can be made partners to compensate for a leader's areas of weakness. However, when two or more people are brought together the potential risk of disagreement and its resolution may be problematic. Common business partners for the HIM department are the billing office, compliance, and information services. Internal relationships in HIM are discussed in chapter 3.

External Business Partnerships

External business-related partnerships often occur with the various vendors providing services to HIM professionals, whether they are HIM consultants, EHR providers, or off-site storage companies. With external business partnerships, areas of responsibility as well as how success is evaluated and measured for both parties must be determined beforehand. It is imperative that the HIM professional assume a leadership role so the vendor will provide what the facility needs, not what is easiest for the vendor to provide, or what is the bare minimum from the vendor. Often projects fail because vendors want to install what they have already developed rather than meet the deliverables required by the facility. It is important that HIM professionals exert their leadership capabilities for the betterment of the organization as well as their own professional development.

Leadership Roles

While leaders may be managers, not all managers are leaders nor are all leaders managers. A leader can be anyone in a department or organization who may or may not have an organizational title. For example, Sarah works in a large HIM department where she rarely sees the HIM director, who is often in meetings in another part of the medical center. The department is transitioning to computer-assisted coding software and Sarah is running into an issue with the software accurately assigning the right codes when the physician does not articulate the proper documentation required by ICD-10-CM/PCS (*International Classification of Diseases, 10th revision, Clinical Modification/Procedure Coding System*). Rather than go to the department director (who has the title) she instead turns to the Melanie, the coder who sits next to her, who has experienced the same problems in the past and has experience in correcting the errors.

While titles do not necessarily guarantee a leader, it does give a person a platform to develop and exhibit leadership qualities. The titles available to HIM professionals listed in the following section are taken from the interactive Career Map published by the American Health Information Management Association (AHIMA). The Career Map lists the different job titles at various levels of mastery of the HIM profession and divides the jobs into different career paths (for example, compliance and risk management and informatics and data analytics). The following jobs listed are at the advanced and master level—those that best show leadership potential (AHIMA 2015).

Health Information Management

There are many opportunities for developing leadership skills in the HIM profession. HIM professionals are instrumental in compliance and risk management, education and communication, informatics and data analysis, information technology and infrastructure, health information administration, and revenue cycle management.

- *Compliance and risk management:* HIM professionals already hold the positions of compliance auditor, compliance officer, and chief compliance officer. Other positions include chief privacy officer and business analyst. These positions are becoming increasingly important as payers are connecting reimbursement to successful outcomes.

- *HIM education and communication:* Professionals with advanced degrees can teach the next generation of HIM professionals what they need to start a career in addition to the skills needed five years in the future. These positions include the different ranks of professor, program director, or department chairperson. In addition, healthcare facilities are seeking knowledgeable people to train their employees in ICD-10-CM/PCS as well as compliance, the EHR, and privacy and security.

- *Informatics and data analysis:* HIM professionals with additional training and knowledge in project management, data analytics, and mapping between nomenclatures are highly valued. These are leaders who can forecast future needs and see a job through to a successful conclusion.

- *IT and infrastructure:* Data quality managers are needed to ensure that the data collected throughout the healthcare enterprise (not just medical codes) conform to the Data Quality Management Model of AHIMA where 10 characteristics of data quality were identified—accuracy, accessibility, comprehensiveness, consistency, currency, definition, granularity, precision, relevance, and timeliness (AHIMA Task Force on Data Quality Management 1998).

- *Health information administration:* To run an efficient department, managers must also lead. Traditional leadership roles are the director and assistant director, manager and supervisor, and regional director of HIM who oversees multiple facilities. In addition, HIM professionals with special skills in certain areas have taken the lead by becoming consultants who aid organizations with their expertise, for example an HIM professional skilled in auditing may offer consultative services in auditing.

- *Revenue cycle management:* HIM professionals have a unique position within any healthcare organization as the bill cannot be dropped until the HIM medical coder has analyzed the patient chart and assigned both diagnosis and procedure codes prior to submission to the billing department. As such, HIM professionals have an opportunity to demonstrate leadership in positions like director of coding, coding manager, revenue cycle manager, and reimbursement and insurance manager.

All of these positions offer HIM professionals an opportunity to demonstrate leadership to their organization by understanding the organizational strategic plan and ensuring their staff will provide support. However, a title does not guarantee leadership, so the HIM professionals must constantly seek out opportunities by volunteering for assignments that will provide additional leadership skills and build a network of professionals both internal and external to the organization.

Future Roles for HIM

With the encouragement of AHIMA, more HIM professionals are seeking positions that were not in existence or anticipated a decade ago. Each of these positions requires advanced training to have the skill set needed to apply for and be accepted into these new and dynamic positions.

- *Chief learning officer (emerging):* This position is dedicated to the training of employees so their learning is in alignment with the organization's mission, goals, and objectives. Also part of this career is identifying what manpower the organization will need in the near future and ensuring that the organizational resources are used strategically and applied to achieve maximum results.

- *E-MPI manager:* This position is dedicated to resolving issues with the master patient indices (MPIs) when an enterprise decides to combine the MPIs from various facilities into an electronic format. The e-MPI manager works with registration to reduce duplicates and changes, and contributes to the design of the e-MPI to ensure coordination with local facility leadership through the use of improved practices. It is highly recommended that this person have extensive information system programming skills as well as HIM departmental experience.

- *Information governance officer:* This position is dedicated to developing an organization-wide framework for managing information throughout the information's life cycle and ensuring the information collected supports the organization's strategic plan and initiatives. This position requires knowledge of theall health information systems as well as data analytics.

- *Meaningful Use specialist:* This position is focused on end-user issues, workflow processes, issues with the EHR, and requires overall understanding of the issues related to the implementation of the EHR and the federal government's Meaningful Use initiative. Not only must this individual understand the information technology aspects of the EHR but also the regulatory and healthcare reform issues that are focused on payment based on performance.

- *Practitioner consultant:* This position works closely with clinicians and IT specialists to develop and provide solutions that have both a clinical and financial impact. The practitioner consultant needs to be well versed in medical terminology and nomenclature, disease processes, and the billing and revenue cycle.

- *Research and development scientists:* This position helps support the development of solutions for health IT as well as being part of the educational system to help train future IT training capacity. This position normally requires a PhD (doctorate).

- *Vice president of coding:* This position is responsible for managing the different facility coding divisions, establishing performance guidelines, forecasting the needs of the organization and its employees, and participating in process improvement opportunities. Since the organization is dependent on well-trained and knowledgeable medical coders, this position is vital for the financial health of the organization.

- *Vice president of security:* This position provides a workforce focused on the protection of information security focused not only on the EHR but also on the patient-centered health record as typified in patient portal access.

Real-World Case 17.1

Changes in healthcare are impacting all healthcare organizations. The HIM professional is desired for their expertise in reimbursement, HIPAA (Health Insurance Portability and Accountability Act), and the integration of the health record from a paper to an electronic format. Because of an increased demand of the HIM professional's time, leaders need to delegate to staff within the department. Jonathan is the director of the HIM department and is also a member (or leader) of additional committees within his medical center. He is discovering that his workday is now 9 to 10 hours long due to not only being responsible for his day-to-day duties but also the additional committee work.

Therefore, Jonathan has decided to delegate his oversight of the release of information unit to Mary, a credentialed member of the HIM department workforce. Jonathan needs to feel confident that Mary is responsible and has the ability to successfully complete this assignment. He also needs to be aware that even though he is focusing his time on other issues and meetings, he is also ultimately responsible for any task that he delegates to someone else. While Jonathan may be delegating a task to Mary to relieve some of his work pressure, this is also a great opportunity for him to test Mary for future assignment of duties and, potentially, promotion.

Real-World Case 17.2

Networking is an important component in being an effective leader as it provides an introduction to a diversity of thought and practice that a leader may not be exposed to otherwise. Sheila lives in Missouri and decided that she wanted to become more involved in the HIM profession at both the state and national levels. She started by asking to be a member of the Missouri Health Information Management Association's (MoHIMA) committee on EHR implementation. Through this committee she met fellow HIM professionals throughout the state that shared common issues and unique solutions about implementing the her system in their facilities. Satisfied with her growth through her association with MoHIMA,

Sheila next turned to volunteering with AHIMA. She volunteered to be on the question writing committee for the Commission on Certification for Health Informatics and Information Management (CCHIIM). Through this committee she was able to make many contacts nationwide. Being a CCHIIM member also allowed her to be considered for additional volunteer opportunities with AHIMA, again increasing her knowledge outside of her organization. Sheila found out that being involved with both MoHIMA and AHIMA added to others' perceptions of her as both employees and managers appreciated that she was recognized both statewide and nationally as an HIM expert and being a leader.

References

AHIMA Task Force on Data Quality Management. 1998. Practice Brief: Data quality management model. *Journal of AHIMA*. 69(6).

American Health Information Management Association 2015. Career Map. http://hicareers.com/CareerMap/.

Bass, B.M. and R. Bass. 2008. *The Bass Handbook of Leadership: Theory, Research, and Managerial Applications*, 4th ed. New York: Free Press.

Blake, R.R. and J.S. Mouton. 1964. *Managerial Grid: The Key to Leadership Excellence*. Houston: Gulf Publishing Company.

Bridges, W.B. 2009. *Managing Transitions*, 3rd ed. Philadelphia: Da Cappo Press.

Critical Thinking Community, of the Foundation for Critical Thinking. 2015 (May 29). Defining Critical Thinking. https://www.criticalthinking.org/pages/defining-critical-thinking/766.

DeRue, D.S., J.D. Nahrgang, N. Wellman, and S.E. Humphrey. 2011. Trait and behavioral theories of leadership: An integration and meta-analytic test of their relative validity. *Personnel Psychology*. 4(1):7–52.

Establishing Group Norms. 2015. Brushy Fork Institute Berea College. https://www.berea.edu/brushy-fork-institute/establishing-group-norms/.

Fielder, F.E. 1964. A Theory of Leadership Effectiveness. In *Advances in Experimental Social Psychology*. Edited by L. Berkowitz. New York: Academic Press.

French, J. P. R. Jr. and B. Raven. 1960. The Bases of Social Power. Chapter 20 in *Group Dynamics*. Edited by D. Cartwright and A. Zander. New York: Harper and Row.

Galton, F. 1869. *Hereditary Genius*. New York: Appleton.

Gratton, L. and T.J. Erickson. 2007 (November). *Eight Ways to Build Collaborative Teams*. Boston, MA: Harvard Business Review.

Groysberg, B., L.K. Kelly, and B. MacDonald. 2011 (March). *The New Path to the C-Suite*. Boston, MA: Harvard Business Review.

Hartnett, T. 2015 (June 26). The Basics of Consensus Decision-Making. http://consensusdecisionmaking.org/Articles/Basics%20of%20Consensus%20Decision%20Making.html.

Hartnett, T. 2011. *Consensus-Oriented Decision-Making: The CODM Model for Facilitating Groups to Widespread Agreement*. Gabriola Island, BC: New Society Publishers.

Hoffman, B.J., D.J. Woehr, R. Maldagen-Youngjohn, and B.D. Lyons. 2011. Great manor great myth? A quantitative review of the relationship between individual differences and leader effectiveness. *Journal of Occupational and Organizational Psychology*. 84(2):347–381.

Kotter, J. 1995. *Leading Change*. Boston, MA: Harvard Business Review.

Lewin, K. 1947. Frontiers of Group Dynamics. *Human Relations*, Vol. 1, pp. 5–41.

Lewin, K., R. Lippitt, and R.K. White. 1939. Patterns of aggressive behavior in experimentally created social climates. *Journal of Social Psychology*. 10:271–301.

Management Study Guide. 2015 (May 28). Trait Theory of Leadership. http://managementstudyguide.com/trait-theory-of-leadership.htm.

Manktelow, J. 2015. What is Leadership? Mindtools.com. http://www.mindtools.com/pages/article/newLDR_41.htm.

McConnell, C.R. 2015. *The Effective Health Care Supervisor*, 8th ed. Burlington, MA: Jones & Bartlett Learning.

McGregor, D. 1960. *The Human Side of Enterprise*. New York: McGraw Hill.

Reynolds, M. 2011. Critical Thinking and Systems Thinking: Towards a Critical Literacy for Systems Thinking in Practice. In *Critical Thinking*. Edited by C.P. Horvath, and J.M. Forte. New York: Nova Science Publishers.

Scott, S. 2015 (May 13). The 10 Effective Qualities of a Team Leader. The Houston Chronicle. http://smallbusiness.chron.com/10-effective-qualities-team-leader-23281.html.

Society for Human Resource Management (SHRM). 2015. http://www.shrm.org/templatestools/samples/jobdescriptions/pages/cms_001618.aspx.

Stogdill, R.M. 1948. Personal factors associated with leadership: A survey of the literature. *Journal of Psychology*. 25:35–71.

Thye, L.K. 2010. Leadership Traits and Behavioral Theories. http://www.slideshare.net/robertsonlee/leadership-traits-and-behavioral-theories.

Tuckman, B. 1965. Developmental sequence in small groups. *Psychological Bulletin*. 63:384–399.

US Department of State. 2015. Active Listening. http://www.state.gov/m/a/os/65759.htm.

Vroom, V.H. and A.G. Jago. 1995. Situation effects and levels of analysis in the study of leader participation. *Leadership Quarterly*. 6:169–181.

18

Performance Improvement

Darcy Carter, DHSc, MHA, RHIA
Miland N. Palmer, MPH, RHIA

In memory of Chris R. Elliott, MS, RHIA who contributed significantly to the original content of this chapter and to the health information management field overall.

Learning Objectives

- Examine performance improvement principles
- Discuss various performance improvement tools and techniques used to facilitate communication, identify root causes, and collect, analyze, and report data
- Explain team-based performance improvement processes
- Examine the concept of quality and its importance in healthcare
- Correlate the importance of patient safety and national patient safety goals
- Apply the elements of a quality assessment program
- Identify major organizations that publish clinical quality standards and guidelines
- Articulate ways in which healthcare organizations manage the prevention and occurrence of infections
- Examine the Medicare requirements for utilization management
- Explain the clinical and administrative use of utilization management information

Key Terms

Accountable Care Organization (ACO)
Affinity grouping
Agency for Healthcare Research and Quality (AHRQ)
Benchmark
Brainstorming
Cause-and-effect diagram
Checksheet
Claims management
Clinical practice guidelines
Clinical protocols
Common-cause variation

Customer
Dashboards
Data abstracts
DNV GL Healthcare
External customers
Financial indicators
Fishbone diagram
Flow charts
Force-field analysis
High Reliability Organization (HRO)
Incident or occurrence report
Inputs

Internal customers
ISO 9000 certification
The Joint Commission
Lean
Lean Six Sigma
Medication Reconciliation
Multivoting technique
National patient safety goals (NPSGs)
Nominal group technique
Opportunity for improvement
Outcome indicators
Outcome measures

Outputs	Risk	Statistics-based modeling
Patient advocacy	Risk management program	Structure indicators
Performance improvement (PI)	Root-cause analysis	Structured brainstorming
Performance indicators	Run chart	Systems thinking
Performance measurement	Scorecards	Time ladders
Potentially compensable event	Sentinel event	Unstructured brainstorming
Process indicators	Six Sigma	method
Process redesign	Special-cause variation	Utilization management (UM)
Productivity indicators	Standard	Virtuoso teams
Quality indicators	Statistical process control chart	

Benjamin Franklin said, "Without continual growth and progress, such words as improvement, achievement, and success have no meaning." These wise words are directly applicable to the healthcare system of the United States today—it is in need of improvement, achievement, and success. This can be accomplished through continual growth and progress guided by quality and process improvement.

Throughout both history and present day we find individuals involved in the provision of healthcare services improving the way services are provided, thereby enhancing outcomes or improving performance. **Performance improvement (PI)** is the continuous study and adaptation of a healthcare organization's functions and processes to increase the likelihood of achieving desired outcomes. To be successful, these improvement activities require the participation of everyone involved at every level of the process.

Performance Measurement and Quality Improvement

Performance measurement is the process of comparing the outcomes of an organization, work unit, or employee against pre-established performance plans and standards. Performance measurement is one of the most important concepts in the introductory discussion of quality improvement. Healthcare professionals have struggled with where to focus their resources for quality improvement. With the assistance of the theoretical writings of general industry quality masters, the key to improvement rests in the measurement of the important characteristics of individual organizations.

Performance is "the execution of an activity or pattern of behavior; the application of inherent or learned capabilities to complete a process according to prescribed specifications or standards" (Meisenheimer 1997). Performance is measured using one or more **performance indicators**—a measure used by healthcare facilities to assess the quality, effectiveness, and efficiency of their services. Examples include **financial indicators**, such as the average cost per laboratory test, or **productivity indicators**, such as the number of patients seen per physician per day. It is important to measure the aspects of performance that reflect quality and point conclusively to the aspects of performance that require improvement. The traditional performance improvement process and sentinel events will be discussed in the next sections.

Traditional Performance Improvement Process

Although a number of terms and acronyms represent the PI concept (for example, continuous quality improvement [CQI] and total quality

Figure 18.1   Organization-wide PI process

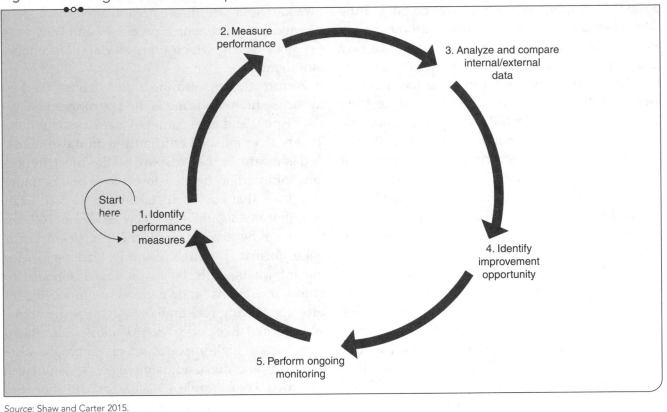

Source: Shaw and Carter 2015.

management [TQM]), this chapter uses PI. The key feature of PI as implemented in today's healthcare organizations is that it is a continuous cycle, starting with identification of the measures, performance measurement, analysis and comparison, opportunities for improvement, and ongoing monitoring as displayed in figure 18.1.

A logical starting point is to identify areas to monitor performance including important organization functions, particularly those that are high-risk, high-volume, or problem-prone (such as discharge not final billed [DNFB], coding compliance, or patient safety issues). Outcomes of care, customer feedback, and the requirements of regulatory agencies are additional areas that organizations consider when prioritizing performance measures. Once the scope and focus of performance monitoring are determined, the data collection requirements for each performance measure are defined (Shaw and Carter 2015).

As shown in step 2 in figure 18.1, measuring performance depends on the identification of performance measures for each service, process, or outcome determined important to track. A performance measure is a quantitative tool (for example, a rate, ratio, index, or percentage) that provides an indication of an organization's performance in relation to a specified process or outcome. Monitoring selected performance measures can help an organization determine process stability or identify improvement opportunities. Specific criteria define the organization's performance measures. Components of an effective performance measure include a documented numerator statement, a denominator statement (such as an error rate in coding with the number of correctly coded charts as the numerator and the total number of charts coded as the denominator), and a description of the population to which the measure is applicable. In addition, the measurement period, baseline goal, data collection method, and frequency of data collection, analysis, and reporting must be identified (Shaw and Carter 2015). An example of this would be managing the DNFB report). A measurement period is set monthly with a baseline goal of the DNFB being under a specific dollar amount (such as $500,000). Data collection would occur weekly and include the value of the charges on the outstanding charts. The health information management (HIM) professional may then analyze (step 3 of figure 18.1) the DNFB weekly and report the monthly figure to the chief financial officer (CFO). Based on the data, performance improvement activities may be initiated. The sum total of the performance measures selected as applicable to a healthcare organization make up the performance measurement system required in the hospital accreditation processes.

Accreditation organizations such as The Joint Commission, Healthcare Facilities Accreditation Program, and DNV GL Healthcare are examples of external resources used to establish the performance measures for a healthcare facility. If a healthcare facility fails to meet the accreditation organization's standards, site surveyors will cite the healthcare organization with a requirement for improvement if the threshold for the measurement is exceeded.

The monthly delinquent health record rate is one important outcome hospitals are required to monitor continuously. To establish this performance measure, the following criteria and formula is used.

$$\frac{\textit{Number of incomplete health records that exceed the established standard}}{\textit{Average monthly discharges}}$$

Tracking this outcome allows the hospital to continuously monitor its deficiency rate or percentage of delinquent health records. If the health record delinquency rate exceeds the hospital's established performance standards (an internal comparison) or nationally established performance standards (external comparison), an **opportunity for improvement** has been identified (step 4 of figure 18.1). Corrective action must be taken when a facility fails to meet a performance indicator.

Step 5 is a culmination of the prior steps. Monitoring performance based on internal and external data is the foundation of all PI activities.

Using its mission, scope of care, and services it provides, each healthcare organization must identify and prioritize which processes and outcomes (in other words, which types of data) are important to monitor.

Performance monitoring is data driven. The key to successful monitoring is the appropriate analysis, display, and application of measurement data. This is accomplished efficiently with **dashboards**. A dashboard is the "display of the most important information needed to achieve one or more objectives that has been consolidated... so it can be monitored at a glance" (Few 2013, 26). A dashboard can be disseminated in either electronic or paper format. The organization's leadership uses the information displayed on the dashboard to guide operations and determine improvement projects. Having real-time data in an easily accessible format like a dashboard allows leaders to keep track of high-impact, high-risk, or high-value processes and make adjustments on a daily basis if needed. For example, a dashboard can show the DNFB at different facilities within an organization. Additional information on data presentation is in chapter 13.

Every department in a healthcare organization should continuously monitor its key performance indicators. The following are tips for identifying and monitoring key performance indicators for HIM functions:

- Collect information at the appropriate level of specificity
- Monitor the overall performance of the department using a number of indicators appropriate for the size and complexity of the department
- Divide the department into the units where specialized work is performed
- Find measures that describe the unit's performance over time, recording on a daily basis and reporting on a weekly basis
- Design a report that can track data over time, including percentage measures to identify problem areas
- Design a dashboard that can be used to monitor key indicators in real-time

Sentinel Events

The Joint Commission requires healthcare organizations to conduct in-depth investigations of occurrences that resulted—or could have resulted—in life-threatening injuries to patients, medical staff, visitors, or employees. The Joint Commission uses the term **sentinel event** for such occurrences.

A sentinel event, therefore, describes an occurrence with an undesirable outcome usually happening only once. The occurrence, however, points to serious issues involved in care processes that must be resolved in order not to suffer the occurrence again.

Examples of sentinel events include medical errors, explosions and fires, and acts of violence. When these occur, the healthcare organization is required to prepare a detailed report of its investigation to explain the root cause of the event in order to avoid recurrence of similar events in the future. The Joint Commission issues sentinel event alerts when it detects a pattern of similar events reported by the healthcare organizations it accredits and uses its sentinel events data as a basis for its National Patient Safety Goals.

Quality Dimensions of Performance Improvement

There are three types of **quality indicators**, or standards against which patient care is measured to identify a level of performance for that standard.

- **Structure indicators** measure the attributes of the healthcare setting, such as number and qualifications of the staff, adequacy of equipment and facilities, and adequacy of organizational policies and procedures.
- **Process indicators** measure steps in a process and tasks people or devices do, from conducting appropriate tests, to making a diagnosis, to carrying out a treatment.
- **Outcome indicators** measure the actual results of care for patients and populations, including patient and family satisfaction (Donabedian 1988).

Quality has both a technical and an interpersonal dimension. The technical dimension recognizes that caregivers must have the knowledge and judgment to arrive at an appropriate strategy for providing service and the technical skills to execute it. The interpersonal aspect recognizes that caregivers must have the communication skills and social attributes necessary to serve patients appropriately. The interpersonal aspect of quality recognizes the importance of empathy, honesty, respectfulness, tactfulness, and sensitivity to others. It is far easier to measure quality's technical dimension than its interpersonal dimension (Donabedian 1988).

Contemporary Approach to Process Improvement

The contemporary approach to process improvement is much more proactive than the traditional quality management approach. Although process improvement uses several traditional quality management techniques such as quality indicators, most often its primary focus is on continually making small, targeted changes for improvement that over time lead to significant overall improvement. Process improvement is a mindset that, when adopted into organizational culture, can produce significant and continuous improvement. Process improvement is a proactive cycle that ensures key processes, products, and services are performed efficiently and within set quality standards. One key to successful process improvement is proactively measuring, monitoring, and improving indicators before the process or indicator is considered broken or unacceptable. An example would be putting an effective coding compliance plan in place that includes measuring, monitoring, and improving the coding in the facility before a negative outside audit or noncompliance fine is assessed and the in-house auditing process or coding product is determined to be unacceptable. Opportunities for improvement are identified by gathering and analyzing data on an ongoing basis. Process improvement assumes that organizations should continuously and systematically identify and test small, planned changes in processes and systems.

As process improvement practices have evolved, an important focus on the opinions of **customers** has developed. Many organizations and quality experts define *quality* as meeting or exceeding customer expectations. **External customers** are those people outside the organization for whom it provides services. For example, the external customers of a hospital would include patients, third-party payers, and the department of health. Organizations also have **internal customers** such as employees. The employees receive services from other areas in the organization that make it possible for them to do their jobs. For example, a nurse in an intensive care unit would be an internal customer of the hospital pharmacy; the nurse depends on the pharmacy to provide the medications needed to fill the physician's orders for his or her patients. As the importance of the perceptions and requirements of external healthcare customers becomes clear, the need for a standardized comparable way to measure their perceptions and opinions is apparent.

The Centers for Medicare and Medicaid Services (CMS) and the Agency for Healthcare Research and Quality (AHRQ) collaborated to develop the Hospital Consumer Assessment of Healthcare Providers and Systems (HCAHPS) survey. This was the first standardized survey used to compare hospital performance and quality at the national level. Hospitals are required to administer and participate in this survey if they provide services to Medicare patients. The results from this survey are informative to process improvement projects within hospitals. Consumers may also access the results of the surveys at the US Department of Health and Human Services (HHS) website and use the information to make informed decisions about which providers and hospitals they would like to use. Depending on the indicators used by the hospital and the information needs to measure those indicators, organizations may use supplemental survey tools to gather that information. Often, contractors or consultants design and administer the surveys; only approved contractors can administer the HCAHPS survey.

Another means by which customers can see how a healthcare organization performs is through the publication of scorecards. As discussed earlier, quality has many dimensions. Healthcare leaders cannot just focus on one aspect of quality (such as financial measures) without also considering other aspects (such as patient satisfaction or clinical quality) or they miss the whole picture. **Scorecards** are tools that present metrics from a variety of quality aspects in one concise report. They may present measures of clinical quality (such as infection rates), financial quality, volume, and patient satisfaction. Several sources, including healthcare organizations as well as local and national agencies provide scorecards.

Check Your Understanding 18.1

Instructions: **Answer the following questions.**

1. The focus of PI should be on which of the following?
   A. Interpersonal skills
   B. Customers
   C. Financial stability of the organization
   D. Employees

2. Fifty percent of the HIM staff has a nationally recognized credential. This is an example of which type of indicator?
   A. Outcome
   B. Process
   C. Structured
   D. Internal

3. Which of the following provides real-time process measure metrics in a consolidated format?
   A. Structured indicator
   B. Outcome indicator
   C. Dashboard
   D. Scoreboard

4. Performance monitoring is driven by which of the following?
   A. The mission of the organization
   B. The process improvement team
   C. Data
   D. Experts

5. True or false: An outcome indicator measures results of care provided to the patient.

6. True or false: Performance monitoring is outcomes driven.

7. True or false: PI is something that is done continuously.

Fundamental Principles of Continuous Performance Improvement

The fundamental principles of performance improvement include the following and are discussed in the next sections.

- The problem is usually the system
- Variation is constant
- Data must support PI activities and decisions
- Support must come from the top down
- The organization must have a shared vision
- Staff and management must be involved in the process
- Setting goals is critical
- Effective communication is important
- Success should be celebrated

The Problem Is Usually the System

Problems in patient care and other areas of the healthcare organization are usually symptoms of shortcomings inherent in a system or a process. A system is a set of related and highly interdependent components that are operating for a particular purpose. Every system has **inputs** or data entered into a hospital system (for example, in the hospital's admitting system, the patient's knowledge of his or her condition, the admitting clerk's knowledge of the admission process, and the computer with its admitting template are all inputs). The system processes the inputs and eventually produces **outputs**, or the outcomes of inputs into a system (for example, the output of the admitting process is the patient's admission to the hospital). One system's outputs may then become inputs for another system. Healthcare organizations are large systems; each department in a healthcare facility is a system with numerous subsystems.

The admitting department in a hospital is a system that exemplifies inputs, outputs, and the interrelationship between processes. When a patient enters the hospital, he or she presents to the admitting clerk. The clerk uses a computer to collect data for the admitting system. Some of the inputs for the admitting system are the patient with knowledge of his or her condition, the admitting clerk with knowledge of the admitting process, and the computer with its admitting template. The process begins with the clerk asking for the patient's address, insurance coverage, and reason for admission, as well as the patient's responses. The output of the process is the patient's admission to the hospital and a completed face sheet (which includes patient information, demographics, insurance information, emergency contact, and such) for his or her health record. These outputs are viewed as inputs into the next system in the hospital, the patient care system.

Systems thinking is a vital part of PI and is an objective way of assessing work-related ideas and processes with the goal of allowing people to uncover ineffective patterns of behavior and thinking and then finding ways to make lasting improvement. This requires individuals to think about patterns and interrelationships between work units in the organization.

Variation Is Constant

Every system has some degree of variation built into it. No system produces the exact same output every time. It is desirable to reduce variation within systems as much as possible so that system output can be more predictable and better controlled (Omachonu 1999). Variation that is inherent within the system is **common-cause variation**. For example, when a nurse takes a patient's blood pressure, she may believe she is performing the procedure in exactly the same way every time, but in practice she will get slightly different readings each time. Although the blood pressure cuff, patient, and nurse are all the same inputs into the system, variations can occur. For example, the cuff may be applied to a different place on the patient's arm. The patient may have a slightly different emotional or physiological status at the time of the measurement. The nurse may have a different level of focus or concentration. Any one of these (or other) factors can affect the values obtained. However, they are potentially present in every single episode of blood pressure measurement in every single patient. It is important to recognize not every variation is a defect. The variation may just be an example of common-cause variation found inherently in the process.

Factors outside of the system may cause variations. This type of variation is **special-cause variation**. If the special cause produces a negative effect, identify the special cause and eliminate it, if possible. If the special cause produces a positive effect, reinforce it so this positive effect will continue and perhaps be expanded into the processes of others in the organization. An example of this type of variation occurs when a patient is diagnosed with hypertension and the physician prescribes a blood pressure medication for the patient. After taking blood pressure medication and there is a substantial drop in the blood pressure measurement. All of the factors (diet, exercise, stress, family history) have remained unchanged demonstrating that the medication caused the decrease in blood pressure values, which is considered a special cause. In this situation, the variation is intentional and desired. In other situations, the variation may produce an undesirable and unintentional effect. For example, if a patient is upset about a phone call he received just before the nurse came in to take his vitals, his blood pressure may register exceptionally high. The change in values occurred due to a special cause (phone call) and resulted in a blood pressure reading much higher than expected.

Similar examples of special-cause variation exist in HIM systems. For example, common-cause variation can be observed in the number of health records that can be coded each day. On a day when one of the regular coders is out sick, the number of records coded might drop significantly because the coder will have no productive work time while home sick leaving the team short staffed. This would be an example of special-cause variation. Ideally, the goal is to remove special causes if they create an undesirable effect. When trying to control and reduce variation in a process it is important to remember there are staff with differing levels of expertise and patients with diverse levels of severity.

Data Must Support Performance Improvement Activities and Decisions

PI activities should be guided and driven by data. In the burgeoning era of big data, organizations and teams must be careful not to become overloaded with data. Data, transformed into information through proper analysis, is a tool key to the success of PI activities. Collection and analysis of appropriate data will provide a solid foundation for PI activities and improve the chances of success (Strome 2013). Before PI was a generally accepted practice, healthcare organizations relied on unsupported assumptions about which processes were functioning well and which ones were not. However, objective and accurate assessment cannot occur without concrete data. Collecting data provides information about the current processes, their effectiveness, and their potential areas for improvement efforts as well as the success of changes already implemented.

PI activities must identify the best method for obtaining timely, accurate, and relevant data.

Examples of data collection methods and instruments include retrospective health record review with specific quality criteria, written surveys, direct observation, and individual or focus group interviews. With the advancement and adoption of electronic health records (EHRs), it is becoming easier to implement and automate data collection within some processes. After adequate data is collected, careful analysis is imperative so that improvement efforts are built on this knowledge gained through accurate and appropriate data analysis.

Support Must Come from the Top Down

PI must become a part of the healthcare organization's culture. It is vital that the executive leaders of the organization believe in its value in order for it to permeate the entire organization. Moreover, they need to ensure their management teams are well versed in the principles and techniques of continuous PI. More information on organizational culture is in chapter 21.

The Organization Must Have a Shared Vision

The organization's executive leaders and board of directors are responsible for developing and communicating a clear vision of the organization's future. The organization's vision, mission, and values set its direction and support the norms it considers important. These statements guide employees as they make their own contributions to the organization in fulfilling their professional responsibilities. See chapter 19 for more information on mission and vision.

Staff and Management Must Be Involved in the Process

PI depends on everyone in the organization actively seeking to meet the spoken or anticipated needs of internal and external customers. This is particularly important for employees who have direct contact with external customers as they may be in the best position to recognize when customer needs are met. Often employees offer helpful ideas for improvement. Staff should be empowered to make a difference for their fellow employees and the patients they serve.

Setting Goals Is Critical

All PI programs must have established goals—targets the organization strives to achieve in a given PI program year. Each goal should be specific and define measurable end results. An example of an organizational goal might be: To provide high-quality patient care that is cost-effective.

After establishing goals, specific, measurable objectives that can be completed within a certain time frame should be identified. An objective associated with the previously mentioned goal might be: By the end of the year, a high-quality, cost-effective care program will be designed for the management of diabetes patients.

Effective Communication Is Important

Effective communication is essential for the PI process to work. Communication must exist at all levels of the organization and in all directions.

Openly identifying and discussing problems is not always comfortable or easy. However, an organization that is committed to serving its customers must view problems as opportunities for improvement. Two-way communication is effective and requires clear, articulate, and tactful speaking. More importantly, it requires careful, attentive listening and understanding. Organizations need to listen to their customers—both internal and external—so they can hear information about which services need improvement.

Success Should Be Celebrated

Although PI demands healthcare organizations focus on identifying and addressing problems, it also must celebrate the organization's successes. A celebration of success communicates to everyone the participants' efforts are applauded, success can result from such efforts, and others should be encouraged to participate in PI initiatives. The people involved in improving the process are recognized and appreciated.

Formal Performance Improvement Activities

Managers should feel empowered to monitor all processes within their supervision and responsibility, making small adjustments where necessary, and identifying when a more in-depth, formal approach is appropriate. Daily monitoring and minor processes adjustments performed by a single manager are informal and more of a maintenance activity. Once a manager identifiess an issue through the monitoring process, it requires a structured, formal PI intervention. The scope of the process, complexity of the problem, and involvement of other systems or departments should influence how formal the process should be and who should be involved.

Data collection and analysis is a vital part of PI; and benchmarking is an important PI data analysis tool. When an organization compares its current performance to its own internal historical data, or uses data from similar external organizations, it helps establish an organizational benchmark. A benchmark is a systematic comparison of one healthcare organization's measured characteristics with those of another similar organization or with internal, regional, or national standards. Often, further study or more focused data collection on a performance measure is warranted when data collection results fall outside the established benchmark. This is the "monitoring and improving customer satisfaction" process (Shaw and Carter 2015, 123). Opportunities for improvement are often discovered when unintended events and patterns are observed during continuous monitoring. This technique is best represented as the "team-based performance improvement process" (Shaw and Carter 2015, 31–32). The interdependency and interrelation of these processes is important and will be discussed later in the chapter.

PI initiatives use a number of tools and techniques. Some of the tools facilitate communication among employees while others help people determine the root causes of performance problems. Some tools indicate areas of agreement or consensus among team members. Others permit the display of data for easy analysis.

Checksheets

A checksheet is a data collection tool that records and compiles observations or occurrences. The checksheet consists of a simple list of categories, issues, or observations on the left side of the chart and a place on the right to record incidences by placing a checkmark (see figure 18.2). When the data collection is finished, the checkmarks are counted to reveal any patterns or trends. A checksheet is a simple way to obtain a clear picture of the basic facts. After data is collected, other tools may be used to display the data and help analyze them more easily.

Data Abstracts

Data abstracts are a defined and standardized set of data points or elements common to a patient population that can be regularly identified in the health records of the population and coded for use and analysis in a database management system. The data abstracts are used in clinical process monitoring where data is collected on each patient from the health record and recorded in the specified fields of an abstract on paper or electronically.

Time Ladders

Time ladders support the collection of data that must be oriented by time; they specify intervals of time necessary to address the problem under consideration listed down the right side of one, two, or three columns. Then, as the data collector observes, he or she records events next to the time of occurrence. For example, a receptionist could record on a time ladder when a patient arrives at his or her workstation and then record again on the same time ladder when the patient goes to an exam room. To visualize how the receptionist's other duties have an impact on his or her interactions with patients, she could also be asked to record timing of phone calls, provider requests for assistance, and other competing tasks. Collecting time ladder data over an appropriate period develops a detailed, clear picture of the workflow or process. Another example is a time ladder created from computer-based data. For example, the EHR could be used to generate a report documenting the time of arrival for patients without appointments. Using this data from a substantial period of a month or more, clinic management could anticipate the need to keep a specific number of appointment slots available for walk-ins. Figure 18.3 shows an example of a time ladder.

Statistics-Based Modeling Techniques

With increased implementation of electronic health records, the amount of data collected by and available to healthcare organizations is growing exponentially. The best way to use and apply this data is through statistics-based modeling. Statistics-based modeling is the use of analytical and graphical techniques to assist in the display and interpretation of raw data. Two common statistical-based modeling techniques are run charts and process control charts. A run chart displays data points for a specific time frame to provide information about performance (see figure 18.4). In a run chart, the measured points of a process

Figure 18.2   Checksheet

Issue Observed	Coders		Total
	1	2	
Missing documentation	||||	||||	9
Missing authentication	|||	||	5
Physician query required	|||	||||	8

Figure 18.3   Time ladder

Patient #1 arrived	9:00	3 calls from patients Request to make call from clinician
Patient #2 arrived Patient #3 arrived	9:15	4 calls from patients Print forms for patient #1
Patient #1 to exam room	9:30	3 calls from patients Print forms for patient #2 Request for specialist consult patient #1
Patient #4 arrived Patient #2 to exam room Patient #5 arrived	9:45	5 calls from patients Print forms for patient #3 Print forms for patient #4
Patient #3 to exam room Patient #4 to exam room	10:00	1 call from patient Print forms for patient #5
Patient #5 to exam room	10:15	Schedule appointment for patient #2

©AHIMA

are plotted on a graph at regular time intervals to help team members identify whether there are substantial changes in the numbers over time. For example, suppose an HIM professional wished to reduce the number of incomplete health records in the HIM department. He or she might first plot the number of incomplete health records each month for the past six months. Based on an analysis of the health records process, he or she then might enact a change designed to improve the process. The data collection should continue after the change is made in order to determine the effect on the process. If the run chart then indicated that the number of incomplete charts had decreased postchange, the HIM professional could attribute the decrease to the improvement effort. A run chart is an excellent tool for providing visual verification of how a process is performing and whether an improvement effort has worked.

A **statistical process control chart** looks like a run chart except that it has reference lines indicating the upper control limit (UCL), and lower control limit (LCL) drawn horizontally at the top and bottom of the chart. The upper

Figure 18.4   Run chart

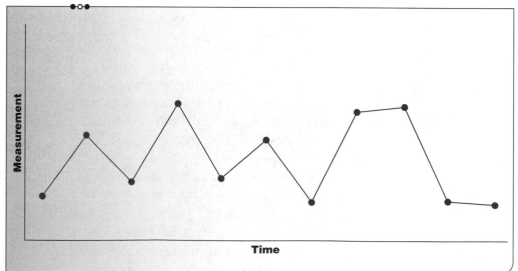

©AHIMA

Figure 18.5 Statistical process control chart

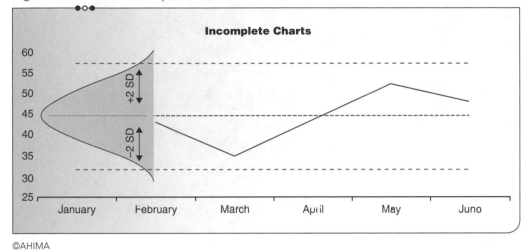

©AHIMA

line represents the UCL, and the lower line represents the LCL. In figure 18.5, the middle line represents the mean and the line above represents two standard deviations above the mean. The line below the mean represents two standard deviations below the mean. Remember that two standard deviations from the mean statistically include 95 percent of the observations of a process and three standard deviations include 99 percent (see chapter 13 for more information on statistical processes). Like the run chart, the statistical process control chart plots points to show how a process is performing over time. However, the two control limit lines permit the evaluator to use the rules of probability to interpret whether the process is stable (in other words, predictable and within the bounds of probability) or out of control (many points of data outside the second or third standard deviations).

The statistical process control chart makes it possible to see whether the variation within a process is the result of a common cause or a special cause. It lets the PI team know whether the team needs to try to reduce the ordinary variation occurring through common cause or to seek out a special cause of the variation and try to eliminate it. Removing the variation will bring the upper and lower control limit lines closer together. Common-cause variation would produce patterns that would stay within the two or three standard deviations of the mean, whereas a special-cause variation is more likely to produce patterns that will exceed the limits of chance of the two or three standard deviations.

Check Your Understanding 18.2

1. Which tool displays performance data over time?
   A. Benchmark
   B. Run chart
   C. Checksheet
   D. Time ladder

2. The nosocomial infection rate for our hospital is 0.2% while the rate at a similar hospital across town is 0.3%. This is an example of which of the following?
   A. Checksheet
   B. Data abstract
   C. Run chart
   D. Benchmark

3. The type of variation caused by factors outside a system is a(n):
   A. Input or output
   B. Processes
   C. Common-cause variation
   D. Special-cause variation

4. True or false: Goals should be measurable.

5. True or false: A checksheet is used to record and complete observations of occurrences.

6. True or false: Effective communication is the responsibility of administration only.

Team-Based Performance Improvement

The combined cognitive ability of teams can be an important tool in PI because of the complex issues faced in healthcare. Team-based PI begins with the assembly of the team. Staff with knowledge and background in the process under examination should be included. In addition, staff members accept change and transition easier when they have been part of the decision-making process.

The team's success depends on the following nine elements, described in detail in the following sections except as otherwise noted.

- Establishing ground rules for the team (see chapter 17)
- Stating the team's purpose or mission (see chapter 17)
- Identifying customers and their requirements
- Documenting current processes and identifying barriers
- Benchmarking
- Collecting current process data
- Analyzing process data
- Process redesign
- Recommendations for process change

Identifying Customers and Their Requirements

The PI team must identify the customers associated with the processes under discussion. Keep in mind customers are both internal (for example, the facility's business office) and external (for example, third-party payers). Once customer groups are identified, their needs related to the process need to be explored and established. The team can then work toward modifying the process to meet the customers' requirements.

Documenting Current Processes and Identifying Barriers

The process improvement team members work together to discuss and document current processes and identify barriers to establishing successful processes. For this step, the team's knowledge is vital because members must answer the following questions:

- What is the current process?
- Where are the start and end points of the process?
- What are the inputs, outputs, and interdependencies?
- What are the barriers to the process?
- What are the gaps to meeting the customer's needs?

Benchmarking

Benchmarking compares an organization's performance against that of external standards. Healthcare organizations routinely use benchmarking as a way to measure their performance.

When benchmarking for PI, a healthcare organization compares its performance data with that of a similar healthcare organization. The findings are used to determine areas in which the healthcare organization needs improvement. Benchmarking also increases motivation to improve processes and outcomes through comparison to potential competitors and similar departments.

Collecting Current Process Data

Once performance monitoring identifies an improvement opportunity, the first task of the PI process team is to research and define performance expectations for the process targeted. For example, performance monitoring of coding productivity identifies that coding staff is consistently not meeting previously set productivity standards.

PI teams have a variety of tools they employ, such as flow charts, brainstorming, diagramming, and force-field analysis (described in the following sections) that make it easier to gather and analyze information; and they help team members remain focused on PI activities and move the process along efficiently. The PI team should also use any information from routinely monitored processes as relevant to the targeted process.

Flow Chart Current Process

A **flow chart** is a graphic tool that uses standard symbols to visually display detailed information, including time and distance of the sequential flow of work of an individual or a product as it progresses through a process. A flow chart should be created to illustrate the current process used because the team must first examine and understand the current process before making improvements. Each team member has a unique perspective on and significant insight into how a portion of the process works. Flow charts help all the team members understand the process in the same way (see figure 18.6).

The work involved in developing the flow chart allows the team to understand every step in the process as well as the sequence of steps. The flow chart provides a visual picture of each decision point and event in the process. It exposes places where there are redundancies and complex and problematic areas.

Figure 18.6 Flow chart

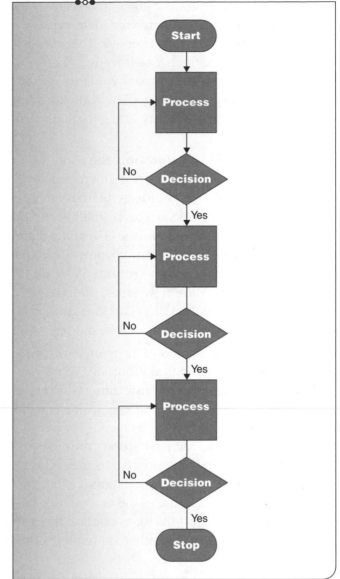

©AHIMA

Brainstorm Problem Areas

Brainstorming is a technique used to generate a large number of creative ideas from a group. It encourages PI team members to think outside the box and offer original ideas to address problems in the process. Brainstorming is highly effective for identifying a number of potential process steps that may benefit from improvement efforts and for generating solutions to specific problems. It helps people to begin thinking in new ways and involves them in the process. It is an excellent method for facilitating open communication. There are a number of approaches to brainstorming.

- The **unstructured brainstorming method** results in a free flow of ideas. The team leader or facilitator writes the ideas on a chart or board when presented. This allows everyone to see the list as it forms. There should be no discussion or evaluation of the ideas at this point. The goal of brainstorming is to encourage creativity and generate many ideas.

- In **structured brainstorming**, the team leader or facilitator asks team members to create their own list of ideas. Team members can work by themselves or in small groups for a specific amount of time. Then, the team members take turns offering a new idea. The process may take several rounds. As team members run out of new ideas, they pass; the next person then offers an idea until no team member can produce a fresh idea.

- **Affinity grouping** allows the team to organize similar ideas into logical groupings. Write ideas generated in a brainstorming session on sticky notes. Without talking to each other, each team member reviews the ideas on the notes and places each in natural groupings that seem related or connected to each other. Each member is empowered to move the ideas in a way that makes the most sense. As team members shift the ideas or place them in other groupings, the other team members

consider the merits of the placements and decide what further action to take. The goal is to have the team become comfortable with the arrangement. Finally, label the natural groupings that emerge. An example of an affinity diagram is in figure 18.7.

- **Nominal group technique** is a process used to reach consensus about an issue or an idea that the team considers most important. Each team member ranks each idea according to importance. For example, if there were six ideas, the most important idea is ranked with the number six (giving it six points); the second most important idea is ranked the number five, and so on. After each individual team member has had a chance to rank the list of ideas, the scores for each idea are totaled. The nominal group technique demonstrates where the team's priorities lie.

- The **multivoting technique** is a variation of the nominal group technique and serves the same purpose. Instead of ranking each issue or idea, team members rate issues by marking them with a distribution of points. In weighted multivoting, a team member distributes his or her allotment of points among as few or as many issues as he or she wants. For example, the team member might give 13 out of 25 points to one issue of

Figure 18.7 Affinity diagram

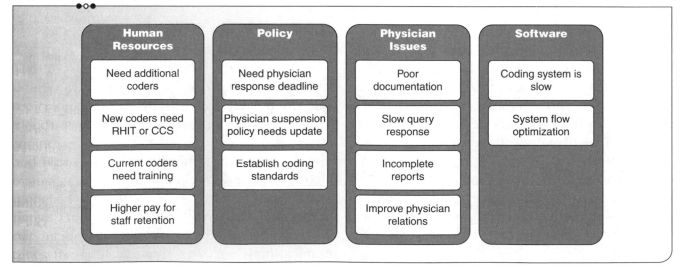

particular importance, 3 points each to four other issues, and no points to the remaining issues. After the voting, the sum of the numbers given to each issue determines the issue with the highest priority. Thus, the team will be able to see which issue emerged as particularly important to the team as a whole.

Cause-and-Effect Diagram

One of the common quality improvement tools used for risk management purposes is the cause-and-effect diagram. A **cause-and-effect diagram**, also known as **fishbone diagram** because of its characteristic fish shape (see figure 18.8), is an investigational technique that facilitates the identification of the various factors that contribute to a problem. It facilitates **root-cause analysis**, or the analysis of an event from all aspects (human, procedural, machinery, material) to identify how each contributed to the occurrence of the event and to develop new systems that will prevent recurrence. The problem or reason for the quality improvement exercise is written clearly in a box on the

right side of the diagram. A horizontal line is drawn and diagonal lines resembling ribs connect the boxes above and below the main horizontal line (or backbone). Each box contains a different category of information.

The categories may represent broad classifications of problem areas. For example, possible categories include people, methods, equipment, materials, policies, procedures, environment, or measurement. The team determines how many categories it needs to classify all the possible sources of the problem.

After constructing the diagram, the team brainstorms the possible root causes of the problem. Brainstorming continues until all the team's ideas about causes are exhausted. The purpose of this tool is to permit the team to explore, identify, and graphically display all of the root causes of a problem.

Force-Field Analysis

Force-field analysis is another tool used to display data generated through brainstorming. Force-field

Figure 18.8 Fishbone diagram

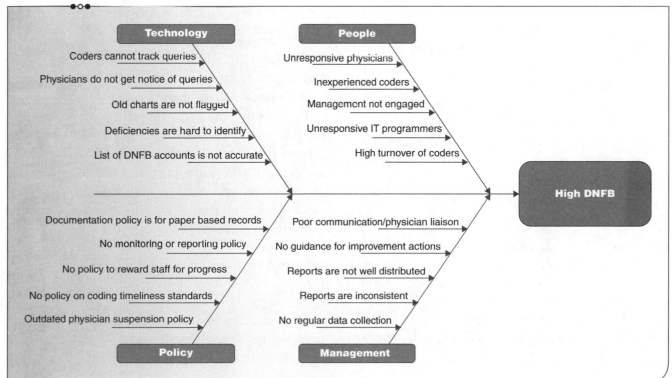

Figure 18.9 Force-field analysis

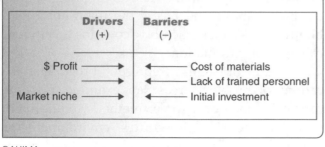

©AHIMA

analysis identifies specific drivers of and barriers to an organizational change, so that positive factors can be reinforced and negative factors reduced (figure 18.9). Team members brainstorm the reasons or factors that would encourage a change for improvement and those that might create barriers. The team leader places the factors in the appropriate column on the chart.

Force-field analysis enables team members to identify factors that support or work against a proposed solution. Often the next step after force-field analysis is to develop ways that would eliminate barriers or reinforce drivers.

Analyzing Process Data

Following the collection of data, it is important for the team to consider the data in a meaningful way. Again, PI tools and techniques can assist the team by providing meaningful documents from which conclusions can be drawn. Teams can use bar graphs, histograms, scatter diagrams, and Pareto charts to better analyze the data. For additional information on these tools and techniques, refer to chapter 13.

Process Redesign

Following in-depth examination of all the data, policies, procedures, and interviews, the team must determine whether the process will receive minor adjustments or a major restructuring to make it meet customers' expectations. If the solution is **process redesign**, the following are the next steps.

- Incorporate findings or changes identified in the research phase of the improvement process.
- If necessary, collect focused data from the prioritized problem areas to further clarify process failure or variation.
- Create a flow chart of the redesigned process.
- Develop policies and procedures that support the redesigned process.
- Educate involved staff about the new process.

Recommendations for Process Change

The process improvement team is responsible for putting the outcome of its work in a report format, along with recommendations for improving the process. Determine the recommendations after receiving and analyzing all data. The data include findings from the appropriate tools and techniques discussed previously. The recommendations should take into account anything that might have an impact on the organization, such as:

- Utilization of staff
- Effect on the budget
- Change in productivity
- Effects on customer requirements

Recommendations are viewed by the appropriate manager or administrator considered by the leadership group and top management for an organization-wide problem or by the management group heading the HIM department if the problem is confined to only that unit.

After implementing the new process, the team continues to measure performance against customers' expectations and established performance standards to determine if there is room for further improvement (refer to figure 18.1). When measurement data indicate the improvement is effective, ongoing monitoring of the process resumes.

The team disbands at this point in the cycle, and routine organizational monitoring of the performance measures resumes. Figure 18.10 illustrates the relationship between organization-wide performance monitoring and team-based PI processes.

Figure 18.10   Organization-wide and team-based PI model

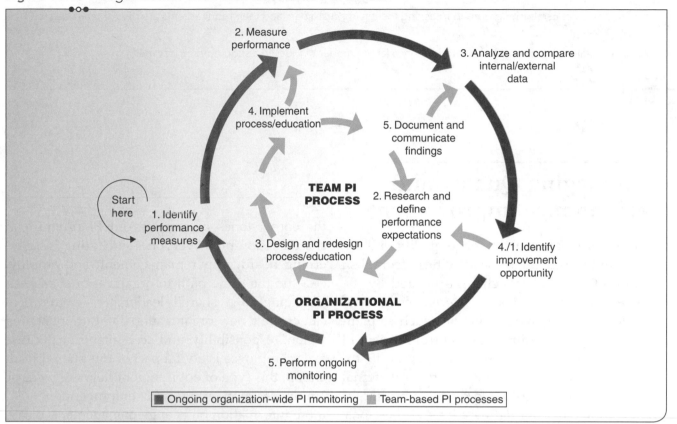

Source: Shaw and Carter 2015.

Check Your Understanding 18.3

1. Which of the following is an investigational technique that facilitates the identification of the various factors that contribute to a problem?
   A. Affinity grouping
   B. Cause-and-effect diagram
   C. Force-field analysis
   D. Nominal group technique

2. Which of the following documents the current process?
   A. Flow chart
   B. Force-field analysis
   C. Unstructured brainstorming
   D. Structured brainstorming

3. In what technique do team members rate issues by distribution of points?
   A. Affinity grouping
   B. Nominal group technique
   C. Multivoting technique
   D. Unstructured brainstorming

4. True or false: Affinity grouping helps to determine what issue is the most important.

5. True or false: Establishing ground rules and identifying customers and their requirements are part of team-based PI processes.

6. True or false: Brainstorming tries to identify a large number of ideas in a short amount of time.

Managing Quality and Performance Improvement

HIM professionals must manage quality and the process of PI to ensure these activities accomplish the important and vital changes needed by the organization's internal and external customers. Traditional management functions such as planning, organizing, leading, and controlling should be applied to PI initiatives. See chapter 19 for information on management functions. External entities should be considered during a healthcare organization's quality deliberations, discussions, and decision making. External entities include agencies that offer voluntary accreditation services, are involved in the reimbursement cycle, administer licensure services, and offer national quality policy and direction. All relevant agencies must be factored into an organization's approach to improving its quality and professional performance to meet the organization's mission and goals as a healthcare organization of superior quality. Components of PI activities include organizational factors, standards of organizational quality, utilization management, and risk management.

Organizational Components of PI

To be successful in implementing PI programs, healthcare organizations may have to restructure and create a new culture to accommodate the vast changes and competition that exist in today's healthcare environment. PI is most successful in organizations that have an interdisciplinary and participative management approach. As discussed previously in this chapter, shared vision is one of the cornerstones of a successful PI program. A shared vision puts everyone—including the governing board, upper management, and employees—on the same path to organizational success. Changing to a shared leadership environment can create a new organizational culture of shared vision, responsibility, and accountability. Because every employee is a vital part of this shared leadership, this type of environment helps to increase employee motivation and empowerment. For more information on change management, please refer to chapter 17.

In addition to an enterprise-wide vision, a shared leadership framework is essential for implementing PI. Shared leadership essentially means organizations ensure all employees participate in an integrated, continuous PI program. When various organizational frameworks or structures are developed, it encourages shared leadership by encouraging employee participation and instilling ownership.

Large healthcare organizations are complex both in size and in geographical location requiring focused effort to standardize and facilitate necessary changes. The organizational structures and processes that constitute a PI program need to be accomplished across the entire healthcare organization, meaning that every location and department within the whole organization takes parts in the PI program. To be effective, the organizational unit responsible for PI must be able to communicate with all areas of the healthcare organization and foster interdisciplinary cooperation. Many healthcare organizations have created a PI department to help the organization pursue its quality efforts. Many PI departments assume leadership in the assessing and tracking of organizational compliance with accreditation standards, focus areas, and national patient safety goals.

The basic responsibilities of the PI department include:

- Helping departments or groups of departments with similar issues to identify potential quality problems
- Assisting determination of the best methods for studying potential problems (for example, survey, chart review, or interview with staff)
- Participating in regular meetings across the organization as appropriate, and training organization members on quality and PI methodology, tools, and techniques

A permanent multidisciplinary committee should coordinate the program and ensure the consistency of clinical quality assessment (QA) processes throughout the organization. The committee should include representatives of the medical staff, nursing staff, and infection control team. Consult representatives from other areas as needed.

Standards of Organizational Quality in Healthcare

A number of private and government entities develop and maintain standards of organizational quality for healthcare. These entities include agencies and departments of the federal government, accreditation organizations, private for-profit organizations, and not-for-profit organizations such as medical societies and organizations dedicated to research on a specific disease or condition. Standards of quality include descriptive statements known as standards of care, quality of care standards, performance standards, accreditation standards, and practice standards.

A **standard** is a written description of the expected features, characteristics, or outcomes of a healthcare-related service. Standards provide a minimum level of performance. Four types of standards relevant within the context of clinical quality assessment are addressed in the following sections:

- Clinical practice guidelines and clinical protocols
- Accreditation standards
- Government regulations
- Licensure requirements

Clinical Practice Guidelines and Protocols

Standards of clinical quality include both clinical practice guidelines and clinical protocols. **Clinical protocols** are detailed, step-by-step instructions used by healthcare practitioners to make knowledge-based clinical decisions directly related to patient care. The **Agency for Healthcare Research and Quality (AHRQ)** is an agency within the Department of Health and Human Services (HHS). AHRQ's mission is to improve the quality, safety, efficiency, and effectiveness of healthcare for all Americans. **Clinical practice guidelines** are developed to standardize clinical decision making. As the word *guideline* suggests, clinical practice guidelines are not meant to be inflexible and do not apply in every case.

In contrast to clinical practice guidelines, clinical protocols are treatment recommendations based on guidelines. They are specific instructions for performing clinical procedures established by authoritative bodies, such as medical staff committees, and intended to be applied literally and universally. One example of a clinical protocol is the step-by-step description of the accepted procedure for preparing intravenous solutions at a specific acute-care hospital.

Accreditation Standards

In the United States, many different organizations monitor the quality of healthcare services and offer accreditation programs for healthcare organizations. All of the programs base accreditation on a data collection and submission process followed by a comprehensive survey process. Participation in accreditation programs is voluntary. (See chapter 3 for a discussion of accreditation.) The

Joint Commission, DNV GL, and other voluntary accreditation organizations are addressed in the following sections.

Joint Commission The Joint Commission (discussed in chapter 8) emphasizes PI in their accreditation standards. All hospitals and long-term care facilities are required to report outcome measures. Outcome measures document the results of care for individual patients as well as for specific types of patients grouped by diagnostic category. For example, an acute-care hospital's overall rate of postsurgical infection is an outcome measure. Outcome and process measures have evolved into quality measures now called accountability measures. Accountability measures focus on four main components: research, proximity, accuracy, and adverse effects. These measures are the key to improving patient care and quality, thus improving patient outcomes. The Joint Commission scores healthcare organizations on compliance with specific national patient safety goals (NPSGs). The NPSGs outlines the areas of organizational practice that most commonly lead to patient injury or other negative outcomes that can be prevented if standardized procedures are used. For example, an NPSG requires healthcare organizations to eliminate wrong-site, wrong-patient, and wrong-procedure surgery. To accomplish this, organizations must create and use a preoperative verification process, such as a checklist, to confirm the patient's identity and that appropriate documents (for example, health records, imaging studies) are available. They also must implement a process to mark the surgical site and involve the patient in the marking process.

The data collected are used to help focus the accreditation survey on patient safety and high-quality patient care and to select specific patients to "trace" during the on-site survey. This approach, known as tracer methodology, consists of following (tracing) a few patients through their entire stay at the hospital in order to identify quality and patient safety issues that might indicate quality problems or patterns of less than optimum care. A trace of a surgical patient, for example, might reveal a missing updated history and physical (H&P) on the patient's health record within 24 hours before surgery. Following this lead, the surveyor might discover that the organization is having an ongoing problem with H&Ps in general; a problem with obtaining the required updated H&P within 24 hours before surgery, or perhaps a problem with just one particular physician.

DNV GL and Other Voluntary Accreditation Organizations DNV GL Healthcare is a voluntary accreditation organization that has operated in the United States since the late 1800s, but is relatively new to healthcare. The organization is recognized by CMS to have *deemed status*, which means healthcare organizations accredited by DNV GL are recognized as meeting the Medicare Conditions of Participation, which are the administrative and operational guidelines and regulations under which healthcare facilities are allowed to take part in the Medicare and Medicaid programs. Medicare and Medicaid is discussed in chapter 15.

Other voluntary accreditation organizations include the National Committee on Quality Assurance, which focuses its accreditation activities on health plans and outpatient provider organizations, and the Commission on the Accreditation of Rehabilitation Facilities, which focuses on long-term and mental health rehabilitation facilities.

Government Regulations and Licensure Requirements

Various agencies and departments of the federal, state, and local governments also review the quality of services provided in healthcare organizations. However, government regulations and licensure requirements are compulsory rather than voluntary.

Medicare Conditions of Participation: To participate in the Medicare program, healthcare providers must comply with federal regulations known as the Conditions of Participation. The Centers for Medicare and Medicaid Services (CMS) develops the Conditions of Participation.

Quality improvement organizations: Quality improvement organizations (QIOs) are responsible for monitoring the quality of care provided to Medicare patients. CMS and the QIOs collaborate with practitioners, beneficiaries, providers, plans, and other purchasers of healthcare services to achieve the following goals:

- Develop quality indicators that are firmly based in science
- Identify opportunities for healthcare improvements through careful measurement of patterns of care
- Communicate with professional and provider communities about patterns of care

- Intervene to foster quality improvement through system improvements
- Conduct follow-up studies to evaluate success and redirect efforts

QIOs use medical peer review, data analysis, and other tools to identify patterns of care and outcomes that need improvement. They then work cooperatively with facilities and individual physicians to improve care. CMS established a comprehensive program in which QIOs use a data-driven approach to monitoring care and outcomes and a shared approach to working with the healthcare community to improve care.

State and local licensure requirements: To maintain its licensed status, each facility must adhere to the state regulations that govern such as quality of care. For additional information, refer to chapter 8.

Check Your Understanding 18.4

1. QIOs use peer review, data analysis, and other tools to:
   A. Evaluate whether or not a healthcare facility is meeting standards for accreditation and licensing
   B. Calculate reimbursement
   C. Penalize healthcare organizations
   D. Identify areas that need improvement

2. Which of the following is a written description of the expected features, characteristics, or outcomes of a healthcare-related service?
   A. Flow chart
   B. Ground rules
   C. Pareto chart
   D. Standard

3. The NPSG scores organizations on areas that:
   A. Affect financial stability of the organization
   B. Affect customers
   C. Affect compliance with state law
   D. Commonly lead to patient injury

4. True or False: Accreditation standards were developed to standardize clinical decision making.

5. True or False: The Conditions of Participation are used to monitor hospitals and other healthcare organizations when becoming licensed by the state.

6. True or False: The mission of AHRQ is to improve quality, safety, efficiency, and effectiveness for all Americans.

Utilization Management

Utilization management (UM) is composed of a set of processes used to determine the appropriateness of medical services provided during specific episodes of care. In most hospitals, UM programs perform three important functions—utilization review, case management, and discharge planning. Utilization management is an important part of quality patient care as it helps to ensure necessary and appropriate care, effectiveness of the services provided to the patient, and timely and safe discharge of patients. See chapter 15 for a complete discussion on utilization management.

Risk Management

In healthcare, **risk** is any occurrence or circumstance that might result in a loss. Loss includes any damage to an entity's person, property, or rights, including physical injury, cognitive injury, emotional injury, wrongful death, and financial loss. In this chapter, the focus is on how risk management relates to quality. For additional information about risk, refer to chapter 10.

The purpose of the **risk management program** is to link risk management functions to the related processes of quality assessment and PI. The aims of the program are to (1) help provide high-quality patient care while also enhancing a safe environment for patients, employees, and visitors, and (2) minimize financial loss by reducing risk through prevention and evaluation.

The basic functions of healthcare risk management programs are similar for most organizations and include:

- Risk identification and analysis
- Loss prevention and reduction
- Claims management

Risk Identification and Analysis

The role of the risk manager is to collect and analyze information on actual losses and potential risks and to design systems that lessen potential losses in the future. Risk managers use information from a variety of sources to identify areas of risk exposure within the organization. Sources of risk management information include:

- Incident reports (sometimes called occurrence reports or occurrence screens)
- Current and past liability claims against the organization
- Performance improvement reports
- Internal inspections of the organization's physical plant and medical equipment
- Reviews conducted by the organization's insurance carriers
- Survey reports from state and local licensing agencies
- Survey reports from accreditation organizations
- Reports of complaints from patients, visitors, medical staff, and employees
- Results of patient satisfaction surveys

An **incident (or occurrence) report** is a structured tool used to collect data and information about any event *not* consistent with routine operational procedures, such as a wrong-side surgery or foreign body left in following surgery. In the language of risk management, the documentation of these events is used to identify **potentially compensable events**. A potentially compensable event is an occurrence, such as an accident or medical error that may result in personal injury or loss of property to patients, staff, visitors, or the healthcare organization.

Incident reports are prepared to help healthcare facilities identify and correct problem areas and prepare for legal defense. An incident report documents the event for operational purposes and is not used for patient care, so it is considered an extremely confidential document that is never filed in the health record and should not be photocopied or prepared in duplicate. The healthcare provider should never document that an incident report was completed. Incident reports are not part of the legal health record and are not discoverable in event of legal action (Farenholz 2011). See figure 18.11 for an example of an incident report.

Loss Prevention and Reduction

The risk manager is responsible for developing systems to prevent injuries and other losses

Figure 18.11 Partial example of incident or occurrence report (including the necessary components for this incident)

Med Rec #: *00-0545*
Name: *Jackson, Julia*
Date of Birth: *06-22-23*
Street: *6401 Fremont Ave*
City: *Western City, CA*

Risk Management use only: _____

Patient ID/Name of individual involved.
Use addressograph for patient.

INSTRUCTIONS: (1) Fill out the first page of the Incident Report Form. (2) Select the type of incident from the bottom of page 2. (3) Fill out all appropriate sections as directed. The report must be dated and filled out by the end of the shift in which the incident occurred or was discovered. **DO NOT COPY THIS FORM.** Please print; this report must be legible. **Please fill out all applicable parts of this form.** Upon completion of this form, route it to your Nurse Manager or Supervisor. Do not leave this form in the patient's chart.

Date of incident: *05/29/03*   Time (2400 Clock): *1645*   Hospital Unit: *Med/Surg*

What day of the week
did it occur?

				Did the incident occur during:		Employee involved worked a(n):	
Sun	[✓]	Thurs	[ ]	Day 0701–1500	[ ]	8 Hour shift	[✓]
Mon	[ ]	Fri	[ ]	Evening 1501–2300	[✓]	10 Hour shift	[ ]
Tues	[ ]	Sat	[ ]	Night 2301–0700	[ ]	12 Hour shift	[ ]
Wed	[ ]					Double shift	[ ]
						Other _____	

Where did the incident occur? *patient room*

Description of incident. Include follow-up care given (i.e., vital signs, x-ray, laboratory tests, etc.).
Pt. developed a macular rash over trunk and extremities after 10 mg

dose of Compazine given for postop nausea. Compazine stopped

and Benadryl given IM.

IMMEDIATE EFFECT OF THE INCIDENT: *Severe macular rash over trunk*
_____

Involved Person Data

Date of Admission: *05/29 03*

What sex is the person?
Male   [ ]
Female [✓]

Inpatient	[✓]
Outpatient	[ ]
Student	[ ]
Employee	[ ]
Visitor	[ ]
Volunteer	[ ]
Other: _____	

What is the person's age? _____

Current Diagnosis/Reason for visit: *Bowel Obstruction*

Is the involved person aware of the incident?   Yes [✓]   No [ ]
Is the family aware of incident?   Yes [ ]   No [✓]

Figure 18.11 (Continued)

**** PLEASE PRINT ****

Person preparing report (Signature): *Gwen Nelson, R.N.*   Print: *Gwen Nelson, R.N.*

Name of individual witnessing incident (Print): *Bob Patterson, R.N.*

Dept/Address: *Med/Surg Team Leader*

Name of employee involved in incident: *Gwen Nelson, R.N.* Dept/Address: *Med/Surg*

Name of employee discovering incident: *Gwen Nelson, R.N.* Dept/Address: *Med/Surg*

**** STAFF TO NOTIFY ATTENDING PHYSICIAN AND/OR DESIGNATED RESIDENT/NURSE PRACTITIONER OF INCIDENT ****

I notified Dr./NP: *Jeff Cook*   at: *1650*   (time).

M.D./NP responded ☐ in person ☑ by phone at: *1705*   (time).

Was the attending physician notified?

Yes [√] Date: *05/29/03* Time: *1650*

No [ ] Why not? _____

Examining Physician/Nurse Practitioner statement regarding condition/outcome of person involved:

Pt. was examined by me at 1700 hours. Trunk and extremities show a macular rash on them. One dose of Benadryl given IM to pt. and rash began to subside. Compazine stopped.

Examining MD/NP signature: *Tom Lander, M.D. House Staff*

Examining MD/NP name (print): *Tom Lander, M.D.*

Date: *05/29/03* Time: *1700*   Clinical Service: *Medicine*

CHOOSE THE TYPE OF INCIDENT YOU ARE REPORTING. Use the index below to locate the type of incident you are reporting, go to that section and mark the appropriate box(es). THERE MAY BE MORE THAN ONE ITEM APPLICABLE IN A SECTION. CHECK BOX(ES) IN APPROPRIATE SECTIONS.

Medication/IV Incident	Page 3, Section 1	Patient Behavioral Incident	Page 5, Section 6
Blood/Blood incident	Page 3, Section 2	Safety Incident	Page 5, Section 9
Burn	Page 5, Section 7	Security Incident	Page 5, Section 8
Equipment Incident	Page 5, Section 10	Surgery Incident	Page 5, Section 4
Fall	Page 4, Section 3	Treatment/Procedure Incident	Page 5, Section 5
Fire Incident	Page 5, Section 11		

CONFIDENTIAL: This material is prepared pursuant to Code Annotated, §26-25-1, et seq., and 58-12-43(7, 8, and 9), for the purpose of evaluating healthcare rendered by hospitals or physicians and is NOT PART of the medical record.

Figure 18.11 *(Continued)*

DO NOT COPY

SECTION 1 MEDICATION/IV INCIDENT

1A. TYPE OF MEDICATION
Fill in specific medication/solution on the adjacent line.
Analgesic _____
Anesthetic agent _____
Antibiotic _____
Anticoagulant _____
Anticonvulsant _____
Antidepressant _____
Antiemetic _*Compazine*_ _____
Antihistamine _____
Antineoplastic _____
Bronchodilator _____
Cardiovascular _____
Contrast media _____
Diuretic _____
Immunizations _____
Immunosuppressive _____
Insulin _____
Intralipids _____
Investigational drug _____
IV solution _____
Laxative _____
Narcotic _____
Oxytocics _____
Psychotherapeutic _____
Radionuclides _____
Sedative/tranquilizer _____
TPN _____
Vasodilator _____
Vasopressor _____
Vitamin _____
Other _____

1B. TYPE OF MEDICATION OR IV INCIDENT
Adverse reaction .... [ ] 1B01
Allergic/contraindication. .... [ ] 1B02
Delayed stat order .... [ ] 1B03
Improper order (MD/NP) .... [ ] 1B04
Incompatible additive .... [ ] 1B05
Incorrect additive .... [ ] 1B06
Incorrect dosage .... [ ] 1B07
Incorrect drug .... [ ] 1B08
Incorrect narcotic count .... [ ] 1B09
Incorrect patient .... [ ] 1B10
Incorrect rate of flow .... [ ] 1B11
Incorrect route. .... [ ] 1B12
Incorrect schedule .... [ ] 1B13
Incorrect solution/type .... [ ] 1B14
Incorrect time .... [ ] 1B15
Incorrect volume .... [ ] 1B16
Infiltration .... [ ] 1B17
Given before culture taken .... [ ] 1B18
Medication given before lab
   results returned .... [ ] 1B19
Medication missing from cart. .... [ ] 1B20

Not documented .... [ ] 1B21
Not prescribed. .... [ ] 1B22
Omitted .... [ ] 1B23
Outdated .... [ ] 1B24
Out-of-sequence .... [ ] 1B25
Patient took unprescribed medication. .... [ ] 1B26
Repeat administration .... [ ] 1B27
Transcription error .... [ ] 1B28
Other_____ 1B29

1C. ROUTE OF MEDICATION ORDERED:
IM .... [ ] 1C01
IV .... [ ] 1C02
PO .... [ ] 1C03
Other_*suppository*_ 1C04

1D. MEDICATION DISPENSING INCIDENT
Meds not sent/delayed from pharmacy. .... [ ] 1D01
Incorrectly labeled .... [ ] 1D02
Incorrect dose .... [ ] 1D03
Incorrect drug sent .... [ ] 1D04
Incorrect IV additive .... [ ] 1D05
Incorrect IV fluid .... [ ] 1D06
Incorrect route (IV, PO, IM, PR) .... [ ] 1D07
Mislabeled .... [ ] 1D08
Other_____ 1D09

SECTION 2
BLOOD/BLOOD COMPONENT INCIDENT

2A. BLOOD/BLOOD COMPONENT TYPE
Albumin. .... [ ] 2A01
Cryoprecipitate .... [ ] 2A02
Factor VIII (AHF). .... [ ] 2A03
Factor IX (Konyne). .... [ ] 2A04
Fresh frozen plasma. .... [ ] 2A05
Packed red blood cells (PRBC) .... [ ] 2A06
Plasmanate®. .... [ ] 2A07
Platelets. .... [ ] 2A08
RhoGAM®. .... [ ] 2A09
Washed red blood cells (WRBC) .... [ ] 2A10
Whole blood .... [ ] 2A11
Other_____ 2A12

**2B. TYPE OF BLOOD/BLOOD COMPONENT
   INCIDENT**
Crossmatch problem .... [ ] 2B01
Improper unit verification. .... [ ] 2B02
Inappropriate IV fluids administered
   with blood components .... [ ] 2B03
Inappropriate documentation .... [ ] 2B04
Inappropriate storage. .... [ ] 2B05
Incomplete patient ID. .... [ ] 2B06
Incorrect patient .... [ ] 2B07
Incorrect rate .... [ ] 2B08
Incorrect type .... [ ] 2B09
Incorrect volume .... [ ] 2B10
Patient refused .... [ ] 2B11
Other_____ 2B12

CONFIDENTIAL: This material is prepared pursuant to Code Annotated, §26-25-1, et seq., and 58-12-43(7, 8, and 9), for the purpose of evaluating healthcare rendered by hospitals or physicians and is NOT PART of the medical record.

Source: Shaw and Carter 2015.

within the organization. Performance improvement actions are often initiated in response to suggestions offered by the risk manager. Education also is an invaluable tool in risk management and sometimes is the only activity required to prevent potential safety problems.

Risk managers in many healthcare organizations also are responsible for developing policies and procedures aimed at preventing accidents and injuries and reducing the organization's risk exposure.

Claims Management

Claims management is the process of managing the legal and administrative aspects of the healthcare organization's response to injury claims (injuries occurring on the facility's property). Different sizes and types of organizations handle it differently. Accordingly, the role of the risk manager in managing claims varies. Many organizations place the entire process in the hands of their liability insurance vendors. In such cases, the risk manager may act as the organization's liaison with the insurance company. However, some organizations are self-insured, meaning that they establish a dedicated fund for financing future liability settlements. Organizations manage claims and risk by incorporating patient advocacy, incorporating regulatory and accreditation requirements, and having an organizational incidence response mechanism in place.

Patient Advocacy

Many large healthcare organizations such as acute-care hospitals have instituted **patient advocacy** programs. In such programs, a patient representative (sometimes called an ombudsperson) responds personally to complaints from patients and their families. Often, patients and their families are looking for nothing more than an explanation of an adverse occurrence or an apology for a mistake or misunderstanding. Patient representatives are able to handle minor complaints and to seek remedies on behalf of patients. They also are able to recognize serious problems that need to be forwarded to performance improvement or risk management personnel.

Accreditation Requirements for Risk Management in Acute-Care Hospitals

Anything that undermines patient safety is a risk issue. According to accreditation standards, all hospital activities must be evaluated as to the potential risk to the patient or the organization. Leadership is responsible for ensuring adequate resources for patient safety.

Incidence Response Patient safety should be of utmost importance to healthcare organizations. Healthcare organizations need to create a culture of safety within their facilities in order to focus on error elimination. Steps must be taken to ensure patient safety and respond to an adverse event occurring within a healthcare organization. Healthcare organizations must be equipped to recognize an adverse event and then have a plan and protocols in place to care for the affected patient and also to mitigate the situation in order to prevent further adverse events. Once the situation has been appropriately resolved, the organization should initiate a PI process to identify what improvements and changes to the systems and processes are needed to prevent future adverse events.

Check Your Understanding 18.5

1. Which of the following is a group of processes that determine the appropriateness of medical services?
    A. Utilization management
    B. Utilization review
    C. Case management
    D. Risk management

2. Which of the following is a basic function of a healthcare risk management program?
   A. Claims management
   B. Discharge plan
   C. Time ladders
   D. Workflow analysis

3. A patient fell out of the bed. What should be done?
   A. Case management
   B. Conduct a continued stay utilization review
   C. Perform claims management functions
   D. Complete an incident report

4. A patient is dissatisfied with his or her care. Who should the patient contact at the hospital?
   A. Utilization review coordinator
   B. Risk manager
   C. Patient representative or advocate
   D. Discharge planner

5. A woman dies in labor and delivery. The Joint Commission would call this type of outcome a(n):
   A. Sentinel event
   B. Clinical protocol
   C. Screening criteria
   D. Occurrence screen

Clinical Quality Management Initiatives

Initiatives and processes seeking to ensure high-quality care and patient safety became a focus in healthcare as the 21st century commenced. Stemming from the Institute of Medicine (IOM) 1999 and 2001 reports on the quality of healthcare in America, a consensus developed around the need to use information technology as both a methodology and a pathway for managing and improving healthcare quality.

The beginning of the 21st century witnessed an increased link between clinical quality and reimbursement for health services. Pay-for-performance initiatives by the federal government, Joint Commission, and private payers began rewarding organizations for quality outcomes. These incentives, such as Meaningful Use, are also encouraging healthcare providers to invest in technology that will improve patient care and safety. For additional information on Meaningful Use, refer to chapter 16.

In recent years, CMS has become an advocate for pay for performance within the Medicare program. One of its efforts requires hospitals participating in the Medicare program to collect and report on proven clinical hospital quality measures to qualify for full inpatient prospective payment. Those that do not report their data on measures such as acute myocardial infarction, heart failure, and pneumonia face a penalty per case. Medicare expects hospitals to compare their own data to national and regional averages in order to identify areas for quality improvement.

The early part of the 21st century witnessed new and creative efforts to encourage medical error reporting. The Patient Safety and Quality Improvement Act of 2005 allows for the voluntary reporting of medical errors, serious adverse events, and their underlying causes (HHS 2015). Subsequent emphasis by The Joint Commission on patient safety issues has resulted in voluminous research and new programs sponsored by The

Joint Commission to assist its accreditation customers in improving this important area of healthcare organization functioning.

Accountable care organizations, PI methodologies, ISO-9000 certification, and medication reconciliation are key components of clinical quality management.

Accountable Care Organizations

Accountable Care Organizations (ACOs) are a part of the Affordable Care Act (2010). ACOs are a network of doctors, hospitals, and other healthcare providers and suppliers working together to coordinate and improve care for patients with Medicare. This coordination of care includes sharing patient information among providers in order to eliminate duplication of tests and prevent medical errors. Participation in an ACO is voluntary. ACOs focus on improving the quality of care of patients and decreasing healthcare spending. As ACOs meet the requirements of the model, they share in the savings. Patients who receive care from an ACO maintain all of their rights as a Medicare beneficiary (CMS 2015). For more information on the Affordable Care Act and ACO, refer to chapter 2.

Robust Process Improvement Methodologies

As discussed earlier, benchmarking is an important quality tool in healthcare quality programs. However, some healthcare organizations have begun to benchmark against other industries (for example, a hospital's hand-off from surgery to intensive care compared against the racecar industry's hand-off during a pit stop) and are selecting models that may be adapted to the healthcare industry. Healthcare organizations have begun applying these methodologies to their PI programs (Karr 2011). Some of these are Lean, Six Sigma, Lean Six Sigma, high reliability organizations, and virtuoso teams.

Lean

Lean is a process improvement methodology focused on eliminating waste and improving the flow of work processes. Healthcare organizations have found ways to apply the Lean methodology. Healthcare has a growing burden to improve the quality of patient care while also decreasing and controlling costs. In many ways, Lean is a good fit for healthcare organizations and many of the principles of Lean are transferrable from its origins in the automotive industry to other industries, including healthcare (Meyer 2010).

Six Sigma

Six Sigma uses statistics for measuring variation in a process with the intent of producing error-free results. Sigma refers to the standard deviation used in descriptive statistics to determine how much an event or observation varies from the estimated average of the population sample. Six Sigma was chosen as a target statistic because even two or three standard deviations would not be acceptable in certain scenarios. A 2.5 percent error rate for making correct change at a movie theater may be acceptable, but that error rate for airlines avoiding fatal crashes is completely unacceptable, because airlines have hundreds of flights in the air on any given day. Even if there were only 100 flights per day, two to three fatal crashes per day would be devastating to the airline industry, not to mention the population as a whole. Therefore, it is important to keep this PI approach in proper perspective when applying it to healthcare. The Six Sigma measure indicates no more than 3.4 errors per 1 million encounters (Kubiak and Benbow 2009). Consider the challenge of achieving no more than 3.4 errors per 1 million prescriptions, surgeries, or diagnoses. In certain areas, this standard may seem unattainable; and in others, it may not be rigorous enough.

Deploying Six Sigma in healthcare requires the identification of elements of a product line that are critical to quality or CTQs. The facility should conduct focus groups or interviews of customers to elicit the CTQs. Typically in healthcare the customers will be the patients and the providers or physicians. All others involved—the corporations, payers, accreditors or licensers—are identified as stakeholders, entities with an important interest in the product that do not have consumer relationships to it. Supporting the CTQs are elements critical to process (CTPs). Techniques such as focus groups or interviews help to determine the CTPs.

Lean Six Sigma

Combining Lean and Six Sigma is a way to combine elements from both techniques into an integrated program to improve process flow and quality (George et al. 2002). This **Lean Six Sigma** methodology utilizes elements of elimination of waste from Lean and critical process quality characteristics from Six Sigma. Using these tools in a combined format allows for quality improvement and overall efficiencies within healthcare organizations—improving both product and process.

High Reliability Organizations

High reliability organizations (HROs) are organizations that focus on creating an environment that eliminates or minimizes error. HRO methodology comes from the airline, wildland firefighting, and nuclear power industries and is also being used in healthcare. HROs are concerned with noticing weak signals in order to prevent a potential negative outcome and these weak signals receive a substantial response within this model. In healthcare, as with other types of industries, there are often small signals that are ignored. Healthcare organizations can become HROs as they pay attention to these small signals. For example, a housekeeper may notice a problem with a patient. Within an organization HRO, that housekeeper would be empowered and motivated to report this concern to a clinician. An important part of this model and one way that HROs notice weak signals is mindfulness—a keen awareness and necessary characteristic for all employees of an HRO. As employees are focused on and mindful of their duties there is less room for error. For example, a distracted physician may be more prone to error. Organizational reliability is improved and errors are reduced when sources of distraction are eliminated and mindfulness is emphasized within a healthcare organization. HROs are preoccupied with failure and use these failures as learning experiences to improve processes and quality in order to eliminate error (Weick and Sutcliffe 2007).

Virtuoso Teams

Virtuoso teams are groups of experts brought together to address an issue or situation. Members of virtuoso teams are selected for their exceptional expertise in a particular field and are given ambitious goals rather than selecting team members according to their availability and experience as is done with traditional teams. Elite experts are most productive when they are put in tight spaces and given strict deadlines (Boynton and Fischer 2005). Leaders of virtuoso teams encourage collaboration and creative confrontation. Instead of relying on e-mail, phone calls, and occasional meetings, virtuoso teams engage in intense, face-to-face conversations. Where politeness and repression of individual egos is the norm in traditional teams, members of virtuoso teams celebrate individual egos, compete, and create opportunities for solo performances (Boynton and Fischer 2005). Virtuoso teams operate on the assumption that members have a stake in their reputation and therefore want to create notable results. Leaders and participants in virtuoso teams are expected to employ different skills and methods of interaction than they have experienced in previous team participation.

ISO 9000 Certification

If healthcare organizations expand into global entities, they are required to deal with the same issues other industries face when doing business outside the United States. **ISO 9000 certification** is part of a PI system required to conduct business in certain foreign countries. The International Organization for Standardization in Geneva, Switzerland, first published ISO 9000 standards in 1987. ISO 9000 sets specification standards for quality management with regard to process management and product control. In the healthcare setting, product control is quality control of patient care activities. Companies that document and demonstrate compliance with ISO 9000 standards can receive certification by independent ISO auditors (Rakhmawati et al. 2014).

Medication Reconciliation

Medication adjustments and changes often occur during patient encounters with health services, as patients are admitted, discharged, transferred to another hospital unit or to another facility. Healthcare providers may not have access to a listing of current medications the patient was taking prior to admission or encounter with health services. As the patient transfers within the facility or to an outside facility, there is potential for missing medication dosage, omitted medications, or information on drug interactions and allergies.

All of these factors put patients at risk for adverse drug events. **Medication reconciliation**, such as ensuring that the patient is receiving the right dose of medication, is the process that monitors and confirms that the patient receives consistent dosing across all facility transfers, such as on admission, from nursing unit to surgery, and from surgery to the intensive care unit. Facilities use the medication reconciliation process to eliminate medication error and improve care for the patient. Medication reconciliation is also part of The Joint Commission's NPSGs.

Shared Governance

Healthcare organizations use measures to determine their level of performance on quality and safety. These measures focus on outcomes, the structure of the healthcare organization, patient surveys, and organizational systems; and are used by healthcare organizations, private payers, and accrediting organizations to ensure they provide exceptional care. Organizations use internal measures as quality standards for their organization. External measures are used by accrediting organizations and private payers for payment based on performance as well as value-based purchasing initiatives. Payment for healthcare services is linked to quality measures. As more and more information is collected and analyzed in relation to quality, the information must maintain integrity. Consumers rely on information regarding quality, such as Hospital Compare data, to make healthcare decisions. This information is an asset and should be governed with accountability (Kloss 2015).

 Real-World Case 18.1

Karen is the regional coding manager for a large healthcare organization. She is responsible for coding compliance and training for three hospitals. Karen creates a dashboard each week with the metrics from each hospital. The metrics are not only specific for each facility, but also by patient type. This dashboard is shared weekly via e-mail with all coding staff and relevant leadership. Although there is some fluctuation from week to week, the metrics have remained relatively consistent for the past two years. Karen notices that the metrics for the past two weeks for Uptown Hospital, the large urban hospital in her region, have shown a significant change. There are a large number of inpatient charts that have not been coded. Karen also receives the results of a recent coding audit for that facility. The audit reveals a coding quality issue with the inpatient coding. Karen contacts Sue, the coding manager at Uptown Hospital, to determine the cause of the recent changes. Sue informs Karen that one of the inpatient coders went on maternity leave three weeks ago and another had surgery two weeks ago and has not returned to work. In order to manage the inpatient coding backlog, Sue was having two outpatient coders fill in. These coders have much lower productivity when coding these inpatient charts and are not properly trained to code this patient type.

These coders' charts were the primary problem in the recent coding audit for inpatient coding. Karen knows from her weekly metrics that the other two facilities are current (up-to-date) on inpatient coding. Karen and Sue brainstormed possible solutions. In an attempt to resolve the problem and formulate a better solution, Karen makes arrangements for inpatient coders at the two other facilities to code charts for Uptown Hospital until their inpatient staffing returns to previous levels. This is possible due to the organization's EHR. Karen monitors that dashboard and coding audits for performance and quality and is pleased with the problem's resolution.

Real-World Case 18.2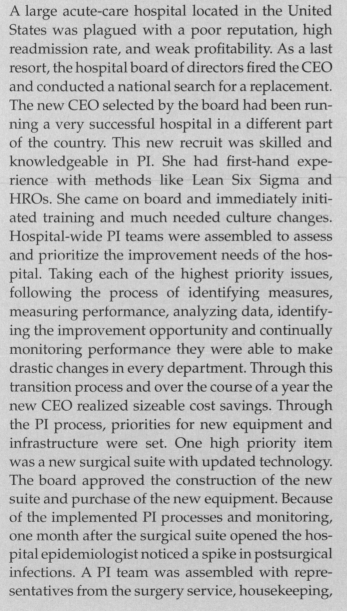

A large acute-care hospital located in the United States was plagued with a poor reputation, high readmission rate, and weak profitability. As a last resort, the hospital board of directors fired the CEO and conducted a national search for a replacement. The new CEO selected by the board had been running a very successful hospital in a different part of the country. This new recruit was skilled and knowledgeable in PI. She had first-hand experience with methods like Lean Six Sigma and HROs. She came on board and immediately initiated training and much needed culture changes. Hospital-wide PI teams were assembled to assess and prioritize the improvement needs of the hospital. Taking each of the highest priority issues, following the process of identifying measures, measuring performance, analyzing data, identifying the improvement opportunity and continually monitoring performance they were able to make drastic changes in every department. Through this transition process and over the course of a year the new CEO realized sizeable cost savings. Through the PI process, priorities for new equipment and infrastructure were set. One high priority item was a new surgical suite with updated technology. The board approved the construction of the new suite and purchase of the new equipment. Because of the implemented PI processes and monitoring, one month after the surgical suite opened the hospital epidemiologist noticed a spike in postsurgical infections. A PI team was assembled with representatives from the surgery service, housekeeping, nursing, infection control, and HIM. The team meticulously evaluated and improved each of the procedures related to the new surgical suite. Continued monitoring only demonstrated minor improvements in postoperative surgeries. Having exhausted the expertise and ideas of the internal PI team, the CEO contacted external experts and assembled a virtuoso team to come and consult with the internal PI team. Both teams were put into a small conference room and given five hours to review the collected data and the changes that had been made with little to no results. The external view of the outside experts, along with a detailed decomposition of the processes related to the suite, pointed to the construction process. Pulling the specifications and reports from the construction process, the virtuoso team had questions for the construction contractors about the grade of materials used in the room. Specifically they were concerned that the walls and flooring were too porous to be properly sterilized. The contractor confirmed the suspicion and came up with a solution to recover the walls and floor with appropriate materials. Monitoring infection rates closely, the suite reopened for use. Weekly dashboard reports were given to all stakeholders and showed no postoperative infections. At a review meeting at one month, the postoperative infection rate had dropped to a level lower than before the new surgical suite was opened. This is an example of how many different PI techniques were used to improve a hospital and solve a difficult problem.

References

Boynton, A. and B. Fischer. 2005. *Virtuoso Teams: Lessons from Teams that Changed Their Worlds.* New York: FT Prentice Hall.

Centers for Medicare and Medicaid Services. 2015. Accountable Care Organizations. http://www.cms.gov/Medicare/Medicare-Fee-for-Service-Payment/ACO/.

Donabedian, A. 1988. The quality of care: How can it be assessed? *Journal of the American Medical Association.* 260(12):1743–1748.

Farenholz, C. 2011. *Documentation for Medical Practices.* Chicago: AHIMA.

Few, S. 2013. *Information Dashboard Design: Displaying Data for At-a-Glance Monitoring,* 2nd ed. Burlingame, CA: Analytics Press.

George, M., D. Rowlands, and B. Kastle. 2002. *What Is Lean Six Sigma?* New York, NY: McGraw-Hill.

Institute of Medicine. 2001. *Crossing the Quality Chasm: A New Health System for the 21st Century.* Washington, DC: National Academies Press.

Institute of Medicine. 1999. *To Err Is Human: Building a Safer Health System.* Washington, DC: National Academies Press.

Karr, T. 2011. Determining what healthcare should be. *Industrial Engineer.* 43(9):45–48.

Kloss, L. 2015. *Implementing Health Information Governance: Lessons from the Field.* Chicago: AHIMA.

Kubiak, T.M. and D. Benbow. 2009. *The Certified Six Sigma Black Belt Handbook,* 2nd ed. Milwaukee, WI: ASQ Quality Press.

Meisenheimer, C. 1997. *Improving Quality: A Guide to Effective Programs,* 2nd ed. Sudbury, MA: Jones and Bartlett.

Meyer, H. 2010. Life in the "lean" lane: Performance improvement at Denver Health. *Health Affairs.* 29(11):2054–2060.

Omachonu, V. K. 1999. *Healthcare Performance Improvement.* Norcross, GA: Engineering and Management Press.

Rakhmawati, T., Sumaedi, S., and N. Astrini. 2014. ISO 9001 in health service sector: a review and future research proposal. *International Journal of Quality and Service Sciences.* 6(1):17–29. http://doi.org/10.1108/IJQSS-12-2012-0025.

Shaw, P. and D. Carter. 2015. *Quality and Performance Improvement in Healthcare: A Tool for Programmed Learning,* 6th ed. Chicago: AHIMA.

Strome, T. 2013. *Healthcare Analytics for Quality and Performance Improvement.* Hoboken, NJ: John Wiley & Sons.

US Department of Health and Human Services. 2015. The Patient Safety and Quality Improvement Act of 2005. http://www.hhs.gov/ocr/privacy/psa/regulation/statute/index.html.

Weick, K. and K. Sutcliffe. 2007. *Managing the Unexpected: Resilient Performance in an Age of Uncertainty.* San Francisco: Jossey-Bass.

19
Management

Leslie L. Gordon, MS, RHIA, FAHIMA
Morley L. Gordon, RHIT

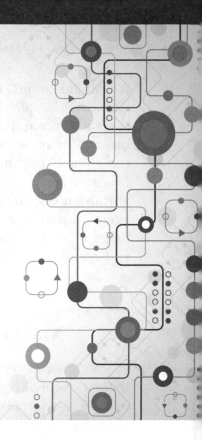

Learning Objectives

- Identify the functions involved in management
- Explain the principles of organization
- Discuss organizational structure in a healthcare organization
- Understand mission, vision, and values statements
- Identify the uses for policies and procedures
- Discuss the process for strategic planning
- Understand the basics and tools of project management
- Explain financial management in healthcare

Key Terms

Accounting
Accrual accounting
Budget
Budget adjustment
Budget management
Budget variance
Cash basis accounting
Change management
Controlling
Corporate compliance
Cultural competence
Enterprise information management
Executive management
Expenses
External analysis
Financial management
Gantt chart

Impact analysis
Internal analysis
Job classification
Job description
Job evaluation
Leading
Management
Market assessment
Mergers
Middle management
Operational planning
Organization
Organizational chart
Organizational structure
Program evaluation and review technique (PERT) chart
Planning
Policies

Principles of organization
Procedures
Project management
Project management life cycle
Resource allocation
Revenue
Risk management
Strategic information systems planning
Strategic plan
Strategic planning
Strategy
Supervisory management
Supply management
SWOT analysis
Variable costs
Work analysis
Workflow

All organizations, from small businesses with a handful of employees to large corporations with several thousand employees, require management. **Management** is the process of planning, controlling, leading, and organizing the activities of a healthcare organization or department within an organization. Securing effective management practices within an organization establishes a positive direction to successfully deliver end results, and to do this strategic planning is necessary. A **strategy** is a course of action designed to produce a desired (business) outcome and a **strategic plan** is the document in which the leadership of a healthcare organization identifies the organization's overall mission, vision, and goals to help define the long-term direction of the organization as a business entity. Successful management practices also encompass work processes and finance, all of which are described throughout this chapter.

Management

Health information management (HIM) ensures the availability, accuracy, and protection of the clinical information needed to deliver healthcare services and to make appropriate healthcare-related decisions. HIM directors and supervisors use four functions of management—planning, controlling, leading, and organizing—in the day-to-day and long-term operations of the HIM department to ensure the healthcare organization is in compliance with laws and regulations that mandate the management of HIM functions.

The HIM director uses the planning function of management to develop goals for the department. **Planning** is the examination of the future and preparation of action strategies to attain goals of the department or healthcare facility; for example, a director in the HIM department may use the planning function to prepare for the future state of the department after the implementation of a new release of information software system installation. The director will anticipate the changes in staffing, processes, and procedures to determine what changes will be necessary in preparing, implementing, and managing the new system. Short-term planning may involve staffing coverage for an employee who is taking leave time.

Controlling is the function in which performance is monitored according to policies and procedures. In HIM, controlling includes monitoring the performance of employees for quality, accuracy, and timeliness of completion of duties. For example, the policy of the department may include a 90 percent accuracy rate for all codes for surgical procedures. The coding supervisor will monitor accuracy for all coders to ensure compliance with this standard. If an employee falls below the stated standard, training will be provided to the employee.

Leading is the function in which people are directed and motivated to achieve the goals of the healthcare organization. In an HIM department, leading involves assigning responsibilities to the tasks the department needs to accomplish. For example, in the case of a disaster where multiple patients are brought to the facility, the HIM director may ask all personnel to report to the emergency staging area to help with record management. The day-to-day operations of the department requires the director to understand the policies and procedures to determine when a change may be needed. Leadership is explained in detail in chapter 17.

The HIM director uses the function of organizing on a daily basis, for both long-term and short-term tasks and goals. **Organization** is coordinating all of the tasks and responsibilities of a department to guarantee the work to be accomplished is completed correctly. A director or supervisor is responsible for the decisions concerning the division of labor for the HIM department. In an HIM coding department, there may be a priority list of chart types needing coding. The coding supervisor ensures certain employees are responsible for specific charts, thus the common goal of chart coding is accomplished by multiple people (Management Study Guide 2015a).

Organization is the planned coordination of activities of multiple people to achieve a common purpose or goal. For a healthcare facility, organization is vital for structure and allows employees at all levels to understand their job duties, to whom they report, and what is expected of them. Managers at all levels use the following **principles of organization** to manage in an effective manner.

- *Specialization:* Each employee has a special qualification or skill that allows that individual to perform his or her designated job to the best of his or her ability; managers who employ this principle assign work among their reporting employees according to their specialization, such as assigning the most complex coding cases to the coder who has the highest quality performance on coding reviews. The manager is able to divide and conquer the work of the department using each employee's strengths, which results in a positive outcome for the organization.

- *Functional definition:* All employee job tasks, responsibilities, and relationships toward each other are clearly defined. Managers who define and adhere to the functions of their department staff provide a healthy working environment. The HIM department employees working in the transcription department know exactly which reports they are responsible for transcribing (for example operations reports) and the time frame expected for completion (within one hour post-dictation). There is a clear understanding of the supervision and direction for the department.

- *Span of control:* The number of employees a person manages is called the span of control and is influenced by the size of the organization (such as a department

with only two employees compared to department with 100 employees), the skill level of the employees (entry-level employees require more supervisor time), and the responsibilities of the supervisor and employees. Span of control can be high, where there are a lot of employees to manage, or low, with few employees to manage. High span of control may cause the manager to be ineffective because too many people report to him or her, or a manager with low span of control may feel he or she is not being used effectively, meaning he or she feels that they are capable of more responsibility.

- *Hierarchical chain:* This is a management principle in which each member is assigned a specific rank that reflects his or her level of decision-making authority within the organization. An HIM director who reports to the chief financial officer (CFO) gives advice and guidance to the CFO; however, ultimately the CFO has a higher authority in making decisions. Reporting structure is described in greater detail later in this chapter.

- *Unity of command:* In this management principle, it is assumed that each employee reports to one manager. The employees in the coding department report to the coding supervisor and the coding supervisor reports to the HIM director (Management Study Guide 2015b).

This chapter discusses management roles as they relate to healthcare organizations. Organizational behavior and structure, the fundamentals of work planning, change management, project management, financial management, resource and vendor management, enterprise information and management of mergers, corporate compliance, patient safety, and risk management are also addressed.

Organizational Behavior

Humans are social by nature and usually live within groups of their own kind. **Cultural competence** is the ability to accept and understand the beliefs and values of other people and groups and is vital to the overall health of an organization. Cultural competence is discussed in detail in chapter 21 and is important for healthcare professionals to understand because they are required to work with different people from diverse backgrounds with varying beliefs, values, and goals. The organizational behavior of a healthcare facility may affect the way its members interact with each other. Organizational behavior involves the ways in which people interact with one another within a healthcare facility. For example, if an HIM director works in a facility that does not have clear lines of supervision defined he or she may be directed by multiple people causing confusion and frustration. A coding supervisor speaking negatively about the HIM director to the people who report to her demonstrates the organizational behavior of that particular department, meaning the coding supervisor is creating a behavior of negativity within the department and the supervisor's direct employees may view such speech as an indication that it is acceptable to speak negatively about others in the department. Supervisors and managers should be aware of the culture of their department and control the organizational behavior to provide positive human interaction.

Organizational Structure

All healthcare organizations have an **organizational structure**—the framework of authority and supervision for the employees within the healthcare organization. The organizational structure defines the hierarchy of reporting and responsibility for each level of decision-making authority and the responsibilities within the institution. The structure follows a chain of command, or the hierarchical structure within an organization. Employees are able to understand to whom they report and to whom their supervisor reports and so forth. A manager may have many reports but an employee only reports to one manager (Management Study Guide 2015c).

Organizational structure at the top starts with the board of directors and ends with line staff throughout the institution. The board of directors is an elected or appointed group of people who bear ultimate responsibility for the successful operation of the organization. Managers are responsible for different aspects of the business and operations of the organization. It is important to understand management levels and organizational tools, including organizational charts; mission, vision, and values; and policies and procedures and how they govern an organization or department.

Management Levels

Management generally includes three levels: executive, middle, and supervisory. **Executive management** is the senior management of a healthcare organization, the people who oversee a broad functional area or group of departments or services. This level of management establishes the organization's future direction and monitors the organization's operations in those areas. An executive manager in HIM may be the chief information officer (CIO) who is responsible for HIM and information technology (IT). CIOs are responsible for the strategic direction for the organization in terms of information governance (IG) and the technology related to IG. **Middle management** involves the people within the organization who oversee the operation of a broad scope of functions; for example, the HIM manager may oversee coding, transcription, and release of information at the departmental level or they may oversee a defined product or line of service, such as in the case of a radiology department manager. **Supervisory management** oversees the staff-level employees and monitors the effectiveness of everyday operations and individual performance against pre-established standards. In HIM a coding supervisor is an example of this level of management—this individual may have inpatient and outpatient coders, discharge analysts, and clerks reporting to him or her. The focus of this chapter is management as a whole, not leadership (for more information on leadership refer to chapter 17).

Organizational Tools

Managers and supervisors rely on tools to help with their functions. These tools include organization charts, policies, procedures, strategic planning and understanding the mission, vision, and values of the business. Each of these is discussed in detail.

Organizational Chart

An **organizational chart**, sometimes called an org chart, is a visual graphic or diagram showing the structure and reporting relationships between positions, departments, and employees of an organization. The org chart shows the relation of one department to another and a department org chart shows the relationships among staff, supervisors, and managers within a single department. Figure 19.1 is a simplistic example of an org chart for a healthcare organization and figure 19.2 is an example of an org chart for an HIM department.

Mission, Vision, and Values Statements

Chapter 1 describes mission, vision, and values—tools healthcare organizations use to set the direction and define their purpose and philosophies. A mission statement is a written statement that identifies the core purpose and philosophies of a healthcare organization; it defines the healthcare organization's general purpose. The vision statement is a short description of an organization's ideal future state,

Figure 19.1 Organizational chart for a healthcare organization

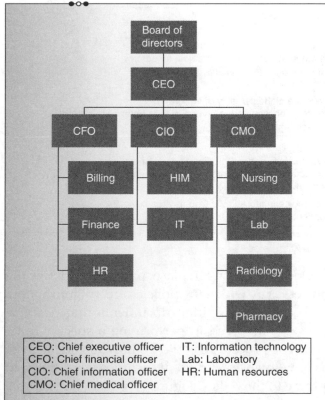

©AHIMA

Figure 19.2 Organizational chart for an HIM department

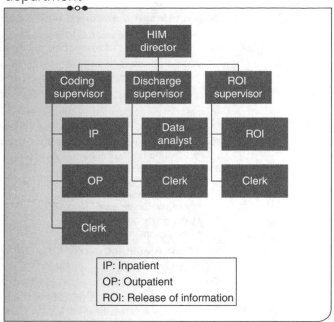

©AHIMA

and the values statement is a short description that communicates an organization's social and cultural belief system. These statements can range from analytical to creative, but they are always a screenshot of what the healthcare organization represents, its goals for the future, and what the healthcare organization believes in (McNamara n.d.).

Healthcare organizations update their mission and vision statements regularly as part of the strategic planning processes (strategic planning is discussed later in this chapter). All employees of the healthcare organization should know and understand the mission and vision of the organization. By understanding the mission and vision, managers are able to determine the direction of their department and if it fits into the overall strategy of the organization. For example, if the mission of a facility includes serving only female patients, managers will not look at expanding services to male patients with prostate cancer. Figure 19.3 provides examples of vision and mission statements from various healthcare organizations.

Policies and Procedures

Policies are the principles describing how a department or an organization will handle a specific situation or execute a specific process. They are clear, simple statements of how an HIM department will

Figure 19.3 Sample mission and vision statements

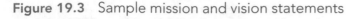

General Hospital Affiliated with a Larger Healthcare System

Lutheran hospital's **mission** is to improve the health of the communities we serve by providing high-quality services in a responsible and caring way.

Our **vision** is to become the leader in promoting healthy lifestyles in an atmosphere of spiritual support, dignity, compassion, and mutual respect for all.

Community General Hospital

Anytown General Hospital's **mission** is to provide quality health services and technology to meet the changing healthcare needs of the people of southwestern Minnesota.

Anytown General Hospital's **vision** is to become the hospital of choice for residents of Polk, Sunny Isle, and Spring counties, a position we strive to strengthen by our long-term commitment to:
- Teamwork
- Service excellence
- Compassionate care
- Cost consciousness
- Continuous improvement

Academic Medical Center

Prairie University Hospital's **mission** is to provide the most up-to-date medical and surgical services available in the three-state area and to train medical students and graduate physicians to meet current and future challenges in healthcare.

Our **vision** is the achievement of healthy communities and progress toward the future of healthcare for Montana, western North Dakota, and northwestern South Dakota.

Specialty Hospital

The **mission** of Women's hospital of Somewhereville is to meet the healthcare needs of our patients and to exceed their service expectations.

Our **vision** is of a hospital:
- Providing services with compassion and kindness
- Striving for performance improvement
- Fostering pride and integrity
- Aiming for increased cost-effectiveness and productivity

Specialty Clinic within an Academic Medical Center

The **mission** of the Midwest Asthma Center is to:
- Provide optimal medical care for persons with asthma and related illnesses
- Develop new knowledge about asthma and its management through medical research programs and materials for our patients, for other healthcare providers, and for the community

The **vision** of the Midwest Asthma Center is to provide the highest quality of integrated comprehensive care for persons with asthma and related illnesses and to be one of the centers of excellence in the world for asthma treatment, research, and education.

Primary Care Physicians' Practice

The **mission** of Coastal Shores Primary Care Associates is to serve the unique needs of individuals and families by providing high-quality, coordinated, primary care medical services through and efficient, accessible, and responsive network of caring providers.

Our **vision** is to be the primary care medical group of choice in the Atlantic County area by delivering high-quality, individualized, and efficient patient care.

Source: Kellogg 2012, 1086–1087.

conduct its services, actions, or business; and a set of guidelines and steps to help with decision making. For example, the American Health Information Management Association (AHIMA) has a privacy policy on their website stating: "AHIMA is committed to honoring the privacy of its members and general users who access the website," (AHIMA 2015). The policy goes on to state what information is collected and for what purpose.

Once policies are in place, **procedures** define the processes by which the policies are put into action. Procedures are written documents that describe the steps involved in performing a specific function. The procedure could be how to code a chart or how to abstract data. It includes steps taken to adhere to the policy. Figure 19.4 gives an example of a policy and procedure for record retention for the Alaska HIM Association.

Figure 19.4   Example policy and procedure for record retention

AKHiMA <AHIMA Affiliate> Alaska Health Information Management Association	Alaska Health Information Management Association Policy and Procedure Manual Record Retention Policy	
Title: Record Retention Policy		Approved Date: 06/23/2015
Subject: Storage and destruction of records related to the management of the AKHIMA Board of Directors and Organization		Effective Date: 07/01/2015
Purpose: AKHIMA is responsible for the maintenance, storage and destruction of business records and activities.		Revised:

Policy:

- The Alaska Health Information Association (AKHIMA) is responsible to maintain and store its business records and records of activity.
- Committees and other groups acting as designees of the Board of Directors will provide records of activity to the AKHIMA Secretary for retention and destruction.
- The AKHIMA Secretary will maintain the AKHIMA records on the AHIMA Engage, AKHIMA Board websites.
- The retention and destruction table in this document will be the guide for retention and destruction.

Procedure:
Media Type:
Records may be contained on a variety of media, including, but not limited to: electronic records, paper, photographs and video files. Additionally, information sets (email, datasets, metadata) stored in document management systems may have record status and require retention to meet administrative, legal or financial needs. A clear and accurate copy or duplicate of an original document may be considered a "final copy" or "original" for the business purposes of AKHIMA.

Responsibility for Record Storage and Archiving:
The AKHIMA Board of Directors is responsible to identify and implement an accessible record storage and archiving methodology that can be utilized by individuals with delegated record storage responsibilities. This storage and archiving solution should allow authorized individuals to access stored and archive records. At the change of the "Board Year", outgoing members of the Board of Directors will relinquish "Board Only" access. Incoming members of the Board will be provided with access as appropriate to their role.
All records will be stored on the American Health Information Management Association (AHIMA) member website Engage, AKHIMA Board Community.
The AKHIMA Secretary is responsible for storage and archiving of all administrative records as defined in the table below. Storage and archiving will use the method identified by the Board of Directors.
The AKHIMA Treasurer is responsible for storage and archiving of all Accounting/Finance records as defined above. Storage and archiving will use the method identified by the Board of Directors.
Committee chairs are responsible to forward to the AKHIMA Secretary records for accessible storage and archiving. The Committee Chair prepares and maintains the following files and forwards them to the AKHIMA Secretary at the end of the Chair's term including committee reports for the current fiscal year.

DESTRUCTION OF RECORDS
The AKHIMA Board of Directors is responsible to identify, implement and maintain a schedule and process for the final disposition/destruction of archived records that have met their defined retention period. Destruction of identified records will take place on or around July 1st of each year and shall be the responsibility of the Secretary and President.

Figure 19.4   (*Continued*)

AKHIMA Policy and Procedure Manual Record Retention		
RECORD DESCRIPTION	**RETENTION PERIOD**	**REFERENCE**
ADMINISTRATIVE		
1 Articles of Incorporation, Bylaws and other foundational	Permanent	AS 29.05
2 Correspondence (general incoming and outgoing letters and memoranda related to the general administration and operation of the agency)	3 years	
3 Policies, procedures, and operational guidelines (manuals for operations including committees)	Permanent	
4 Minutes of meetings of Board of Directors	Permanent	AS 10.06.430
5 Minutes of Committee activities	Permanent	
6 Minutes of Membership Meetings	Permanent	
7 Membership Rosters	Permanent	
8 Position Descriptions	Until obsolete	
9 Legal opinions issued by counsel for AKHIMA	Permanent	
10 Conflict of Interest Statements	6 years	AS 29.20.010
11 Correspondence	2 years except legal or other important matters	
12 Endowments, trusts, bequests	Permanent	
13 Property records (leases)	Term of Lease + 6 years	
ACCOUNTING/FINANCE		
1 Determination of Tax Exempt Status (from IRS)	Permanent	
2 Income Tax returns	Permanent	
3 Letters pertaining to audits or examinations by the	Permanent	
4 Audit reports (Financial statement audit or review)	Permanent	
5 Ledgers and Journals	Permanent	
6 Banking documents	3 years	
Vouchers: Cash vouchers/Capital purchases	7 years	
7 Paid invoices and/or receipts and cancelled checks	3 years	
8 Records of receipt of cash, check, or credit card	3 years	
9 Approved Budgets	5 years	
10 Contracts (signed)	Permanent	
11 Bonding Documents or Insurance Policies	Expiration + 3 years	
12 Insurance Claims and related documents	7 years	
13 Asset Inventories	Permanent	
14 Grant and subcontract records	7 years	7AAC 78.250(a)(4)
NOMINATING COMMITTEE		
1 Ballots	Until election results finalized by Board	
MARKETING/COMMUNICATIONS COMMITTEE		
1 Publications	Permanent	
2 Research and surveys	Permanent	
3 Photographs	Permanent	
4 Marketing Materials	6 years	
PROGRAM COMMITTEE		
1 Training programs and classes provided to members	Current year + 3 years	
2 Committee Reports to Board of Directors and Membership	6 years	
3 Documentation regarding reprint requests and the authorization to reprint.	Permanent	

Note: AAC= Alaska Administrative Code; AS= Alaska Statutes;

Source: AKHIMA 2014.

Check Your Understanding 19.1

Instructions: **Answer the following questions by matching the term with the definition.**

1. _____ Written statement that sets forth the core purpose and philosophies of an organization

2. _____ Principle that describes how a department or an organization will handle a specific situation or execute a specific process

3. _____ A description of an organization's future

4. _____ A document that describes the steps involved in performing a specific function

5. _____ A description that communicates an organization's social and cultural belief system

   A. Values statement
   B. Mission statement
   C. Policies
   D. Procedure
   E. Vision statement

Strategic and Operational Planning

The strategic plan of a healthcare organization is a map to the future state of the company. The plan outlines the outcomes and goals for the long range. **Strategic planning** involves how the organization will react to changes in the external environment in the foreseeable future. Usually the time frame is three to five years in the future. In the healthcare environment a strategic plan must take into consideration the regulatory environment, meaning federal, state and local regulations, because healthcare legislation changes regularly. Strategic planning involves specific steps and includes participants from all levels of management in the organization (Gartenstein 2015). The steps for creating a strategic plan will be explored in more detail in this chapter and includes internal and external analysis of the environment in which the healthcare organization is functioning.

By analyzing the environment every few years, executive management should stay abreast of the changes in regulation, technology, culture, and direction of the organization. The strategic plan

process will help keep a healthcare organization in business because everyone associated with it will understand the changes the organization must make to stay in compliance with regulation, and determine the future state of the organization.

Operational planning is the specific day-to-day tasks required in operating a healthcare organization or an HIM department. The operational plan is the road map to guide a healthcare organization or department toward the goals of the strategic plan. The operational plan is a shorter and more defined time frame than the strategic plan. Department managers are involved in creating an operational plan for their department to propose how to staff and accomplish the work tasks for the coming year. Supervisors use operational planning on a daily basis to organize the work of their teams to keep up with department workload.

An **internal analysis** involves reviewing the inner working of the healthcare organization to determine strengths and weaknesses of the business practice and process. For example, an internal analysis of the coding department may reveal that

10 of the coders are credentialed and have at least 10 years of experience; however, the top five coders are all leaving their employment within the next three months. An **external analysis** includes development of the **market assessment** to determine opportunities and threats to the future of the organization. For example, an external analysis is performed by facility A within the service area in which it operates. The analysis determines that at facility B, operating within the same service area, coders are paid 25 percent more than what facility A is paying. Facility A concludes that the reason experienced coders are not applying for open coding positions is because they can be paid more at facility B. Facility A has the external analysis information needed to understand it must increase the wages of coder to be competitive within its' service area. An assessment of the market would involve determining the number of coding positions on the market and the eligible workforce looking for work (Buchbinder 2012).

Developing Strategic and Operational Plans

The process to develop a strategic and operational plan begins with a SWOT (acronym for strengths, weaknesses, opportunities, and threats) analysis. In a **SWOT analysis**, key leadership personnel determine the strengths of the organization (what the company does well), the weaknesses (needs for improvement), and establishes future opportunities (and evaluates threats to those opportunities). An example SWOT analysis performed by an HIM department found the following:

Strengths: Fully staffed long-term employees are all credentialed.
Weaknesses: Staff is not trained in the technology being implemented.
Opportunities: New technology will increase productivity in the department by 45 percent.
Threats: There are members of the staff that are opposed to change and there is a time delay with implementing new technology (Buchbinder 2012)

By exploring SWOT in detail an organization's management is able to determine what the future state of the organization could and should be.

It gives an honest portrayal of the current and future state of the healthcare organization. The strengths and weakness are usually internal to the organization with opportunities and threats being external (Buchbinder 2012). Healthcare organizations have information management strategic plans to guide the overall enterprise management of information and information systems.

Information Management Strategic Plan

Information is a strategic asset and requires a high level of oversight in order to be able to effectively use it for organizational decision making, performance improvement, cost management, and to lower risk to the company A strategic plan for information management is vital to stay within the guidelines of legal and regulatory laws and is described in terms of strategic plans in the next section.

Strategic Information Systems Planning

Strategic information systems planning is the process of identifying and prioritizing various upgrades and changes that might be made in an organization's information systems. The Office for the National Coordinator (ONC) for Health Information Technology released a Federal Health IT Strategic Plan for the years 2015 through 2020 with the main goals to collect, share, and use healthcare information. The following describes the strategies to reach these goals:

- Collect
  Expand adoption of Health IT by increasing the adoption, use, and consumer confidence of IT products and systems
- Share
  Advance secure and interoperable health information by enabling providers and patients to send, receive, find, and use electronic health information
- Use
  o Strengthen healthcare delivery by improving healthcare quality, access and experience in healthcare

- Advance the health and well-being of individuals and communities by empowering individual, family, and caregiver health management and engagement
- Advance research, scientific knowledge, and innovation by increasing access to and usability of high-quality electronic health information services (ONC 2015)

Healthcare organizations should use the ONC strategic plan in the development of their own IT strategic plan to ensure compliance with federal guidelines. The organization should include representation from all stakeholders who use health IT. For example, a laboratory manager may want to implement a new technology to perform lab tests that does not submit data to the EHR. The HIM manager may want to implement a release of information software system but it does not keep an audit trail of releases, which is required by law. Strategic planning for IT development includes planning, analysis, design, implementation, maintenance, and evaluation. Figure 19.5 shows a graphical representation of the life cycle of information technology within a healthcare organization. The process starts with planning which involves examination of what is needed in the future and includes a SWOT analysis of the IT systems currently in place. After planning, an analysis of how the IT systems work together (interoperability, discussed in chapter 11) of different systems. The design phase includes consideration of all the options available in the selection of a new information system. If the planning analysis and design phases were completed properly, the implementation phase will be easier for the end

Figure 19.5 Life cycle of information technology development

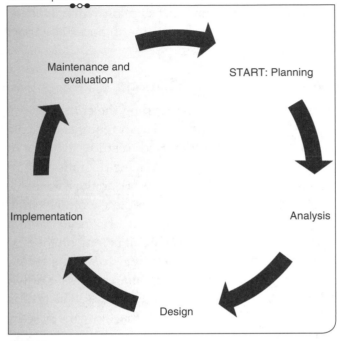

©AHIMA

users. Implementation involves development of a comprehensive plan which is instituted to ensure the new information system is effectively implemented within the healthcare organization. The maintenance and evaluation phase helps to ensure adequate technical support staff and resources are available to maintain or support the system. The organization is not finished with the life cycle at this point; the cycle starts again at the planning phase to allow for continuous quality improvement.

After the strategic and operational plans are developed and in place, a healthcare organization will analyze the work flow and process and determine ways for improvement.

Work Analysis, Change Management, and Project Management

It is important for healthcare organizations to understand what it takes to accomplish the tasks involved in everyday **workflow**—the process and steps it takes to complete a task. With new technology and advances in healthcare delivery and processes, healthcare managers are required to manage change. Knowledge of the workflow makes changes easier to identify. **Work analysis** is the process of gathering information about what it takes to get a job done. **Change management** is the formal process of introducing change, adopting the change, and diffusing it throughout the organization. This section will explain work analysis and design, change management, and the impact of change on processes.

Work Analysis and Design

Work analysis involves mapping the entire process from start to finish for a task that requires multiple steps. It is the technique used to study the flow of operations and is sometimes called operations analysis or workflow analysis. A work analysis for completing a trauma registry for the state would include many steps from running a report on all trauma codes, analyzing the records that belong on the registry, completing the trauma registry, and sending the report to the state. A work analysis breaks down the workflow into its component parts. The goal is to determine if there are areas that slow the process of the job task under review. It should be completed by detailing every single step of a process.

After analyzing the workflow, a job description, job classification, and job evaluation are created. A **job description** is a list of duties, reporting relationships, working conditions, and responsibilities for a particular job. **Job classification** is a method of evaluating a job description against written descriptions of various classification grades. **Job evaluation** is the process of applying predefined compensable factors to determine their worth. It allows the company to have guidelines and clear boundaries of the scopes of individual jobs. The company is able to measure the work being done, and also place employees in a position that best fits the needs of the company. In healthcare, advances in technology and information systems means that employees are constantly changing their processes or job tasks.

Change Management

Healthcare is continually improving and changing, and managing change is a challenging yet necessary task for healthcare supervisors. Healthcare rules, regulations, and laws are passed with each congressional session in the United States. Changes in payment methodologies, privacy, and security guidelines and other regulations directly affect HIM professionals regularly.

The key to having a smooth transition is in the planning. By thoroughly analyzing how change is going to affect the workflow and work procedures, the organization will be able to determine the best course of action. **Impact analysis** is a collective term used to refer to any study that determines the benefit of a proposed project, including cost-benefit analysis, return on investment, benefits realization study, qualitative benefit study, or how change affects workflow.

Project Management

Project management is a formal set of principles and procedures to help control the activities associated with implementing a large undertaking to achieve a specific goal (such as an information system implementation) and has a definitive beginning and end. There is never a shortage of projects to manage in healthcare. There are small projects like the implementation of a new software system in the HIM department to track release of information data, and much larger projects such as implementing International Classification of Diseases, Tenth Revision, Clinical Modification (ICD-10-CM)—a multidiscipline, hospital-wide, technological challenge. The project management life cycle, methodologies, tools and techniques, and the project management profession are discussed in the following sections.

Project Management Life Cycle

The **project management life cycle** is the period in which the processes involved in carrying out a project are completed, including the definition, planning and organization, tracking and analysis, revisions, change control, and communication. The following is an example of a project management life cycle as applied to HIM.

An HIM department in small community health clinic uses an alphabetic filing system for their paper charts and decides to start using the patient health record number as their filing system. The department manager assembles a project team to manage the conversion to the new filing system. The following terms are defined for this project:

- Definition: This outlines the project that is being accomplished by determining the objectives, activities, assumptions, estimated cost, and schedule such as:
  - Objectives: To convert the filing system from alphabetic to numerical
  - Activities: Identify health record number for each patient, create new filing system, convert all charts
  - Assumptions: Assume project will be straightforward with no delays
  - Cost estimate: Cost of supplies and staff time
  - Anticipated schedule: Schedule for completion is two weeks
- Planning and organization: A project plan lists the steps needed to complete the project with an estimated time frame for each step.
- Tracking and analysis: The project team members follow the steps in the plan to determine where there are time delays or problems.
- Revision: As the team monitors the project they can determine if changes need to take place in the project plan.
- Change control: As changes occur to the plan the team manages these changes. In the chart filing example, the team determines in the middle of the project that the filing system for the charts should be terminal digit filing and not straight numeric and ask to change the project accordingly (more information on filing systems can be found in chapter 3).
- Communication: All team members are informed and aware of the exact status of the project (Seidl 2013).

Project Management Tools

Project management is made easier by utilizing tools to track and analyze the steps and tasks within the overall project. Tools needed for project management include a project plan, Gantt charts, and PERT charts.

A detailed project plan identifies the individual steps to complete the project. Gantt and PERT charts are visual tools used to manage the elements or steps of a project. A **Gantt chart** is a graphic tool used to plot tasks and shows the duration of project tasks and overlapping tasks; in other words it is used as a method to illustrate the time needed for each task. A **program evaluation and review technique (PERT) chart** is a project management tool that diagrams a project's timelines and tasks as well as its interdependencies. Gantt charts focus on the percentage completion of each task and do not show a link between one or more tasks. In the example mentioned earlier, the charts will indicate the time it takes to complete the task of converting the filing system for records. Figure 19.6 is a display of a Gantt chart; figure 19.7 is a display of a PERT chart.

Project Management Professional

A project management professional (PMP) certification is a credential offered by the Project Management Institute (PMI). Individuals with this certification demonstrate competency in the project manager role and lead and direct projects and teams. The certification examination covers the areas of initiating, planning, executing, monitoring, controlling, and closing the project (PMI 2015). The HIM professional needs to understand project management to manage the implementation of new software systems, EHR systems, or new processes mandated by laws; for example, the implementation of the Health Insurance Portability and Accountability Act (HIPAA) mandated new privacy and security policies for healthcare organizations. The PMP certification is a highly desirable and valued certification that could benefit HIM professionals looking to ether work as a project manager or wanting the knowledge and background of a PMP.

Figure 19.6 Gantt chart

	Task	Start	Complete	6/1 - 6/7 1	6/8 - 6/14 2	6/15 - 6/21 3	6/22 - 6/28 4	6/29 - 7/5 5	7/6 - 7/12 6	7/13 - 7/19 7	7/20 - 7/26 8
Phase 1	**Design**										
1.1	Identify Requirements	1	1								
1.2	Acquire Software	2	2								
1.3	Test Software	3	3								
Phase 2	**Construct**										
2.1	Develop Training Program	3	4								
2.2	Train Coders	4	4								
2.3	Test Application	4	5								
2.3.1	Unit Testing	5	5								
2.3.2	System Testing	6	7								
Phase 3	**Pilot**										
3.1	Implement Software	7	8								
3.2	Conduct System Training	7	8								
3.3	Support Pilot	8	8								
Ongoing	**Pre / Post Production**										
	Weekly Team Meetings	1	8								
	Engage Stakeholders	2	8								

Implementation of New Coding Software Hospital Wide

Source: Najduch 2015a. Used with permission.

Figure 19.7 PERT chart

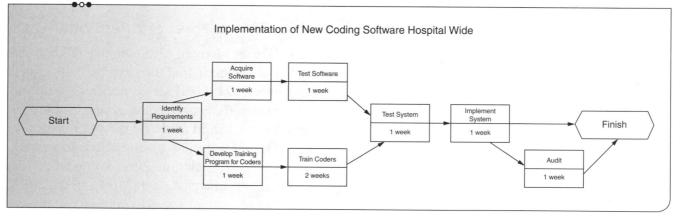

Implementation of New Coding Software Hospital Wide

Source: Najduch 2015b. Used with permission.

 Check Your Understanding 19.2

Instructions: **Answer the following questions.**

1. What analysis shows the honest portrayal of the current and future state of the healthcare organization?
   A. External analysis
   B. Workflow analysis
   C. Supply management analysis
   D. SWOT analysis

2. What is a useful general tool for guiding day-to-day decisions?
   A. Operational plan
   B. SWOT
   C. Strategies
   D. Strategic plan

3. What are the specific plans to accomplish and achieve short-term and long-term goals called?
   A. Internal analysis
   B. Strategic plan
   C. SWOT
   D. Operational plan

4. Which of the following is the management and control of the supplies used within an organization?
   A. Work analysis
   B. Staffing
   C. Supply management
   D. Strategic plan

5. What is the formal process of introducing change, adopting the change, and diffusing it throughout the organization?
   A. SWOT
   B. Change management
   C. Supply management
   D. Workflow

Financial Management

Financial management is the mechanism that all organizations and businesses use to fully comprehend and communicate their financial activities and status. It is usually managed by top-level executives in the organization with input from department leaders. It is important to understand the basics of accounting and budgets.

Accounting

Accounting is the process of collecting, recording, and reporting an organization's financial data including the assets, expenses, and liabilities of the company. It is important for the HIM professional to understand accounting methodologies and budgets so they are prepared to manage a department. The viability of a healthcare organization relies on financial management and the revenues that enter the institution rely heavily on the functions of the HIM department (for example, correct coding for reimbursement). Assets include the human, financial, and physical resources of an organization such as the employees, financial holdings, and physical buildings owned by the organization. Expenses are the amount of money charged as a cost to the organization, such as the cost of utilities. Liabilities include the amounts the organization owes to others, like loans.

The financial stability of the healthcare organization depends on the ability to understand the revenue and overall expenses each year. **Revenue** is the recognition of income earned and the use of appropriated capital from the rendering of services during the current period (CMS 2016), while **expense** is the amount that is charged as cost by an organization to the current year's activities of operation. Revenue is earned through coding and billing for healthcare services. Management must take into consideration they will not receive the entire amount billed for services due to adjustments to claims. More information on reimbursement adjustments is found in chapter 15. An HIM manager may choose to hire an independent coding consultant who can audit unpaid Medicare claims, which can result in higher revenue for the organization. Expenses are either variable or fixed costs with variable costs including resources that change like supplies, while fixed costs remain constant like rent, wages, and equipment rental.

There are two ways to record the transactions in the financial books—cash basis accounting and accrual accounting. **Cash basis accounting** is registering the transaction when it occurs, meaning when money is actually received for services provided, or paid for expenses incurred. This type of accounting is usually used in small businesses, because it is easier to manage. A small health clinic operating in a remote village in Alaska may use cash basis accounting for healthcare services rendered because they do not bill health insurance and patients pay for services as they are delivered. **Accrual accounting** involves recording known transactions in the appropriate time period before cash payment (receipts) are expected or due. A company records the revenue when it is earned and records expenses as the transactions happen, not when it receives the cash or makes a payment. For example, a large rehab center will write on their books the exercise classes that they provide, even if they have not been paid for those classes yet. In healthcare, most facilities use accrual accounting where cash or revenue reflects the amount the organization expects to receive for the services provided. The HIM department may use the accrual accounting system for the release of information function, charging for the service of coping records with revenue reflecting the amount expected from the patient.

Budgets

A **budget** is a plan that converts the organization's goals and objectives into targets for revenue and spending. A comprehensive organization master budget includes forecasted revenue (amount of money expected for the year) and forecasted expenses (cost of doing business for the year). In reality, the budget of a healthcare organization is several budgets, each addressing a specific need. For example, the budget for an HIM department includes what is needed to staff and manage the required functions of the department. The HIM department manager can use the budget to provide information that allows her to forecast success or difficulty for the department by analyzing the projected staff available to work during the upcoming holiday season when many employees are requesting time off. There are many types of budgets including operating, salaries, capital, and allocated costs.

- Operating budget: Allocates and controls resources to meet an organization's goals and objectives for a fiscal year

- Salaries and benefits: Allocates all of the employee wages and benefits taking into consideration salary and cost of living increases

- Capital budget: Schedules the purchase of assets that will be purchased in the future (for example, a new piece of radiology equipment)

- Allocated cost: Takes into account departments that are not revenue-producing but are necessary for operation—for example, maintenance, utilities, and insurance (Harrison and Harrison 2013)

Budget management involves the process of maintaining financial viability by ensuring operating revenues for the year are sufficient to cover the operating expenditures (Harrison and Harrison 2013). Managers control their budget throughout the year by making adjustments or amendments when needed. A **budget adjustment** is the approval to move funds from one budget to another. For example, an HIM department manager has a coding employee vacancy for a period of time. The amount of money budgeted to pay for that employee is not used, so a budget adjustment could be made to move the unused money into a different fund to cover the cost of something else such as overtime pay for employees who are covering for the unmanned position. A **budget variance** is a difference in the budgeted revenue or expense amount; for instance, an HIM manager budgeted $10,000 for training coders during the current year and training actually cost the department $11,500. Therefore, the department has a negative budget variance of $1,500. Ideally, a positive variance occurs when the projected revenue is higher or the expenses are lower than projected, meaning the expenditures are within or below the amount that was budgeted. Part of the budgeting process involves supplies and staffing management.

Supply management

Supply management is the management and control of the supplies used within an organization. It can be physical goods, services, information, or any resources needed to run the organization. Knowing the supplies needed to run the healthcare organization vastly improves and helps in managing a successful organization. In an HIM department it is important for the manager to anticipate and include in the budget the costs that the department incurs with supplies, pens, paper, copy costs, coding books, and regulation documentation requirements.

Staffing

Staffing is the managerial function that involves proper and effective selection, appraisal, and training of personnel. The HIM manager must be aware of (and budget for) the staffing needs of the department and take into consideration employee paid time off, leave, and illness. When it comes to staffing, the manager should keep in mind the following:

- Staff recruitment and selection
- Performance management
- Staff retention
- Employee relations and fair treatment
- Staffing planning and scheduling
- Productivity
- Training and development

For additional information on staffing, see chapter 20.

Management of Resources and Allocation

Healthcare organizations have limited resources that include money, people, tools, and technology. **Resource allocation** is a process and strategy of deciding where resources should be used to achieve the mission, values, and goals of the organization. For example, in an HIM department the budget includes an amount of money to be used for information technology systems and the manager must decide between a software system to help with clinical documentation improvement or a system to track information needed for various registries. The manager must prioritize the needs of the department with legal and regulatory issues that may affect the choice of resources. For example, the coding department must have the current coding guidelines each year and cannot work with outdated codes; thus they must purchase updated code books each year.

Management of Vendors and Contracts

A vendor is a company outside the healthcare organization with which an HIM department conducts business; for example, coders may use an encoding system that is owned and operated by an external company (vendor). A contractor is an outside company or individual who provides or performs a service for the HIM department; for example, the coding functions could be contracted to a company that specializes in coding. HIM professionals must understand the process for selection, implementation, and managing of outside vendors and contractors. A contract is a legal document that details the relationship between two entities—for instance, the contracted coders mentioned earlier and the department manager enter into a contract to provide coding services to the HIM department. In this case the vendor is the outside coding department and the HIM department manager is contracting with the vendor for coding services. Choosing a vendor or contractor includes identifying the need, designing the system, submitting a request for information (ROI), analyzing the ROI, submitting a request for proposal (RFP), and establishing a contract for services with the chosen proposal.

Enterprise Information Management

Enterprise information management (EIM) ensures the value of information assets, requiring an organization-wide perspective of information management functions; it calls for explicit structures, policies, processes, technology, and controls. It also includes the infrastructure and processes to ensure the information is trustworthy and actionable. EIM is the set of functions used by organizations to plan and organize, and coordinate people, processes, technology, and content for managing information as a corporate asset that ensures data quality, safety, and ease of use (Johns 2014). With executive-level management decisions relying on the data and information found within its own health information systems, the importance of accurate, complete, and quality data becomes clear. Management of information from the entire enterprise perspective is vital to quality patient care and business viability.

Management of Mergers

Mergers are business situations where two or more companies combine—one of them continues to exist as a legal business entity while the other(s) cease to exist legally and their assets and liabilities become part of the continuing company. Mergers commonly occur in healthcare with healthcare providers and organizations attempting to streamline their operations and improve their competitive positions. AHIMA Practice Brief, 2012A merger may entail a consolidation where two entities combine to form one new entity (the surviving entity), or it may be an asset acquisition where one entity acquires part or all of the assets of the other; or a stock acquisition where one entity acquires the stock of the other entity. All organizations must determine the licensure, regulatory, and accreditation requirements before the operational issues of a merger (AHIMA 2012). Information on licensure, regulatory requirements and accreditation can be found in chapter 16.

The HIM professional understands the operational issues related to the management of information and the functions of the department and how they will be affected by the merger. Operational issues for the HIM manager include the following:

- Single or multiple locations for HIM functions
- Integration of information systems
- Completion of current records
- Merging of department employees
- How will the master patient index (MPI) be handled (MPI information is found in chapter 2)
- How release of information will be handled

The function of the HIM department must be reviewed to guarantee compliance with state licensure and regulatory requirements (AHIMA 2012).

Management of Corporate Compliance and Patient Safety

Corporate compliance is the process of establishing an organizational structure that promotes the prevention, detection, and resolution of instances of conduct that do not conform to federal, state, or private payer healthcare program requirements nor to the healthcare organization's ethical and business policies. In HIM, compliance includes managing a coding or billing department according to the laws, regulations, and guidelines that govern it. A compliance officer is a designated individual who monitors the compliance process at a healthcare facility. (For more information on compliance see chapter 16.) The HIM manager is responsible for knowing and obeying laws that govern the management of HIM functions including coding and billing. A formal compliance program plan is the process that helps an organization accomplish its goal of providing high-quality healthcare and efficiently operating a business under various laws and regulations. The plan will include internal controls that promote adherence to applicable federal and state guidelines. Improving the quality and safety of healthcare delivery should be a goal of all healthcare organizations; risk management and analysis determines how the healthcare organization is reaching the goal of quality healthcare and safety of patients. Customer satisfaction is critical to the health of an organization—when customers are not happy the organization will not stay solvent.

Risk Management and Risk Analysis

Risk management is a comprehensive program of activities intended to minimize the potential for injuries to occur in a facility and to anticipate and respond to ensuring liabilities for those injuries that occur. Risk management includes the processes that are in place to identify, evaluate, and control risk, defined as the organization's risk of accidental financial liability. A healthcare organization as a whole has a risk management director or department to evaluate and manage the potential for injuries that happen during the course of doing business—for example, patient falls, patient infections occurring while being treated, or surgery on the wrong body part. HIM managers must handle risk in terms of coding and billing fraud and abuse. Managers must know the laws and regulations governing HIM functions and educate staff on those items. For more on risk management programs see chapter 10.

Risk managements begins with a risk analysis which includes identifying weaknesses in an organization's operations and determining how likely it is that any given threat may occur. An HIM manager performs a risk analysis of the HIM functions and procedures (such as coding and billing) to ensure the functions are being performed properly. For more on risk analysis see chapter 10.

Customer Satisfaction

Customer satisfaction is important to healthcare organizations. Customer satisfaction is a measurement of a customer's expectation, either by falling short, meeting, or exceeding the expectation. Customer satisfaction is usually determined using surveys that measure satisfaction with services provided. In an HIM department, the manager may want to assess customer satisfaction with the process of attaining copies of patient immunization records. Customers can be considered internal or external based on the relationship to the service. An internal customer needing a copy of immunization records could be the surgeon who works for the facility. An external customer is the parent of the patient who needs the records for their child to start playing baseball at the local community center. A sample satisfaction survey is displayed in figure 19.8.

Figure 19.8 Customer satisfaction survey

Customer Satisfaction Survey
City Community Hospital
123 Main Street
Your City, ST 00111
800-555-5555

Who received services at City Community Hospital?

☐ Me

☐ My dependent

Were your important questions answered regarding your condition or treatment by your healthcare providers (doctor, nurses)?

☐ Yes, always

☐ Yes, sometimes

☐ No

☐ I didn't have any questions

Were the answers you were given presented in a way that you could understand?

☐ Yes, always

☐ Yes, sometimes

☐ No

☐ I do not have any questions

How would you rate the skills of our staff in meeting or exceeding your expectations?

☐ Excellent

☐ Very good

☐ Good

☐ Fair

☐ Poor

How would you rate how well the staff worked together on your behalf?

☐ Excellent

☐ Very good

☐ Good

☐ Fair

☐ Poor

Overall, how satisfied were you with the treatment and care you received at City Community Hospital?

☐ Excellent

☐ Very good

☐ Good

☐ Fair

☐ Poor

Overall, how satisfied were you with your provider?

☐ Excellent

☐ Very good

☐ Good

☐ Fair

☐ Poor

Would you recommend City Community Hospital to your family or friends?

☐ Yes, definitely

☐ Yes, probably

☐ No

If no, why not?

Comments:

©AHIMA

 Check Your Understanding 19.3

Instructions: **Answer the following questions.**

1. What process should an organization use to see if there are resources available to help accomplish the mission, values, and goals of the organization?

   A. Measuring

   B. Process improvement

   C. Resource allocation

   D. PERT chart

2. What is a formal set of principles and procedures that help control the activities associated with implementing a large undertaking?
   A. Resource allocation
   B. Project management
   C. Project improvement
   D. Financial management

3. What project management tool focuses on the percentage completion of a task but does not show a link between one or more tasks?
   A. PERT chart
   B. Project management
   C. Planning and design
   D. Gantt

4. Which of the following is the process that all organizations and businesses use to fully comprehend and communicate financial activities and status?
   A. Financial management
   B. Cash basis accounting
   C. Budgets
   D. Resource allocation

5. The process of maintaining financial viability by ensuring operating revenues for the year are sufficient to cover the operating expenditures is called what?
   A. Budge adjustment
   B. Budget management
   C. Budget variance
   D. Accrual accounting

6. Which of the following are amounts charged as costs by an organization to the current year's activities of operation?
   A. Budgets
   B. Accrual accounting
   C. Revenue
   D. Expenses

Real-World Case 19.1

Central Community Hospital hired Susan Davis as the new manager to work in the health information management (HIM) department. One of the first items Susan reviewed was the workflow process for how documents were handled between the intake department and HIM. The intake department is responsible for assuring all documentation needed for a new admission to the hospital is received from the clinic that is admitting the patient. She noticed that the two departments were managing a lot of the same work, which created duplicate documents in patient charts. She noticed that intake would send documents to HIM that they (intake) already scanned. HIM would then see the documents come through, and scan them as well, but also created a copy to send to the utilization nurse who is responsible for ensuring that reimbursement authorizations are in place and managed. When Susan asked intake about why they sent the documents to HIM, the answer was "because that's how it has always been done." When thinking about other ways the situation could be handled, Susan came up with the following ideas:

- Have intake scan the documents into the EHR, and then hand the copy to the utilization review nurse, leaving HIM out of the process for this particular situation all together; or

- Once intake is done with the document, do not scan into the chart, rather hand it directly over to HIM, and continue with the rest of the process.

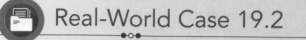

Real-World Case 19.2

A small community hospital in a rural area of Alaska is seeing an increase in their patient population in both the inpatient and outpatient setting. In reviewing the data for the increase the chief executive officer (CEO) noticed that it is due to a large project—the construction of a dam on a nearby lake. In speaking with the city administrator it was determined that an additional 2,000 people are in the town for the two-year duration of this project. The hospital CEO determines that by midyear the operating units of the hospital need to make adjustments to their budgets. They have the need for an increase in employee overtime, supplies, equipment, and part-time hires.

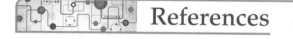

References

American Health Information Management Association. 2015. Privacy Statements for AHIMA's websites. http://www.ahima.org/privacy.

American Health Information Management Association. 2012. Identifying issues in Facility and Provider Mergers and Acquisitions. *Journal of AHIMA.* 83(2):50–53.

AKHIMA Record Retention Policy and Procedure. 2014. AKHIMA Policy and Procedure Manual. Alaska Health Information Management Association. www.akhima.org.

Buchbinder, S.B. and N.H. Shanks. 2012. *Introduction to Health Care Management,* 2nd ed. Burlington, MA: Jones & Bartlett Learning.

Centers for Medicare and Medicaid Services. 2016. https://www.cms.gov/apps/glossary/Gartenstein, D. 2015. Why Is Strategic Planning Important to an Organization? http://yourbusiness.azcentral.com/strategic-planning-important-organization-4103.html.

Harrison, C. and W. Harrison. 2013. *Introduction to Health Care Finance and Accounting.* Clifton Park, NY: Cengage.

Johns, M.L. 2014. *Enterprise Information Management and Data Governance.* Chicago: AHIMA.

Kellogg, D. 2012. Principles of Organization and Work Planning. Chapter 18 in *Health Information Management Technology: An Applied Approach,* 4th ed. N.B. Sayles, ed. Chicago: AHIMA.

Management Study Guide. 2015a. Functions of Management—Planning, Organizing, Staffing, Directing, and Controlling. http://www.managementstudyguide.com/management_functions.htm.

Management Study Guide. 2015b. Levels of Management. http://www.managementstudyguide.com/management_levels.htm.

Management Study Guide. 2015c. Principles of Organizing. http://www.managementstudyguide.com/organizing_principles.htm.

McNamara, C. n.d. Basics of Developing Mission, Vision, and Values Statements. http://managementhelp.org/strategicplanning/mission-vision-values.htm.

Najduch, A. 2015a. GANTT Chart. Implementation of New Coding Software Hospital Wide.

Najduch, A. 2015b. PERT Chart. Implementation of New Coding Software Hospital Wide.

Office of the National Coordinator for Health Information Technology (ONC). 2015. Federal Health IT Strategic Plan. https://www.healthit.gov/sites/default/files/9-5-federalhealthitstratplanfinal_0.pdf.

Project Management Institute. 2015. PMI Certifications. http://www.pmi.org/certification.aspx.

Seidl, P. 2013. Project Management. Chapter 27 in *Health Information Management Concepts, Principles and Practice,* 4th ed. Edited by K.M. LaTour, S. Eichenwald Maki, and P. Oachs. Chicago: AHIMA.

20

Human Resources Management and Professional Development

Valerie S. Prater, MBA, RHIT, FAHIMA

Learning Objectives

- Define human resources management using a health information management example
- Explain major provisions of equal opportunity employment laws
- Apply knowledge of labor laws and the principle of autonomy to a union-organizing scenario
- Analyze the role of job analysis in the employee recruitment and selection process
- Compare and contrast performance appraisal methods using examples
- Recommend employee engagement strategies to reduce turnover
- Assess approaches to conflict management in a given scenario
- Examine staffing issues and approaches to developing staff scheduling arrangements
- Differentiate benchmarking and work measurement approaches to development of performance standards
- Recommend training delivery methods given training content, budget, and audience
- Create an annual employee training and development plan

Key Terms

Accommodation
ADDIE model
Age Discrimination in Employment Act of 1967
Americans with Disabilities Act (ADA)

Asynchronous
Authorization cards
Autonomy
Avoidance
Bargaining unit
Behaviorally anchored rating scale

Benchmarking
Bias
Bona fide occupational qualification
Business process
Career development

555

Career planning
Civil Rights Act (CRA) of 1991
Classroom-based learning
Coaching
Collective bargaining
Competencies
Compressed workweek
Computer-based training
Consolidated Omnibus Budget
   Reconciliation Act (COBRA)
Contingent or contract work
Critical incident method
Development
Disciplinary action
Discipline without punishment
Discrimination
Dismissal
Disparate impact
Disparate treatment
Distributional errors
Downsizing
Dysfunctional conflict
Employee engagement
Employee relations
Employee Retirement Income
   Security Act (ERISA)
Employment at will
Equal employment opportunity law
Equal Pay Act
Exempt employees
Exit interview
Fair Labor Standards Act (FLSA)
Family and Medical Leave Act
   (FMLA)
Flextime

Forced distribution
Full-time equivalent
Genetic Nondiscrimination Act
   (GINA)
Graphic rating scale
Grievance
Halo-horns effect
Harassment
Hostile work environment
Human capital
Human resources management
   (HRM)
Job analysis
Job description
Job interview
Job sharing
Job specifications
Justice
Layoff
Line authority
Mentoring
National Labor Relations Act
   (NLRA)
National Labor Relations Board
   (NLRB)
Negligent hiring
New employee orientation
Nonexempt employees
Occupational Safety and Health Act
Offshoring
Onboarding
Online learning
On-the-job training
Outsourcing
Parallel work division

Part-time employee
Performance appraisal
Performance management
Performance measurement
Pregnancy Discrimination Act
Progressive penalties
Protected class
Quid pro quo
Ranking method
Recruitment
Reliability
Right-to-work laws
Selection
Selection test
Self-directed learning
Serial work division
Sexual harassment
Simulation
Staffing
Strike
Synchronous
Taft-Hartley Act
Telecommuting
Termination
Title VII of the Civil Rights Act of
   1964
Training
Turnover
Union
Validity
Variance
Work measurement
Workflow analysis
Workforce planning
Wrongful discharge

The healthcare industry is the largest employer in the United States (BLS 2014a). This represents a dramatic change from 1990, when manufacturing was dominant, and 2003 when retail was the largest employer in most states. Further, the healthcare sector is projected to add the largest number of jobs to the US economy to the year 2022, a trend supported by the aging US population, continued advances in technology, impact of the Affordable Care Act (ACA) and growth in outpatient services (Henderson 2013). The healthcare practitioners and technical occupations group is projected to grow 21.5 percent to 2022 (Richards and Terkanian 2013). The workforce need in healthcare is clear.

With this employment growth and opportunity comes challenges. The healthcare industry is complex and is experiencing rapid change. In addition to the factors noted as drivers of employment growth, healthcare organizations must deal with pressures to reduce costs, demonstrate evidence of quality and safety improvement, manage a growing volume of data, and meet the needs of a variety of internal and external customers, while facing increased competition.

Given this backdrop, the need to fill positions with qualified candidates and effectively handle the people aspects of management, the management of human resources has never been more important in healthcare than it is today. Despite the emphasis on technology, healthcare remains a service industry with people as its most necessary and valuable asset. In financial accounting terms, an asset is something of value to an organization that appears on the positive side of the balance sheet. The people asset is often referred to as **human capital**, the sum of the knowledge, skills, and abilities of an organization's workforce (SHRM 2015a). Yet, salaries are shown on the other side of the balance sheet (liabilities) as costs to the organization. While this is not a chapter on finance, in terms of human resources management it can be useful to consider how managers view people, as either assets or costs. Organizations are more productive (and profitable) when people are managed and treated as assets to be developed, versus as costs to be cut (Paton 2000). Discussion about assets and liabilities is discussed in chapter 19.

Human resources management (HRM) has been defined as "the process of acquiring, training, appraising, and compensating employees, and of attending to their labor relations, health and safety, and fairness concerns" (Dessler 2014, 2). Another practical way to look at human resource management is as an organization's formal structure encompassing responsibility for the decisions, strategies, principles, practices, and functions related to the management of people (SHRM 2015a).

This chapter begins with a foundation in employment law, ethical principles, and labor relations. Next, HRM functions of importance to healthcare organizations and to the health information management (HIM) profession are reviewed including staff recruitment, selection, performance management, and retention; employee relations; and staff scheduling, productivity reporting, training, and development. Principles of fairness and respect are applied across topics. The focus is on responsibilities and roles of HIM team leaders, supervisors, and middle managers. Intended as an overview, the chapter is not a comprehensive review of all aspects of HRM.

Supervisory-level leaders can contribute directly to effective and efficient management of an organization's human resources. They also support the organization's mission and financial health by helping to make the organization a place where people want to work.

Employment Law, Ethics, and Labor Relations

As a basis for HRM responsibilities, major United States employment laws addressing the employer-employee relationship are reviewed in this section. The focus is on federal **equal employment opportunity law**— government efforts to ensure equal access to and fairness in employment without regard to race, religion, age, disability, gender, or other characteristics not related to a job. While state law will not be reviewed here, managers should be aware that most states have laws in one or more of the areas noted. It is important for supervisory and middle-level managers to have a basic understanding of employment law for these major reasons:

- Compliance is the right thing to do.
- People want to work where they are treated fairly.
- Violations of law can result in significant legal and financial liability for the organization.

Ethical principles are introduced in this section and referenced throughout the chapter as related to HRM. For more on ethics and ethical principles, see chapter 21. Labor law and aspects of labor relations are also addressed in the following sections.

Ethical Principles

Ethics refers to a formal, intentional process used to make clear and consistent decisions involving personal and professional values (Harman 2006). Ethical principles used in this decision-making process complement equal opportunity law, and help guide managers to make fair and respectful decisions while working with employees. Two ethical principles stand out as particularly applicable to human resources management in the healthcare field:

- The principle of **justice** recognizes the importance of treating people fairly, applying rules consistently, and fairly distributing cost and risk.

- Recognizing that employees need a voice in what happens to them in the workplace is consistent with the ethical principle of **autonomy**, or respect for an individual's voluntary choice (Beauchamp and Childress 2013).

The American Health Information Management Association (AHIMA) Code of Ethics obligates HIM professionals to demonstrate actions that reflect ethical principles, including to "respect the inherent dignity and worth of every person" (AHIMA 2011). Showing respect for employees, without favoritism or discrimination, is consistent with the intent of equal opportunity laws, and is essential to ethical human resources management. **Discrimination** refers to treating a person differently based on individual characteristics or group membership; if in violation of a law, it is illegal.

In making fair hiring and supervisory decisions managers should "avoid making employment decisions on the basis of personal attributes, characteristics, or behaviors unless they can be shown to be directly related to job performance" (Filerman et al. 2014, 192).

In each section of the chapter, the reader is encouraged to consider specific ways a manager can uphold the ethical principles of justice and autonomy in effectively carrying out HRM responsibilities.

Fair Labor Standards Act of 1938

Amended several times since its passage and continuing to evolve, the **Fair Labor Standards Act (FLSA)** of 1938 sets the minimum wage, requirements for overtime pay, and child labor standards; it is administered and enforced by the Wage and Hour Division of the US Department of Labor (DOL) and applies to most work settings (DOL 2014). The Patient Protection and Affordable Care Act amended the FLSA in 2010 to provide required break time for nursing mothers holding nonexempt positions (DOL 2008).

Nonexempt employees are covered by FLSA minimum wage and overtime provisions. Employees classified as **exempt employees** based on job title, duties, and salary level are not covered by these provisions, for example, professional and managerial personnel who are expected to work as needed to keep operations running. Top executive positions are clearly exempt, clerical hourly-paid jobs are nonexempt. Administrative, professional, and technical positions should be carefully analyzed to determine if overtime pay rules apply; check updated definitions published by the Department of Labor.

Equal Pay Act of 1963

According to the Equal Employment Opportunity Commission (EEOC), the federal **Equal Pay Act** requires that men and women in the same workplace receive equal pay for performing equivalent work. Comparison of job content, rather than job title, is used to determine whether one job is substantially equivalent to another (EEOC 2015a). An amendment to the FLSA, the Equal Pay Act covers essentially all employers and all forms of pay including salary, overtime, bonuses, vacation and holiday pay, reimbursement for business travel expenses, and benefits (EEOC 2015a).

Title VII of the Civil Rights Act of 1964

Title VII of the Civil Rights Act of 1964 and its amendments represent perhaps the most important and sweeping of the federal antidiscrimination laws. Commonly referred to simply as Title VII, this act applies to employers with 15 or more

Figure 20.1 Title VII of the Civil Rights Act of 1964: unlawful employment

From the text of Title VII of the Civil Rights Act of 1964 (Pub. L. 88-352) (Title VII)
Unlawful employment practices SEC. 2000e-2. *[Section 703]*

(a) Employer practices

It shall be an unlawful employment practice for an employer—

(1) to fail or refuse to hire or to discharge any individual, or otherwise to discriminate against any individual with respect to his compensation, terms, conditions, or privileges of employment, because of such individual's race, color, religion, sex, or national origin; or

(2) to limit, segregate, or classify his employees or applicants for employment in any way which would deprive or tend to deprive any individual of employment opportunities or otherwise adversely affect his status as an employee, because of such individual's race, color, religion, sex, or national origin.

Source: EEOC 2015b.

employees and prohibits employment decisions, including those involving hiring and compensation (pay and benefits) based on an individual's race, color, religion, sex, or national origin (Gomez-Mejia et al. 2012). Key provisions of this law are noted in figure 20.1.

Title VII established the EEOC as the federal agency to administer and enforce equal opportunity employment laws; under an amendment (the Equal Opportunity Act of 1972), this includes not only complaint investigation, but the power to file discrimination charges in court.

Definitions important to human resources management that have developed from court cases based on Title VII include the following.

- **Protected class**: Identified groups, such as racial minorities and women, that are protected by law based on past employment discrimination

- **Disparate treatment**: Employment discrimination based on intentional unequal treatment of an individual who is a member of a protected class

- **Disparate (adverse) impact**: Unequal effect of a discriminatory employment practice on a protected class, even if unintentional (Gomez-Mejia et al. 2012)

Hiring managers and supervisors should be aware that employment discrimination based on a characteristic associated with a racial or ethnic group—such as hair feature, manner of dress, or cultural practice—is illegal unless the characteristic can be shown to directly interfere with job performance (EEOC 2015c). Amendments to Title VII that address issues surrounding harassment and pregnancy discrimination in the workplace are described in the sections that follow.

Harassment

Harassment, including sexual harassment, is covered as a form of illegal discrimination under Title VII. **Harassment** involves unwelcome workplace conduct based on an individual's race, color, religion, sex or gender, national origin, age, disability, or genetic information (EEOC 2015d). To be considered illegal, enduring the offensive conduct becomes a condition of the individual's continued employment, or is severe enough to create a hostile work environment (EEOC 2015d). A **hostile work environment** is a setting in which intimidating and abusive conduct takes place that interferes with an employee's job performance; the unwanted conduct goes beyond a minor or occasional annoyance.

A type of harassment based on sex is known as **sexual harassment**; this may include verbal comments, unwanted physical contact, sexual advances, or requests for sexual favors (EEOC 2015d). Sexual harassment complaints can arise based on a hostile work environment where repeated and unwelcome sexually-oriented conduct occurs, or may be based on direct *quid pro quo* advances where sexual favors are requested in exchange for a job benefit or continued employment (McWay 2016). Sexual harassment can apply to workers regardless of gender and can be perpetrated by supervisors, other workers, or even nonemployees. In a 2003 example, a hospital settled a case brought by a group of women alleging they were sexually harassed by a physician during employment-related medical examinations. The hospital had received complaints but had failed to take action (McNair et al. 2007).

Management strategies to address workplace harassment are best focused on prevention, featuring clear policies, open communication, and anti-harassment training. It is important to inform employees of the organization's complaint procedure, take all complaints seriously, and document prompt follow-up action on complaints.

Pregnancy Discrimination Act of 1978

Title VII was amended with the **Pregnancy Discrimination Act of 1978** to protect women from sex discrimination based on pregnancy, and conditions related to pregnancy or childbirth (EEOC 2015e). It further specifies that women should be treated the same as other employees with respect to eligibility for health plan benefits and with regard to their ability to work.

Supervisors and managers with responsibility for staff scheduling, hiring, and performance appraisal (addressed later in the chapter) should be familiar with the major provisions of this legislation, and with other antidiscrimination laws.

Age Discrimination in Employment Act of 1967

The federal **Age Discrimination in Employment Act of 1967** prohibits age discrimination against job applicants or workers, protecting those age 40 and older, and making hiring, compensation, and other employment decisions based on age illegal (EEOC 2015f). Age presents an area of legal risk for managers and supervisors particularly in the candidate selection process and when a staff layoff is necessary. To avoid violation of this law, hiring and continued employment decisions should focus on job requirements and performance standards. On the positive side, hiring and retaining older workers can add experience and help maintain stability within an organization's workforce.

While this law essentially ended the practice of mandatory retirement, in narrowly-interpreted situations employers may still be able to defend this practice if age is shown to be a **bona fide occupational qualification (BFOQ)**. With a BFOQ, a factor (age in this case) has been shown to be related directly to job performance based on documented job analysis. A well-known example is the age requirement for retirement of airline pilots based on safety.

Occupational Safety and Health Act of 1970

The **Occupational Safety and Health Act 1970**, as amended 2004, states as its purpose:

> To assure safe and healthful working conditions for working men and women; by authorizing enforcement of the standards developed under the Act; by assisting and encouraging the States in their efforts to assure safe and healthful working conditions; by providing for research, information, education, and training in the field of occupational safety and health. (OSHA 2004)

This legislation created the Occupational Safety and Health Administration (OSHA) agency within the Department of Labor to administer and enforce the law and provide education on workplace safety. Employers are expected to provide a physically safe work environment and to report all job-related illnesses, injuries, and fatalities. Supervisors and managers should be mindful of potential workplace safety hazards, knowledgeable of OSHA injury and illness reporting requirements, and work with the organization's human resources department and safety officer to ensure that employees receive required safety orientation and training.

While HIM managers are not expected to be benefits experts, background knowledge of the laws described in the following sections can be helpful in understanding the legal basis of benefit plans and in supporting employees who may leave the organization for a variety of reasons.

Employee Retirement Income Security Act of 1974

Title I of the **Employee Retirement Income Security Act (ERISA)** covers most private employers; the intent is to set standards to protect employee benefit and retirement plans. The Department of Labor's Employee Benefits Security Administration (EBSA), working with the Internal Revenue Service (IRS), has regulatory authority to enforce the ERISA to ensure plans are established and administered in a financially sound manner (SHRM 2008).

The **Consolidated Omnibus Budget Reconciliation Act (COBRA)** applies to employers with 20 or more employees and gives workers who lose their health benefits, due to voluntary or involuntary job loss, the right to choose temporary continuation of group health benefits (DOL 2013). COBRA was enacted as part of Title I of ERISA. Provisions for continuation of health coverage were improved to address pre-existing conditions when the Health Insurance Portability and Accountability Act of 1996 (HIPAA) amended ERISA (SHRM 2008). The next section will further explore areas of concern with respect to discrimination in the workplace.

Americans with Disabilities Act of 1990

The **Americans with Disabilities Act (ADA)** prohibits discrimination against people with disabilities in employment. The ADA applies to employers with 15 or more workers and is enforced primarily by the EEOC (DOL 2015a).

The ADA applies to qualified job applicants and to current employees; its scope continues to evolve as courts rule on complaints. A complaint would involve a disabled individual's allegation that an employer failed to provide a reasonable **accommodation**, or adjustment, and that this failure interfered with the qualified individual's being hired for a job or with her ability to perform in the workplace. In order to comply with this law and demonstrate fair employment practices, managers should have an appreciation of the key terms and concepts explained in figure 20.2, and work closely with the organization's human resources department.

Civil Rights Act of 1991

The **Civil Rights Act of 1991 (CRA)** amended Title VII of the Civil Rights Act of 1964 and the Americans with Disabilities Act. CRA made it easier for the plaintiff (complaining party, such as a former employee or job applicant in a protected class) to sue for damages claiming disparate impact or disparate treatment. Driving its passage were several US Supreme Court decisions in the 1980s interpreted as limiting the impact of earlier

Figure 20.2   Americans with Disabilities Act of 1990: key terms for compliance

Disability: This refers to a physical or mental impairment that substantially limits one or more major life activities, such as the ability to see, hear, stand, walk, or learn.

Essential job functions: These are duties required to be performed by every person in a job in order to meet job performance standards. During an interview, an employer can legally ask a disabled (or any) job applicant about their ability to perform essential job functions. Thorough job analysis and a clearly-written job description define the essential functions of a job. An example of an essential function for a coder: Accurately assign diagnostic codes using International Classification of Diseases, Tenth Revision, Clinical Modification (ICD-10-CM).

Reasonable accommodation: This is reasonable action taken by an employer to allow a disabled applicant or employee access to a work opportunity. The disabled person is typically expected to request the accommodation. Examples of accommodations might include altering their work schedule, modifying office equipment or software. A coder with a vision impairment, for example, may need additional workspace lighting and a larger computer monitor installed with adjustments to screen contrast and magnification.

Undue hardship: An accommodation that would result in a significant expense, cause extreme difficulty, or have negative impact on an organization may be an undue hardship. Cost to the employer is a major consideration in defining what is reasonable. Each situation is evaluated by the employer, the EEOC and by the courts when there is a legal challenge, based on the circumstances.

Adapted from Gomez-Mejia et al. 2012 and McWay 2016

antidiscrimination laws. The CRA made this clear: It is the employer's responsibility to prove that hiring and workplace discrimination did not occur.

Family and Medical Leave Act of 1993

The **Family and Medical Leave Act (FMLA)** of 1993 covers all public agencies, as well as private employers with 50 or more employees working 20 or more workweeks in a calendar year. It is administered and enforced by the Department of Labor's Wage and Hour Division (except for federal employers it is enforced under US Office of Personnel Management or Congress jurisdiction) (SHRM 2013). Provisions of the law include the following.

- Eligible employees who have worked at least 12 months are entitled to take unpaid, job-protected leave of up to 12 work weeks with continuation of benefits for specified family and medical reasons
- Reasons include birth or adoption of a child, care of a seriously ill family member or the employee's own serious health condition, or for an emergent issue related to a family member's active military status
- Employees are required to comply with an employer's existing policies regarding request for leave, including advance notice or for use of accrued sick leave and vacation time (DOL 2012)

Managers should be familiar with this law, with related organizational policies and requirements for communicating rights and responsibilities to staff, such as in employee handbooks.

Genetic Nondiscrimination Act of 2008

The ability to conduct genetic tests and generate sensitive genetic information resulted from the Human Genome Project. This major public research project identified and mapped a complete set of DNA, the chemical compound with genetic code that provides building blocks for the human body (NIH 2013). Concerns that highly personal information, such as the potential to develop a particular disease, could be used by insurers to deny health coverage, or by employers to screen out candidates for hire, rule out an employee for promotion, or terminate employment led to passage of the **Genetic Nondiscrimination Act (GINA)** of 2008. Genetic discrimination by health insurers and employers is prohibited.

- Title I of GINA provides "that health plans may not use genetic information to make eligibility, coverage, underwriting, or premium-setting decisions," or impose "pre-existing condition exclusions on the basis of genetic information" (Brodnik and Sharp 2012, 345).
- Title II of GINA is administered by the EEOC; it prohibits use of genetic information in employment decisions and restricts disclosure by employers, employment agencies, and labor organizations of genetic information about applicants, employees, or members (Brodnik and Sharp 2012).

Some states also have laws regarding use of genetic information in employment and health insurance, with which managers should be aware.

 Check Your Understanding 20.1

Instructions: **Answer the following questions.**

1. Which of the following refers to the people asset of an organization, the sum of the knowledge, skills, and abilities of its workforce?
   A. Labor
   B. Management
   C. Human capital
   D. Employees

2. The ethical principle of _____ recognizes the importance of treating people fairly and applying rules consistently.
   A. Autonomy
   B. Justice
   C. Respect
   D. Morality

3. Which of the following laws established the EEOC as the federal agency to administer and enforce equal opportunity employment laws?
   A. Equal Pay Act of 1963
   B. Title VII of the Civil Rights Act of 1964
   C. Age Discrimination Act of 1967
   D. Civil Rights Act of 1991

4. In defining illegal harassment in the workplace, a setting in which intimidating and abusive conduct takes place that interferes with an employee's job performance is known as:
   A. Discrimination
   B. Sexual harassment
   C. Hostile work environment
   D. Unsafe work environment

5. Title VII of the Civil Rights Act of 1964 prohibits discrimination in employment based on an individual's membership in which of the following?
   A. Disparate group
   B. Professional association
   C. Union
   D. Protected class

6. Which of the following statements is true of the federal Age Discrimination in Employment Act of 1967?
   A. The act prohibits employment discrimination against individuals with disabilities.
   B. The intent is to set standards to protect benefit and retirement plans of older workers.
   C. Discrimination against workers age 40 and older is illegal.
   D. The practice of mandatory retirement based on age can never be defended.

7. The HIM department's receptionist is paid an hourly rate and is eligible for overtime pay, consistent with the Fair Labor Standards Act of 1938. According to this law, her position is classified as which of the following?
   A. Exempt
   B. Nonexempt
   C. Full-time
   D. Professional

8. An employer should offer reasonable accommodation, such as by modifying office equipment, to an applicant or employee based on impairment is a provision of the:
   A. Genetic Nondiscrimination Act of 2008
   B. Occupational Safety and Health Act of 1970
   C. Civil Rights Act of 1991
   D. Americans with Disabilities Act of 1990

Labor Relations

While unions are not present in all work settings, it is worthwhile to examine what a union is and to consider some of the major laws and principles involved in the labor–management relationship. A union is an organization formed by employees for the purpose of acting as a unit when dealing with management regarding work issues (Fried and Fottler 2011). Research from a variety of sources indicates that pay and benefits, along with employee concerns regarding employer fairness, job security, and lack of recognition, are among the factors that drive interest in labor unions. When employees feel strongly that they need to work as a group when meeting with management about a workplace issue, believing they will benefit from strength in numbers, someone in the employee group may contact a labor union for assistance (Carrell and Heavrin 2013).

The right of workers to unionize is recognized from an ethical perspective as a human right consistent with the principle autonomy. "Everyone has the right to form and to join trade unions for the protection of his interests" (United Nations 1948, 6). In the United States, workers' right to unionize and to bargain collectively with management is protected by law. Union membership in the United States was just above 11 percent of the total workforce in 2014, down from 20 percent in 1983; however, union membership is higher in the public sector and the rate varies across states (BLS 2015). In 2007, the Service Employees International Union (SEIU) formed SEIU Healthcare to target workers in hospitals, long-term care, clinics, and other health organizations (Fried and Fottler 2011). A brief overview of the union-organizing process, major labor laws, and key concepts for supervisors in union settings are presented in this section.

Union Organization

In the initial phase of union development within a workplace, labor union officials attempt to gauge the level of employee interest in joining a union. Union representatives provide employees information (outside of scheduled work hours) about unionization and solicit signing of **authorization cards**. An authorization card is a document that indicates an employee's interest in having a union represent him or her. The next step is then for the union to petition the **National Labor Relations Board (NLRB)** for an election to become the employees' representative. The NLRB verifies the signed authorization cards and recognizes a group of employees within the organization to be the **bargaining unit**, those who will be represented by the union. By law, supervisors and managers are excluded from

the employee bargaining unit. Major labor laws are addressed in the next section of this chapter.

Once the bargaining unit is certified, an election is scheduled to decide whether the union will represent the employee group (the bargaining unit). Prior to the vote, a campaign period ensues where both management and the union can make appeals to employees, consistent with law. A simple majority of votes cast by workers in the bargaining unit is required to win the election. If the union does win the right to represent employees, **collective bargaining** begins. The NLRB describes collective bargaining as a mutual obligation of the employer and union "to meet at reasonable times to bargain in good faith about wages, hours, vacation time, insurance, safety practices and other mandatory subjects" and negotiate agreement (NLRB 2015a). Labor law defines the types of items that must be included in collective bargaining (for example, wages) vs. those that are voluntary. The concept of good-faith bargaining assumes that both sides are participating and willing to negotiate an agreement. Ultimately, if there is failure to agree after repeated attempts, unionized employees may initiate a **strike**, a temporary work stoppage called in an effort to express an employment contract negotiation demand. A strike obviously represents a low point in labor–management relations; while distressing for all parties, including patients served, the prospect of a strike should be considered in a unionized healthcare organization. Managers should work with the human resources department to understand the rules for communication with employees and plan for worker replacement in case a strike scenario develops.

Major Labor Laws

In 1935, Congress passed the Wagner Act, known as the **National Labor Relations Act (NLRA)**, prohibiting employers from interfering with employees' rights to form labor unions and bargain collectively, outlining labor organization obligations, and forming the NLRB as the federal agency to enforce the law (NLRB 2015a). Major provisions of this important act include that it is unlawful for employers to:

- Threaten employees with loss of jobs based on union vote or activity

- Question employees about their union views
- Promise special benefits to employees to discourage union support
- Punish employees for engaging in legal union activity, as by firing or by transferring to a more difficult job (NLRB 2015a)

Labor organizations are prohibited under the NLRA from such things as using threatening or coercive tactics in an effort to gain employees' support for the union or striking over issues not related to employment terms or conditions (NLRB 2015a).

The NLRA differentiates employees from supervisors, excluding managerial and supervisory staff from protections of the act and from participation in a bargaining unit. A supervisor is defined in the NLRA as one who has authority and uses independent judgment "in the interest of the employer, to hire, transfer, suspend, lay off, recall, promote, discharge, assign, reward, or discipline other employees, or responsibly to direct them, or to adjust their grievances, or effectively to recommend such action" (NLRA 1935, 152–11).

The definition of who is a supervisor or manager in a healthcare organization, and therefore who can or cannot be a member of a union collective bargaining unit, has also been addressed by the courts as case law. Summarized as follows, the ruling in a landmark case provides an example where nurses were considered managers, not part of the bargaining unit.

> The facility had classified six nurses as supervisors, excluding them from the union bargaining unit. The NLRB disagreed, indicating that the nurses' exercise of professional judgment did not place them in a supervisory role; the employer was cited for unfair labor practice. The US Supreme Court disagreed with the NLRB's definition, saying it contradicted the wording of the NLRA statute describing use of independent judgment by supervisors; the nurses could in fact be classified as managers. (*NLRB v. Kentucky River Community Care, Inc.* 2001, 1)

The **Taft-Hartley Act** amended the NLRA, focusing on rights of employers by:

- Allowing the US president to issue a temporary ban on strikes that might impact national health and safety

- Prohibiting unfair labor practices by unions
- Giving states permission to enact right-to-work laws
- Giving employers specific freedom to express their views regarding unionization (Dessler 2014)

The 1974 Healthcare Amendments to the Taft-Hartley Act clarified that employees of private, not-for-profit hospitals are covered under federal labor law and that a special provision applicable to healthcare unions requires 10-day advance notice of strike (Fried and Fottler 2011). Since the Taft-Hartley amendment, **right-to-work laws** have been enacted in approximately half of the states. These laws prohibit forced union membership as a condition of employment.

Supervising Employees in a Union Environment

Many organizations, including healthcare, see labor unions as interference with management. Top management may take an opposing view during a union-organizing effort, actively presenting its "side" to employees using a variety of communication methods. Once a union officially represents employees, the collective bargaining process may become contentious.

Demonstrating respect for employees' right to join unions, along with knowledge of the laws in place, provides a foundation for front-line managers to best work with their employees in a union environment. Managers and supervisors facing union-organizing campaigns are advised to be truthful in providing information to employees and to avoid interfering with legal unionizing activity. Managers should be aware of and consistently enforce employer policies regarding solicitation and distribution of union (or other) literature during paid work hours. As offered by the National Labor Relations Board in explaining employee rights:

> Working time is for work, so your employer may maintain and enforce nondiscriminatory rules limiting solicitation and distribution, except that your employer cannot prohibit you from talking about or soliciting for a union during non-work time, such as before or after work or during break times (NLRB 2015b).

Table 20.1 Useful acronyms for supervisors during a union-organizing drive

Term	Example
Threaten	Do not threaten loss of job, reduced hours, or discipline because of employees' union election or other union activity. Intimidating behavior risks long-term damage to the employer–employee relationship.
Interrogate	Do not ask an employee, "How are you going to vote?" Or, "Have you signed a union authorization card?" Do not schedule mandatory one-on-one meetings with employees to discuss union representation.
Promise	Do not promise a pay increase, promotion, or favor in exchange for a union vote.
Spy	Do not go to union meetings or try to listen in on conversations about the union during employee breaks.
Facts	Do state facts, such as that signing an authorization card makes the union an employee's legal representative. Review current human resource policies related to solicitation. Do this in a way that is informative, avoids distortion, and is not intimidating.
Opinion	When asked your opinion by an individual employee or in a staff meeting, do voice your professional opinion on the value of a union, without telling the employee(s) what to do. Be honest.
Rules	Do accurately review what the law permits, such as regarding worker replacement in the event of a strike. Again, be informative as opposed to threatening. Consistently enforce rules on solicitation and distribution of any non-work related information during work hours, not just during a union drive.
Experience	Do share your personal experience, positive or negative, in working with or as a member of a labor union. Be honest and factual.

Source: Adapted from Carrell and Heavrin 2013, 1.

Being nondiscriminatory as a supervisor would mean, for example, allowing employees to talk about the union during work time if they are ordinarily allowed to talk about other personal, non-work topics during work hours. Sets of easy-to-recall acronyms have been developed to help managers remember what to do and not do, consistent with respect for employees' ethical right to unionize and labor law compliance. To remember things a manager may not do, or can do, in a union environment, recall the acronyms TIPS and FORE, explained with examples in table 20.1.

 ## Check Your Understanding 20.2

Instructions: **Answer the following questions.**

1. The _____ Act formed the National Labor Relations Board (NLRB) as the federal agency to enforce labor law.
   A. National Labor Relations
   B. Taft-Hartley
   C. Equal Opportunity Employment
   D. Fair Labor Standards

2. Respecting employees' free choice to join a labor union, and upholding labor laws, it is appropriate for a manager to do which of the following during a union-organizing drive?
   A. Threaten reduced hours or loss of job based on employee's union vote.
   B. Interrogate employees regarding union activity.
   C. Promise a party, pay raise, or other favor based on union vote.
   D. State facts, such as the organization's policy on solicitation.

3. True or false: By law, supervisors are included in the employee union bargaining unit.

4. True or false: Right-to-work laws prohibit forced union membership as a condition of employment.

5. True or false: An employee signs an authorization card to indicate interest in having a union represent him.

Human Resources Management Roles and Responsibilities

HRM is critical as healthcare organizations seek to improve financial and quality performance, operating in a competitive environment. Effective management of personnel can have a huge impact on an organization's success. But, what specifically is involved in HRM, and why are these functions so important?

Unless very small, most healthcare organizations have a human resources department with a manager. What, then, is the relationship between the human resources department and a line manager in a healthcare organization with assigned HRM responsibilities? Managers who have **line authority** in an organization are those who supervise one or more employees, have decision-making authority, can give orders, and are responsible for getting work done by directing the work of others (Dessler 2014). There are many HIM line manager roles across all types and sizes of healthcare organizations; examples of titles include HIM director, release of information manager, and coding supervisor. HRM functions performed by these managers can vary, but typically include direct, day-to-day involvement in one or all of the areas addressed in this chapter—from staff selection to performance management to training.

The human resources department serves line managers in an advisory role, supporting performance of HRM functions. In a large hospital, for example, the human resources department might include employees who specialize in recruiting, compensation, training, or another area; these staff assist both individual employees and line managers. The human resources department is responsible for organization-wide functions such as human resource strategic planning, payroll, and benefits administration, and for ensuring compliance with personnel policies and procedures consistent with the organization's mission. In a smaller healthcare business, a single human resource manager may handle a variety of human resource responsibilities. In some settings, certain human resources department functions, such as employee recruiting and training, have been outsourced or automated as the result of restructuring, with line managers taking on more HRM tasks; this trend is expected to continue given pressure to reduce healthcare costs (Fried and Fottler 2011).

A cooperative relationship among the organization's human resources manager, department, and line managers is essential for effective overall HRM in an organization. Key functions for which HIM line managers may have HRM roles and responsibilities are explored in the sections that follow.

Staff Recruitment and Selection

As noted previously, growth in the healthcare field and in HIM presents both opportunity and challenge. An effective (and cost-effective) staff recruitment and selection process begins with an understanding of the positions to be filled. In some cases, new position creation or position redesign is necessary as the result of changes in HIM or in the regulatory environment. For example, clerks that used to assemble paper records now prepare and scan documents into an electronic health record and perform quality control. A thorough understanding of the qualifications for a position is essential to support the selection process. Then the objective is to find the best person for the job using effective selection tools. These steps, outlined in table 20.2 may seem straightforward, but knowledge, skill, and preparation are required in order for the process to be effective. This section of the chapter will present additional detail on the HRM functions listed in table 20.2, including job analysis, job description, job specifications, employee recruiting, and testing.

Job Analysis

Job analysis is collecting and analyzing information about a job in order to better understand the significant component duties of the job, and

Table 20.2 Overview: staff recruitment and selection process

Opportunity or challenge	HRM functions
Understand position to fill	Conduct, review, and revise job analysis Prepare, review, and revise job description
Know job requirements such as skills and education required	Prepare, review, and revise job specifications
Develop a pool of qualified candidates	Attract and recruit candidates, both internally and externally
Select the right candidate	Check, test, interview, select, and hire the best candidate
Comply with legal and regulatory requirements	Stay informed on applicable laws and consult human resources department as needed

to identify the skills and characteristics required of an employee who can successfully perform the job. Job analysis supports not only employee recruitment and selection, but other HRM functions addressed later in the chapter such as performance appraisal, staffing, and training.

Steps in conducting a job analysis are as follows:

1. *Clarify the purpose of the analysis.* Identify the job to be analyzed. If the current job is being redesigned or the unit or department is undergoing restructure, consider that more than one job may be involved. Comparison of a sample of jobs by type may be appropriate in order to identify similarities and relationships among jobs and determine which jobs to analyze. A **workflow analysis** may be needed prior to the job analysis, if this has not already been conducted. Workflow analysis is a detailed step-by-step assessment of how work moves from one task to the next and from one employee to the next within a work process. A chart or workflow diagram is typically used to show the beginning-to-end process. An example of a workflow diagram can be found in chapter 18.

2. *Collect information about the job.* Sources of information for an existing job include documents such as organization charts, job descriptions, and job procedures. An interview with an employee in the position who knows the job, as appropriate, can be a valuable method for gathering details. The manager conducting the analysis should develop a list of specific interview questions, such as what are your primary job duties? Where do you work (physical location)? What equipment do you use? What education, skill, or certification is required to perform your job? How is your work evaluated? Other data collection methods include observing the job being performed, conducting a survey, having an employee keep a log of job activity for a period of time, or consulting a relevant website. A reliable source of information for job analysis is in the US Department of Labor's O*NET online (DOL 2015b)

   o Use of a variety of data sources and collection methods is recommended; see examples of sources of data and methods of data collection in figure 20.3.

3. *Identify the job's primary duties or tasks and the competencies required to perform them.* Based on data collected, what essential work is done? Are some duties or tasks more important than others? If so, indicate priority among job duties such as by showing rank order, a scaled value, or amount of time spent on each duty. What is required to competently perform these primary job components? **Competencies** are "do" statements identifying measurable skills, abilities, behaviors, or other characteristics required of an individual in order to successfully do the work (Office of Personnel Management 2015). HIM example for a release of information specialist might read like this: Apply policies and procedures for disclosure of health information to process requests with 98 percent accuracy.

Figure 20.3 Sources of data and methods of data collection for job analysis

Sources of data
- Organizational chart (discussed in chapter 19)
- Job description
- Job procedures
- Workflow analysis (discussed in chapter 19)
- Employee
- Supervisor

Methods of data collection
- Interviews (employee, supervisor)
- Direct observation of work (best for jobs involving physical tasks)

- Survey questionnaire (to employee, delivered in person or online)
- Diary or log (by employee)
- External sources:
  - Online databases for job analysis
  - Professional association websites (research and practice briefs, sample job descriptions, sample survey, and interview questions for job analysis)
  - Proprietary websites (sample descriptions and set-up wizards)

Adapted from: Fried and Fottler 2011.

Upon completion of the job analysis, information is then available on which to base (revise or redesign) a job description and specifications for the job, critical to the staff recruitment and selection process. In addition to support for staff recruitment and selection, information in a job analysis provides a basis for performance appraisal, discipline, training, and staffing functions discussed later the chapter.

Job Description and Specifications

A **job description**, sometimes called a position description, is a written explanation of a job and the duties it entails and is based on information provided by the job analysis. A job description helps the human resources department, hiring manager, the employee's direct supervisor and the employee understand the job duties and expectations. While formats may vary across organizations, most job descriptions contain section headings similar to these:

- Job title or identification
- Job summary
- Reporting relationships (reports to, supervises as applicable)
- Duties (or responsibilities)
- Working conditions

The most useful job descriptions are very clear and concise. The relationships section can include not only internal reporting and supervisory relations, but significant contacts outside of the unit (for example, medical staff committee chairs, vendors). Clarity as to which job duties are more or less essential can be indicated in various ways on a job description, such as by showing percentage of time typically spent on a duty or by ranking responsibilities in order of importance. Standards of performance are valuable to include and indicate a volume and quality expectation (for example, code an average of X inpatient records per week with Y or fewer errors). Statements on working conditions address health or safety issues.

In the rapidly changing field of HIM, job descriptions should be updated often and always when a new procedure or technology is introduced. The annual (or more frequent) performance appraisal provides an opportunity for job description review and update.

Some job description formats include a section on job specifications or may be provided as a separate document. **Job specifications** describe the individual qualifications required to perform the job outlined in the job description. If included as part of the job description document, the section may be titled something such as "required knowledge, skills, and experience." Based on job analysis, specifications list the education level, experience, skills, personal characteristics, physical strength requirements, licensure, or credential needed to do the job (for example, associate's degree required, RHIT [registered health information technician] preferred).

Specifications must be job related. If a skill, attribute, or education level is required in order to do the job, it must be justified by job analysis data. This is necessary to support fair hiring decisions, consistent with the principle of justice and equal employment opportunity law as discussed earlier in the chapter. An HIM example of job specifications: For a clinical documentation improvement specialist position, a healthcare organization could justify an associate's degree as the required minimum education level based on job analysis. A bachelor's degree and the clinical documentation improvement professional (CDIP) credential could be listed as preferred or desired specifications (AHIMA 2013a).

Figure 20.4 provides an example of a job description with job specifications included.

Figure 20.4 Release of information specialist job description

Release of information specialist job description

Job title: Release of information (ROI) specialist
Department: Medical Records/Health Information Management
Department supervisor's title: Release of information manager

General summary
Purpose: To provide coverage for release of health information functions, including written and verbal requests for health information. Duties include: managing incoming requests, verification of proper authorization for requests, using master patient index to obtain health record numbers, using chart location system to locate paper charts, using EHR system to locate electronic health information, copying health information, billing for copies of health information when applicable, entering all releases into correspondence tracking system, answering telephone calls related to the ROI function, and numerous other small associated duties.

Decision-making authority: Routine decisions include verification of appropriate authorization, prioritizing requests, problem solving record locations, problem solving in customer service for internal and external departmental personnel.

Supervisory responsibility: No formal supervisory responsibility.

Essential duties:

Duty A	**Processes incoming requests for the ROI area with 98% accuracy.**	**Time % 15%**	**Relative Importance = 5 (1–5 scale)**

Task #1: Opens and date stamps 100% of all requests received each day.
Task #2: Screens each request for release of information requirements and verifies proper authorization.
Task #3: Utilizes facility computer system to obtain health record numbers and dates of service.
Task #4: Enters health record number, name, requestor, requestor type, date received, and other data items into correspondence tracking system.

Duty B	**Identifies locations of and retrieves health records needed to complete ROI request with 98% accuracy.**	**Time % 20%**	**Relative Importance = 5**

Task #1: Locates patient charts, utilizing the chart tracking system.
Task #2: Locates older charts on microfilm using the microfilm system.
Task #3: Locates and obtains records from other departments not housed in the health records or HIM department.

Duty C	**Tracks health records during ROI request processing with 98% accuracy.**	**Time % 5%**	**Relative Importance = 4**

Task #1: Transfers location of chart in the chart location system.
Task #2: Returns all health records to correct location.

Duty D	**Processes authorizations and subpoenas with 98% accuracy.**	**Time % 25%**	**Relative Importance = 5**

Task #1: Determines information requested on authorization.
Task #2: Communicates with requestor regarding possible charges.
Task #3: Photocopies requested information.
Task #4: Calculates invoice and determines whether prepayment is required.
Task #5: Determines disposition and mails out copies (pick-up, mail, overnight).
Task #6: Completes request in correspondence tracking system, entering date processed, documents sent, and such.

Figure 20.4 (Continued)

Duty E	Processes STAT (needed immediately) and walk-in requests same day with 98% accuracy.	Time % 10%	Relative Importance = 4

Task #1: STAT requests are completed according to the need of the patient for patient care purposes.
Task #2: Assist walk-in requestors in filling out authorization for release of confidential medical information form.

Duty F	Processes problem requests.	Time % 5%	Relative Importance = 4

Task #1: Researches request.
Task #2: Returns request with letters stating reason for return.
Task #3: Sends final notices on requests pending more than two months.
Task #4: Cancels unpaid prepayment requests after three to four months.

Duty G	Answers phone calls related to release of information.	Time % 20%	Relative Importance = 4

Task #1: Assists requestors with verbal continuity of care requests.
Task #2: Assists callers concerning status of requests.

Required knowledge and skills (job specifications):

Component	Description
Knowledge	Working knowledge of health records functions to include chart order and assembly, terminal digit order filing, and record flow of department. Required for completely satisfactory performance in this job is knowledge of health record format, computerized registration inquiry process and back-up manual registration system, as well as admissions process. Working knowledge of computerized access systems. Knowledge of policies and procedure surrounding disclosure of protection health information preferred.
Skills	Required for completely satisfactory performance in this job is the ability to communicate effectively, provide good customer service, problem solve routine health record issues, prioritize tasks, be punctual and dependable regarding work tasks, work independently, and pay attention to detail. Must utilize well-organized work habits along with good written and verbal communication skills, utilize electronic messaging, and perform accurate data entry, verification, and updating. Able to learn and apply detailed policies and procedures. Computer skills proficiency.
Formal education and experience	The formal education normally associated with completely satisfactory performance in this job is a high school diploma or the equivalent. A minimum of two years of experience in health record department or equivalent is required. Experience processing release of information requests preferred.

Working conditions: Conditions that differ from the normal work environment include stress when communicating with parents, patients, physicians, attorneys, telephones constantly ringing, meeting deadlines, and frequent distractions.

These statements are intended to describe the essential responsibilities being performed by people assigned to this job. They are not intended to be an exhaustive list of the responsibilities assigned to these people.

APPROVED BY
NAME:
TITLE:

Source: AHIMA 2013b.

Recruitment

With a job clearly described, recruitment for an open position can begin. **Recruitment** is the way an organization attracts a pool of qualified applicants from whom to select. The best way to recruit talent is to build an environment where people want to work; factors supporting this include treating employees with respect, and offering opportunities for growth (AHIMA 2013a).

An HIM manager typically works in cooperation with the human resources department to effectively recruit. Sources of qualified job candidates can be broadly classified as internal and external. Internal sources of candidates include promotion or transfer of employees from within the organization. Internal candidates have the advantage of being individuals who know, and are known by, the healthcare organization. The internal candidate will

Figure 20.5   Internal versus external job candidate: advantages and disadvantages

Internal candidate

Advantages

- Known individual (strengths, weaknesses)
- Morale boost with new opportunity, promotion
- Needs less orientation
- Knows organization and the culture
- Faster, less costly hiring process

Disadvantages

- Strong candidates may not be available or have not been developed
- Morale problem may develop among applicants not selected
- Can lead to stagnation, lack of new ideas
- May need specialized training
- Another vacancy to fill

External candidate

Advantages

- Represents a larger, more diverse pool of applicants
- Brings fresh ideas from outside
- May already have specialized training (saving time and money)
- Not involved in organizational politics

Disadvantages

- Reliance on references for information about candidate
- Working relationships with internal applicants not selected may be strained
- Requires orientation
- Needs time for socialization into organization (may not fit culture)
- More complex, costly hiring process

©AHIMA

need less orientation, though may need additional special training. Promotion from within can be a motivator. On the other hand, the healthcare organization is not bringing in new talent and by hiring from one position to another, may in turn create an open position to fill. A rejected internal applicant may harbor hard feelings that negatively impact individual performance or team morale. A summary of the pros and cons of internal vs. external recruiting is presented in figure 20.5.

Methods to identify qualified candidates include internal job posting, employee referral, the Internet (an organization's homepage, online job boards, social media sites), and print advertising (local newspaper, professional journals). Job fairs and other college recruiting efforts can be valuable to fill entry-level positions, but can be time-consuming to staff. Employment agencies are another option, including those run by government agencies. Use of private agencies involves a fee to the organization, an option typically reserved for top executive or hard-to-recruit technical positions.

Use of online recruiting methods, including targeted use of social media, has become prevalent across many organizations, with advantages and disadvantages. Internet-based recruiting typically generates more responses faster and at a lower cost than other methods. However, many of the applicants may not be qualified, and fewer minority applicants may be captured. Therefore, more than one recruiting method is recommended, with the message offering clear information about the job duties and job specifications.

Selecting Employees

Recruitment, selection, and training of employees is costly to an organization so making the most of this investment of time and dollars is important. Successful recruiting efforts provide a pool of qualified job candidates; selection is then the process of choosing the best individual to hire from among those prospects. This step deserves careful attention for a number of reasons; hiring the right person for a job can positively impact the department in the following ways:

- Productivity
- Teamwork and staff morale
- The organization's competitive edge (Mondy 2015).

Careful selection is also necessary to avoid the negative impact of placing the wrong person in the job. For example, an underqualified or over-qualified individual may perform poorly on the job, or may not fit with the organizational culture, leading to a need for replacement after a short time. Ruling out candidates with a history of prob-lematic behavior can help to avoid disciplinary issues, as well as turnover (employees leaving the organization). Hiring managers must avoid ille-gal discrimination in selection practices, applying the previously noted concept of job-relatedness in the selection process. Courts have held employers liable for **negligent hiring**; this can occur where crimes are committed and employees with prior criminal records were not subjected to thorough pre-employment screening (Dessler 2014, 141). The importance of verifying candidate work his-tory and of conducting reference and background checks cannot be underestimated in a field where employees have access to protected health infor-mation; hiring managers should work closely with human resource managers on this aspect of selection. Additional techniques common to the employee selection process, and critical to its suc-cess, are selection testing and job interviews, dis-cussed as follows.

Testing

When used as one component of the candidate selection process, a well-constructed **selection test** can assess job skills and abilities or identify job-related attitudes that may not surface in an interview. Disadvantages of tests include inabil-ity to measure motivation to work, as well as risk of discrimination. The federal *Uniform Guidelines on Employee Selection Procedures* provide regula-tory standards for the selection process to assist employers in avoiding discriminatory practices; testing is specifically addressed, focusing on the importance of test validity based on job analysis (SHRM 2015b).

To be fair, legal, and effective, selection tests should be designed to meet standards for valid-ity and reliability. **Validity** refers to the ability of a selection test to accurately measure the job skill, knowledge, or behavior it was meant to measure. One common method of test valida-tion is content validity. Tasks or questions are

linked directly to knowledge, skills, and abilities required on the job, as supported by job analysis and job description (Mondy 2015). For example, a selection test for a coder might include perfor-mance on an encoder application exercise or on a pencil-and-paper coding test. Other types of selection tests include cognitive (mental) ability, physical ability, occupational interest, and per-sonality tests. The type of test(s) used should be consistent with the types of skills and abilities required of the job.

Reliability refers to the degree to which a selec-tion test produces consistent scores on test and retest. Using the coding example, if a candidate scored 150 on a coding test, then on a retake of the same test the following day scored 70, test reliabil-ity could be questioned. Other selection testing considerations include consistency of environmen-tal conditions (namely, temperature) under which a test is given, determination of statistical norms (reference points) for test scoring, and cost of test development or purchase. Given the numerous important factors in employee selection testing, hiring managers are advised to work closely with the human resources department in determining testing tools and approaches.

Interviewing

A **job interview** is a conversation in which a hir-ing manager and a job applicant exchange infor-mation. It is goal oriented and designed to support the selection process based on the candidate's oral responses. Job interviews can be classified as structured (specific) or unstructured (open-ended). Interview types, common question types, and major advantages and disadvantages of each are summarized in table 20.3.

Methods of interviewing include the famil-iar one-on-one candidate meeting with an inter-viewer, arranged as a single event or as a sequence of individual interviews, group interviews where several candidates meet with one or more inter-viewers, and a panel where one candidate is inter-viewed by several interviewers at the same time. Phone and video interviews have become com-mon, especially for initial screening interviews. Advantages of phone interviews include time

Table 20.3 Types of job interviews and questions

Interview types	Interview question types	Advantages and disadvantages
Unstructured: Interviewer asks questions that come to mind	Open-ended, probing (for example, What is your greatest professional strength, and how have you used it to advance your career?)	• Flexible; may uncover information missed in structured interview • Not standardized; different information obtained across job candidates cannot be rated or scored • Candidate encouraged to talk, may volunteer information not related to job • Potentially discriminatory • Time consuming
Structured: Each candidate for a job is asked the same questions planned in advance	*Situational*: Ask how candidate would handle a given scenario (for example, How would you handle an employee who is chronically late? What would you do if a physician becomes angry when you query her about documentation in a record?) *Behavioral*: Ask candidate to relate behavior from the past to a job situation (for example, Describe a situation where you had to deal with a subordinate's chronic tardiness, and explain how you handled it.) *Knowledge*: Straightforward job knowledge or experience questions (for example, What type of encoder software have you used?)	• Standardized • Answers can be rated or scored • Questions are job related, based on job analysis • More objective and consistent than unstructured interview • Legally defensible • Time efficient

saving and greater focus on content. Lack of visual or body language cues and emphasis on voice can be disadvantages for which interviewees need to prepare (Sutton 2013). Mock interviews help to increase interviewees' comfort level and effectiveness, especially if these practice sessions are videotaped for review.

Used for nearly all positions, interviews unfortunately have not always proven to be a reliable predictor of candidate success. Factors contributing to this include hiring managers' reliance on generic "tell me about yourself" questions (HR Specialist 2011). Ways hiring managers can improve effectiveness of job interviews include:

- using structured interviews, asking all interviewees the same questions;
- using job-related situational or behavioral questions based on job description; and by
- participating in interviewer training (or by providing training for hiring managers).

Combined with other techniques, such as selection testing, interviewing can be useful in evaluating job candidates. However, planning and preparation are required to support an effective interviewing process.

Performance Management

Performance management is an ongoing, goal-oriented process focused on productivity and continuous improvement of employees and teams. Performance appraisal, presented in this section of the chapter, is a key component of performance management. But performance management is not a single, scheduled review; it is a process continually fed by and related to other important HRM functions. For example, job analysis, previously discussed, provides information and standards needed for the appraisal of job performance. Information from performance appraisal can in turn help management assess the effectiveness of recruitment and selection activities (Fried and Fottler 2011). Both job analysis and performance appraisal help to identify employee training needs. Performance management provides the big picture context for the relationships among these important HRM functions. For a visual representation of HRM functions within the performance management process, see figure 20.6.

Figure 20.6 Relationship of HRM functions within performance management

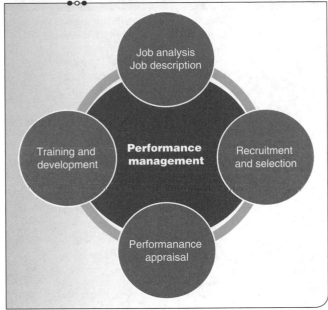

Source: Adapted from Fried and Fottler 2011.

The next section provides further detail on the performance appraisal component of performance management.

Performance Appraisal

Performance appraisal refers to the formal system of review and evaluation methods used to assess employee and team performance (Mondy 2015). Performance appraisal serves critical data collection and communication roles in performance management. Organizations need legally defensible performance data to support decisions such as employee pay rate, promotion, or dismissal; to develop training and career development plans; and to help forecast recruitment needs. Most employees want to know where they stand and can handle constructive feedback. In a recent survey, 92 percent of those surveyed responded positively to the statement, "Negative feedback, if delivered appropriately, is effective at improving performance" (Folkman 2014).

Planning and implementation of an effective and fair appraisal system involves attention to the following factors:

- Use of job-related criteria for employee assessment, supported by job analysis; criteria should be objective and measurable,

such those based on behaviors, knowledge, skills, and achievement of goals

- Clear performance expectations, agreed on in advance on between manager and subordinate

- Standardization of methods, instruments, and time periods (at least annual) for data collection with formal documentation for legal protection

- Training of appraisers in areas such as how to provide unbiased ratings and how to give effective feedback

- A formal appraisal interview with time for each individual employee to review results

- Continuous communication and feedback before and after the appraisal interview to support performance improvement and avoid surprises

- A formal grievance (complaint) procedure available to support due process should the need for appeal of appraisal results arise (Mondy 2015)

An employee's immediate supervisor is traditionally the primary evaluator (appraiser) of performance. The supervisor has authority over and is ultimately responsible for performance of a unit, and typically is in a good position to observe an individual employee's performance. Additional sources of performance data include subordinates, peers or team members, multiple raters, and self-appraisal. Gathering performance data from additional sources allows the supervisor to take into account input from others in close contact with the employee, and helps the supervisor to avoid bias, also referred to as favoritism, partiality, or prejudice. The supervisor typically remains involved, even when additional sources are included. Pros and cons of sources of responsibility for performance appraisal data are outlined in table 20.4.

Performance Appraisal Methods

Methods used in performance appraisal must meet criteria for validity and reliability, as described previously for selection testing. Management decisions on pay, promotion, or dismissal based on a

Table 20.4 Responsibility for performance appraisal: pros and cons of performance data sources

Appraiser	Pros	Cons
Immediate supervisor	• Often in best position to know and observe employee's work • Typically responsible for unit performance to which employee is a contributor • Appraisal data supports unit's employee training and development plan	• May not be familiar with all aspects of employee's job or projects (may lack technical expertise; employee may work in a different geographic location or with multiple units in the organization) • Potential for bias (positive or negative) if supervisor is the only appraiser
Subordinates	• Offers insight into manager's strengths and weaknesses • Feedback can be useful for manager development	• May be perceived as "popularity" rating of limited value • If not anonymous (difficult to achieve in small unit or organization), subordinates may fear reprisal and not offer honest input
Peers or team members	• Provides close-up view of employee performance • Multiple opinions reduce bias • Peer pressure of evaluation can motivate team members to be more productive	• Reluctance to criticize teammates or peers • Evaluator may focus on one specific problem or conflict that occurred and provide an unbalanced overall assessment
Multiple sources (also called multi-rater, 360-degree rating)	• Bias is reduced by including multiple perspectives from inside and outside the organization (that is, managers, subordinates, peers, customers; may also include self-appraisal) • Development-focused; less useful for promotion, compensation • Emphasizes team and customer relationships	• If not anonymous (difficult to achieve in small unit or organization), raters may not offer honest input • Can be expensive to include multiple parties; use of an online rating system recommended • Appraiser and employee training on purpose, procedures of the process essential
Self	• Encourages employee involvement in appraisal process • Employees in ideal position to evaluate their own performance, and identify their own development goals • Provides opportunity for employee to keep supervisor informed of accomplishments, issues	• Can be manipulated by employee to overstate good performance or minimize negatives • Not recommended for compensation decisions

performance appraisal are subject to defense in discrimination lawsuits. The human resources department provides guidance as to an organization's accepted performance appraisal method(s). Some common methods are briefly described as follows.

- **Graphic rating scale**: A checklist is used to numerically rate employees on general traits related to job performance, like teamwork. While simple and easy to use, because this method often lacks specifics, its validity and reliability and value for employee development may be limited (Schermerhorn 2014).

- **Behaviorally anchored rating scale (BARS)**: This more sophisticated rating system links specific examples of job-related performance

to each rating. For example, excellent, acceptable, and poor team behavior is described in terms that can be observed and rated at each level (for instance, employee consistently volunteers to lead project teams; all projects are completed on time and exceed quality expectations). Validity and reliability are improved and training benchmarks are provided (Schermerhorn 2014).

- **Critical incident method**: An ongoing written log of examples of an employee's job-related behavior during the appraisal period is used. It offers specific examples for development and is important that a manager documents both positive actions and negative incidents. This method can be used to supplement rating methods.

- **Ranking method**: Appraiser ranks all employees in a group or unit from highest to lowest based on overall performance. This is difficult to apply where several employees have performed at a similar level, but it can be useful to identify who receives the top pay increase (Mondy 2015).

- **Forced distribution**: This ranking method is similar to grading on a curve, where managers place subordinates into predetermined performance categories. For example, 15 percent are at the top, 75 percent at the average, 10 percent at the bottom. While this helps to avoid inflated ratings, the system can negatively impact employee morale (Dessler 2014).

Ensuring performance appraisal fairness can be challenging for managers and supervisors. One problem area, as noted before, is bias. Bias is clearly illegal when a manager allows race, color, religion, age, gender, or disability to influence performance ratings. More subtle forms of bias include a manager's tendency to rate an employee higher or lower based on a trait, such as personal appearance or punctuality, regardless of the trait's actual effect on performance. Another risk area is placing more weight on a behavior immediately preceding the appraisal meeting vs. considering the entire review period. A ratings fairness trap for managers, the **halo-horns effect** occurs when an employee is strong or weak in one rated area, such as communication, and the supervisor unfairly generalizes that performance to rate the employee high or low across all other areas on the performance appraisal (SHRM 2014). **Distributional errors** in ratings are also seen—central tendency, where all employees are rated satisfactory regardless of performance in order to avoid conflict; or leniency or strictness where some managers are overly generous or strict compared to other raters (Fried and Fottler 2011). Manager training is the best strategy to address these rating inequities.

In the appraisal interview, supervisor and employee meet to review the performance appraisal. The following steps help the appraising supervisor successfully plan and implement the interview.

1. Preparation is important. Provide the employee with advance notice (at least one week) and set a mutually agreed-upon time to meet. Identify a private place for the interview; set aside enough time (at least 30 minutes) so that the meeting is not rushed.

2. Make sure the appraisal is objective and defensible. This means the appraisal has been based on job-related criteria and performance standards and on more than one source of data; an effort has been made to avoid challenges to fairness.

3. During the interview, reinforce positive performance. Where improvement is needed, offer clear, specific examples. Allow the employee time to speak. Agree on an action plan going forward (Dessler 2014).

Check Your Understanding 20.3

***Instructions:* Answer the following questions.**

1. Information in _____ can be used as the basis for development of a job description.
   A. a job interview
   B. an employee performance appraisal
   C. job specifications
   D. a job analysis

2. The statement of duties responsibilities required of a job would be found in which of the following?
   A. Job summary
   B. Job description
   C. Job specifications
   D. Job interview

3. Which of the following refers to the ability of a selection test to measure the job skill, knowledge, or behavior the test was intended to measure?
   A. Reliability
   B. Impact
   C. Performance
   D. Validity

4. "Describe a situation in the past where there was team conflict and how you handled it" would be an example of which type of interview question?
   A. Open-ended
   B. Behavioral
   C. Situational
   D. Knowledge

5. The performance appraisal method that links specific job-related performance to each rating level is the:
   A. Graphic rating scale
   B. Critical incident method
   C. Behaviorally-anchored rating scale
   D. Ranking method

6. Which of the following is a positive aspect of using employee self-appraisal as a source of data for performance appraisal?
   A. Employees are in the best position to provide objective review without overstatement.
   B. The supervisor is kept informed of the employee's accomplishments.
   C. Appraiser and employee training on the purpose and procedures of this process is essential.
   D. Peer pressure of evaluation can motivate team members to be more productive.

Staff Retention

Given the investment in job analysis, employee recruitment, selection, and performance appraisal, retention of employees is important to an organization. **Turnover** reflects the rate at which employees leave a firm and have to be replaced, and is typically calculated per year. The rate includes voluntary exits and **dismissal** (involuntary termination of employment). The cost of turnover includes the costs of recruitment, the interview and testing process, pay during an employee's orientation period when productivity may be low, and the cost of management time needed for orientation and on-the-job training.

A survey of 262 US companies revealed the top five reasons that high-performing employees left organizations were pay, promotion opportunity, work–life balance, career development, and health benefits (Dessler 2014). This section will explore areas where line managers, particularly immediate supervisors, can help to influence employee engagement with the organization and reduce employee turnover.

Employee Engagement

Employee engagement refers to the level of commitment employees demonstrate, their willingness to continue working for the organization, and to go above and beyond the minimum expectations (Frauenheim 2009). Disengaged employees have been described as those who have mentally quit, but remain on the job working at a low level. Engagement is especially important in healthcare, an industry where cost-containment, concern regarding quality of care, and competition are major forces. The link between an organization's productivity and profitability and its employee engagement has been reported in consulting firm studies (Frauenheim 2009).

The following are top reasons why employees disengage and then leave, along with brief explanations.

- Job or workplace was not as expected—Unrealistic expectations of the applicant on hire, hiring managers' rush to hire, or failure to present the job realistically

- Mismatch between the job and the person—Failure to check references, use behavioral interview questions, or assume that training will correct talent gaps

- Too little coaching and feedback provided—Lack of effective training for managers on how to provide effective feedback, then infrequent and inadequate feedback to employees

- Too few career development and advancement opportunities—Managers' failure to discuss and provide development opportunities, or even efforts to block career advancement

- Feeling devalued and unrecognized—Employees feeling disrespected, treated unfairly, or even ignored

- Stress due to overwork and work–life imbalance—Constant push to do more (Branham 2005)

While the employee shares responsibility for remaining engaged, line managers are in a position to influence engagement and impact turnover, as discussed in the next section.

Reducing Turnover

Managers can employ the following strategies to enhance engagement, reduce voluntary turnover, and retain strong performers:

- *Investigate the scope of the issue*: Work with the human resources department to identify and review the unit's turnover rate, analyze exit interviews (addressed later in this chapter) and employee survey data for issues or trends. Are new hires leaving quickly? Are top performing employees leaving? Consider that along with loss of talent, some turnover is healthy for an organization; a very low turnover rate may signal lack of promotion opportunity.

- *Improve employee selection*: Tighten-up testing and interviewing to improve effectiveness (see selection process earlier in the chapter). Provide realistic previews of a job to applicants; include negative aspects of a job such as dealing with demanding customers.

- *Provide clear expectations and feedback*: This emphasizes clear job descriptions and effective performance appraisals, previously discussed, supported by ongoing employee communication and feedback.

- *Provide professional growth opportunities*: Training and career development programs, addressed later in this chapter, demonstrate management's investment in employees.

- *Improve compensation and recognition*: Advocate for appropriate pay rates for employees using job analysis data. Create opportunities to recognize employees for good work, for example, employee recognition awards.

- *Recognize the need for work–life balance*: Consider alternative work scheduling options for employees, where feasible (addressed later in this chapter). (Dessler 2014)

Employee Relations and Fair Treatment

Employee relations is a broad term referencing the general management and planning of activities related to developing and improving employee relationships through communication and fair handling of disputes (SHRM 2015a). Strategies for dealing with some of the least appealing aspects of management often start with reflections on how a negative situation, such as a grievance, could have been avoided. Communication, fairness, and respect are themes of positive employer–employee relationships and of handling difficult situations.

Communication Strategies

Without a communication system in place, managers may be unaware of suggestions for improvement or of problems until a crisis has brewed. Employees like to be informed about what goes on in the healthcare organization, feel they are involved, and have a means to voice their ideas and complaints. A 2007 survey by the Ethics Resource Center indicated most employees prefer to go to someone they know, like a supervisor, to voice a complaint or to report misconduct (Hirschmann 2008). Line managers often need training on ways to gather employee feedback, and to listen openly and respectfully to complaints. Practical suggestions of ways to foster communication include:

- An open-door policy to send the message that a manager is accessible and to encourage an open flow of communication; approaches can include a physical open door, use of a website, e-mail, and other communication tools

- Management by walking around to informally connect with staff, asking open-ended questions about how things are going

- Conducting staff meetings and focus groups to encourage two-way communication

- Making sure employees are aware of organizational options, such as hotlines or suggestion boxes, to voice concerns

Reviewing results of employee surveys and exit interviews conducted by the human resources department can also help managers better understand employee attitudes and concerns. **Exit interview** refers to the final meeting an employee has with his or her employer; the meeting provides an opportunity to collect feedback on issues or problem areas, including what may have caused the employee to leave (LeBlanc 2016).

Most employees want to make suggestions. An active approach to increase employee involvement in problem solving is appointment of a temporary suggestion team focused on a specific work-related assignment (Dessler 2014). The team is given a charge, such as to improve workflow in an area to reduce costs, meeting space, or a website and asked to propose ideas by a target date.

Conflict Management

Despite efforts at employee communication, some conflict is to be expected where people work together, especially in teams. The type and intensity of conflict are of concern to managers. Some level of healthy disagreement is necessary to encourage new ideas and creativity in an organization but too much conflict becomes distracting and harmful. **Dysfunctional conflict** is a destructive type of struggle that becomes emotionally draining and harms productivity.

Sources of conflict are many, from individual personalities and beliefs to organizational issues such as role confusion, scarce resources, and tasks that are interdependent across employees or departments. As healthcare organizations become more culturally, racially, and gender diverse, the potential for greater creativity increases as does the risk of employee conflict. Healthcare organizations that have been most successful in managing diversity and minimizing conflict have several factors in common—a culture of inclusion and respect, a commitment to valuing diversity, a diversity training program, accommodation of family needs, offering of employee support groups and alternative scheduling options (Gomez-Mejia et al. 2012).

When dysfunctional conflict does occur, **avoidance** or denial of the disruption may be a natural response, but this approach does not resolve the issue. Determining the best approach to conflict management involves consideration of time, budget, the importance and complexity of the issues at play, and the potential for long-term damage if conflict is not resolved. Table 20.5 identifies common conflict management strategies and when each should be used.

Disciplinary Action

When an employee fails to abide by rules, policies, and procedures, or fails to meet performance standards, organizations have processes in place for **disciplinary action**—applying a reprimand or penalty (SHRM 2015a). Efforts to ensure fairness of the discipline process and to show respect for employees are critical in supporting positive employee relations. Supervisors support this by thoroughly investigating facts and gathering evidence before taking disciplinary action, not acting when angry, applying penalties without bias, and clearly explaining the consequences of discipline and right of appeal to an employee (Dessler 2014).

Table 20.5   Approaches to conflict management

Method	When to apply
Accommodation: Downplays differences, focuses on similarities to reduce conflict	Use when the issue is minor and more important to the employee than to the manager or organization and when seeking harmony and moving on is the goal.
Compromise: Bargaining; each side gives up something, gains something	Useful for complex issues where a temporary or rapid resolution is needed. There is a risk that conflicts may reoccur.
Collaboration: Addresses the problem, differences, and underlying conflict to arrive at a mutually beneficial resolution	Ideal for long-term problem-solving and conflict resolution, but takes time (which is costly) and depends on the willingness of all parties to participate openly and invest in the process.
Command: Authority figure issues a directive to resolve the issue	Used by management when quick action is needed, as in a crisis, or when a law or policy must be enforced.
Structural change: Provide additional budget or training, transfer personnel, change roles, physical workspace, procedures, and such.	Use when interpersonal conflict is not involved, or when interpersonal differences cannot be resolved, and where resources permit.

Source: Adapted from Schermerhorn 2014, 320–322.

Keeping focus on the behavior not the person is important, as is clear documentation.

Approaches to fair discipline used in most organizations include:

- **Progressive penalties**, which ensures that the minimum penalty appropriate to the level of offense is applied. Penalties may include but are not limited to oral warning for first unexcused tardiness, written warning for the second instance; serious rule violations, such as bringing a weapon to work, may result in immediate dismissal.

- **Discipline without punishment** includes a step where the employee is given a one- to two-day paid decision-making leave following oral and written warnings and attempts to problem solve. On return from leave, the employee agrees to abide by expectations or leave the company if the issue occurs again (Mondy 2015, 340).

Avoidance of decisions in other areas of HRM can compound the disciplinary process. For example, overly lenient annual performance appraisal ratings of a poor performer provide weak background documentation when a manager is ultimately forced to discipline the employee for low productivity. The employee may claim, perhaps justly, that no feedback was provided. A manager's failure to consistently apply disciplinary policies across all employees may lead to EEOC charges and even lawsuits from employees in protected groups. As with conflict management, avoidance does not address the problem.

Handling Grievances

Disciplinary issues and problems related to promotions and transfers top the list of sources for employee grievance, followed by performance appraisal, wages, work assignment, and scheduling issues (Dessler 2014). A **grievance** is a formal complaint by an employee or group of employees alleging unfair treatment or (where applicable) a violation of union contract terms (SHRM 2015a). Facing an employee grievance can be daunting for a manager, but most larger (and all unionized) organizations have a multistep system in place for handling grievances to make the process clear for both employee and employer. Line managers should be familiar with the process.

Guidelines for handling grievances start with prevention efforts, by developing open communication with employees and fair performance appraisal and disciplinary processes as noted earlier. Less formal appeals processes are important to avoid escalation of complaints. The opportunity for employees to voice their views, such as on performance rating decisions, may be handled using channels like the open-door policy described previously.

Points to keep in mind when handling a formal grievance include:

- Inform the next level of management of the grievance
- As applicable, work with the union representative
- Investigate the situation thoroughly
- Review the employee's personnel file and any prior grievance reports
- Meet with the employee in private to discuss the grievance and listen to what he or she says
- Respond within time limits specified by policy or labor contract and keep responses focused on facts and consistent with policy or contract (Dessler 2014)

Managers should be prepared to work through any next steps in the grievance process, which may include working on a solution with the employee (and union representative where applicable) or appealing the grievance decision. Ineffective handling of grievances can put a healthcare organization at risk for costly legal action.

Dismissal

Employees leave an organization voluntarily for a variety of reasons, including a career or job change, retirement, or family circumstances. **Termination** of employment is a broad term encompassing voluntary separation by the employee, as well as dismissal of the employee by the employer. Dismissal, or involuntary separation, is the involuntary termination of employment.

The legal concept of **employment at will** (employment can be terminated by the employer or the employee for any reason, absent a written contract) has been recognized in the US legal system since the 19th century; however, changing economics and views of the balance of power between employer and employee have led to exceptions (Muhl 2001). Employees now have protections against wrongful discharge based on statutes (for example, Title VII) and court decisions. **Wrongful**

discharge is unfair dismissal of employment due to failure of the employer to comply with law, organizational policy, or a contract.

Appropriate reasons for dismissal of an employee fall into these four general groups:

- *Performance*: Consistent failure to perform assigned job duties, or to meet specified performance standards, as documented
- *Conduct*: Intentional violation of the organization's policies or rules
- *Qualifications*: Inability to perform skills or to meet other specified qualifications of the assigned job; training and job transfer have been explored
- *Elimination* of work or job

Dismissal for the first three reasons is obviously a very serious action. This step should be taken when needed, but only after careful planning and consultation with the human resources department to ensure that all documentation is in order and that law, company policy, and union contract (where applicable) are followed. The employee should not be surprised by the decision if clear feedback and support have been provided via performance appraisal and in the progressive disciplinary process. However, involuntary loss of employment can be traumatic for employees who may feel fear, failure, disappointment or anger, and react emotionally or even violently (Mondy 2015).

Best practices recommend that a dismissal interview should be scheduled early in the week to allow the dismissed employee to begin an immediate job search. Demonstrate respect by avoiding dates of special significance to the employee, such as a birthday or religious holiday. These guidelines are recommended for the dismissal interview:

- Conduct the meeting in person, scheduled for about 10 minutes.
- Use a conference room or other neutral location (not the manager's office). Have a phone and the number for security available in case of emergency (for example, medical attention is needed or a threatening situation develops).

- Consider having a witness join the interview; introduce this individual to the employee.
- Get to the point. Briefly describe the situation, then state the decision. Be clear, use facts.
- Listen to the employee, but leave no options.
- Provide severance information, final paycheck, and such (arranged in advance with the human resources department).
- Close the interview, tell the employee where they should go next (Dessler 2014).

The experience of firing for cause is difficult on the manager, as well as the employee. Solid hiring decisions as discussed earlier in this chapter are the best strategy for reducing disciplinary-based dismissals.

For economic reasons, an employer may initiate nondisciplinary dismissal of one or more employees in the form of a layoff or downsizing. A **layoff** is a temporary dismissal where employees are told there is no work available now, but that they may be recalled; there is no guarantee of being recalled. When **downsizing**, the workforce is permanently reduced through elimination of positions, processes, and functions (SHRM 2015a).

Senior management makes the strategic layoff or downsizing decision and is responsible for compliance with any applicable law. Supervisors may have roles in determining which employees stay on the job and of informing staff of the outcome. Layoff and downsizing decisions can have a negative effect on morale, for those out of work as well as those remaining, and a negative impact on the organization's image. While not pleasant, handling the situation with fairness and respect is important. This involves keeping employees informed, providing advance notice of termination, and basing decisions as to who stays on solid performance appraisal information or on seniority.

Check Your Understanding 20.4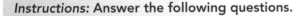

Instructions: **Answer the following questions.**

1. True or false: Some turnover is good for an organization.

2. True or false: Recommended guidelines for a manager handling an employee's dismissal interview include holding the interview in the manager's private office.

3. True or false: Grievance prevention strategies include having fair performance appraisal and disciplinary processes.

4. A mismatch between the job and the individual and feelings of being devalued or treated unfairly are among reasons why employees:
   A. Disengage and then leave an organization
   B. File a grievance
   C. Are disciplined without punishment
   D. Are dismissed

5. Actions of management to develop and improve employee relationships through communication and fair handling of disputes are at the heart of which of the following?
   A. Employee relations
   B. The disciplinary process
   C. Handling grievances
   D. Employee engagement

6. A conflict occurred within a workgroup. The issue was minor, but had become a distraction. The leader felt it was important to resolve the issue, get the group back on track, and move on. Which of the following would be the best approach to conflict management here?
   A. Avoidance
   B. Accommodation
   C. Compromise
   D. Command

7. Which policy ensures that the minimum penalty appropriate to the level of employee offense is applied?
   A. Employment at will
   B. Downsizing
   C. Progressive penalties
   D. Discipline without punishment

Staffing, Planning, and Scheduling

Staffing involves decisions about the types of employees needed, how many employees are needed, how work will be organized, and how employees are scheduled. Addressing the types of employees needed by knowledge, skills, and experience, as well as the number of employees required, starts with the job analysis process. Work volume projections provided by the organization are used in supporting the number of staff needed. Also useful for staffing planning is analysis of environmental workforce data and trends.

Organizing Work

A process is a way to organize work and resources to accomplish a result. A **business process** is a collection of interrelated activities, initiated by a triggering event, that achieves a specific result for the customer and other stakeholders (Sharp and McDermott 2009). Much of the work in HIM involves business processes; activities in the revenue cycle or in release of information (ROI) provide examples.

Two major ways that process-type work is organized in HIM organizations are:

- **Serial work division**: Tasks or steps in a process are handled separately in sequence by individual workers, as with a factory assembly line, to complete a process
- **Parallel work division**: The same tasks are handled simultaneously by several workers; each completes all steps in the process from beginning to end, working independently of the other employees (Oachs 2016)

As an example, the triggering event in the ROI business process would be receipt of a request for release of information. In serial work division, a clerk might open the mail and log a request in a tracking system. An ROI specialist would then complete the remaining steps to validate and process the request unless a paper record must be retrieved, in which case that step would be completed by request to a file clerk. With parallel work division, several ROI specialists are each responsible for receiving, logging, tracking, validating, and processing requests including retrieving the necessary records. The specialists' work may be divided in various ways, such as by type of request (for example, attorneys, insurers, medical providers, patients). Volume of work and skill level of employees should be considered in determining which pattern of work division is the best fit.

To view the efficiency of work in a process, managers can conduct a workflow analysis, (discussed earlier in the chapter and in chapter 19) as identifying each step in a process sequence and how steps relate to each other. A diagram is typically used to visualize a business process. Results can help identify redundancies or roadblocks in the process.

A work distribution analysis can also be conducted. This is a process of data collection to determine the type and appropriateness of a unit's work assignments, the time allowed for the tasks, and the employees doing the work. This analysis can be accomplished by having employees log time spent on key tasks or functions (as outlined in job descriptions) during a given period of time. Results of work distribution analysis can be used to create a chart or spreadsheet to help a manager identify whether:

- Enough time is being spent on priority job functions vs. minor tasks
- Some employees are working over capacity, and others are underutilized
- There is duplication of work (Oachs 2016)

Based on workflow analysis and work distribution analysis, job descriptions, procedures, physical space plans, or staff schedules may be revised to improve work quality and productivity.

Scheduling Work

After the type, amount, and distribution of work have been determined, an effective plan for staff scheduling can be developed that provides coverage of services and is fair to employees.

Understanding the organizational definition of the workday and workweek is important in the development of standard scheduling. General rules are as follows: one **full-time equivalent (FTE)** employee is expected to work 8 hours per day, 5 days per week, 40 hours per week, 52 weeks per year, 2,080 hours in a year. There are variations, such as a 7.5 hour day and alternative scheduling arrangements. The workweek typically beginning Sunday or Monday, with nonexempt employees paid at a higher rate for work on weekends and holidays. HIM services often cover daytime business hours, Monday through Friday. Evening and weekend hours may also be needed, or even 24-hour, seven day per week coverage for specific functions or in larger organizations. The organization's hours of operation and the types and volume of services provided drive decisions regarding the number of FTEs needed to cover required HIM job functions on a typical-volume day, and for lighter weekends or holidays.

An equitable system of staff rotation is important to have in place where evening, weekend, and holiday coverage is required so that staff feel the burden is shared, although some facilities hire staff to work solely on the weekend. It is necessary for managers to be familiar with vacation policy and to plan staff vacation schedules in advance. Options for work coverage during vacations, or for other absences such as illness, include using float employees who are cross-trained to perform several jobs, hiring temporary workers, or distributing work across other staff during the absence (Oachs 2016). Anticipating work disruptions when new systems are introduced is also important; it may be necessary to make scheduling adjustments or hire supplemental temporary workers while full-time staff attends training.

Beyond standard schedules, alternative work schedule designs can allow employees more control over their schedules, offer a response to employee and family needs, may result in a morale boost and improved productivity, and can provide a recruitment feature. Adjustment to orientation and training offerings may be needed where employees are not on a standard schedule or at a single location. Alternatives described by various sources include the following.

- **Flextime**, or flexible work hours: An employee is able to choose his or her start and departure times, completing a set number of hours each day (typically 7 to 8) so long as the hours worked overlap a core busy time period (for example, 10 a.m. to 3 p.m.) required for unit or shift coverage.
- **Compressed workweek**: An employee works longer days to complete 40 hours of work in less than five days, perhaps on a 10-hour, four-day schedule. The downside to this strategy is that the long days may lead to fatigue.
- **Job sharing**: Two or more employees split one full-time job over a day, a week, or a month. Employees in the arrangement must be compatible. A significant scheduling challenge can arise if one employee leaves

the organization and a match to the sharing arrangement is not available.

- **Part-time employee**: An employee regularly works fewer hours than the standard full-time 40-hour week. The number of hours varies but may be 20 or 32 hours.

- **Contingent or contract work**: In these arrangements, temporary workers supplement full-time employees, often as part-time workers. This offers flexibility to both parties, but the temporary workers do not usually qualify for benefits.

- **Telecommuting**: Also called remote or virtual work, the employee uses technology to perform work and link with the organization from home or another out-of-office location. The organization usually provides a computer and the required software. Coding, transcription, and ROI are HIM examples of where telecommuting can work. Advantages for the employee include reduced expense of commuting and increased productivity as there will be fewer distractions. However, separating work from personal time and social isolation can be challenges. Lack of frequent communication with the employee and security concerns are challenges for the employer. An approach is to have the employee sign a telecommuting agreement with the supervisor that outlines mutual expectations for location, hours, communication frequency, security, confidentiality, and such (LeBlanc 2016).

- **Outsourcing**: The organization contracts with a vendor firm having expertise in an area to provide the staff and assume responsibility for a function such as transcription, release of information, or coding. The HIM manager's job then becomes vendor relationship management (LeBlanc 2016). The hired firm provides the services on-site or via telecommuting. Advantages include not having to manage recruitment and selection or to supervise the individual employees. Disadvantages for the manager include less hands-on control over quality of work and the need to develop methods to monitor vendor performance.

- **Offshoring**: Offshoring is where employees of the vendor firm are based outside of the United States. Cost savings is a benefit due to lower wages; whereas quality control, privacy, and security are among concerns to address. Transcription, coding, and billing are areas where offshoring is used. Before considering offshoring, an HIM department should already have experience with remote work arrangements, have a solid technology infrastructure, and strong privacy and security policies in place (Gurrieri and Karban 2013).

Creative approaches to staff scheduling have become more commonly used to meet a variety of human resource and business needs. In studies of US businesses in 2007 and 2010, flextime was the most prevalent alternative work schedule option used, followed by telecommuting, and job sharing was least often used (Fried and Fottler 2015). Given changing needs in healthcare settings (for example, introduction of new technology), scheduling to provide workforce capability and flexibility calls for use of permanent full-time, part-time, and contingent workers.

Workforce Analysis and Planning

Attempting to predict, prevent and respond to workforce shortages and oversupply is a challenge for healthcare organizations. Reviewing national demographic, social, and economic data and trends and relating these to an organization's local staffing needs is central to **workforce planning**. While workforce planning (deciding what positions are needed) is a top management responsibility, HIM managers can contribute by staying abreast of data and trends relevant to our profession that may impact staffing, recruitment and selection, turnover, and training.

Sources of HIM workforce data include government reports provided by the Department of Labor and the Health Resources and Services Administration's Bureau of Health Professions. Reports produced by the American Health Information Management Association (AHIMA) and other professional associations are also important sources of workforce analysis. For example, the AHIMA House of Delegates 2015 Environmental Scan noted the following shifts expected to impact staff scheduling and other aspects of HRM:

- As of 2015, millennials (those born in the 1980s or 1990s) were projected to make up the largest percentage of the workforce; this generation's demand for greater work–life balance has and will continue to place priority on alternative schedule options and mobile work environments.

- Baby-boomer generation (those born following World War II through the mid-1960s) retirement continues at a faster rate than the rate of new HIM professionals entering the workforce; when vacant positions stay open longer, staff workloads and scheduling are impacted.

- Change in market demand for HIM skills in areas such as clinical documentation improvement, data and information governance, data analysis, and management of regulatory requirements calls for more education, analytical and critical thinking skills, and clinical knowledge. (Desai 2015)

Staying current on external workforce data can assist managers and the organization in forecasting and planning for the right number and types of workers needed to cover HIM functions.

Measuring Performance

Managers must be able to report on the amount, efficiency, and quality of work being done in a unit. Employees need to know what is expected of them, and how they are doing relative to expectations. Setting performance standards and measuring performance can address the needs of both. Analysis of employee performance data based on standards can support:

- Productivity and quality improvement initiatives
- Staffing decisions
- Employee performance appraisals
- Job analysis and job description redesign

Developing Standards

Two methods of developing performance standards commonly used in HIM are benchmarking and work measurement. **Benchmarking** is based on comparison of external performance data on similar functions performed in similar organizations, collected through research. Sources of data for benchmarking include reports and articles published by national, state, and local professional associations, or through contact with peer institutions. To initiate benchmarking, a manager should first identify the work function to be benchmarked (such as coding or release of information), the type of performance measure (for example, number of records coded or requests for information processed) and a time period (per hour or day) (Oachs 2016). The search for relevant performance standards can then be conducted. As an example, 40 records per day was published as a baseline productivity standard by the AHIMA e-HIM Coding Benchmark Workgroup for coding of ambulatory and outpatient invasive procedures (DeVault 2012). Any external standard should be assessed as a match to the unit's job function. Consider organization size, patient type and volume, classification system, health record system, and so forth, and adjust as appropriate. Internal performance data collected on the same measure can be compared to the external data to support validity of the standard. Upper management should approve the selected performance standard.

Work measurement is based on assessment of internal data collected on actual work performed within the organization and the calculation of time it takes to do the work. The process can start by identifying certain work functions to be measured, or all can be included. There are several techniques that can be used to gather this information:

- *Analyze historical performance data*: Total hours worked on a job can be obtained from payroll records; this does not provide detailed task information.

- *Have the supervisor perform the work, logging the time spent*: This gives management an understanding of the work, but the clocked time-on-task will likely be slower than that of an employee who performs the work daily, and it may not be the best use of management time.

- *Ask employees to self-report data:* Employees log what they do and the time spent on tasks and units of work received and processed each day. This can be done for a defined period of time as a study, such as over two weeks excluding any holidays. A log or tracking form should be provided to each participating employee for consistency of data capture. For example, a daily log entry for ICD-10-CM/PCS coding might contain: 8 hours worked, 24 records received, 24 coded. A basic unit/ and time productivity statistic can then be calculated, dividing the number of units produced by the time worked; for example 24 charts coded divided by 8 hours equals 3 charts coded per hour. Where multiple employees are performing the same job, average the rate across employees to determine a reasonable productivity standard for that job.

- *Observe a sample of job functions for a period of time*: Identify the job functions to be observed and the time period (for example, number of days or weeks) of the work observation study. Identify and train observers on what information is to be gathered, when, and how it should be collected (for example, observation schedule, forms). Inform the employees selected to be observed of the purpose of the study and how the information will be used and shared. (Oachs 2016)

Determining which work measurement technique to use involves considering time and budget, and personnel available and willing to participate.

Monitoring and Measuring HIM Performance

Once standards have been established, the manager can then develop a plan for ongoing monitoring and measuring of performance. **Performance measurement** compares work outcomes to the established performance standards and results are typically expressed in quantifiable terms, such as rates (Oachs 2016). Not every task needs to be monitored (that is, tracked and reviewed). The manager and the healthcare organization decide on outcomes to monitor, such as volume, turnaround time, or accuracy of key services. Data on actual practice in the identified performance areas are then collected and reviewed.

Collecting accurate productivity data is important. Routine methods of data collection and review should be established. Suggestions for managers include the following:

- Require employees to complete a weekly or monthly productivity report; use an electronic format such as a spreadsheet for efficiency. See figure 20.7 for a sample productivity report.

- Review work volume reports available from organizational systems, such as payroll, or from computer applications used by HIM employees (for example, encoders) to supplement or to validate employees' individual productivity reports.

- Meet with each supervised employee regularly (namely, weekly or monthly) to review the data collected and discuss any issues related to standards not met.

A word of caution: Do not become so task-focused or time conscious in productivity monitoring that quality is forgotten. Focusing on daily volume statistics or turnaround time can distract from other variables that matter to customers. Consider including performance measures that address quality of services, such as accuracy benchmarks or completing error-free work (Sharp and McDermott 2009).

Finally, reported performance data are regularly analyzed for **variance**. Variance—where actual performance does not meet, varies, or is significantly different from the standard—should be further assessed. Questions the manager should first consider in analyzing variances include: Does the figure represent a trend? Is there an obvious explanation, as with a temporary staffing shortage, a holiday, or a spike in work volume? Is more information or additional monitoring needed to fully assess the variance? After further review, then consider if action is needed; for example, change in procedure or physical space, workflow analysis, staffing adjustment, or training. Review table 20.6 and consider how a manager might interpret this report.

Figure 20.7 Sample productivity report for release of information specialist

Name: Best Employee	Mon.	Tue.	Wed.	Thur.	Fri.	Sat.	Sun.	Weekly total	Comments
Date									
Hours worked									
Mail requests: (#)									
Total opened and date stamped									
Logged into system by type									
Authorization verified									
Processed and records sent									
Invoice sent									
Unable to process and letter sent									
Fax requests for patient care (#)									
Received and verified									
Cover sheets prepared									
Patient records faxed									
Walk-in requests (#)									
Phone requests (#)									
Records (# pages)									
Paper copied									
Electronic printed									
Misc. time (hours)									
Meetings									
Training									
Other (explain)									

Adapted from: Tooley 2007.

Table 20.6 Sample inpatient health information management services report

Indicator: Standard	January 2015	February 2015	March 2015
Discharges (actual)	5,000	5,400	5,360
Incomplete record delinquency rate: < 50%	35%	45%	50%
Days in accounts receivable due to uncoded records: < 5 days	3	5	5
Charts coded per day: ≥ 24	26	22	23
Coding accuracy: 99%	99%	95%	98%
Turnaround transcribed history and physical (H&P): < 24 hours	12	16	24
ROI routine requests received (actual)	200	245	300
ROI routine request turnaround: < 4 days	3*	3	6
Budgeted FTEs: 50 (actual)	50	50	48
Resignations: < 1%	0	0	4% (2)
Training hours (required)	4	16	8

*Background: This figure shows the average number of days it took to respond to routine ROI requests in January based on these data: 100 requests responded to within 2 days; 100 responded to within 4 days; 200 total routine requests. Calculate turnaround: [(100 x 2 days) + (200 x 4 days)]/200 = 3 days average response rate. Average response meets the standard of less than four days, although many requests took up to four days for a response.
Adapted from: Oachs 2016.

Check Your Understanding 20.5

Instructions: **Answer the following questions.**

1. One ROI specialist handles requests from insurance and managed care companies. Another handles requests from attorneys and courts. Each completes all steps in the business process from beginning to end. This is an example of which of the following?
   A. Serial work division
   B. Job sharing
   C. Job rotation
   D. Parallel work division

2. Mary is able to start work at her office between 8 and 10 a.m. and work an 8-hour day Monday through Friday. This is an example of what type of alternative staffing design?
   A. Compressed workweek
   B. Flextime
   C. Telecommuting
   D. Floater

3. Coding is done by a vendor whose employees are located in China. This is an example of which of the following?
   A. Contingent workers
   B. Job sharing
   C. Outsourcing
   D. Offshoring

4. To develop performance standards for release of information turnaround time, the manager conducted a literature search and contacted peer institutions. Which method did she use?
   A. Workflow analysis
   B. Benchmarking
   C. Work measurement
   D. Productivity analysis

5. The manager calculated a unit and time productivity statistic based on employee self-reported data. He used the ____ method to develop this performance standard.
   A. Benchmarking
   B. Work distribution analysis
   C. Work measurement
   D. Workflow analysis

6. Results of which of the following can help a manager assess prioritization of work, duplication of work, and underutilization of employees?
   A. Work distribution analysis
   B. Work measurement
   C. Benchmarking
   D. Workflow analysis

7. When reviewing the monthly performance report, a manager noticed the coding accuracy rate was below standard. She considered whether this difference might be related to a recent change in systems or attributed to another factor. This manager is performing which of the following?
   A. Performance measurement
   B. Workforce planning
   C. Work observation study
   D. Variance analysis

Training and Development

HIM roles are changing, becoming more complex, and demanding higher skill levels. This change impacts HRM functions from staff recruitment and selection to training and development. Strategies to address worker shortages and talent gaps include hiring new workers, retraining existing workers for new roles, bringing back and retraining retirees, or shifting workers into different roles within the unit or the organization (Fried and Fottler 2015). These workers need training in order to be successful. In healthcare, the training function is typically decentralized. Departments are responsible for their specific needs and the human resources department manages education programs required for employees organization-wide (for example, OSHA, HIPAA privacy) and management training (for example, equal employment opportunity law compliance, leadership). Accrediting agencies such as the Joint Commission require documentation of staff training that may be managed centrally to ensure compliance. The process of connecting employees to the organization and initiating training begins with new employee orientation, discussed in the next section.

New Employee Orientation

New employee orientation includes a group of activities that welcome new employees and introduce them to the healthcare organization; to the assigned department, unit, or workgroup; and to the specific job to be performed. It is the first step in helping the employee to feel knowledgeable, competent, and satisfied (Patena 2016). Formats vary, though large healthcare organizations often have a formal process for new employee orientation. Some activities may be conducted one-on-one, others in a group of new employees, and some activities may be computerized. An aspect of successful orientation is **onboarding**, or socialization into the values and culture of an organization. An example of a best practice that demonstrates this approach is shown in figure 20.8.

Because there is so much for the new employee to absorb, orientation typically takes places over several days or even weeks. While orientation responsibility is typically shared between the human resources department staff and the line manager, peers can also play a role. Some organizations assign a buddy (current employee) to each new employee to help them get adjusted. Each healthcare organization and job has unique new employee orientation content, but there are some common topics addressed, as outlined in table 20.7.

Regardless of the specific schedule or content of orientation, obtaining evaluation feedback from new employees is essential to support improvement of the orientation process. Orientation sets the stage for further employee training and development, discussed next.

Figure 20.8 New employee orientation best practice

New employee orientation and onboarding at The Mayo Clinic, Rochester, Minnesota

The following approach has been referenced as a best practice model:

New employees are welcomed with balloons, upbeat music, and breakfast. A multidisciplinary team introduces the organization's mission and values. New employees are engaged in role-playing exercises focused on diversity and mutual respect. A resource fair is set up during lunch; employees can network while obtaining information on benefits, parking, and such. Small groups conduct tours of the facilities. The goal is to introduce the organization's culture, provide a positive first impression, and keep the momentum going on the job.

Source: Hicks et al. 2006.

Table 20.7 Common types of content covered in new employee orientation

Employee-centered
• Compensation t(pay, holidays) and benefits (insurance, retirement)
• Career development opportunities, career planning resources
Organization-centered
• Organization overview: history, mission, structure, services, customs, culture
• Health and safety information and procedures
• Privacy and security policies and procedures
• Employment policies and procedures (sick leave, vacation, discipline and grievance processes)
• How to file a discrimination or harassment complaint
• Information on employee activities and events
• Tour of facility
• Time for networking
• Evaluation of organization and employee-centered orientation
Job- or department-centered
• Job description, job duties, schedule, performance standards
• Department policies and procedures
• Introduction to workspace and equipment
• Department tour
• Time for socialization with co-workers
• Meet with supervisor, question and answer session, feedback on job- or department-centered orientation

Source: Adapted from Fried and Fottler 2015, 377.

Employee Training and Development

Training provides new or current employees with knowledge, skills, and abilities related to specific competencies needed to perform their present jobs. Training can also fulfill legal requirements or support organizational goals, as with diversity awareness training that educates employees on specific cultural and gender differences and how to respond to these in the workplace (Gomez-Mejia et al. 2012). **Development** refers to educational programs with a longer-term focus, designed to stimulate an individual's professional growth by increasing or enhancing his or her skills, knowledge, or abilities (SHRM 2015a). Both training and development are learning strategies that support employee recruitment, productivity, performance improvement and engagement, and serving organizations well in a competitive environment. Investment in employee training and development is necessary, but comes at a cost to the organization. Therefore, careful planning and implementation are required to support its effectiveness.

Planning and Implementation

The analyze-design-develop-implement-evaluate (ADDIE) model has been recommended by numerous experts in the HRM and instructional design fields as a general guide to planning and implementation of employee training programs. The **ADDIE model** steps are as follows.

1. *Analyze:* Assess and document a need for the training. Identify the learning gap to be addressed. Sources of information for this step include, but are not limited to, job analyses, performance reports, performance appraisals, external requirements of law or accreditation, trends identified in literature and employee surveys, focus groups, and exit interviews.

2. *Design:* Establish objectives for the training as well as criteria for evaluating the training. Evaluation criteria may include employee reactions (for example, did employees like the training and find it valuable) as well as measurement of improvement is job performance following the training. During this step, the target employee audience should be identified and the training method(s) selected. A realistic budget must be developed and any required approvals should be obtained.

3. *Develop:* Create the program content and lesson plans, and identify facilitator(s), equipment, and supplies needed. (Alternately,

purchase from a vendor a packaged training program that meets the identified need, objectives, and budget, and that fits the target audience.) Consider a pilot or test run of the training program before full implementation.

4. *Implement:* Schedule, publicize and provide the training to the identified employee audience.

5. *Evaluate:* Conduct evaluation of the training and then analyze evaluation results. If evaluation identifies additional training needs, the planning process can restart at step 1.

The nature of the audience—adult learners—is important to consider in planning effective employee training. Most adults are challenged to some degree with balancing work, home, and personal demands and time is valuable. Concepts to consider in helping adults learn, and that can contribute to successful training activities, include:

- *Motivation:* Adults are more likely to remember material that is relevant and has practical value to them. Positive training participation and outcomes are more likely to occur from employees who see a direct connection between the training and an interesting work goal that provides opportunity for growth.

- *Knowledge of results:* Adults appreciate feedback, ideally immediately, on their performance.

- *Reinforcement:* Ways to increase motivation to participate in training include incentive pay, providing a convenient schedule that saves time, and offering immediate feedback on performance (Patena 2016).

Additional considerations regarding training include attention to learning styles and needs of the target audience. Some workers and groups respond more enthusiastically than others to social interaction. A mix of methods can be used to address sensory needs of learners: use of sound for the auditory learner, reading material for the visual learner, and simulated practice for the hands-on learner (Patena 2016). As required by the ADA, employers must make reasonable accommodations for access to training by employees with disabilities. For example, to accommodate trainees with limited visual acuity, use larger font and clear color contrast in presentations and handouts and for the hearing impared, include captioning in videos.

Delivery Methods

Multiple delivery options are available to the training planner. The one(s) selected should be based on training objectives, audience, content, and budget. Major training delivery methods and approaches are described in the next section.

Self-Directed Learning **Self-directed learning** allows learners to control their own education at their own pace; a trainer or instructor does not participate. This can be accomplished by the learner reading a textbook, listening to audiotapes, or through multimedia **computer-based training** modules delivered using DVDs or the Internet (see also online learning). Training can be offered to one or multiple learners. Costs of self-directed learning vary but are usually relatively low (for example, price of a book with web-access code). Scheduling flexibility is an advantage for the self-directed learner. Computer-based training allows the learner to receive immediate answer feedback and to repeat content. The self-paced online certification exam preparation courses offered by AHIMA are an example of this delivery method (AHIMA 2015a).

Classroom-Based Learning **Classroom-based learning** refers to instructor-led, face-to-face training such as traditional lectures, workshops, and seminars. This method is commonly used by managers because it is familiar and content is relatively quick, easy, and inexpensive to develop. However, the delivery budget for classroom-based learning increases where room rental and food are included, even more so for travel costs of employees not in the same location. This method is efficient for offering facts to a large group at the same time. Small group discussion can be added to encourage learner interaction, as appropriate to the learning topic. Scheduling the face-to-face classroom-based training can present challenges for employer and employees. The training should be conducted during the employee's regular working hours. Classroom sessions can be videotaped for playback to those unable to attend the live meeting due to work schedule conflict. Presentation of a new policy and procedure, such as a new time reporting system for all nonexempt HIM department employees, would represent an example where classroom-based delivery would be an appropriate training method. Where face-to-face interaction is needed, such as for team-building, live classroom training that includes small group work would be an effective choice.

Online Learning Online learning, or e-learning, is a broad term referring to the use of electronic media instead of classroom-based learning to deliver training; a trainer or instructor typically leads the training. Approaches include use of videoconferencing, webinars, learning management systems, web-based vendor portals and mobile learning using mobile devices such as smartphones and tablets (also called m-learning). Asynchronous online learning is self-paced; the students and instructor can communicate, but not in real-time. Synchronous delivery involves students and instructor meeting online at a specified time, such as for a scheduled webinar. The online learning method has grown in popularity due to convenience, flexibility of scheduling for employees and trainers, and the ability to customize content to workers' needs. Cost savings on travel is a major advantage of online learning where employees are not in the same location. Disadvantages are that some skills, such as team-building, interpersonal skills, and conflict resolution, are not easily taught outside of the face-to-face classroom and technical problems with connectivity, browsers, or operating systems can occur (Fried and Fottler 2011). Webinars to help coders stay current are examples of synchronous online learning.

Simulation Simulation training uses physical devices, computer-based scenarios, and video gaming. The learner interacts with a fictional experience as if it were real, chooses actions. and

answers questions. AHIMA's VLab is an online environment that provides simulations and actual practice with HIM applications such as use of an electronic health record (AHIMA 2015b). The feedback provided in simulation training enhances motivation to learn.

On-the-Job Training On-the-job training refers to an employee learning his or her job by actually doing it, ideally as part of a structured training plan. On-the-job training can apply to new employees, as well as to current employees learning a new job or system. Trainers can be the supervisor or an experienced peer employee. The steps outlined in figure 20.9 can be used by the trainer to help structure the training and support the employee receiving training.

For on-the-job training where employees work remotely, a team of experienced employees can be assigned to answer call-in questions from new off-site employees learning an operation (Dessler 2014).

Other approaches to on-the-job training include use of job rotation, where an employee moves from one job to the next, learning aspects of each job; this is applicable to supervisors needing to learn various functions within a department or organization. Shadowing is used to show one employee what another does on a daily basis, such as attend meetings and make decisions. This method provides a quick job review, can be useful when an employee is leaving and needs to prepare her replacement (Fried and Fottler 2011). Cross-training refers to an employee learning to do several jobs within a unit or department. This method provides scheduling flexibility helpful to management, and offers high-performing employees an opportunity to develop new skills.

Career Development

Given the changing healthcare landscape—consolidations, mergers, new technology and regulations, globalization, pressure to reduce costs—workers may find the need to develop, or redevelop, themselves to fit in. Coders' auditing skills have increased in importance within a computer-assisted

Figure 20.9 Steps for on-the-job training

Step 1	**Prepare the employee**
	Put the employee at ease.
	Explain the job and find out what the individual already knows about it.
	Get the employee interested in learning the job.
	Explain why the job is important.
	Clarify standards of performance.
	If using equipment, assure the employee is in the correct position for use.
	Familiarize the employee with equipment and materials needed.
Step 2	**Present the operation**
	Explain and show one important step at a time.
	Stress each key point slowly.
	Instruct clearly, completely, and patiently, but no more than the employee can master.
	Have the employee explain what has been demonstrated.
Step 3	**Try out performance**
	Have the employee do the job and correct any errors.
	Have the employee explain each key point as he or she does the job again.
	Make sure the employee understands the steps and answer any questions.
	Continue until the employee demonstrates confidence.
	Put the employee on his or her own.
Step 4	**Follow-up**
	Designate who the employee is to go to for help.
	Check frequently and encourage questions.
	Compliment good work and offer constructive feedback.
	Taper off close supervision but continue monitoring work against standards.
	Check back periodically.

Adapted from: Juran 1995.

coding environment; managers of electronic health record systems now need more advanced technical skills; data analysis skills are needed as healthcare organizations collect and store more health data (Caviart Group 2015). This section of the chapter examines the roles of employer and employee in meeting the need for HIM career development in the changing healthcare world.

Career development is the process by which individuals assess their existing skills, knowledge and experience; explore and establish current and future career objectives; and develop an appropriate course of action (SHRM 2015a). **Career planning** is the complementary, but more specific process of establishing career objectives and determining the appropriate educational and development programs required to achieve

short- or long-term career objectives (SHRM 2015a). The outcome of these processes is an employee career development plan.

As noted earlier, training is focused on skills for immediate job performance. But components of training can be included parts of an employee's career development plan. The career development process and plan can support both the employer and the employee. "Development supports longer-term career aspirations for the individual and benefits the organization in building workforce strength. Doing this well means building an effective process to guide individual development, linked to organizational needs" (Elsdon 2010, 43).

Effective career development practices help to establish this mutual employer—employee benefit link and guide planning of training and development activities that will be most valuable to the individual employee and to the organization. Examples of career development practices and roles of employer and employee are discussed in the following sections.

Employer Role

Managers can use the performance appraisal process as a career development practice, connecting an employee's job performance, training needs, and career interests. Use of the existing appraisal process is efficient (versus creating a new process), and serves to link the organization's needs to employee career development and career planning. The performance appraisal interview provides a time to discuss the employee's training and development needs and career plans, and then agree on action steps. This can work especially well if self-appraisal is a component of the performance appraisal process, is completed in advance of the appraisal interview, and includes specific questions or reflections on the employee's career development needs and objectives. Documenting the manager–employee agreed-upon career development plan and a timeline for tracking progress are important. See figure 20.10 for an example of a format that can be used to support documentation of a combined employee training and career development plan.

Other career development practices are coaching and mentoring, applicable to both new and experienced employees. **Coaching**, the ongoing process of educating, training, and communicating with subordinates, is a managerial or supervisory skill (Dessler 2014). In addition to offering specific job-related training, an effective coach provides an employee with feedback and support, serving as a professional role model and as a sounding board for career advice. HIM department managers and

Figure 20.10 Sample annual employee training and development plan

Sample annual employee training and development plan

Employee: | Job title:
Supervisor: | Department or unit:
Start date: | Next review target date:

Employee strengths:
- Strong leadership potential, volunteers to lead teams and projects
- Consistently meets project deadlines
- Detail-oriented, focused on quality of work

Training and development needs:
- Learn to better manage conflicts among team members
- Increase understanding of cultural differences in work settings
- Develop supervisory skills
- Strengthen public speaking and presentation skills
- Consider next steps in professional education

Learning assignments

Training activities	Timeline
• Complete self-paced module on managing team conflict	By x date
• Attend an internal or external seminar on cultural competency	By mid-year

Coaching and mentoring

Meet with assigned mentor once a month for next six months	Start to end dates

Special projects or assignments

Present at a local or state professional meeting	By end of year

Other professional development

• Practice supervisory skills as team leader, delegating more tasks to team members to make time for own professional development	Now; review progress by x date
• Gather information on three schools offering bachelor's degree completion programs; review with mentor	By end of next quarter

Adapted from Elsdon 2010.

supervisors who demonstrate interest in their employees' career development, and who are willing to invest the time to provide thoughtful advising, can be effective career coaches. **Mentoring** also involves career advising and counseling, and can be performed by a manager, but more often is a role for a senior employee. Mentors may be assigned to an employee as part of a formal mentoring program, or chosen informally by the employee. A mentor can assist the employee in making professional connections within the organization and in professional associations, and may be in a position to point the employee toward special project opportunities that assist in skill-building (for example, public speaking). A mentoring relationship can be valuable to an employee for sharing of career challenges and aspirations he or she might not yet be ready to discuss with a supervisor.

Referral of employees to internal and external resources can be useful to support a career development plan. Large organizations may have a career center, career planning workshops, or a budget to support an employee's access to outside continuing education. Best practice for managers is to have a list of internal organizational, as well as government and professional association resources available when providing career development advising to employees.

The employer's career development practices include the need to remain aware of healthcare industry and HIM professional employment trends. HIM managers can obtain online access to professional resources, such as the most recently published AHIMA workforce study and the Bureau of Labor Statistics Occupational Outlook Handbook for Medical Records and Health Information Technicians published by the US Department of Labor (BLS 2014b). Reports such as these are valuable for the manager's reference, as well as for sharing with employees during career development advising.

Employee Role

While employer guidance is important, employees need to take personal responsibility for career decisions and be active in their own career planning. Managers can challenge employees to take charge of in their own career development and career planning by suggesting employees regularly ask themselves (and answer) these questions:

- Who am I?
- What can I do?
- Where do I want to go?
- How do I get there? (Schermerhorn 2014, 249)

Managers can encourage and support employees' career development by pointing out available career assessment tools and making time to answer employees' follow-up questions. As examples, the Department of Labor's O*Net offers a free online occupational and career assessment system that helps users sort interests, skills, and career options (DOL 2015b). AHIMA's Career and Student Center offers online career mapping and other information for HIM professionals (AHIMA 2015c). Assigning visits to these sites, or asking an employee to write a short essay on his or her dream job, can serve as specific career planning exercises in advance of a scheduled performance appraisal interview or other career development discussion. Employees should be expected to follow through on timelines as part of a career development plan, and to be proactive in seeking advice when barriers to accomplishing agreed-upon learning assignments are encountered.

Return on Investment: Training and Development

Given the cost of employee training and development (time and dollars), and pressure within the healthcare industry to reduce cost, is training worth the investment? Consider a brief summary of thoughts offered across this chapter:

- Organizations are more productive (and profitable) when people are managed and treated as assets to be developed, versus as costs to be cut (Paton 2000, 95).

- Managers' basic understanding of employment law can help ensure compliance and avoid costly legal and financial liability for the organization.

- The best way to recruit talent is to build an environment where people want to work; factors supporting this include treating employees with respect and offering opportunities for growth (AHIMA 2013a).
- Among top reasons why high-performing employees leave organizations is the lack of career development opportunity.

After investing in recruitment, selection, and orientation of employees, administration of a fair and performance appraisal system, designing equitable staffing plans, and productivity analysis, it seems only logical that an organization should invest in training and development to help retain its best employees. Hiring new employees is costly and involves risk. Keeping and developing proven staff and retraining as the HIM workforce needs change is the best and most cost-effective strategy.

 Check Your Understanding 20.6

Instructions: **Answer the following questions.**

1. True or false: Training refers to educational programs with a longer-term focus, designed to stimulate an individual's professional growth by enhancing his or her skills, knowledge, or abilities.

2. True or false: Onboarding refers to the socialization of new employees into the values and culture of an organization.

3. True or false: Due to many demands on their time, adult learners are not interested in feedback.

4. In the ADDIE model for the training, planning, and implementation process, setting objectives and preparing a budget for training occur during:
   A. Step 1
   B. Step 2
   C. Step 3
   D. Step 4

5. In the ADDIE model for the training, planning, and implementation process, conducting an assessment to identify learning needs occurs at:
   A. Step 1
   B. Step 2
   C. Step 4
   D. Step 5

6. A need for conflict management training for supervisors has been identified. Which of the following would be the training delivery method of choice?
   A. Self-paced learning
   B. Video-conference
   C. Classroom-style learning
   D. Computer-based learning

7. In a structured on-the-job-training process, "Check frequently and encourage questions" would occur during which of the following?
   A. Step 1: Prepare the employee
   B. Step 2: Present the operation
   C. Step 3: Try out performance
   D. Step 4: Follow up

8. An example of an employee's role in the career development and career planning process would be to:
   A. Complete the Department of Labor's O*Net online occupational and career assessment
   B. Provide coaching and mentoring
   C. Connect job performance, training needs, and career interests during performance appraisal
   D. Refer to organizational career planning resources

Real-World Case 20.1

A busy HIM supervisor with a limited understanding of what a release of information (ROI) specialist does was asked to make a hiring decision for the position at his hospital. A bright woman interviewed well, her references checked out, and she was hired. The new employee participated in general hospital orientation. In a rush to get the employee started, she was given a brief introduction to the job. The normal high-volume of requests for information continued over her first three months on the job, but the processing rate slowed dramatically. Complaints came in to the HIM supervisor's manager. During her 90-day probationary interview, the new employee was given a written warning to speed up. She complained that she did not receive the same training on ROI processing procedures or systems as provided to other staff. She threatened to file a grievance then abruptly quit. A job opening notice is once again posted.

Real-World Case 20.2

Maxine has been a coder with the hospital for nearly 15 years. She has been exceedingly loyal and hard working. Her performance record had been outstanding, until this past year. The transition to computer-assisted coding has not gone well for her. Other coders in the department have made the shift in job duties to auditing and clinical documentation improvement. She has not been comfortable with these changes, particularly the new technology, and her productivity has decreased compared to coding quality and quantity performance benchmarks. The manager went easy on Maxine during the last performance appraisal cycle due to the change in job description and in light of her outstanding personal qualities. Recently, another coder came to the manager to voice concern that she might be expected to pick up the slack for Maxine. Something will need to be done soon to address the performance issue and prevent additional staff issues. Maxine is getting older; she has seniority with the organization, but is not yet at retirement age.

References

American Health Information Management Association. 2015a. Certification Exam Prep. http://www.ahima.org/education/onlineed/Programs/examprep.

American Health Information Management Association. 2015b. VLab Overview. http://www.ahima.org/education/vlab?tabid=overview.

American Health Information Management Association. 2015c. Career and Student Center. http://www.ahima.org/careers.

American Health Information Management Association. 2013a. Recruitment, Selection, and Orientation for CDI Specialists. *Journal of AHIMA.* 84(7):58–62 [expanded web version]. http://library.ahima.org/doc?oid=106800#.Vxk06PkrK9I.

American Health Information Management Association. 2013b. Release of Information Toolkit. http://library.ahima.org/doc?oid=106371#.Vxk00vkrK9I.

Appendix I Release of Information Specialist Job Description, 56–58. http://library.ahima.org/doc?oid=106371#.Vxk0tfkrK9I.

American Health Information Management Association. 2011. American Health Information Management Association Code of Ethics. http://library.ahima.org/doc?oid=105098#.Vxk0nfkrK9I.

Beauchamp, T.L. and J.F. Childress. 2013. *Principles of Biomedical Ethics,* 7th ed. New York: Oxford University Press.

Branham, L. 2005 (February). The Seven Hidden Reasons Employees Leave. *Executive Update.* American Society of Association Executives (ASAE). http://www.asaecenter.org/Resources/EUArticle.cfm?ItemNumber=11514.

Brodnik, M.S. and M. Sharp. 2012. Chapter 12 in *Fundamentals of Law for Health Informatics and Information Management,* 2nd ed., revised reprint. Edited by M.S. Brodnik, L.A. Rinehart-Thompson, and R.B. Reynolds. Chicago: AHIMA.

Bureau of Labor Statistics (BLS). 2015 (January 23). Union Membership (Annual) News Release. http://www.bls.gov/news.release/union2.htm.

Bureau of Labor Statistics (BLS). 2014a. The Economics Daily. Largest industries by state, 1990–2013. http://www.bls.gov/opub/ted/2014/ted_20140728.htm.

Bureau of Labor Statistics (BLS). 2014b. Occupational Outlook Handbook, Medical Records and Health Information Technicians. http://www.bls.gov/ooh/healthcare/medical-records-and-health-information-technicians.htm.

Carrell, M. and C. Heavrin. 2013. Chapter 4 in *Labor Relations and Collective Bargaining: Private and Public Sectors,* 10th ed. Upper Saddle River, NJ: Pearson.

Caviart Group, LLC. 2015. A Workforce Study of the Future Direction and Skill Set for HIM Professionals. Prepared for AHIMA. http://bok.ahima.org/PdfView?oid=300801.

Desai, A. 2015. Scanning the HIM Environment: AHIMA's 2015 report offers insight on emerging industry trends and challenges. *Journal of AHIMA.* 86(5):38–43.

Dessler, G. 2014. *Fundamentals of Human Resource Management,* 3rd ed. Upper Saddle River, NJ: Pearson.

DeVault, K. 2012. Best Practices for Coding Productivity: Assessing Productivity in ICD-9 to Prepare for ICD-10. *Journal of AHIMA.* 83(7):72–74.

Elsdon, R. 2010. Building Workforce Strength: Creating Value through Workforce and Career Development. Santa Barbara, CA, USA: ABC-CLIO. ProQuest ebrary.

Equal Employment Opportunity Commission (EEOC). 2015a. Equal Pay/Compensation Discrimination. http://www.eeoc.gov/laws/types/equalcompensation.cfm.

Equal Employment Opportunity Commission (EEOC). 2015b. Title VII of the Civil Rights Act of 1964. http://www.eeoc.gov/laws/statutes/titlevii.cfm.

Equal Employment Opportunity Commission (EEOC). 2015c. Facts About Race/Color Discrimination. http://www.eeoc.gov/eeoc/publications/fs-race.cfm.

Equal Employment Opportunity Commission (EEOC). 2015d. Harassment. http://www.eeoc.gov/laws/types/harassment.cfm.

Equal Employment Opportunity Commission (EEOC). 2015e. The Pregnancy Discrimination Act of 1978. http://www.eeoc.gov/laws/statutes/pregnancy.cfm.

Equal Employment Opportunity Commission (EEOC). 2015f. The Age Discrimination in Employment Act of 1967. http://www.eeoc.gov/laws/statutes/adea.cfm.

Filerman, G.L., A.E. Mills, and P.M. Schyve, eds. 2014. *Managerial Ethics in Healthcare: A New Perspective.* Chicago: Health Administration Press.

Folkman, J. 2014 (February 19). "Should I Tell You The Good News First?" The Feedback Employees Most Want To Hear. http://www.forbes.com/sites/joefolkman/2014/02/19/should-i-tell-you-the-good-news-first-the-feedback-employees-most-want-to-hear/.

Frauenheim, E. 2009. Downturn Puts New Emphasis on Engagement. *Workforce*. http://www.workforce.com/articles/downturn-puts-new-emphasis-on-engagement.

Fried, B.J. and M.D. Fottler, eds. 2015. *Human Resources in Healthcare: Managing for Success*, 4th ed. Chicago: Health Administration Press.

Fried, B.J. and M.D. Fottler, eds. 2011. *Fundamentals of Human Resources in Healthcare*. Chicago: Health Administration Press.

Gomez-Mejia, L.R., D. Balkin, and R. Cardy. 2012. *Managing Human Resources*, 7th ed. Upper Saddle River, NJ: Pearson.

Gurrieri, J.J. and K.M. Karban. 2013. The good, bad, and reality of offshore coding: Some turn to distant shores to fill US coding demands. *Journal of AHIMA*. 84(9):44–48.

Harman, L.B. 2006. *Ethical Challenges in the Management of Health Information*, 2nd ed. Sudbury, MA: Jones & Bartlett Learning.

Henderson, R. 2013. Industry Employment and Output Projections to 2022. *Monthly Labor Review*. US Department of Labor, Bureau of Labor Statistics. http://www.bls.gov/opub/mlr/2013/article/industry-employment-and-output-projections-to-2022.htm#top.

Hicks, S., M. Peters, and M. Smith. 2006. Orientation redesign. *T + D* 60, (7) (07): 43-45,4.

Hirschmann, C. 2008. Giving Voice to Employee Concerns. *HR Magazine*. 53(8). http://www.shrm.org/publications/hrmagazine/editorialcontent/pages/0808hirscman.aspx.

HR Specialist. 2011 (September 6). The 5 worst interview questions … and what to ask instead. *Business Management Daily*. http://www.thehrspecialist.com/print.aspx?id=39435&cat=.

Juran, J. M. 1995. *Managerial Breakthrough: The Classic Book On Improving Management Performance*. Universals for Breakthrough and Control. New York: McGraw-Hill.

LeBlanc, M.M. 2016. Chapter 22 in *Health Information Management: Concepts Principles and Practice*, 5th ed. Edited by P.K. Oachs and A.L. Watters. Chicago: AHIMA.

McNair, J.H., W. Anglade, and R. Smith. 2007 (March 23). Litigating non-economic compensatory damages: How do you piece together lives shattered by workplace discrimination? Compensatory damages—Maybe, maybe not. *ABA National Conference on EEO Law*. http://www.americanbar.org/content/dam/aba/administrative/labor_law/meetings/2007/2007_eeo_mcnair.authcheckdam.pdf.

McWay, D. 2016. Chapter 15 in *Legal and Ethical Aspects of Health Information Management*, 4th ed. Clifton Park, NY: Cengage Learning.

Mondy, R.W. 2015. *Human Resource Management*, 13th ed. Upper Saddle River, NJ: Pearson.

Muhl, C.J. 2001 (January). The Employment-at-Will Doctrine: Three Major Exceptions. *Monthly Labor Review*. http://www.bls.gov/opub/mlr/2001/01/art1full.pdf.

National Institutes of Health (NIH). 2013. Human Genome Project. http://report.nih.gov/nihfactsheets/ViewFactSheet.aspx?csid=45.

National Labor Relations Act (NLRA). 1935. USC 151-169. https://www.nlrb.gov/resources/national-labor-relations-act.

National Labor Relations Board (NLRB). 2015a. Employer/Union Rights and Obligations. http://www.nlrb.gov/rights-we-protect/employerunion-rights-and-obligations.

National Labor Relations Board (NLRB). 2015b. Your Rights During Union Organizing. http://www.nlrb.gov/rights-we-protect/whats-law/employees/i-am-not-represented-union/your-rights-during-union-organizing.

National Labor Relations Board v. Kentucky River Community Care, Inc. 532 US 706; 121 S. Ct. 1861; 149 L. Ed. 2d 939 (2001).

Oachs, P.K. 2016. Chapter 24 in *Health Information Management: Concepts Principles and Practice*, 5th ed. Edited by P.K. Oachs and A.L. Watters. Chicago: AHIMA.

Occupational Safety and Health Administration (OSHA). 2004. Occupational Health and Safety Act of 1970, Public Law 91-596. https://www.osha.gov/pls/oshaweb/owadisp.show_document?p_table=OSHACT&p_id=2743.

Office of Personnel Management. 2015. Assessment and Selection, Job Analysis. Six Steps to Conducting a Job Analysis. http://www.opm.gov/policy-data-oversight/assessment-and-selection/job-analysis/.

Patena, K.R. 2016. Chapter 23 in *Health Information Management: Concepts Principles and Practice,* 5th ed. Edited by P.K. Oachs and A.L. Watters. Chicago: AHIMA.

Paton, R. 2000. *The Human Equation: Building Profits by Putting People First* by Jeffrey Pfeffer, reviewed. *Human Resource Management Journal.* 10(2):91–92.

Richards, E. and D. Terkanian. 2013. Occupational Employment Projections to 2022. Bureau of Labor Statistics, US Department of Labor. http://www.bls.gov/opub/mlr/2013/article/occupational-employment-projections-to-2022.htm.

Schermerhorn, J.R. 2014. *Exploring Management,* 4th ed. Hoboken, NJ: John Wiley & Sons.

Sharp, A. and P. McDermott. 2009. *Workflow Modeling: Tools for Process Improvement and Applications Development,* 2nd ed. Norwood, MA: Artech House, ProQuest ebrary.

Society for Human Resource Management (SHRM). 2015a. Glossaries. http://www.shrm.org/templatestools/glossaries/hrterms/pages/h.aspx.

Society for Human Resource Management (SHRM). 2015b. Uniform Guidelines on Employee Selection Procedures of 1978. http://www.shrm.org/legalissues/federalresources/federalstatutesregulationsandguidanc/pages/uniformguidelinesonselectionprocedures.aspx#sthash.IXL6wtRR.dpuf.

Society for Human Resource Management (SHRM). 2014. Managing Employee Performance. Toolkits. http://www.shrm.org/templatestools/toolkits/pages/managingemployeeperformance.aspx.

Society for Human Resource Management (SHRM). 2013. Family and Medical Leave Act (FMLA) of 1993. http://www.shrm.org/legalissues/federalresources/federalstatutesregulationsandguidanc/pages/familyandmedicalleaveactof1993.aspx.

Society for Human Resource Management (SHRM). 2008. Employee Retirement Income Security Act (ERISA) of 1974. http://www.shrm.org/legalissues/federalresources/federalstatutesregulationsandguidanc/pages/employeeretirementincomesecurityact%28erisa%29of1974.aspx.

Sutton, V. 2013. Acing Your Interview with Valerie Sutton. Understanding Interview Formats. Video course. Lynda.com, Inc.

Tooley, P. 2007. Release of information: Strategies to maximize customer service, productivity, and revenue with release of information activity tracking Form. *Proceedings of AHIMA's 79th National Convention and Exhibit.* Philadelphia, PA.

United Nations. 1948. The Universal Declaration of Human Rights. Article 23. http://www.un.org/en/universal-declaration-human-rights/index.html.

US Department of Labor (DOL). 2015a. Disability Resources, Laws, and Regulations. http://www.dol.gov/dol/topic/disability/laws.htm.

US Department of Labor (DOL). 2015b. Employment and Training Administration. O*NET OnLine. http://www.onetonline.org.

US Department of Labor (DOL), Wage and Hour Division. 2014. Handy Reference Guide to the Fair Labor Standards Act. http://www.dol.gov/whd/regs/compliance/hrg.htm.

U.S. Department of Labor (DOL). 2013. Employee Benefits Security Administration (EBSA) Fact Sheet. Consolidated Omnibus Budget Reconciliation Act (COBRA). http://www.dol.gov/ebsa/newsroom/fscobra.html.

US Department of Labor (DOL), Wage and Hour Division. 2012. Fact Sheet #28: The Family Medical Leave Act. http://www.dol.gov/whd/regs/compliance/whdfs28.pdf.

US Department of Labor (DOL), Wage and Hour Division. 2008. Fact Sheet #17A: Exemption for Executive, Administrative, Professional, Computer and Outside Sales Employees under the Fair Labor Standards Act (FLSA). http://www.dol.gov/whd/overtime/fs17a_overview.pdf.

21

Ethical Issues in Health Information Management

Leslie L. Gordon, MS, RHIA, FAHIMA
Morley L. Gordon, RHIT

Learning Objectives

- Explain ethics and ethical dilemmas
- Interpret the concepts of morality, code of conduct, and moral judgment
- Explain the AHIMA Code of Ethics
- Differentiate how cultural issues affect health and healthcare quality, cost, and health information management

- Evaluate the consequences of a breach of healthcare ethics
- Identify ethical issues related to research
- Identify the process of ethical decision making
- Evaluate cultural diversity policies and programs

Key Terms

Autonomy
Beneficence
Bias
Blanket authorization
Breach
Code of ethics
Confidentiality
Culture
Cultural audit
Cultural competence
Cultural diversity

Cultural competence
Double billing
Ethical principles
Ethics
Ethics committee
Integrity
Leadership
Managed care
Medical identity theft
Moral values
Need-to-know principle

Nonmaleficence
Prejudice
Privacy
Quality
Respect
Retrospective documentation
Security
Stereotyping
Unbundling
Upcoding
Values

The phrase "first do no harm" is well known in healthcare as a long standing code of conduct for medical professionals. First and foremost, the goal of a healthcare professional is to not cause harm to those being treated; the legal term is **nonmaleficence**. Health information management (HIM) professionals are guided by a similar code of conduct and adhere to a professional **code of ethics**, a set of principles regarding business practices and professional behavior (described in detail in this chapter). HIM professionals do not have direct patient care contact but they do interact with patients in terms of coding, release of information, data quality, and so forth. **Ethics** is a field of study dealing with moral principles, theories, and values. In healthcare, ethics involves formal decision making needed to deal with competing perspectives and obligations of the people who have an interest in a common problem.

An individual has the right to determine what does or does not happen to him or her in terms of healthcare. **Autonomy** is a core ethical principle centered on this fact, meaning a patient has the right to choose his or her course of treatment. A clinical application of this concept is a cancer patient's right to refuse chemotherapy, radiation, or surgical treatment. **Beneficence** is a legal term that means promoting good for others or providing services that benefit others, such as releasing health information that will help a patient receive care or will ensure payment of services received.

People are guided by their own sets of values and ethical principles according to their personal beliefs and cultural upbringing. It is important for HIM professionals to understand cultural competency and diversity to help guide their interactions in the workplace as well as when associating with patients. Understanding a person's background, culture, beliefs, and values makes it possible to comprehend why they act in a certain way and can help guide professional interactions. This chapter explores the individual moral values and ethical principles of people and defines cultural competence in the healthcare environment. The ethical foundations of HIM include ethical issues related to medical identify theft, ethical decision making, and breach of healthcare ethics. Finally, important HIM specific ethical problems are addressed. Ethical issues related to labor and employment laws can be found in chapter 20.

Moral Values and Ethical Principles

Moral values are a system of principles, usually with regard to right or wrong, by which an individual guides his or her life (AHIMA 2015). In healthcare, employees need to be mindful of the moral values of the people with whom they work, including fellow employees and patients. The moral values people hold can be deeply seeded in who they are as a person which can cause conflict with others who hold opposing values. As an HIM professional it is also important to understand **ethical principles** to help with decision making and understand why others may make the decisions they do. The following principles explain the ways in which ethical decisions are made.

- *Altruism:* This is the belief that other people are more important than an individual person, wherein a personal sacrifice must take place. An example would be donating a kidney to a complete stranger (Allen 2013).

- *Autonomy*: Autonomy is an individual's right to self-determination, or a patient having the right to decide what does or does not happen to him or her (AHIMA 2015).

- *Beneficence*: Beneficence is promoting good for others or providing services that benefit others; for example, releasing health information to help a patient receive further care (AHIMA 2015).

- *Consequentialism*: Consequentialism considers the consequences before making a decision and is based on the end result; for example, when documenting in a patient chart, a provider understands that certain medical codes receive higher reimbursement, but the consequence of miscoding could result in legal charges against the provider.

- *Deontology*: Deontology is the duty or responsibility guiding the decision based on action and not the end result; for example, a department policy may indicate that an original signed court order must be obtained before health records can be released and a release of information (ROI) clerk is presented with a copy of the court order and not the original. The clerk knows that some employees will process the release without question, however she denies the request without the original court order. She believes it is her duty to follow the exact policy of the department (Allen 2013).

- *Egoism:* Instead of taking others into consideration, egoism involves only considering oneself in the decision-making process; for example, a person donating blood plasma for money during a financial emergency, not to help people in need.

- *Least harm:* Least harm occurs with situations where two choices may be less than ideal. One should choose the situation that will do the least amount of harm to the fewest number of people; for example, a physician choosing to treat the patient in the emergency room with the greatest chance for survival instead of the patient with more severe or life threatening injuries.

- *Utilitarianism:* Utilitarianism deals with situations that may provide the greatest benefit to the most people; for example one person's organ donations can benefit many (Allen 2013).

Ethical decision making involves consideration of what is right and what is wrong based on a code of conduct or behavior. An ethical dilemma occurs when one is faced with a choice between two or more situations—for example, should life support be discontinued or continued, or who decides which patient will receive a single kidney. An HIM professional who has strong beliefs against assisted suicide may not be comfortable working in a state where it is legal and at an organization where it is practiced.

Many ethical decisions are based on one's **culture**, which include the values, beliefs, attitudes, languages, symbols, rituals, behaviors, and customs unique to a particular group of people (Simmers et al. 2014). **Values** include the social and cultural belief system of a person or a healthcare organization. Culture is learned, shared, social in nature, dynamic, and changing, meaning people generally have similar beliefs and values based on their upbringing—what they were taught by parents, peers, and surroundings. The values of an individual can change over time based on varying environments and social networks. For example, a student who leaves home for the first time to go away to college will be exposed to new and different experiences, and as a result the values developed at home may shift and reflect those from his or her college environment.

Cultural Competence in the Healthcare Environment

Cultural competence is the ability to accept and understand the beliefs and values of other people and groups and is vital to the overall health of an organization, whereas **cultural diversity** is the perceived or actual difference among people. For example, to express cultural competence is the ability to accept a transgender person by the pronoun (he or she) by which the individual identifies. Accepting diversity and the inclusion of all people is important to cultural competence and acceptance. Culture includes the following:

- Ethnicity (classification of people based on national origin or culture)
- Socioeconomic status (classification of people based on economic or social welfare status)
- Religion

- Gender or gender identity
- Sexual orientation
- Age
- Education
- Occupation

Attitudes that affect one's cultural competence include prejudice, stereotyping, and bias. **Prejudice** occurs when a person is judged solely based on one of the cultural factors listed previously, for example liking a person because she has green eyes. **Stereotyping** is an assumption that everyone within a certain group are the same; for example, believing surgeons are difficult to communicate with. A **bias** prevents a person from having an impartial judgment; for example, only watching news from one side of the political spectrum.

Healthcare professionals should be mindful of the differences in culture, beliefs, and values of other people particularly co-workers and patients, and avoid prejudice, stereotyping, and bias. This can be done by exploring different cultures, values, and beliefs; trying to understand why people believe and act the way they do; and being sensitive to other cultures (Simmers et al. 2014). The following sections will introduce HIM professionals to cultural issues and the effects on health, healthcare quality, and cost. They introduce cultural competence by helping to identify self-awareness of one's own culture perception, describing training programs related to expanding culture in the workplace, and exploring regulations in regard to cultural competence.

Cultural Disparities in US Healthcare

Many factors have an effect on health and healthcare including health status, disease risk factors, and access to healthcare, and all are influenced by the culture in which people live. The World Health Organization (WHO) defines the social determinants of health as the conditions into which persons are born, grow, live, work, and age (WHO 2012). Health disparities exist disproportionately in certain populations. Data shows that residents in mostly minority communities have lower socioeconomic status, greater barriers to healthcare access, and greater risks for disease compared with the general population (Meyer et al. 2013).

The United States Department of Health and Human Services Office of Minority Health established national standards for culturally and linguistically appropriate services (CLAS) in health and healthcare with the intention to advance health quality, improve quality of care, and help eliminate healthcare disparities in the United States. The principal standard is to provide effective, equitable, understandable, and respectful quality care while being responsive to diverse cultural beliefs and practices, preferred languages, health literacy and other communication needs (HHS n.d.).

Healthcare Professionals and Cultural Competence

Healthcare professionals nationally are struggling to respond to the needs of people from diverse groups and incorporating cultural competence in healthcare settings has many benefits to patients (Goode and Dunne 2003). The following are some of the reasons to incorporate cultural competence into organizational policies and procedures.

- To reflect the current and projected demographic changes in the United States.

- To eliminate long-standing disparities in the health status of people of diverse racial, ethnic, and cultural backgrounds. The disparities in the incidence of illness and death among people of certain ethnicities is related to the bias, stereotyping, and prejudice on the part of healthcare providers; and incorporation of cultural competence can help improve the disparities (Goode and Dunne 2003).

- To improve the quality of health services and outcomes. Healthcare providers who are culturally competent provide a higher level of patient satisfaction, health outcomes, and higher levels of preventative care (Goode and Dunne 2003).

- To meet legislative, regulatory, and accreditation mandates.
- To gain a competitive edge in the market place.
- To decrease the likelihood of liability or malpractice claims (NCCC 2015).

Cultural competence for an entire healthcare organization means the institution and its employees have the capacity to:

- Value diversity
- Conduct self-assessments to determine the attitudes, practices, and policies of the organization, meaning both the organization as a whole conducts a self-assessment and employees individually assess themselves to align with the culture and attitude of the organization
- Manage the dynamics of difference
- Acquire and institutionalize cultural knowledge
- Adapt to the diversity and cultural context of the communities served (Goode et al. 2002).

Assessing the cultural awareness and competence of a healthcare organization's employees involves training to help employees understand their own attitudes and practices toward cultural awareness, as well as understanding and practicing the policies of the organization. Healthcare organizations conduct ongoing assessments of their progress toward reaching the goals of CLAS-related activities with the purpose of assessing performance, monitoring progress, obtaining information about the organization and customers, and assessing the value of activities that fulfill governance, leadership, and workforce responsibilities (HHS n.d.). One of the assessments an organization measures includes the accessibility of interpreters for people who speak a language other than English, including American sign language. Many organizations maintain lists of interpreters who can be called to help communicate with patients. The assessment is part of an organization's continuous quality improvement activities. Table 21.1 is a sample of measures in performance improvement and outcomes assessments.

Healthcare Organization Cultural Competence Awareness

Addressing how one views language, communication style, belief systems, customs, attitudes, perceptions, and values in others is a way to assess personal cultural competence. Each employee of the healthcare organization should honestly determine if he or she has biases and assess if those biases affect his or her actions and thinking toward fellow employees, patients, healthcare providers, and vendors.

Healthcare professionals should also assess their department's strengths and weaknesses in the area of accepting diversity. It is important for healthcare organizations to educate and train employees in the areas of diversity and cultural competence. For example, the manager of an HIM department should provide training to employees on acceptance, understanding, and tolerance for others. They can do this by exploring a specific culture or ethnicity and helping to

Table 21.1 Assessment of culture and linguistic competency

Continuous quality improvement program assessment of cultural and linguistic competency			
Monitor and assess the organization's performance for the prior year in the areas listed	Outcome	Assessment	Plan
Accessibility of interpreter services	Interpreter needed 100 times	Sign language interpreter was not available five times	Hire sign language interpreter
Effectiveness of culture and linguistic competency training for providers	Training provided twice per year	Five healthcare providers did not attend training	Follow up with all providers once per year to confirm training is completed

Adapted from: HHS n.d.

understand why people may act the way they do (for instance, in some cultures a person will not make eye contact with a member of the opposite sex unless it is a close family member). The following are examples of how an organization can encourage employees and everyone who does business with the organization to improve the cultural acceptance with all who are in contact with the organization.

- Challenge colleagues when they make racial, ethnic, or sexually offensive comments or jokes; for example, if a fellow employee is overheard telling a racially-toned joke, other co-workers should let the employee know the behavior is unacceptable.

- Humans by nature are social beings and strive to be with others, and people tend to socialize with those similar to them. Actively seek to connect with people who are different and include diversity in social circles. For example, many people are comfortable with the same group of co-workers and friends while having lunch. Inviting new people to the group increases cultural competence of the group, which positively affects the organization.

- Do not make assumptions about a person before the facts are verified. For example, if a new person is hired in the HIM department and speaks broken English, a co-worker without cultural awareness may assume the new person is not able to perform the job functions because of the language barrier, when in fact he or she may be able to perform the job well.

An understanding and sensitivity to the beliefs and cultures of others can help alleviate misunderstanding and offenses that may happen because someone has not been trained to be sensitive. For example, a cultural miscommunication may occur when a supervisor accentuates the positive attributes of an employee and minimizes the negatives, which leads the employee who is accustomed to direct and honest (even when negative) feedback to think he or she is doing a comprehensively great job.

Training Programs

Cultural awareness training for all employees is an important component of an organization's overall cultural competence. By providing training, healthcare professionals will gain the knowledge, skills, and abilities to understand peoples' beliefs and culture. A **cultural audit** is a strategy to define an organization's values, symbols, and routines, and identify areas for improvement. To perform a cultural audit an organization assesses the availability of interpreter services, the effectiveness and availability of cultural training provided to staff, and determines if there are differences in the services provided to diverse populations. The organization may also evaluate the health outcomes and health status of diverse populations to determine if cultural competency training and awareness helps change the outcomes for patients over time. This list is not comprehensive and organizations may use others methods to perform a cultural audit.

Healthcare organizations have established continuous quality improvement programs to measure the quality of a service or product through systems or process evaluation and implementation of revised processes that result in better healthcare outcomes. (Quality improvement is discussed in greater detail in chapter 18). Organizations incorporate CLAS measures into their ongoing quality improvement activities to determine how well they assess cultural competence.

Regulations for Cultural Awareness

Legal responsibilities of healthcare organizations, as determined by federal law, prohibit discrimination based on ethnicity, religious faith, physical disability, or age. By incorporating cultural awareness training and monitoring across the spectrum of business, a healthcare organization abides by the laws prohibiting discrimination of employees, patients, vendors, or anyone who may have contact with the organization. The Equal Employment Opportunity Commission (EEOC) was established to help provide equal employment opportunities for minority groups, women, people with disabilities, and veterans. Healthcare organizations must follow federal regulations and laws to remain in compliance. Chapter 20 contains more information on employment law.

Check Your Understanding 21.1

Instructions: **Answer the following questions by matching the term with the definition.**

1. _____ Duty or responsibility guiding the decision based on action and not the end result
2. _____ The socioeconomic or religious differences in people
3. _____ The individual's right to determine what does or does not happen to him or her in terms of healthcare
4. _____ Only considering oneself instead of taking others into consideration
5. _____ System of principles by which an individual guides his or her life, usually with regards to right and wrong
6. _____ Field of study dealing with moral principles, theories, and values
7. _____ To not cause harm
8. _____ Promoting good for others or providing services that benefit others

A. Egoism
B. Moral value
C. Nonmalificence
D. Deontology
E. Beneficence
F. Autonomy
G. Ethics
H. Cultural diversity

Ethical Foundations of Health Information Management

Ethical principles and values have been important to the HIM profession since its inception in 1928. The first ethical pledge was presented in 1934 by Grace Whiting Myers, a visionary leader who recognized the importance of protecting information in medical records. The HIM profession was launched with recognition of the importance of privacy and the requirement of an authorization for the release of health information:

> I pledge myself to give out no information from any clinical record placed in my charge, or from any other source to any person whatsoever, except upon order from the chief executive officer of the institution which I may be serving. (Huffman 1972, 135)

Today, it is the patient who authorizes the release of his or her health information and not the chief executive officer (CEO) of the healthcare organization, as stated in the original pledge. The most important values embedded in this pledge are to protect patient privacy and confidential information and to recognize the importance of the HIM professional as a moral agent in protecting patient information. The HIM professional has a clear ethical and professional obligation not to give any information to anyone unless the release has been authorized (Harman 2012). Release of information is discussed in detail in chapter 3.

HIM professionals are responsible for the protection of patient privacy, confidentiality, and maintaining the security and control of health records. It is important to understand these terms, as they are sometimes used interchangeably (Harman 2012).

- **Privacy** is the right of a patient to control the disclosure of protected health information (PHI) and includes the freedom from unauthorized intrusion in healthcare.
- **Confidentiality** is a legal and ethical concept that requires healthcare providers to protect health records and other personal and private information from unauthorized use or disclosure.
- **Security** is the means to control and protect access of health information and records (AHIMA 2015).

Professionals working in the HIM field are guided by the ethical foundations of privacy, confidentiality, and security that are detailed in a professional code of ethics that outlines values and obligations for HIM professionals. Ethical issues related to medical identity theft, ethical decision-making questions, and specific ethical problems encountered by HIM professionals are explored in detail in the following sections.

Professional Code of Ethics for the Health Information Management Professional

A professional code of ethics is adopted by an organization to guide the members in determining right and wrong conduct when performing the duties of their job. The American Health Information Management Association (AHIMA) Code of Ethics applies to all AHIMA members and is based on the core values of the association. The preamble to the AHIMA Code of Ethics states:

> The ethical obligations of the HIM professional include the safeguarding of privacy and security of health information; disclosure of health information; development, use, and maintenance of health information systems and health information; and ensuring the accessibility and integrity of health information.

> Healthcare consumers are increasingly concerned about security and the potential loss of privacy and the inability to control how their personal health information is used and disclosed. Core health information issues include what information should be collected; how the information should be handled, who should have access to the information, under what conditions the information should

be disclosed, how the information is retained and when it is no longer needed, and how is it disposed of in a confidential manner. All of the core health information issues are performed in compliance with state and federal regulations, and employer policies and procedures.

> Ethical obligations are central to the professional's responsibility, regardless of the employment site or the method of collection, storage, and security of health information. In addition, sensitive information (for example, genetic, adoption, drug, alcohol, sexual, health, and behavioral information) requires special attention to prevent misuse. In the world of business and interactions with consumers, expertise in the protection of the information is required (AHIMA 2011).

HIM professionals have access to sensitive information contained within the health record. Patients trust the information they share with their healthcare provider will be protected. When a celebrity or well-known person receives care, his or her protected health information has a value to the media and may be sold by people without ethical values.

The HIM professional is obligated to demonstrate actions that reflect values, ethical principles, and the ethical guidelines. The seven purposes listed in table 21.2 are descriptions of the values and principles used to guide the conduct of HIM professionals. The code includes enforceable core principles and guidelines. Alleged violation of ethical principles is taken very seriously by AHIMA and reviewed by a team dedicated to that purpose.

Professional Values and Obligations

HIM professionals are ethically responsible for preserving, protecting, and securing health information in all mediums. The professional values AHIMA identifies as important are quality, integrity, respect, and leadership and are demonstrated as follows.

- **Quality:** An abiding commitment to innovation, relevance, and continuous improvement in programs, products, and services
- **Integrity:** Openness in decision making, honesty in communication and activity, and ethical practices that command trust and support collaboration

Table 21.2   AHIMA Code of Ethics

The Code of Ethics serves seven purposes
1. Promote high standards of HIM practice
2. Identify core values on which the HIM mission is based
3. Summarize broad ethical principles that reflect the profession's core values
4. Establish a set of ethical principles to be used to guide decision making and actions
5. Establish a framework for professional behavior and responsibilities when professional obligations conflict or ethical uncertainties arise
6. Provide ethical principles by which the general public can hold the HIM professional accountable
7. Mentor practitioners new to the field to HIM's mission, values, and ethical principles

Principles and guidelines form the foundation of the Code of Ethics	
Principle	**Example**
1. Advocate, uphold, and defend the individual's right to privacy and the doctrine of confidentiality in the use and disclosure of information.	Safeguard all confidential patient information to include, but not limited to, personal, health financial, genetic, and outcome information
2. Put service and the health and welfare of persons before self-interest and conduct oneself in the practice of the profession so as to bring honor to oneself, peers, and to the health information management profession.	Act with integrity, behave in a trustworthy manner, elevate service to others above self-interest and promote high standards of practice in every setting
3. Preserve, protect, and secure personal health information in any form or medium and hold in the highest regards health information and other information of a confidential nature obtained in an official capacity, taking into account the applicable statutes and regulations.	Take precautions to ensure and maintain the confidentiality of information transmitted to other parties through the use of any media, transferred, or disposed of in the event of termination, incapacitation, or death of a healthcare provider
4. Refuse to participate in or conceal unethical practices or procedures and report such practices.	Act in a professional and ethical manner at all times
5. Advance health information management knowledge and practice through continuing education, research, publications and presentations.	Develop and enhance continually professional expertise, knowledge, and skills (including appropriate education, research, training, consultation, and supervision); contribute to the knowledge base of health information management and share one's knowledge related to practice, research, and ethics
6. Recruit and mentor students, staff, peers, and colleagues to develop and strengthen professional workforce.	Provide directed practice opportunities for students
7. Represent the profession to the public in a positive manner.	Be an advocate for the profession in all settings and participate in activities that promote and explain the mission, values, and principles of the profession to the public
8. Perform honorably health information management association responsibilities, either appointed or elected, and preserve the confidentiality of any privileged information made known in any official capacity.	Perform responsibly all duties as assigned by the professional association operating within bylaws and policies and procedures of the association and any pertinent laws
9. State truthfully and accurately one's credentials, professional education, and experiences.	Claim only those relevant professional credentials actually possessed and correct any inaccuracies occurring regarding credentials
10. Facilitate interdisciplinary collaboration in situations supporting health information practice.	Foster trust among group members and adjust behavior in order to establish relationships with teams
11. Respect the inherent dignity and worth of every person.	Treat each person in a respectful fashion, being mindful of individual differences and cultural and ethnic diversity

Adapted from: AHIMA 2011.

- **Respect**: Appreciation of the value of differing perspectives, enjoyable experiences, courteous interaction, and celebration of achievements that advance our common cause

- **Leadership**: Visionary thinking, decisions responsive to membership and mission, and accountability for actions and outcomes (AHIMA 2015)

An HIM professional's ethical obligations as out-lined by the AHIMA standards include duty to the patient and the healthcare team to protect health information, provide service to those who seek access to their information, preserve and secure health information, promote the quality and advancement of healthcare, and function within the scope of responsibility and restrain from pass-ing clinical judgment (AHIMA 2011). Obligations also include those to the employer such as loyalty; protection of committee deliberations (for exam-ple, a committee may make decisions related to who will receive an organ donation from a dona-tion list, and those deliberations are protected much like patient information); compliance with all laws, regulations, and policies that govern the health information system; recognizing the authority and power of the job responsibilities; and to accept compensation only in relationship to work responsibilities. Ethical obligations to

the public include advocating change when pat-terns or system problems are not in the best inter-est of the patients, reporting violations of practice standards to the proper authorities, and promot-ing interdisciplinary cooperation and collabora-tion. Finally, ethical obligations to self, peers, and professional associations include being honest about degrees, credentials, and work experiences; bringing honor to oneself by committing to life-long learning; strengthening HIM membership in AHIMA and state associations; representing the HIM profession to the public; and promoting and participating in HIM research (Harman 2012).

HIM professionals are ethically obligated to give back to the HIM community by providing practice opportunities for students, such as being involved in student professional practice experience opportuni-ties. HIM professionals also have a responsibility to pass on knowledge to and mentor new health infor-mation management professionals and students.

Ethical Issues Related to Medical Identity Theft

Identity theft is illegally obtaining another person's personal information and using it to commit theft or fraud, usually for the purpose of financial trans-actions. **Medical identify theft** is the fraudulent use of an individual's identifying information in a healthcare setting. This fraudulent information in a health record corrupts the record with erroneous information and can lead to incorrect diagnosis and treatment (McNabb and Rhodes 2014). The two primary ways medical identity theft happens is (1) consensual, or knowingly sharing information, and (2) nonconsensual, when someone unknown to the victim, or without the victims permission, uses his or her information. A thief may use another person's insurance information, including Social Security numbers, to see a doctor, obtain prescrip-tion drugs, or fraudulently bill for healthcare ser-vices. Medical identity theft can be difficult to detect because people do not always pay close attention to their medical bills and insurance claims. If health-care professionals do not recognize this impact on

patient records and do not fix the error, the theft can remain on the record of the patient, potentially causing misdiagnosis or treatment (McNabb and Rhodes 2014). For example, consider a thief using a patient's insurance card to obtain prescription drugs from multiple providers and pharmacies. The patient is unaware of this use; months later the patient returns to his provider and needs medi-cation but his record has been flagged as "drug seeking" and his provider will not prescribe the medication he needs. It can take some time for the patient to identify where and when his information was stolen and to clear his record. The patient and the HIM professional each have a unique perspec-tive on medical identity theft and are each respon-sible for identifying, reporting, and combating the crime. HIM professionals serve patients well by educating them about what to look for in terms of medical identity theft. For example, HIM pro-fessionals should work with patients and explain what to look for if they receive a bill for medical ser-vices they do not recognize, and instruct that they should check for fraudulent behavior in their name on their medical bills and credit reports. Patients can detect medical identity theft by reviewing their credit reports annually. A credit report will indicate accounts opened in the patient's name by healthcare organizations; if the patient does not recognize the organization, he or she can begin the steps to rectify the situation and identify the fraud.

It is important for HIM professionals to help find and correct fraudulent information within a health record. The California Attorney General's Office created an information sheet for consumers—First Aid for Medical Identify Theft: Tips for Consumers (OAG, CA DOJ 2013). The information sheet describes five signs of possible medical identify theft and provides tips on what to do in response to each.

- If a patient receives a Receipt of a Breach Notice from a healthcare organization it indicates that the patient's protected health information was involved in a data breach. Depending on the type of information involved in the breach, a security freeze on the patient's credit records may be required. Breach notifications will be discussed in more detail later in this chapter.

- If a patient notices an unknown item in the Explanation of Benefits he or she receives from an insurance company and does not recognize the service being paid for, the patient must contact the insurer and the provider who billed for the services to correct the information.

- If a patient receives a notification from the insurance provider that he or she is close to, or has reached the benefit limit for a service (for example, a patient is notified the limit to the number of refills for a certain medication has been reached), the patient may need to obtain a complete list of all benefits paid on his or her behalf to determine erroneous charges.

- A call from a debt collector for medical services not received indicates the patient should contract the service provider and obtain a copy of all bills and related documentation of care, to determine where the fraud came from and determine if the health record needs to be changed.

- Patients should listen carefully to the questions asked of them when they are registering for a healthcare visit, meaning they should always verify their own demographic information when being seen by a provider and should always address and correct erroneous information (OAG, CA DOJ 2013).

HIM professionals are able to assist patients with the process of finding out what happened in cases of medical identity theft and help guide patients to fixing errors that may be in their health record.

Ethical Decision Making

When a healthcare professional is faced with ethical decisions and dilemmas, several factors are included in the decision-making process including but not limited to: cost, technological feasibility, federal and state laws, medical staff bylaws, accreditation and licensing stands, and employer policies, rules and regulations (Harman 2012).

An example of an ethical decision-making process for a healthcare organization would be an elderly patient who is not able to make his own healthcare decisions and has a limited chance of long-time survival. The patient has a daughter who wants the facility to do everything possible to keep her father alive and her brother wants to remove all care and let the patient pass. The ethics committee would consider the cost to the organization, the technological feasibility to care for the patient, the bylaws of the organization, and such in order to make the decision.

HIM professionals should be guided by the AHIMA Code of Ethics in making ethical decisions because they relate directly to the HIM profession. Most professional organizations are guided by a code of ethical standards of practice for the profession; the American Medical Association (AMA)

Figure 21.1 Ethical decision making process

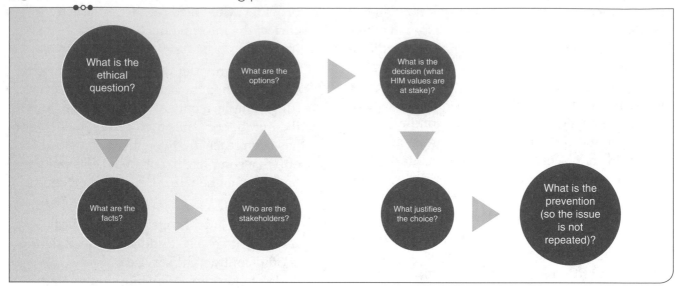

subscribes to a body of ethical statements for a physician to recognize responsibility to the patient first, as well as to society, other health professionals, and to self (AMA 2015). Figure 21.1 shows seven considerations that should be deliberated by HIM professionals faced with an ethical decision.

For example, Sarah—a new graduate of a health information technology program—sits for the registered health information technician (RHIT) examination and fails. She does not want her employer to know she failed and tells all her co-workers she passed the examination. Sarah then starts using the RHIT credential after her name in work correspondence. A co-worker, Nancy, discovers that Sarah is using the RHIT credential fraudulently and notifies the supervisor, Joan. It is the responsibility of both Nancy and Joan as HIM professionals to prevent this activity from happening. Joan should contact AHIMA and report the abuse. Sarah's ethical dilemma is outlined in figure 21.2.

Figure 21.2 Sarah's ethical dilemma outline

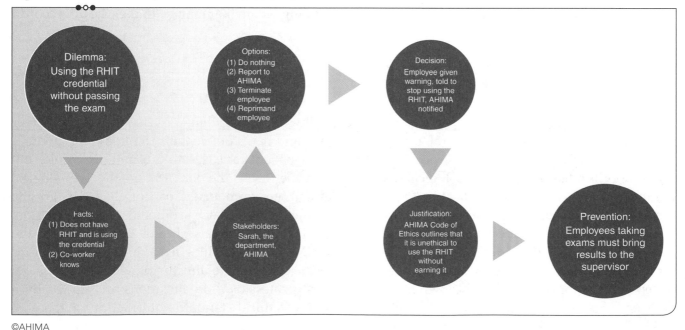

Breach of Healthcare Ethics

A breach of healthcare ethics is a situation in which ethics are either intentionally or accidentally violated. As discussed in detail in chapter 9, organizations must disclose when a breach of PHI is disclosed erroneously; as part of the organization's ongoing monitoring of disclosures it also tracks ethical violations. For example, a security breach of PHI would occur if a patient asks for a copy of a payment made by her insurance company for a surgery she had last month and the business office copies the remittance advice (RA) notice the organization received but fails to delete or remove the PHI for 10 other patients listed on the same RA. An example of a healthcare ethics breach would be a physician choosing to perform a clinical procedure that has not been tested or approved for the purpose of interest or study. Healthcare facilities may choose to establish an ethics committee, a committee tasked with reviewing clinical ethics violations to determine the course of action required to remedy the violations. Most ethics committees involve people from varied backgrounds and have three major functions: (1) providing clinical ethics consultation, (2) developing policies pertaining to clinical ethics, and (3) facilitating education on topical issues in clinical ethics (Pearlman 2013). The goals of the ethics committee include identifying and ensuring the rights of patients, establishing processes to ensure shared decision making between patients and clinicians, and ensuring the processes do not interfere with ethical practices of the facility (Pearlman 2013). Breach of healthcare ethics not related to clinical situations are the responsibility of the supervisor or manager where the breach occurred. The example of the breach of PHI would be the addressed by the business office manager.

Important Health Information Ethical Problems

Some areas in health information management have specific ethical problems. Documentation, privacy, coding, ROI, quality management, decision support, and public health are described in the following sections.

Ethical Issues Related to Documentation and Privacy

It is the responsibility of the HIM professional to ensure patient documentation is accurate, timely, and created by authorized parties. This is accomplished by developing policies and procedures in accordance with laws and regulations to ensure the integrity of patient information is upheld by the organization. The policies and procedures to ensure integrity of patient information is described in detail in chapter 9. Healthcare providers are required to document their decision-making processes; educational sessions are important to provide training on documentation, which can help protect against unethical behaviors and the healthcare organization from malpractice claims.

An example of unethical documentation in healthcare is retrospective documentation—when healthcare providers add documentation after care has been given, possibly for the purpose of increasing reimbursement or avoiding a medical legal action. The HIM professional is responsible for maintaining accurate and complete records and is able to identify the occurrence and either correct the error or indicate that the entry is a late entry into the health record.

Ethical Issues Related to Release of Information

ROI specialists should embody the value of integrity. The HIM professional must "release information only with valid authorization from a patient or a person legally authorized to consent on behalf of a patient" (AHIMA 2011). There are two primary ethical issues that arise from ROI: the need-to-know-principle and blanket authorizations. The **need-to-know principle** is based on the minimum necessary standard. For example, in responding to a request to verify an admission for lap-band surgery, if the ROI specialist gives out the history and physical, labs, discharge summary, and operative report to an insurance company, the documentation could reveal more information than requested—which in turn results in a violation of the patient's privacy. An ROI specialist must only disclose the need-to-know or the least amount of information necessary, in this case only the admission information.

The other ethical concern for ROI is misuse of the **blanket authorization**, which is when the patient signs an authorization allowing the ROI specialist to release any and all information from that point forward. This is an issue because under a blanket authorization the patient is giving authorization for future diagnosis and treatment, one of which he or she may not want authorized. For example, if the patient signs the blanket authorization today to release annual examination results to his or her employer and in five years the patient is diagnosed with cancer, the employer could find out about the cancer because the information was automatically released to the employer (and the patient may not remember signing the blanket authorization five years prior). Most authorizations will state a set amount of time and for a specific reason, diagnosis, date range, provider, and such. This can be prevented by a blanket authorization having an end date, usually after one year, and will need to be signed again the next year.

Ethical Issues Related to Coding

Codes are associated with reimbursement rates and, therefore, there are inherent incentives to code so the healthcare facilities will receive the highest reimbursement dollar amount possible. Coding professionals need to be guided by ethical coding practices because they may be asked by a provider to fraudulently code to receive

higher payment for services rendered. It is important for a coder to only assign codes where data is clearly stated in the health record. If more information is needed, or the information needs to be clarified, a query to the physician should be used. This process for a physician query is discussed in chapter 16.

The standards of ethical coding, based on AHIMA's Code of Ethics, are guidelines outlining 11 standards for ethical coding.

- Apply accurate, complete, and consistent coding practices for the production of high-quality healthcare data
- Report all healthcare data elements required for external reporting purposes completely and accurately, in accordance with regulatory and documentation standards and requirement and applicable official coding conventions, rules, and guidelines
- Assign and report only the codes and data that are clearly and consistently supported by health record documentation in accordance with applicable code set and abstraction conventions, rules, and guidelines
- Query provider for clarification and additional documentation prior to code assignment when there is conflicting, incomplete, or ambiguous information in the health record regarding a significant reportable condition or procedure or other reportable data element dependent on health record documentation
- Refuse to change reported codes or the narratives of codes so that meanings are misrepresented
- Refuse to participate in or support coding or documentation practices intended to inappropriately increase payment, quality for insurance policy coverage, or skew data by means that do not comply with federal and state statues, regulations, and official rules and guidelines
- Facilitate interdisciplinary collaboration in situations supporting proper coding practices

- Advance coding knowledge and practice through continuing education
- Refuse to participate in or conceal unethical coding or abstraction practices or procedures
- Protect the confidentiality of the health record at all times and refuse to access protected health information not required for coding-related activities
- Demonstrate behavior that reflects integrity and shows a commitment to ethical and legal coding

Upcoding, unbundling, and double billing are coding ethical dilemmas. **Upcoding** is the practice of assigning diagnostic or procedural codes that represent higher payment rates than the codes that truly reflect the services provided to patients via the documentation. For example, a physician examines a patient briefly for the flu, but the bill submitted for the visit includes an hour long, complex exam that did not occur. **Unbundling** is the practice of using multiple codes to bill for the various individual steps in a single procedure rather than using a single code that includes all of the steps. For example, a patient goes in for a new cast on a broken leg and instead of billing for one bundled visit (all of the services related to treating the fracture are billed as one service), the bill lists codes for each step as individual procedures resulting in a larger reimbursement. **Double billing** is when two providers bill for one service provided to one patient. An example of this is a surgeon who was an assistant for an operation bills Medicare as if she were the primary surgeon, with the primary surgeon also billing Medicare for the same surgery on the same patient.

Ethical Issues Related to Quality Management, Decision Support, and Public Health

Healthcare costs are increasing and organizations are trying to find ways to keep costs down while still providing quality services, which can be a difficult task. Some examples of quality outcome problems due to this trend include:

- Healthcare organizations falsifying their performance information to the public

- Negative patient outcomes, such as inattentive patient care
- Failure to ensure a physician's license is valid
- When accreditation or licensure surveys occur, health records are hidden or not available to the surveyors
- Repetition of unsuitable healthcare (Harman 2012)

The HIM professional is put in an advocate position so the interest of both the public and the individual patient can be served. An example of this is global infections, or bioterrorism, where it is pertinent to keep the balance between protecting the privacy of those injured or affected and delivering information to the government and healthcare professionals so the medical crisis can be resolved.

Ethical Issues Related to Managed Care

Managed care helps control the cost of healthcare by providing services at a fixed cost. It does this by minimizing variation in clinical practice; for example, all patients seen for hypertension receive the exact same standard of care and service, with little variation for individual patients. Ethical issues that arise with this type of care involve physicians missing a clinical indication a patient needs more than what the standard care provides. In some managed care settings the goal is to increase productivity while keeping costs the same, where physicians have less time with patients, creating an opportunity for the physician to miss some key information.

Managed care incentives may affect provider behavior or have a negative effect on patient care. Incentives include providing rewards to physicians who provide the lowest cost care or withholding bonuses for physicians who have too many costly diagnostic procedures. A physician may be worried about having too many costly procedures so the physician may not order a needed procedure because he or she wants to save money. These incentives can have a negative effect on patient care because if a physician is worried about having too many costly procedures, patient care can be compromised (Jecker and Braddock 1998).

Ethical Issues Related to Sensitive Health Information

All health information must be protected; however, there is some information that requires special attention because it is considered sensitive health information such as genetic, adoption, drug, alcohol, sexual health, and behavioral information. This type of information not only has strict rules and regulations, but also provides an ethical gray area when it comes to releasing and providing records. For example, Benjamin is being treated for mental health and behavioral problems and upon turning age 18 chooses to receive a copy of all of his medical information. Benjamin has the right to receive a copy of his medical information but it may not be in his best interest to read the medical notes from his teenage years. The mental health clinic where he was treated has a policy that states before the patient is given a copy of their record the clinic psychiatrist reviews the record with the patient to explain it to him or her.

When developing policies and procedures for ROI that contain substance abuse, sexually transmitted disease, and mental health information, extra caution is required on the HIM professional's part because there may be competing interests between public safety and patient privacy. Federal and state legislation provides some guidance, but often extra legal counsel may be needed.

Ethical Issues Related to Research

Research is important for the growth and advancement of the healthcare profession. The Institutional Review Board for the Protection of Human Subjects (IRB) oversees the clinical research that is conducted for healthcare, and has the responsibility over the ethical application of research (Adams and Callahan 2013). Without research, common medications or cures would not exist. However, with research comes an ethical obligation to provide patient safety and protection. This obligation is cited in the Belmont Report, which provides the foundation for ethical research. The Belmont Report protects "the autonomy, safety, privacy, and welfare of human research subjects" (Adams and Callahan 2013). There are three primary ethical principles the Belmont Report provides.

- *Autonomy:* Autonomy includes the informed consent process for human research subjects and starts with a full disclosure of the nature of the study; the risks and benefits; and gives the participant the opportunity to back out of the study. The idea behind this is that the potential participant has full knowledge of what he or she is doing, and can confidently say yes or no.

- *Beneficence:* Beneficence occurs when a researcher determines what the maximum potential is for society, compared to the minimum risk of harm done to the participants in the research. An example would be a researcher looking at a trial for finding the cure for the common cold. The risk to the research participants would be low and the maximum potential for the trial is high because the common cold affects a large number of people each year.

- *Justice:* This principle involves impartial selection of participants in a research study, as it is important to avoid unfairly coercing participants; for example, prisoners have historically been coerced into taking part in medical research against their will (Adams and Callahan 2013).

The HIM department is involved in the IRB process by making the health records of patients enrolled in a research study available to external monitors and auditors. Agreements between the HIM department and researchers assure patient consent and policies and procedures are followed. In the case of electronic health information there are agreements outlining the exact information to be released to researchers. The HIM department offers training to researchers and HIM staff for the procedures in place for the consent process and maintenance of the records. Research is often provided at large teaching hospitals but is sometime case specific; for instance, a rare disease is being researched and a small facility is seeing one patient for follow-up treatment. In this case the HIM professionals of that facility may not have the policies and procedures for research established and would need to create the process and training.

Ethical Issues Related to Electronic Health Record Systems

The access of electronic health record (EHR) systems is a complex challenge in regards to record integrity, information security, linkage of information for continuum of care within different e-health systems, and the development of software for HIM purposes. HIM professionals need to be part of the implementation team to provide their unique understanding of the federal rules and regulations regarding privacy and security, and can help facilitate a successful core in the implementations of these issues. More information on EHR implementation is found in chapter 11.

Healthcare professionals are trained in the ethical issues related to EHR systems because staff may have access to more information than what is needed to do their jobs. Employees accessing the record should not explore information out of curiosity, as this would be unethical. When a patient's health information is shared or linked within an EHR without his or her knowledge the patient's autonomy is breached. Providers sometimes may use the copy and paste option to copy information from one patient record to another and may inadvertently add incorrect information into a record. Understanding ethical issues in documentation and HIM processes help the HIM professional to prevent unethical behaviors and train others in the code of ethics in HIM. HIM professionals must follow the AHIMA Code of Ethics in their work as well as strive for cultural competence in their dealings with others.

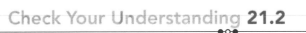

Check Your Understanding 21.2

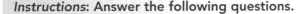

Instructions: **Answer the following questions.**

1. Which of the following is the authorization that allows the release of information from the time of signing forward to include future information?
   A. Disclosure authorization
   B. Blanket authorization
   C. Need-to-know authorization
   D. Consent authorization

2. What is the practice of assigning diagnostic or procedural codes that represent higher payment rates?
   A. Upcoding
   B. Unbundling
   C. Utilization
   D. Managed care

3. What is the practice of using multiple codes to bill for various individual steps in a single procedure, rather than using a single code that includes all of the steps of the comprehensive procedure?
   A. Utilization
   B. Upcoding
   C. Need-to-know
   D. Unbundling

4. The minimization of variation in a clinical practice is used in what setting?
   A. Need-to-know
   B. Utilization
   C. Managed care
   D. Quality assurance

5. Which of the following types of information include areas like genetics, adoption, and drug use that require special attention?
   A. Special information
   B. Scientific information
   C. Sensitive information
   D. Super information

6. Which of the following considers risk vs. benefit in regards to ethical principles?
   A. Beneficence
   B. Justice
   C. Autonomy
   D. Vulnerable population

7. The participant in a research group has been given full disclosure on what the study entails and the choice to opt out of the study. This falls under what ethical principle?
   A. Justice
   B. Autonomy
   C. Vulnerable population
   D. Beneficence

8. Which of the following has created ethical issues based on security, interoperability, and record integrity?
   A. HIPAA
   B. Advocate
   C. Sensitive data
   D. Electronic health record

 Real-World Case 21.1

Kelly was a new coder who had never held an HIM job before. She had just graduated from college and passed her RHIT when she was hired by a local clinic and was so excited to start working. A few weeks later, her manager asked to meet with her. The manager closed the door and told Kelly that she wanted her to code charts for a particular procedure using two codes instead of one so the reimbursement would be higher. The manager then proceeded to divulge information that the clinic was struggling financially so anything extra would help. Kelly got the impression that if she did not comply they would let her go; and she really needed this job. Also, since it was her boss asking, she felt obligated to do as she was told.

 Real-World Case 21. 2

A woman was found unresponsive on a desert highway and brought to the emergency room of a local hospital. After five days in a coma, the woman awoke and did not know her name, where she was from, her history, or have any recollection of her past. She was given the name Jane Brown and eventually released from the hospital. After many years working with social service agencies, she built a new life but never regained memories of her past. Eventually, she graduated from college, moved to the Pacific Northwest, married, and had two sets of twins one year apart. One day a man recognized her as a missing woman from Arizona and contacted authorities. The police notified Ms. Brown of her past life and informed her she has family members who want to meet her. With the hope of remembering her past, she met with them. With the case receiving national news coverage and attention, the local hospital noticed a marked increase in the number of people requesting access the health records of Ms. Brown and her children.

References

Adams, L. and T. Callahan. 2013. Research Ethics. Ethics in Medicine, University of Washington School of Medicine. https://depts.washington.edu/bioethx/topics/resrch.html.

Allen, J. 2013. *Health Law & Medical Ethics for Healthcare Professionals*. Upper Saddle River, NJ. Prentice Hall.

American Health Information Management Association. 2015. Mission Vision and Values. http://www.ahima.org/about/aboutahima?tabid=mission.

American Health Information Management Association. 2011. Code of Ethics. http://library.ahima.org/doc?oid=105098#.Vxk2qPkrK9I.

American Medical Association. 2015. Principles of Medical Ethics. http://www.ama-assn.org/ama/pub/physician-resources/medical-ethics/code-medical-ethics/principles-medical-ethics.page?.

Goode, T.D. and C. Dunne. 2003 revision. Policy Brief 1: Rational for Cultural Competence in Primary Care. Washington, DC: National Center for Cultural Competence, Georgetown University Center for Child and Human Development. http://nccc.georgetown.edu/documents/Policy_Brief_1_2003.pdf.

Goode, T.D., W. Jones. and J. Mason. 2002. A Guide to Planning and Implementing Cultural Competence Organization Self-Assessment. Washington, DC: National Center for Cultural Competence, Georgetown University Child Development Center. http://nccc.georgetown.edu/documents/ncccorgselfassess.pdf.

Harman, L.B. 2012. Ethical Issues in Health Information Management. Chapter 12 in *Health Information Management Technology: An Applied Approach*, 4th ed. Edited by N.B. Sayles. Chicago: AHIMA.

Huffman, E.K. 1972. *Manual for Medical Record Librarians*, 6th ed. Chicago: Physician's Record Company.

Jecker, N.S. and C.H. Braddock III. 1998. Managed Care. Ethics in Medicine, University of Washington School of Medicine. https://depts.washington.edu/bioethx/topics/manag.html.

McNabb, J. and H.B. Rhodes. 2014. Combating the privacy crime that can kill. *Journal of AHIMA*. 85(4): 26–29.

Meyer, P., P. Yoon, and R. Kaufmann. 2013. Introduction: CDC Health Disparities and Inequalities Report. http://www.cdc.gov/mmwr/preview/mmwrhtml/su6203a2.htm?s_cid=su6203a2_w.

National Center for Cultural Competence. 2015. Georgetown University. http://nccc.georgetown.edu/foundations/need.html.

Office of the Attorney General, California Department of Justice. 2013. First Aid For Medical Identity Theft Tips for Consumers. http://www.oag.ca.gov/sites/all/files/agweb/pdfs/privacy/cis_16_med_id_theft.pdf.

Pearlman, R. 2013. Ethics Committees, Programs and Consultation. Ethics in Medicine, University of Washington School of Medicine. https://depts.washington.edu/bioethx/topics/ethics.html.

Simmers, L., K. Simmers-Nartker, and S. Simmers-Kobelak. 2014. *Simmers DHO Health Science*, 8th ed. Boston, MA: Cengage Learning.

US Department of Health and Human Services, Office of Minority Health (HHS). n.d. National Standards for Culturally and Linguistically Appropriate Services. https://www.thinkculturalhealth.hhs.gov/pdfs/EnhancedNationalCLASStandards.pdf.

World Health Organization. 2012. Social Determinants of Health. http://www.who.int/social_determinants/sdh_definition/en/.

Appendix A
Check Your Understanding Answer Key

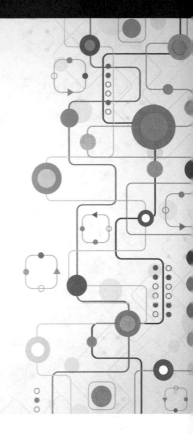

Chapter 1

1.1

1. B
2. C
3. A
4. A
5. A
6. B

1.2

1. B
2. A
3. B
4. C
5. B

Chapter 2

2.1

1. D
2. D
3. B
4. D
5. D
6. B
7. A
8. False
9. True
10. True

2.2

1. B
2. C
3. C
4. C
5. B
6. E
7. D
8. B
9. C
10. A

2.3

1. D
2. A
3. A
4. C
5. A
6. True
7. True
8. True
9. False
10. True

2.4

1. D
2. D
3. B
4. A
5. A
6. E
7. B
8. A
9. C
10. D

2.5

1. D
2. B
3. C
4. A
5. B
6. True
7. False
8. False
9. True
10. True

Chapter 3

3.1
1. D
2. C
3. A
4. C
5. B

3.2
1. A
2. C
3. C
4. B
5. A
6. A
7. B
8. C
9. B
10. B

3.3
1. A
2. D
3. B
4. C
5. B

3.4
1. C
2. A
3. B
4. B
5. A

Chapter 4

4.1
1. D
2. B
3. A
4. B

4.2
1. B
2. True
3. True
4. False
5. False

4.3
1. C
2. A
3. A
4. C
5. A
6. B
7. D
8. C
9. A
10. A
11. C
12. C
13. B
14. True
15. True
16. True

4.4
1. B
2. B
3. B
4. B

4.5
1. C
2. False
3. False
4. False
5. True

Chapter 5

5.1
1. False
2. True
3. False
4. True
5. False

5.2
1. E
2. C
3. D
4. B
5. A

5.3
1. A
2. C
3. B
4. A
5. C

5.4
1. False
2. False
3. True
4. False
5. False

Chapter 6

6.1
1. True
2. B
3. B
4. C
5. False
6. False

6.2
1. False
2. D
3. True
4. True
5. A

6.3
1. False
2. D
3. C
4. True
5. C

6.4
1. B
2. False
3. C

6.5
1. True
2. C
3. True
4. B
5. False

Chapter 7

7.1

1. A
2. D
3. A
4. True
5. False
6. True
7. False

7.2

1. B
2. D
3. A
4. A
5. C
6. B
7. A
8. A
9. C

Chapter 8

8.1

1. A
2. B
3. B
4. D
5. C
6. B
7. A
8. D
9. C
10. A
11. B
12. A
13. D
14. A
15. D

8.2

1. C
2. B
3. C
4. B
5. C
6. C
7. C
8. B
9. A
10. C
11. B
12. A
13. A
14. C
15. D

Chapter 9

9.1

1. B
2. C
3. B
4. B
5. B
6. C
7. B
8. C
9. C
10. C

9.2

1. A
2. C
3. D
4. B
5. D
6. A
7. B
8. B
9. B
10. A

9.3

1. B
2. A
3. C
4. B
5. D
6. C
7. A
8. D
9. C
10. D

9.4

1. B
2. A
3. D
4. C
5. B
6. A
7. A
8. A
9. D
10. C

Chapter 10

10.1

1. C
2. C
3. D
4. C
5. C
6. A
7. B
8. D
9. A
10. C

10.2

1. B
2. D
3. B
4. B
5. A
6. B
7. A
8. B
9. C
10. C

10.3
1. D
2. A
3. D
4. A
5. D
6. C
7. A
8. D
9. B
10. B

Chapter 11

11.1
1. B
2. A
3. A
4. A
5. C
6. True
7. True
8. False
9. False
10. True

11.2
1. B
2. A
3. B
4. B
5. True
6. False
7. False
8. False
9. False

11.3
1. B
2. B
3. C
4. B
5. D
6. C
7. A
8. B
9. A
10. D

Chapter 12

12.1
1. A
2. D
3. B
4. E
5. C

12.2
1. True
2. False
3. True
4. True
5. False

12.3
1. C
2. A
3. C
4. D
5. A

Chapter 13

13.1
1. True
2. False
3. A
4. C
5. A

13.2
1. False
2. True
3. B
4. C
5. A

13.3
1. False
2. True
3. False
4. C
5. B
6. B
7. A

13.4
1. False
2. False
3. True
4. False
5. True
6. C
7. B

13.5
1. E
2. I
3. J
4. C
5. D
6. G
7. B
8. F
9. H
10. A

13.6
1. True
2. True
3. False
4. D
5. B

13.7
1. False
2. True
3. True
4. B
5. B
6. A

Chapter 14

14.1

1. D
2. C
3. D
4. C
5. D
6. D
7. C
8. D
9. C
10. D
11. D
12. C
13. D
14. D
15. C

14.2

1. Ratio
2. Proportion
3. Percentage
4. Ratio
5. Proportion

14.3

1. a. 165 [(160+20) − 15]
   b. 167 [160 + (20 − 15) + 2]
   c. 167 [160 + (20 − 15) + 2]

2. a. 12 [(10 + 5) − 3]
   b. 13 [10 + (5 − 3) + 1]

3. a. 14 [(12 + 1) + (1 + 1 − 1)]
   b. 15 [(12 + 1) + (1 + 1 − 1) + 1]

14.4

1. Medicine 59.6% 680/(38 × 30) × 100
   Surgery 71.2% [790/(37 × 30) × 100]
   Pediatric 39.2% [235/(20 × 30) × 100]
   Psychiatry 77.3% [927/(40 × 30) × 100]
   Obstetrics 70.0% [252/(12 × 30) × 100]
   Newborn 22.1% [252/(16 × 30) × 100]

2. 50.8% [2,884/(163 × 30) × 100]

3. 86.1%: Jan–June
   31+28+31+30+31+30 = 181; 181 × 165= 29865; 25720/29865×100
   75.7%: July–Dec 31 + 31 + 30 + 31 + 30 + 31 = 184; 184 × 200 = 36800; 27852/36800 × 100
   80.4% Total for the year

14.5

1. 831
2. 125
3. 6.6 days
4. 6.47 days
5. 7.52 days

14.6

1. 1.59% [(43/2703) × 100] = 4300/2703
2. 1.52% [(43 − 2)/(2703 − 2) × 100] = 4100/2701
3. 0.57% [(1/175) × 100] = 0.57%
4. 2.78% [(5/(175 + 5) × 100]
5. 1.53% [(43 +1)/(2703 +175) × 100] = 4400/2878
6. 0.57% [(1/175) × 100]
7. 1.46% {[(43 +1) − 2]/(2703 + 175) − 2] × 100} = 4200/2876

14.7

1. 25.7%
2. 27.3%
3. 29.4%
4. 20.0%
5. 8.30%

14.8

1. A. 4.32% (12/278 × 100)
   B. 2.16% (6/278 × 100)
2. A. 7.32% (15/205 × 100)
   B. 1.48% (3/203 × 100)

14.9

1. 8.8% [(6/68) × 100]
2. 44.9% [(57/127) × 100]
3. Answers in table 14.19
4. Hospital acquired
5. Nosocomial

Table 14.19 Community Hospital number of patients Dr. Green discharged by MS-DRG, August, 20XX

MS-DRG	MS-DRG title	Relative weight	Number of patients	Total weight
179	Respiratory infections and inflammations w/o CC/MCC	0.9693	5	4.8465
187	Pleural effusion w/ CC	1.0691	2	2.1382
189	Pulmonary edema and respiratory failure	1.2136	3	2.1382
194	Simple pneumonia and pleurisy w/ CC	0.9688	1	0.9688
208	Respiratory system diagnosis w/ ventilator support < 96 hours	2.2969	1	2.2969
280	Acute myocardial infarction, discharged alive w/ MCC	1.7289	3	5.1867
299	Peripheral vascular disorders w/ MCC	1.4094	2	2.8188
313	Chest pain	0.6138	4	2.4522
377	G.I. hemorrhage w/ MCC	1.7775	1	1.7775
391	Esophagitis, gastroenteritis. and miscellaneous digestive disorders w/ MCC	1.1976	1	1.1976
547	Connective tissue disorders w/o CC/ MCC	0.7985	1	0.7985
552	Medical back problems w/o MCC	0.8698	1	0.8698
684	Renal failure w/o CC/ MCC	0.6085	1	0.6085
812	Red blood cell disorders w/o MCC	0.8182	2	1.6364
872	Septicemia w/o MV 96+ hours w/o MCC	1.0528	1	1.0528
918	Poisoning and toxic effects of drugs w/o MCC	0.6412	1	0.6412
Total				16; 32.9342
Case-mix index =				32.9342/16 = 2.0584

14.10

1. B
2. D
3. I
4. J
5. E
6. C
7. F
8. H
9. G
10. A
11. K

14.11

1. a. 83.9% (1,305,939/155,651,602) × 10,000
   b. 80.4% (1,290,922/160,477,237) × 10,000
   c. 82.2% [(1,305,939 + 1,290,922)/(155,651,602 + 160,477,237)] × 10,000 = (2,596,861/316,128,839) × 10,000
   d. 9.3% (20,864/22,525,155) × 10,000
   e. 3.6% (7,622/21,429,247) × 10,000
2. 7 births per 1,000 population (4,899/750,000) × 1,000
3. 2 deaths per 1,000 live births (8/4,899) × 1,000
4. 3 deaths per 1,000 live births minus the neonatal deaths [14/4,899 − 8) × 1,000
5. 5 infant deaths per 1,000 live births ((8 + 14)/4,899) × 1,000
6. 5.6 deaths per 1,000 population (4,225/750,000) × 1,000
7. 16.7 deaths of lung cancer per 100,000 population (125/750,000) × 100,000
8. (4/37) × 100 = 10.8 deaths due to *Clostridium difficile*.
9. (4/4,225) × 100 = 0.09 proportionate death rate.
10. (2/4,012) × 100,000 = 50 maternal deaths per 100,000 population.

14.12

1. Incidence rate: A computation that compares the number of new cases of a specific disease for a given time period to the population at risk for the disease during the same time period

   Prevalence rate: The proportion of people in a population who have a particular disease at a specific point in time or over a specified period of time
2. Notifiable disease: A disease that must be reported to a government agency so that regular, frequent, and timely information on individual cases can be used to prevent and control future cases of the disease
3. $(189,000/301,623,157) \times 100,000 = 62.7$ new cases of coronary artery disease per 100,000 population
4. $(4/50,000) \times 10,000 = 0.8$ cases per 10,000 population
5. $(8 + 3)/50,000 \times 10,000 = 2.2$ cases per 10,000 population

Chapter 15

15.1

1. C
2. F
3. A
4. H
5. G
6. D
7. B
8. E

15.2

1. C
2. A
3. D
4. B
5. A
6. C
7. A

15.3

1. C
2. C
3. D
4. E
5. A
6. B

Chapter 16

16.1

1. C
2. C
3. C
4. C
5. B

16.2

1. D
2. A
3. False
4. True
5. True

16.3

1. B
2. A
3. True
4. True
5. False

Chapter 17

17.1

1. B
2. C
3. A
4. C
5. A
6. D
7. A
8. False
9. True
10. True

17.2

1. A
2. B
3. D
4. B
5. D
6. C
7. D
8. True
9. False
10. False

17.3

1. A
2. D
3. B
4. B
5. A
6. C
7. B
8. True
9. False
10. True

Chapter 18

18.1

1. B
2. C
3. C
4. C
5. True
6. False
7. True

18.2

1. B
2. D
3. D
4. True
5. True
6. False

18.3

1. B
2. A
3. C
4. False
5. True
6. True

18.4
1. A
2. D
3. D
4. False
5. False
6. True

18.5
1. A
2. A
3. D
4. C
5. A

Chapter 19

19.1
1. B
2. C
3. E
4. D
5. A

19.2
1. D
2. A
3. B
4. C
5. B

19.3
1. C
2. B
3. D
4. A
5. C
6. D

Chapter 20

20.1
1. C
2. B
3. B
4. C
5. D
6. C
7. B
8. D

20.2
1. A
2. D
3. False
4. True
5. True

20.3
1. D
2. B
3. D
4. B
5. C
6. B

20.4
1. True
2. False
3. True
4. A
5. A
6. B
7. C

20.5
1. D
2. B
3. D
4. B
5. C
6. A
7. D

20.6
1. False
2. True
3. False
4. B
5. A
6. C
7. D
8. A

Chapter 21

21.1
1. D
2. H
3. F
4. A
5. B
6. G
7. C
8. E

21.2
1. B
2. A
3. D
4. C
5. C
6. A
7. B
8. D

Glossary

A

Abbreviated Injury Scale (AIS): An anatomically-based, consensus-derived global severity scoring system that classifies each injury by region according to its relative importance on a 6-point ordinal scale (1 = minor and 6 = maximal). AIS is the basis for the Injury Severity Score (ISS) calculation of the multiply injured patient

Abstracting: 1. The process of extracting information from a document to create a brief summary of a patient's illness, treatment, and outcome 2. The process of extracting elements of data from a source document or database and entering them into an automated system

Abuse: Describes practices that, either directly or indirectly, result in unnecessary costs to the Medicare Program. Abuse includes any practice that is not consistent with the goals of providing patients with services that are medically necessary, meet professionally recognized standards, and are fairly priced

Accept assignment: A term used to refer to a provider's or a supplier's acceptance of the allowed charges (from a fee schedule) as payment in full for services or materials provided

Access control: 1. A computer software program designed to prevent unauthorized use of an information resource 2. As amended by HITECH, a technical safeguard that requires a covered entity must in accordance with 164.306(a)(1) implement technical policies and procedures for electronic information systems that maintain electronic protected health information to allow access only to those persons or software programs that have been granted access rights as specified in 164.308(a)(4) (45 CFR 164.312 2003)

Access report: Report that provides a list of individuals who accessed patient information during a given period

Access safeguards: Identification of which employees should have access to what data; the general practice is that employees should have access only to data they need to do their jobs.

Accession number: A number assigned to each case as it is entered in a cancer registry

Accession registry: A list of cases in a cancer registry in the order in which they were entered

Accommodation: An employer providing a reasonable adjustment for an employee

Accountable care organizations (ACOs): A legal entity that is recognized and authorized under applicable state, federal, or tribal law, is identified by a Taxpayer Identification Number (TIN), and is formed by one or more ACO participant(s) that is (are) defined at 425.102(a) and may also include any other ACO participants described at 425.102(b) (42 CFR 425.20 2011)

Accounting: 1. The process of collecting, recording, and reporting an organization's financial data 2. A list of all disclosures made of a patient's health information

Accreditation: 1. A voluntary process of institutional or organizational review in which a quasi-independent body created for this purpose periodically evaluates the quality of the entity's work against preestablished written criteria 2. A determination by an accrediting body that an eligible organization, network, program, group, or individual complies with applicable standards 3. The act of granting approval to a healthcare organization based on whether the organization has met a set of voluntary standards developed by an accreditation agency

Accreditation organizations: A professional organization that establishes the standards against which healthcare organizations are measured and conducts periodic assessments of the performance of individual healthcare organizations

Accredited Standards Committee X12 (ASC X12): A committee accredited by ANSI responsible for the development and maintenance of EDI standards for many industries. The ASC "X12N" is the subcommittee of ASC X12 responsible for the EDI health insurance administrative transactions such as 837 Institutional Health Care Claim and 835 Professional Health Care Claim forms

Accrual accounting: Recording known transactions in the appropriate time period before cash payment (receipts) are expected or due

Acknowledgments: A form that provides a mechanism for the resident to recognize receipt of important information

Active listening: The application of effective verbal communication skills as evidenced by the listener's restatement of what the speaker said

Active membership: Individuals interested in the AHIMA purpose and willing to abide by the Code of Ethics are eligible for active membership. Active members in good standing shall be entitled to all membership privileges including the right to vote

Addendum: A late entry added to a health record to provide additional information in conjunction with a previous entry. The late entry should be timely and bear the current date and reason for the additional information being added to the health record

ADDIE model: Recommended by numerous experts in the HRM and instructional design fields as a general guide to planning and implementation of employee training programs; the steps in this model are analyze-design-develop-implement-evaluate

Adjudication: Refers to the process of paying, denying, and adjusting claims based on the patient's health insurance coverage benefits

Administrative data: Coded information contained in secondary records, such as billing records, describing patient identification, diagnoses, procedures, and insurance

Administrative law: A body of rules and regulations developed by various administrative entities empowered by Congress; falls under the umbrella of public law

Administrative safeguards: Under HIPAA, are administrative actions and policies and procedures, to manage the selection, development, implementation, and maintenance of security measures to protect electronic protected health information and to manage the conduct of the covered entity's or business associate's workforce in relation to the protection of that information (45 CFR 164.304 2013)

Administrative simplification: As amended by HITECH, authorizes HHS to: (1) adopt standards for transactions and code sets that are used to exchange health data; (2) adopt standard identifiers for health plans, health care providers, employers, and individuals for use on standard transactions; and (3) adopt standards to protect the security and privacy of personally identifiable health information (45 CFR Parts 160, 162, and 164 2013)

Admissibility: The condition of being admitted into evidence in a court of law

Adoption: Reflects the fact that the organization has implemented all of the major components of technology, although there may be some available technology that is more specialized, costly, or time-consuming to implement that has not yet been implemented

Affinity grouping: A technique for organizing similar ideas together in natural groupings

Affordable Care Act: A federal statute that was signed into law on March 23, 2010. Along with the Health Care and Education Reconciliation Act of 2010 (signed into law on March 30, 2010), the act is the product of the healthcare reform agenda of the Democratic 111th Congress and the Obama administration

Age Discrimination in Employment Act of 1967: The federal act that states, it is unlawful for an employer to discriminate against an individual in any aspect of employment because that individual is 40 years old or older, unless one of the statutory exceptions applies. Favoring an older individual over a younger individual because of age is not unlawful discrimination under the ADEA, even if the younger individual is at least 40 years old. However, the ADEA does not require employers to prefer older individuals and does not affect applicable state, municipal, or local laws that prohibit such preferences (72 FR 36875 2007)

Agency for Healthcare Research and Quality (AHRQ): The branch of the US Public Health Service that supports general health research and distributes research findings and treatment guidelines with the goal of improving the quality, appropriateness, and effectiveness of healthcare services

Aggregate data: Data extracted from individual health records and combined to form de-identified information about groups of patients that can be compared and analyzed

Alert fatigue: When an excessive number of alerts are used in an information system, users get tired of looking at the alerts and may ignore them

Allied health professional: A credentialed healthcare worker who is not a physician, nurse, psychologist, or pharmacist (for example, a physical therapist, dietitian, social worker, or occupational therapist)

All patient refined diagnosis-related groups (APR-DRGs): An expansion of the inpatient classification system that includes four distinct subclasses (minor, moderate, major, and extreme) based on the severity of the patient's illness

Alphabetic filing system: A system of health record identification and storage that uses the patient's last name as the first component of identification and his or her first name and middle name or initial for further definition

Alphanumeric filing system: Both alphabetic and numeric characters are used to sort health records in this system

Alternative dispute resolution: Methods of resolving legal disputes outside of the court system such as arbitration or mediation

Ambulatory: Treatment provided on an outpatient basis

Ambulatory care: Preventive or corrective healthcare services provided on a nonresident basis in a provider's office clinic setting, or hospital emergency setting

Ambulatory payment classification: Hospital outpatient prospective payment system (OPPS). The classification is a resource-based reimbursement system

Ambulatory surgery center/ambulatory surgical center (ASC): Under Medicare, an outpatient surgical facility that has its own national identifier; is a separate entity with respect to its licensure, accreditation, governance, professional supervision, administrative functions, clinical services, recordkeeping, and financial and accounting systems; has as its sole purpose the provision of services in connection with surgical procedures that do not require inpatient hospitalization; and meets the conditions and requirements set forth in the Medicare Conditions of Participation

Ambulatory surgery center (ASC) payment rate: The Medicare ASC reimbursement methodology system referred to as the ambulatory surgery center (ASC) payment system. The ASC payment system is based on the ambulatory payment classifications (APCs) utilized under the hospital OPPS

Amendment: A clarification made to health care documentation after the original document has been signed; it should be dated, timed and signed

American Academy of Professional Coders: The American Academy of Professional Coders provides certified credentials to medical coders in physician offices, hospital outpatient facilities, ambulatory surgical centers, and in payer organizations

American Association for Accreditation of Ambulatory Surgery Facilities (AAAASF): An organization that provides an accreditation program to ensure the quality and safety of medical and surgical care provided in ambulatory surgery facilities

American Association of Medical Record Librarians (AAMRL): The name adopted by the Association

of Record Librarians of North America in 1944; precursor of the American Health Information Management Association

American College of Surgeons (ACS): The scientific and educational association of surgeons formed to improve the quality of surgical care by setting high standards for surgical education and practice

American College of Surgeons (ACS) Commission on Cancer: Established by the American College of Surgeons (ACoS) in 1922, the multidisciplinary Commission on Cancer (CoC) establishes standards to ensure quality, multidisciplinary, and comprehensive cancer care delivery in healthcare settings

American Health Information Management Association (AHIMA): The professional membership organization for managers of health record services and healthcare information systems as well as coding services; provides accreditation, advocacy, certification, and educational services

American Medical Record Association (AMRA): The name adopted by the American Association of Medical Record Librarians in 1970; precursor of the American Health Information Management Association

American Recovery and Reinvestment Act (ARRA): The purposes of this act include the following: (1) To preserve and create jobs and promote economic recovery. (2) To assist those most impacted by the recession. (3) To provide investments needed to increase economic efficiency by spurring technological advances in science and health. (4) To invest in transportation, environmental protection, and other infrastructure that will provide long-term economic benefits. (5) To stabilize state and local government budgets, in order to minimize and avoid reductions in essential services and counterproductive state and local tax increases

American Society for Testing and Materials (ASTM) International: An international organization whose purpose is to establish standards on materials, products, systems, and services

Americans with Disabilities Act (ADA): Federal legislation which ensures equal opportunity for and elimination of discrimination against persons with disabilities (Public Law 110-325 2008)

Analysis: Review of health record for proper documentation and adherence to regulatory and accreditation standards

Analytics: Refers to statistical processing of data to reveal new information

Ancillary services: 1. Tests and procedures ordered by a physician to provide information for use in patient diagnosis or treatment 2. Professional healthcare services such as radiology, laboratory, or physical therapy

Ancillary systems: Systems that serve primarily to manage the department in which they exist, while at the same time providing key clinical data for the EHR

Anesthesia report: The report that notes any preoperative medication and response to it, the anesthesia administered with dose and method of administration, the duration of administration, the patient's vital signs while under anesthesia, and any additional products given the patient during a procedure

Anti-Kickback Statute: A statute that establishes criminal penalties for individuals and entities that knowingly and willfully offer, pay, solicit or receive remuneration in order to induce business for which payment may be made under any federal healthcare program

Appeal: 1. A request for reconsideration of a denial of coverage or rejection of claim decision 2. The next stage in the litigation process after a court has rendered a verdict; must be based on alleged errors or disputes of law rather than errors of fact

Appellate courts: Courts that hear appeals on final judgments of the state trial courts or federal trial courts

Application controls: Security strategies, such as password management, included in application software and computer programs

Application safeguards: Controls contained in application software or computer programs to protect the security and integrity of information

Application service provider (ASP): A third-party service company that delivers, manages, and remotely hosts standardized applications software via a network through an outsourcing contract based on fixed, monthly usage, or transaction-based pricing

Arbitration: A proceeding in which disputes are submitted to a third party or a panel of experts outside the judicial trial system

Assembly: The process of ensuring that each page in the health record is organized in a standardized order

Association for Healthcare Documentation Integrity (AHDI): Formerly the American Association for Medical Transcription (AAMT), the AHDI has a model curriculum for formal educational programs that includes the study of medical terminology, anatomy and physiology, medical science, operative procedures, instruments, supplies, laboratory values, reference use and research techniques, and English grammar

Association of Record Librarians of North America (ARLNA): Organization formed 10 years after the beginning of the hospital standardization movement whose original objective was to elevate the standards of clinical recordkeeping in hospitals, dispensaries, and other healthcare facilities; precursor of the American Health Information Management Association

Asynchronous: Self-paced learning; students and instructor can communicate, but not in real-time

Audit: 1. A function that allows retrospective reconstruction of events, including who executed the events in question, why, and what changes were made as a result 2. To conduct an independent review of electronic system records and activities in order to test the adequacy and effectiveness of data security and data integrity procedures and to ensure compliance with established policies and procedures

Audit controls: The mechanisms that record and examine activity in information systems

Audit trail: 1. A chronological set of computerized records that provides evidence of information system activity (logins and logouts, file accesses) used to determine security violations 2. A record that shows who has accessed a computer system, when it was accessed, and what operations were performed

Authentication: 1. The process of identifying the source of health record entries by attaching a handwritten signature, the author's initials, or an electronic signature 2. Proof of authorship that ensures, as much as possible, that log-ins and messages from a user originate from an authorized source 3. As amended by HITECH, means the corroboration that a person is the one claimed

Authoritarian leadership: Domineering leadership style where decisions are made at a distance from those affected

Authorization: 1. As amended by HITECH, except as otherwise specified, a covered entity may not use or disclose protected health information without an authorization that is valid under section 164.508 2. When a covered entity obtains or receives a valid authorization for its use or disclosure of protected health information, such use or disclosure must be consistent with the authorization (45 CFR 164.508 2013)

Authorization card: A document that indicates an employee's interest in having a union represent him or her

Auto-authentication: 1. A procedure that allows dictated reports to be considered automatically signed unless the health information management department is notified of needed revisions within a certain time limit 2. A process by which the failure of an author to review and affirmatively either approve or disapprove an entry within a specified time period results in authentication

Auto-analyzer: Device that analyzes the specimen

Automated drug dispensing machines: System that makes drugs available for patient care

Automated reviews: Reviews performed electronically rather than by humans

Autonomy: A core ethical principle centered on the individual's right to self-determination that includes respect for the individual; in clinical applications, the patient's right to determine what does or does not happen to him or her in terms of healthcare

Autopsy report: Written documentation of the findings from a postmortem pathological examination

Average daily census: The mean number of hospital inpatients present in the hospital each day for a given period of time

Average length of stay (ALOS): The mean length of stay for hospital inpatients discharged during a given period of time

Avoidance: In business, a situation where two parties in conflict ignore that conflict

B

Balance billing: A reimbursement method that allows providers to bill patients for charges in excess of the amount paid by the patients' health plan or other third-party payer (not allowed under Medicare or Medicaid)

Balanced Budget Act of 1997: Public Law 105-33 enacted by Congress on August 5, 1997, that mandated a number of additions, deletions, and revisions to the original Medicare and Medicaid legislation; the legislation that added penalties for healthcare fraud and abuse to the Medicare and Medicaid programs and also affected the hospital outpatient prospective payment system (HOPPS) and programs of all-inclusive care for elderly (PACE) (Public Law 105-33 1997)

Bar chart: A graphic technique used to display frequency distributions of nominal or ordinal data that fall into categories

Barcode medication administration record (BC-MAR): System that uses barcoding technology for positive patient identification and drug information

Bargaining unit: Those individuals who will be represented by the union

Bed count: The number of inpatient beds set up and staffed for use on a given day

Bed count day: One inpatient bed, set up and staffed for use in a 24-hour time period

Bed turnover rate: The average number of times a bed changes occupants during a given period of time

Behavior theory: Theory in which proponents believe that leaders can be made and that successful leadership is based on definable, learnable behavior

Behaviorally anchored rating scale: Rating system that links specific examples of job-related performance to each rating

Bench trial: A trial in which a judge reviews the evidence and makes a determination, without a sitting jury

Benchmark: The systematic comparison of the products, services, and outcomes of one organization with those of a similar organization; or the systematic comparison of one organization's outcomes with regional or national standards

Benchmarking: The systematic comparison of the products, services, and outcomes of one organization with those of a similar organization; or the systematic comparison of one organization's outcomes with regional or national standards

Beneficence: A legal term that means promoting good for others or providing services that benefit others, such as releasing health information that will help a patient receive care or will ensure payment for services received

Beneficiary: An individual who is eligible for benefits from a health plan

Benevolent autocracy: The leader wields absolute power but is generally kind and sincere in the use of the team for the good of the organization

Best of breed: A vendor strategy used when purchasing an EHR that refers to system applications that are considered the best in their class

Best of fit: A vendor strategy used when purchasing an EHR in which all the systems required by the healthcare facility are available from one vendor

Bias: Favoritism, partiality, or prejudice

Big data: Very large volume of data that offers greater reliability and validity

Billing system: Information system that generates a bill for healthcare services performed

Biometrics: The physical characteristics of users (such as fingerprints, voiceprints, retinal scans, iris traits) that systems store and use to authenticate identity before allowing the user access to a system

Blanket authorization: The patient signs an authorization allowing the release of information specialist to release any and all information from that point forward

Board of directors: The elected or appointed group of officials who bear ultimate responsibility for the successful operation of a healthcare organization

Bona fide occupational qualification: A factor (for example, age) is shown to be directly related to job performance based on documented job analysis

Brainstorming: A group problem-solving technique that involves the spontaneous contribution of ideas from all members of the group

Breach: Under HITECH, the acquisition, access, use, or disclosure of protected health information in a manner not permitted under subpart E of this part that compromises the security or privacy of the protected health information (45 CFR 164.402 2013)

Breach notification: As amended by HITECH, a covered entity shall, following the discovery of a breach of unsecured protected health information, notify each individual whose unsecured protected health information has been, or is reasonably believed by the covered entity to have been, accessed, acquired, used, or disclosed as a result of such breach (45 CFR 164.404 2013)

Breach of contract: Failure to perform any term of a contract by any party involved in the contract

Bubble chart: A type of scatter plot with circular symbols used to compare three variables; the area of the circle indicates the value of a third variable

Budget: A plan that converts the organization's goals and objectives into targets for revenue and spending

Budget adjustment: The approval to move funds from one budget to another

Budget management: The process of maintaining financial viability by ensuring operating revenues for the year are sufficient to cover the operating expenditures

Budget variance: A difference in the budgeted revenue or expense amount

Bureaucracy: A formal organizational structure based on a rigid hierarchy of decision making and inflexible rules and procedures

Business associate (BA): 1. A person or organization other than a member of a covered entity's workforce that performs functions or activities on behalf of or affecting a covered entity that involve the use or disclosure of individually identifiable health information 2. As amended by HITECH, with respect to a covered entity, a person who creates, receives, maintains, or transmits PHI for a function or activity regulated by HIPAA, including claims processing or administration, data analysis, processing or administration, utilization review, quality assurance, patient safety activities, billing, benefit management, practice management, and repricing or provides legal, actuarial, accounting, consulting, data aggregation, management, administrative, accreditation, or financial services (45 CFR 160.103 2013)

Business associate agreement (BAA): As amended by HITECH, a contract between the covered entity and a business associate must establish the permitted and required uses and disclosures of protected health information by the business associate and provides specific content requirements of the agreement. The contract may not authorize the business associate to use or further disclose the information in a manner that would violate the requirements of HIPAA, and requires termination of the contract if the covered entity or business associate are aware of noncompliant activities of the other (45 CFR 164.504 2013)

Business continuity plan: A program that incorporates policies and procedures for continuing business operations during a computer system shutdown

Business intelligence (BI): The end product or goal of knowledge management

Business process: A set of related policies and procedures that are performed step by step to accomplish a business-related function

Business records exception: A rule under which a record is determined not to be hearsay if it was made at or near the time by, or from information transmitted by, a person with knowledge; it was kept in the course of a regularly conducted business activity; and it was the regular practice of that business activity to make the record

Business-related partnerships: An agreement between two parties to cooperate for the advancement of their mutual interests and the entity's strategic goals

Bylaws: Operating documents that describe the rules and regulations under which a healthcare organization operates

C

Capitation: A specified amount of money paid to a healthcare plan or doctor, used to cover the cost of a healthcare plan member's services for a certain length of time

Care area assessments (CAAs): The patient is assessed and reassessed at defined intervals as well as whenever there is a significant change in his or her condition

Care plan: The specific goals in the treatment of an individual patient, amended as the patient's condition requires, and the assessment of the outcomes of care; serves as the primary source for ongoing documentation of the resident's care, condition, and needs

Career development: The process by which individuals assess their existing skills, knowledge and experience, explore and establish current and future career objectives, and develop an appropriate course of action

Career planning: Looking beyond simply getting a job to position oneself for more challenging and diverse work in the long term

Case definition: A method of determining criteria for cases that should be included in a registry

Case fatality rate: Rate that measures the total number of deaths among the diagnosed cases of a specific disease, most often acute illness

Case finding: A method of identifying patients who have been seen or treated in a healthcare facility for the particular disease or condition of interest to the registry

Case management: 1. A process used by a doctor, nurse, or other health professional to manage a patient's healthcare (CMS 2013) 2. The ongoing, concurrent review performed by clinical professionals to ensure the necessity and effectiveness of the clinical services being provided to a patient

Case mix: 1. A description of a patient population based on any number of specific characteristics, including age, gender, type of insurance, diagnosis, risk factors, treatment received, and resources used 2. The distribution of patient into categories reflecting differences in severity of illness or resource consumption

Case-mix index (CMI): The average relative weight of all cases treated at a given facility or by a given physician, which reflects the resource intensity or clinical severity of a specific group in relation to the other groups in the classification system; calculated by dividing the sum of the weights of diagnosis-related groups for patients discharged during a given period by the total number of patients discharged

Cash basis accounting: Registering the transaction when it occurs, meaning when money is actually received for services provided, or paid for expenses incurred

Causation: In law, a relationship between the defendant's conduct and the harm that was suffered

Cause-and-effect diagram: An investigational technique that facilitates the identification of the various factors that contribute to a problem

Cause-specific mortality rate: The rate of death due to a specified cause

Cause of action: Theories under which lawsuits are brought that are related to professional liability such as breach of contract, intentional tort, and negligence

Census: The number of inpatients present in a healthcare facility at any given time

Centers for Disease Control and Prevention (CDC): A federal agency dedicated to protecting health and promoting quality of life through the prevention and control of disease, injury, and disability. Committed to programs that reduce the health and economic consequences of the leading causes of death and disability, thereby ensuring a long, productive, healthy life for all people

Centers for Medicare and Medicaid Services (CMS): The Department of Health and Human Services agency responsible for Medicare and parts of Medicaid. Historically, CMS has maintained the UB-92 institutional EMC format specifications, the professional EMC NSF specifications, and specifications for various certifications and authorizations used by the Medicare and Medicaid programs. CMS is responsible for the oversight of HIPAA administrative simplification transaction and code sets, health identifiers, and security standards. CMS also maintains the HCPCS medical code set and the Medicare Remittance Advice Remark Codes administrative code set

Centralized unit filing system: All of the patient's encounters are filed together in a single location

Certificate authority: An organization that verifies a person's credentials and can revoke the certificate if the credentials are revoked

Certification: 1. The process by which a duly authorized body evaluates and recognizes an individual, institution, or educational program as meeting predetermined requirements 2. An evaluation performed to establish the extent to which a particular computer system, network design, or application implementation meets a prespecified set of requirements

Certified EHR technology: EHRs that have been approved for use in the MU program by organizations hired by CMS to evaluate EHRs

Certified tumor registrar (CTR): Credential for a cancer registrar achieved by passing an examination provided by the National Board for Certification of Registrars (NBCR); eligibility requirements for the certification examination include a combination of experience and education

Change control program: Assures that there is documented approval for the change to be made and evidence that all elements of implementation, testing, rollout, training, and such are performed

Change management: The formal process of introducing change, getting it adopted, and diffusing it throughout the organization

Charge capture: The process of collecting all services, procedures, and supplies provided during patient care

Charge description master: A financial management form that contains information about the organization's charges for the healthcare services it provides to patients; *Also called a chargemaster*

Chargemaster: A financial management form that contains information about the organization's charges for the healthcare services it provides to patients; *Also called charge description master (CDM)*

Chart: 1. (noun) The health record of a patient 2. (verb) To document information about a patient in a health record

Chart conversion: An EHR implementation activity in which data from the paper chart are converted into electronic form

Chart tracking: A process that identifies the current location of a paper record or information

Checksheet: A data collection tool that records and compiles observations or occurrences

Chief executive officer (CEO): The senior manager appointed by a governing board to direct an organization's overall long-term strategic management

Chief financial officer (CFO): The senior manager responsible for the fiscal management of an organization

Chief information officer (CIO): The senior manager responsible for the overall management of information resources in an organization

Chief medical informatics officer (CMIO): A salaried physician (most often part time so that he or she retains credibility with other practicing physicians) who is heavily involved in policy development, workflow and process improvement, and ongoing maintenance of CDS and other systems requiring significant physician input

Chief nursing officer (CNO): The senior manager (usually a registered nurse with advanced education and extensive experience) responsible for administering patient care services

Chief operating officer (COO): An executive-level role responsible at a high level for day-to-day operations of an organization

Children's Health Insurance Program: Provides health coverage to eligible children through both Medicaid and individual state CHIP programs; like all Medicaid programs, CHIP is administered by states according to federal requirements and is funded jointly by states and the federal government

Civil Rights Act of 1991 (CRA 1991): The federal legislation that focuses on establishing an employer's responsibility for justifying hiring practices that seem to adversely affect people because of race, color, religion, sex, or national origin (Public Law 102-166 1991)

Civilian Health and Medical Program—Veterans Administration (CHAMPVA): The federal healthcare benefits program for dependents (spouse or widow[er] and children) of veterans rated by the Veterans Administration (VA) as having a total and permanent disability, for survivors of veterans who died from VA-rated service-connected conditions or who were rated permanently and totally disabled at the time of death from a VA-rated service-connected condition, and for survivors of persons who died in the line of duty

Claim: A request for payment for services, benefits, or costs by a hospital, physician or other provider that is submitted for reimbursement to the healthcare insurance plan by either the insured party or by the provider

Claim attachment: Any of a variety of hardcopy or electronic forms needed to process a claim in addition to the claim itself, such as a copy of the emergency department note

Claims data: Information required to be reported on a healthcare claim for service reimbursement

Claims management: The process of managing the legal and administrative aspects of the healthcare organization's response to injury claims (injuries occurring on the facility's property)

Claims status inquiry and response: Used to determine if a health plan has ended a claim for additional information or is processing the claim

Classifications: A clinical vocabulary, terminology, or nomenclature that lists words or phrases with their meanings, provides for the proper use of clinical words as names or symbols, and facilitates mapping standardized terms to broader classifications for administrative, regulatory, oversight, and fiscal requirements

Classroom-based learning: Instructor-led, face-to-face training including traditional lectures, workshops, and seminars

Client/server system: System in which the healthcare organization has commercial software installed on servers housed and maintained within the organization itself, housed within the organization and managed by an outsourced company, or housed and maintained by a contractor for the healthcare organization

Clinic outpatient: A patient who is admitted to a clinical service of a clinic or hospital for diagnosis or treatment on an ambulatory basis

Clinical coding: Assigning codes to represent diagnoses and procedures

Clinical data: The information that reflects the treatment and services provided to the patient as well as how the patient responded to such treatment and services

Clinical data analytics: The process by which health information is captured, reviewed, and used to measure quality

Clinical data repository (CDR): A central database that focuses on clinical information

Clinical data warehouse (CDW): A database that makes it possible to access data from multiple databases and combine the results into a single query and reporting interface

Clinical decision support (CDS): The process in which individual data elements are represented in the computer by a special code to be used in making comparisons, trending results, and supplying clinical reminders and alerts

Clinical decision support system (CDSS): CDS that requires the combination of data from more than one sources and the ability to deliver the alert back to the appropriate system or systems

Clinical Document Architecture (CDA): An HL7 XML-based document markup standard for the electronic exchange model for clinical documents (such as discharge summaries and progress notes). The implementation guide contains a library of CDA templates, incorporating and harmonizing previous efforts from HL7, Integrating the Healthcare Enterprise (IHE), and Health Information Technology Standards Panel (HITSP). It includes all required CDA templates for Stage I Meaningful Use, and HITECH final rule. It is commonly referred to as Consolidate CDA or C-CDA

Clinical documentation: Any manual or electronic notation (or recording) made by a physician or other healthcare clinician related to a patient's medical condition or treatment

Clinical documentation improvement (CDI): The process an organization undertakes that will improve clinical specificity and documentation that will allow coders to assign more concise disease classification codes

Clinical documentation system: System that supplies templates to the user to be completed primarily via point-and-click, drop-down, type-ahead, and other data-entry tools

Clinical Laboratory Improvement Amendments (CLIA) of 1988: Established quality standards for all laboratory testing to ensure the accuracy, reliability, and timeliness of patient test results regardless of where the test is (Public Law 90-174 1967)

Clinical observations: The observations of physicians, nurses, and other caregivers in order to create a chronological report of the patient's condition and response to treatment during his or her hospital stay

Clinical practice guidelines: A detailed, step-by-step guide used by healthcare practitioners to make knowledge-based decisions related to patient care and issued by an authoritative organization such as a medical society or government agency

Clinical privileges: The authorization granted by a healthcare organization's governing board to a member of the medical staff that enables the physician to provide patient services in the organization within specific practice limits

Clinical protocols: Specific instructions for performing clinical procedures established by authoritative bodies, such as medical staff committees, and intended to be applied literally and universally

Clinical terminology: A set of standardized terms and their synonyms that record patient findings, circumstances, events, and interventions with sufficient detail to support clinical care, decision support, outcomes research, and quality improvement

Clinical transformation: A fundamental change in how medicine is practiced using health IT systems to aid in diagnosis and treatment

Clinical trial: 1. The final stages of a long and careful research process that tests new types of medical care to see if they are safe (CMS 2013) 2. Experimental study in which an intervention or treatment is given to one group in a clinical setting and the outcomes compared with a control group that did not have the intervention or treatment or that had a different intervention or treatment

Closed-loop medication management: Information systems used to provide patient safety when ordering and administering medications

Cloud computing: A practice that uses a vendor to archive data, and in some cases also provide application software, including an EHR, on multiple, disparate servers

Coaching: 1. A training method in which an experienced person gives advice to a less-experienced worker on a formal or informal basis 2. A disciplinary method used as the first step for employees who are not meeting performance expectations

Code of ethics: A statement of ethical principles regarding business practices and professional behavior

Code systems: An accumulation of numeric or alphanumeric representations or codes for exchanging or storing information

Coding: The process of assigning numeric or alphanumeric representations to clinical documentation

Coding compliance plan: A component of an HIM compliance plan or a corporate compliance plan modeling the OIG Program Guidance for Hospitals and the OIG Supplemental Compliance Program Guidance for Hospitals that focuses on the unique regulations and guidelines with which coding professionals must comply

Coercive power: Power in which a team leader uses threats and punishments to get his or her way

Coinsurance: Cost sharing in which the policy or certificate holder pays a pre-established percentage of eligible expenses after the deductible has been met; the percentage may vary by type or site of service

Collaborative Stage Data Set: A new standardized neoplasm-staging system developed by the American Joint Commission on Cancer

Collective bargaining: A process through which a contract is negotiated that sets forth the relationship between the employees and the healthcare organization

Commission for the Accreditation of Birth Centers: A group that surveys and accredits birth centers in the United States

Commission on Accreditation of Rehabilitation Facilities (CARF): An international, independent, nonprofit accreditor of health and human services that develops customer-focused standards for areas such as behavioral healthcare, aging services, child and youth services, and medical rehabilitation programs and accredits such programs on the basis of its standards

Commission on Accreditation for Health Informatics and Information Management Education (CAHIIM): An independent accrediting organization whose mission is to serve the public interest by establishing and enforcing quality accreditation standards for health informatics and health information management educational programs

Commission on Certification for Health Informatics and Information Management (CCHIIM): An independent body within AHIMA that establishes and enforces standards for the certification and certification maintenance of health informatics and information management professionals

Common-cause variation: The source of variation in a process that is inherent within the process

Common Clinical Data Set: A common set of data types and elements and associated standards for use across several certification criteria

Comorbidity: 1. A medical condition that coexists with the primary cause for hospitalization and affects the patient's treatment and length of stay 2. Pre-existing condition that, because of its presence with a specific diagnosis, causes an increase in length of stay by at least one day in approximately 75 percent of the cases (as in complication and comorbidity [CC])

Comparative data: Individual data that is organized numerically and collated to make some comparisons against standards or benchmarks

Competencies: Demonstrated skills that a worker should perform at a high level

Complaint: In litigation, a written legal statement from a plaintiff that initiates a civil lawsuit

Complex review: In a revenue audit contractor (RAC) review, this type of review results in an overpayment or underpayment determination based on a review of the health record associated with the claim in question

Compliance: 1. The process of establishing an organizational culture that promotes the prevention, detection, and resolution of instances of conduct that do not conform to federal, state, or private payer healthcare program requirements or the healthcare organization's ethical and business policies 2. The act of adhering to official requirements 3. Managing a coding or billing department according to the laws, regulations, and guidelines that govern it

Compliance program: A process that helps an organization, such as a hospital, accomplish its goal of providing high-quality medical care and efficiently operating a business under various laws and regulations

Complication: 1. A medical condition that arises during an inpatient hospitalization (for example, a postoperative wound infection) 2. Condition that arises during the hospital stay that prolongs the length of stay at least one day in approximately 75 percent of the cases (as in complication and comorbidity [CC])

Component state associations (CSAs): Component state associations are part of the volunteer structure of AHIMA and are organized in every state, the District of Columbia, and the Commonwealth of Puerto Rico. The purpose of each Component State Association shall be to promote the mission and purpose of AHIMA in its state

Compressed workweek: A work schedule that permits a full-time job to be completed in less than the standard five days of eight-hour shifts

Computer-assisted coding (CAC): The process of extracting and translating dictated and then transcribed free-text data (or dictated and then computer-generated discrete data) into ICD-10-CM and CPT evaluation and management codes for billing and coding purposes

Computer-based training: A type of training that is delivered partially or completely using a computer

Computerized provider order entry (CPOE): Electronic prescribing systems that allow physicians to write prescriptions and transmit them electronically. These systems usually contain error prevention software that provides the user with prompts that warn against the possibility of drug interaction, allergy, or overdose and other relevant information

Concept: A unique unit of knowledge or thought created by a unique combination of characteristics

Concurrent review: Screening for medical necessity and the appropriateness and timeliness of the delivery of medical care from the time of admission until discharge

Conditions for Coverage: Standards applied to facilities that choose to participate in federal government reimbursement programs such as Medicare and Medicaid

Conditions of Participation: The administrative and operational guidelines and regulations under which facilities are allowed to take part in the Medicare and Medicaid programs; published by the Centers for Medicare and Medicaid Services, a federal agency under the Department of Health and Human Services

Confidentiality: 1. A legal and ethical concept that establishes the healthcare provider's responsibility for protecting health records and other personal and private information from unauthorized use or disclosure 2. As amended by HITECH, the practice that data or information is not made available or disclosed to unauthorized persons or processes (45 CFR 164.304 2013)

Conflict management: A problem-solving technique that focuses on working with individuals to find a mutually acceptable solution

CONNECT: Open-source software that implements health exchange specifications; it enables discovery of where there may be information as well as directly retrieving it from the source

Consensus building: A decision-making method that seeks consent of all participants to resolve differences so an acceptable result can be found

Consensus-oriented decision-making model: A seven-step progression that allows groups to be flexible enough to come to a consensus by starting important topics with open discussion rather than by presenting a preformulated proposal; gathering a list of all the needs and concerns expressed by the group to form a list of conditions for possible proposals to address; taking turns in a unified attempt to build each proposal idea into the best possible proposal before choosing among them; and using empathy in the closure stage to address any unresolved feelings from the process. The seven CODM steps are: (1) framing the topic, (2) open discussion, (3) identifying underlying concerns, (4) collaborative proposal building, (5) choosing a direction, (6) synthesizing a final proposal, and (7) closure

Consent: 1. A patient's acknowledgment that he or she understands a proposed intervention, including that intervention's risks, benefits, and alternatives 2. The document signed by the patient that indicates agreement that protected health information (PHI) can be disclosed

Consent directive: A process by which patients may opt in or opt out of having their data exchanged in the HIE

Consent management systems: Systems that help maintain patient preferences about who may have access to their health information

Consent to treatment: Legal permission given by a patient or a patient's legal representative to a healthcare provider that allows the provider to administer care and treatment or to perform surgery or other medical procedures

Consolidated Clinical Document Architecture (C-CDA): HL7-created document templates

Consolidated Omnibus Budget Reconciliation Act (COBRA): The federal law requiring every hospital that participates in Medicare and has an emergency room to treat any patient in an emergency condition or active labor, whether or not the patient is covered by Medicare and regardless of the patient's ability to pay; COBRA also requires employers to provide continuation benefits to specified workers and families who have been terminated but previously had healthcare insurance benefits (Public Law 99-272 1986)

Constitutional law: The body of law that deals with the amount and types of power and authority that governments are given

Consultation rate: The total number of hospital inpatients receiving consultations for a given period divided by the total number of discharges and deaths for the same period

Consultation report: Documentation of the clinical opinion of a physician other than the primary or attending physician

Consultative leadership: The leader remains open to input from members of the team but still retains full decision-making authority

Consumer-directed health plans: Managed care organization characterized by influencing patients and clients to select cost-efficient healthcare through the provision of information about health benefit packages and through financial incentives

Context-based access control (CBAC): An access control system which limits users to accessing information not only in accordance with their identity and role, but to the location and time in which they are accessing the information

Contingency plan: 1. Documentation of the process for responding to a system emergency, including the performance of backups, the line-up of critical alternative facilities to facilitate continuity of operations, and the process of recovering from a disaster 2. A recovery plan in the event of a power failure, disaster, or other emergency that limits or eliminates access to facilities and electronic protected personal health information (ePHI)

Contingency theory: Theory that states leadership exists between persons in social situations, and persons who are leaders in one situation may not necessarily be leaders in other situations

Contingent or contract work: Temporary workers supplement full-time employees, often as part-time workers

Continuing education units (CEUs): Training that enables employees to remain current with advancing knowledge in their profession; activities that qualify for CEUs include such things as attending workshops and seminars, taking college courses, participating in independent study activities, and engaging in self-assessment activities

Continuity of care document (CCD): The result of ASTM's Continuity of Care Record standard content being represented and mapped into the HL7's Clinical Document Architecture specifications to enable transmission of referral information between providers; also frequently adopted for personal health records

Continuity of care record (CCR): Is a core data set of the most relevant administrative, demographic, and clinical information about a patient's healthcare, covering one or more healthcare encounters. It provides a means for one healthcare practitioner, system, or setting to aggregate all of the pertinent data about a patient and forward it to another practitioner, system, or setting to support the continuity of care

Continuous data: Data that represent measurable quantities but are not restricted to certain specified values

Continuous variables: Discrete variables measured with sufficient precision

Continuum of care: A system that guides and tracks patients over time through a comprehensive array of health services spanning all levels and intensity of care

Contraindication: Medication should not be prescribed due to another medication or condition

Controlling: The management function in which performance is monitored according to policies and procedures

Coordination of benefits: Process for determining the respective responsibilities of two or more health plan that have some financial responsibility for a medical claim

Copayment: Cost-sharing measure in which the policy or certificate holder pays a fixed dollar amount (flat fee) per service, supply, or procedure that is owed to the healthcare facility by the patient. The fixed amount that the policyholder pays may vary by type of service, such as $20.00 per prescription or $15.00 per physician office visit

Core measures: Standardized performance measures developed to improve the safety and quality of healthcare

Coroner: The official (elected or appointed, physician or nonphysician) who is responsible for determining the cause, time, and manner of death in unattended, violent, or unexplained deaths, or a case where a law may have been broken

Corporate compliance: 1. A facility-wide program that comprises a system of policies, procedures, and guidelines that are used to ensure ethical business practices, identify potential fraudulence, and improve overall organizational performance 2. A program that became common after the Federal Sentencing Guidelines reduced fines and penalties to organizations found guilty of fraud if the organization has a prevention and detection program in place

Correction: Edit made to the health record by drawing a single line through the erroneous information and writing the word "error" above the mistake; the practitioner should sign, date and time the correction

Correlational studies: A design of research that determines the existence and degree of relationships among factors

Cost sharing: The cost for medical care that patients pay for themselves, like a copayment, coinsurance, or deductible

Counterclaim: In a court of law, a countersuit

Court of Appeal: A branch of the federal court system that has the power to hear appeals on the final judgments of district courts

Court order: An official direction issued by a court judge and requiring or forbidding specific parties to perform specific actions

Covered entity (CE): As amended by HITECH, (1) a health plan, (2) a health care clearinghouse, (3) a health care provider who transmits any health information in electronic form in connection with a transaction covered by this subchapter (45 CFR 160.103 2013)

Credential: A formal agreement granting an individual permission to practice in a profession, usually conferred by a national professional organization dedicated to a specific area of healthcare practice; or the accordance of permission by a healthcare organization to a licensed, independent practitioner (physician, nurse practitioner, or other professional) to practice in a specific area of specialty within that organization. Usually requires an applicant to pass an examination to obtain the credential initially and then to participate in continuing education activities to maintain the credential thereafter

Credentialing: The process of reviewing and validating the qualifications (degrees, licenses, and other credentials) of physicians and other licensed independent practitioners, for granting medical staff membership to provide patient care services

Critical access hospitals: 1. Hospitals that are excluded from the outpatient prospective payment system because they are paid under a reasonable cost-based system as required under section 1834(g) of the Social Security Act 2. Under HITECH incentives, a facility that has been certified as a critical access hospital under section 1820(e) of the Act and for which Medicare payment is made under section 1814(l) of the Act for inpatient services and under section 1834(g) of the Act for outpatient services (42 CFR 495.4 2012)

Critical incident method: An ongoing written log of examples of an employee's job-related behavior during the appraisal period

Critical thinking: Refers to the process of analyzing, assessing, and reconstructing a situation to provide enhanced solutions and outcomes to a problem

Cross-claim: 1. In law, a complaint filed against a codefendant 2. A claim by one party against another party who is on the same side of the main litigation

Crude birth rate: The number of live births divided by the population at risk

Crude death/mortality rate: The total number of deaths in a given population for a given period of time divided by the estimated population for the same period of time

Cryptography: 1. The art of keeping data secret through the use of mathematical or logical functions that transform intelligible data into seemingly unintelligible data and back again 2. In information security, the study of encryption and decryption techniques

Culture: The values, beliefs, attitudes, languages, symbols, rituals, behaviors, and customs unique to a particular group of people

Cultural audit: A strategy to define an organization's values, symbols, and routines and identify areas for improvement

Cultural competence: Skilled in awareness, understanding, and acceptance of beliefs and values of the people of groups other than one's own

Cultural diversity: The perceived or actual difference among people

Customer: An internal or external recipient of services, products, or information

D

Daily inpatient census: The number of inpatients present at census-taking time each day, plus any inpatients who were both admitted and discharged after the census-taking time the previous day

Dashboards: Reports of process measures to help leaders follow progress to assist with strategic planning

Data: The dates, numbers, images, symbols, letters, and words that represent basic facts and observations about people, processes, measurements, and conditions

Data abstraction: The identification of data elements by an individual through health record review

Data abstracts: A defined and standardized set of data points or elements common to a patient population that can be regularly identified in the health records of the population and coded for use and analysis in a database management system

Data analytics: The science of examining raw data with the purpose of drawing conclusions about that information. It includes data mining, machine language, development of models, and statistical measurements. Analytics can be descriptive, predictive, or prescriptive

Data availability: The extent to which healthcare data are accessible whenever and wherever they are needed

Data capture: The process of recording healthcare-related data in a health record system or clinical database

Data collection tool: A paper or electronic form that contains all of the data elements to be collected in the audit

Data consistency: The extent to which the healthcare data are reliable and the same across applications

Data conversion: The task of moving data from one data structure to another, usually at the time of a new system installation

Data definition: The specific meaning of a healthcare-related data element

Data dictionary: A descriptive list of the names, definitions, and attributes of data elements to be collected in an information system or database whose purpose is to standardize definitions and ensure consistent use

Data element: 1. An individual fact or measurement that is the smallest unique subset of a database 2. Under HIPAA, the smallest named unit of information in a transaction

Data governance: The overall management of the availability, usability, integrity, and security of the data employed in an organization or enterprise

Data integrity: 1. The extent to which healthcare data are complete, accurate, consistent, and timely 2. A security principle that keeps information from being modified or otherwise corrupted either maliciously or accidentally

Data interchange standards: Standards developed in order to support and create structure with data exchanges to support interoperability; the goals of the data interchange standards are to facilitate consistent, accurate, and reproducible capture of clinical data

Data management: The combined practices of HIM, IT, and HI that affect how data and documentation combine to create a single business record for an organization

Data mapping: 1. Data mapping allows for connections between two systems. This connection allows for data initially captured for one purpose to be translated and used for another purpose. One system in a map is identified as the source while the other is the target. 2. Process by which two distinct data models are created and a link between these models is defined. 3. A process used in data warehousing by which different data models are linked to each other using a defined set of methods to characterize the data in a specific definition. This definition can be any atomic unit, such as a unit of metadata or any other semantic. This data linking follows a set of standards, which depends on the domain value of the data model used. Data mapping serves as the initial step in data integration

Data mining: The process of extracting and analyzing large volumes of data from a database for the purpose of identifying hidden and sometimes subtle relationships or patterns and using those relationships to predict behaviors

Data model: 1. A picture or abstraction of real conditions used to describe the definitions of fields and records and their relationships in a database 2. A conceptual model of the information needed to support a business function or process

Data quality: The reliability and effectiveness of data for its intended uses in operations, decision making, and planning

Data security: The process of keeping data, both in transit and at rest, safe from unauthorized access, alteration, or destruction

Data set: A list of recommended data elements with uniform definitions that are relevant for a particular use or are specific to a type of healthcare industry

Data stewardship: The responsibilities and accountabilities associated with managing, collecting, viewing, storing, sharing, disclosing, or otherwise making use of personal health information

Data Use and Reciprocal Support Agreement (DURSA): A trust agreement entered into when exchanging information with other organizations using an agreed upon set of national standards, services and policies developed in coordination with the Office of the National Coordinator for Health Information Technology

Data warehouse: A database that makes it possible to access data from multiple databases and combine the results into a single query and reporting interface

Data warehousing: The acquisition of all the business data and information from potentially multiple, cross-platform sources, such as legacy databases, departmental databases, and online transaction-based databases, and then the warehouse storage of all the data in one consistent format used to analyze data for decision-making purposes

Database: An organized collection of data, text, references, or pictures in a standardized format, typically stored in a computer system for multiple applications

Database life cycle: A system consisting of several phases that represent the useful life of a database, including initial study, design, implementation, testing and evaluation, operation, and maintenance and evaluation

Decision support system: A computer-based system that gathers data from a variety of sources and assists in providing structure to the data by using various analytical models and visual tools in order to facilitate and improve the ultimate outcome in decision-making tasks associated with nonroutine and nonrepetitive problems

Decryption: Data decoded and restored back to original readable form

Deductible: 1. The amount of cost, usually annual, that the policyholder must incur (and pay) before the insurance plan will assume liability for remaining covered expenses. 2. Under Medicare, the amount a beneficiary must pay for healthcare before Medicare begins to pay, either for each benefit period for Part A, or each year for Part B, these amounts can change every year

Deemed status: An official designation indicating that a healthcare facility is in compliance with the Medicare Conditions of Participation

Default: 1. The status to which a computer application reverts in the absence of alternative instructions 2. Pertains to an attribute, value, or option that is assumed when none is explicitly specified

Defendant: In civil cases, an individual or entity against whom a civil complaint has been filed; in criminal cases, an individual who has been accused of a crime

Deficiency slip: Notification when a document or signature is missing that identifies the pertinent document and what needs to be done (dictated, completed, and signed)

Deidentified information: Information where personal characteristics have been stripped from it in such a way that it cannot be later constituted or combined to reidentify an individual; it is commonly used in research

Delinquent record: An incomplete record not finished or made complete within the time frame determined by the medical staff of the facility

Democratic leadership: Participative leadership style that supports collective decision making by offering choices to the group members and facilitating discussion and member involvement

Demographic data: Information used to identify an individual, such as name, address, gender, age, and other information linked to a specific person

Demographics: Information used to identify an individual, such as name, address, gender, age, and other information linked to a specific person; *also known as demographic data*

Department of Health and Human Services (HHS): The cabinet-level federal agency, and principal agency for protecting the health of all Americans and providing essential human services, especially for those who are at least able to help themselves

Deposition: A method of gathering information to be used in a litigation process

Derived classification: Classification based on a reference classification such as ICD or ICF by adopting the reference classification structure and categories and providing additional detail or through rearrangement or aggregation of items from one or more reference classifications

Descriptive statistics: A set of statistical techniques used to describe data such as means, frequency distributions, and standard deviations; statistical information that describes the characteristics of a specific group or a population

Descriptive studies: Research that is exploratory in nature and generate new hypotheses from the data that is collected

Designated record set (DRS): As amended by HITECH: (1) A group of records maintained by or for a covered entity that is: (i) The medical records and billing records about individuals maintained by or for a covered health care provider; (ii) The enrollment, payment, claims adjudication, and case or medical management record systems maintained by or for a health plan; or (iii) Used, in whole or in part, by or for the covered entity to make decisions about individuals (2) For purposes of this paragraph, the term means any item, collection, or grouping of information that includes protected health information and is maintained, collected, used, or disseminated by or for a covered entity (45 CFR 164.501 2013)

Deterministic algorithm: Algorithm that requires exact matches in data elements such as the patient name, date of birth, and social security number

Development: Refers to educational programs with a longer-term focus, designed to stimulate an individual's professional growth by increasing or enhancing his or her skills, knowledge, or abilities

Diagnosis-related group: 1. A unit of case-mix classification adopted by the federal government and some other payers as a prospective payment mechanism for hospital inpatients in which diseases are placed into groups because related diseases and treatments tend to consume similar amounts of healthcare resources and incur similar amounts of cost; in the Medicare and Medicaid programs, one of more than 500 diagnostic classifications in which cases demonstrate similar resource consumption and length-of-stay patterns. Under the prospective payment system (PPS), hospitals are paid a set fee for treating patients in a single DRG category, regardless of the actual cost of care for the individual. 2. A classification system that groups patients according to diagnosis, type of treatment, age, and other relevant criteria. Under the prospective payment system, hospitals are paid a set fee for treating patients in a single DRG category, regardless of the actual cost of care for the individual

Diagnostic studies: All diagnostic services of any type, including history, physical examination, laboratory, x-ray or radiography, and others that are performed or ordered pertinent to the patient's reasons for the encounter

Digital certificate: An electronic document that establishes a person's online identity

Digital Imaging and Communications in Medicine (DICOM): An ISO standard that promotes a digital image communications format and picture archive and communications systems for use with digital images

Digital signature: An electronic signature that binds a message to a particular individual and can be used by the receiver to authenticate the identity of the sender

Direct Project: Launched in March 2010 to offer a simpler, standards-based way for participants to send authenticated, encrypted health information directly to known recipients over the Internet

Disability: A physical or mental condition that either temporarily or permanently renders a person unable to do the work for which he or she is qualified and educated

Disaster recovery plan: The document that defines the resources, actions, tasks, and data required to manage the businesses recovery process in the event of a business interruption

Discharge summary: A summary of the resident's stay at a healthcare facility that is used along with the postdischarge plan of care to provide continuity of care upon discharge from the facility

Disciplinary action: Action taken to improve unsatisfactory work performance or behavior on the job

Discipline without punishment: A step where the employee is given a one- to two-day paid decision-making leave following oral and written warnings and attempts to problem solve

Disclosure: As amended by HITECH, the release, transfer, provision of access to, or divulging in any manner of information outside the entity holding the information (45 CFR 160.103 2013)

Discovery: The pretrial stage in the litigation process during which both parties to a suit use various strategies to identify information about the case, the primary focus of which is to determine the strength of the opposing party's case

Discrete data: Data that represent separate and distinct values or observations; that is, data that contain only finite numbers and have only specified values

Discrete reportable transcription (DRT): Transcription system that combines speech dictation with natural language processing

Discrete variable: A dichotomous or nominal variable whose values are placed into categories

Discrimination: Treating a person differently based upon individual characteristics or group membership

Disease index: A listing in diagnosis code number order of patients discharged from the facility during a particular time period

Disease registry: A centralized collection of data used to improve the quality of care and measure the effectiveness of a particular aspect of healthcare delivery

Dismissal: Involuntary termination of employment

Disparate impact: Unequal effect of a discriminatory employment practice on a protected class, even if unintentional

Disparate treatment: Employment discrimination based on intentional unequal treatment of an individual who is a member of a protected class

Disproportionate share hospital: Healthcare organizations that meet governmental criteria for percentages of indigent patients. Hospital with an unequally (disproportionately) large share of low-income patients. Federal payments to these hospitals are increased to adjust for the financial burden

Distal attributes: Division of leadership traits that includes personality, cognitive abilities, motives, and values that surround the leader as a person

Distributional errors: Errors of inequity like central tendency, where all employees are rated satisfactory regardless of performance in order to avoid conflict, or leniency or strictness where some managers are overly generous or strict compared to other raters

District court: The lowest tier in the federal court system, which hears cases involving felonies and misdemeanors that fall under federal statute and suits in which a citizen of one state sues a citizen of another state

DNV GL Healthcare: An international certification body and classification society with main expertise in technical assessment, advisory, and risk management created in 2013 with the merger of Det Norske Veritas (Norway) and Germanischer Lloyd (Germany)

Documentation: The recording of pertinent healthcare findings, interventions, and responses to treatment as a business record and form of communication among caregivers

Documentation standards: Within the context of healthcare, describe those principles, codes, beliefs, guidelines, and regulations that guide health record documentation

Document management system: System commonly used when transitioning from paper-based to electronic health record that scans the paper record and stores it digitally

Document imaging: 1. The practice of electronically scanning written or printed paper documents into an optical or electronic system for later retrieval of the document or parts of the document if parts have been indexed; 2. The process by which paper-based documentation is captured, digitized, stored, and made available for retrieval by the end-user

Do-not-resuscitate (DNR) order: An order written by the treating physician stating that in the event the patient suffers cardiac or pulmonary arrest, cardiopulmonary resuscitation should not be attempted

Double billing: Occurs when two providers bill for one service provided to one patient

Downsizing: A reengineering strategy to reduce the cost of labor and streamline the organization by laying off portions of the workforce

Drug knowledge database: A subscription service that provides current information about drugs and is accessible to users and CDS

Dual eligible: An individual covered by both Medicare and Medicaid

Due diligence: The actions associated with making a good decision, including investigation of legal, technical, human, and financial predictions and ramifications of proposed endeavors with another party

Duplicate health record: Occurs when the patient has two or more health record numbers issued; the patient's medical information becomes fragmented with some information under the first number and the remainder under the second

Durable power of attorney for healthcare decisions (DPOA-HCD): A legal instrument through which a principal appoints an agent to make healthcare decisions on the principal's behalf in the event the principal becomes incapacitated

Dysfunctional conflict: A destructive type of struggle that becomes emotionally draining and harms productivity

E

E-discovery: Refers to Amendments to Federal Rules of Civil Procedure and Uniform Rules Relating to Discovery of Electronically Stored Information; wherein audit trails, the source code of the program, metadata, and any other electronic information that is not typically considered the legal health record is subject to motion for compulsory discovery

Edit check: Helps to ensure data integrity by allowing only reasonable and predetermined values to be entered into the computer

eHealth Exchange: A group of federal agencies and non-federal organizations that came together under a common mission and purpose to improve patient care, streamline disability benefit claims, and improve public health reporting through secure, trusted, and interoperable health information exchange. Participating organizations mutually agree to support a common set of standards and specifications that enable the establishment of a secure, trusted, and interoperable connection among all participating Exchange organizations for the standardized flow of information

Electronic health record (EHR): An electronic record of health-related information on an individual that conforms to nationally recognized interoperability standards and that can be created, managed, and consulted by authorized clinicians and staff across more than one healthcare organization

Eligibility: Verification that the patient is currently covered by the plan on the date of service and the services being provided are covered by the plan

Eligibility verification: Verification that determines if a patient's health plan will provide reimbursement for services to be performed, and sometimes prior-authorization management systems where a health plan requires review and approval of a procedure (or referral) prior to performing the service

Eligible professional: Under HITECH, specific to the Medicare program, means a physician as defined in section 1861(r) of the Act, which includes, with certain limitations, all of the following types of professionals: (1) a doctor of medicine or osteopathy, (2) a doctor of dental surgery or medicine, (3) a doctor of podiatric medicine, (4) a doctor of optometry, (5) a chiropractor (45 CFR 495.100 2012)

Emergency Medical Treatment and Active Labor Act (EMTALA): A 1986 law enacted as part of the Consolidated Omnibus Reconciliation Act largely to combat "patient dumping"—the transferring, discharging, or refusal to treat indigent emergency department patients because of their inability to pay (Public Law 99-272 1986)

Emergency mode of operations: A plan that defines the processes and controls that will be followed until the operations are fully restored

Emergency patient: A patient who is admitted to the emergency services department of a hospital for the diagnosis and treatment of a condition that requires immediate medical, dental, or allied health services in order to sustain life or to prevent critical consequences

Emeritus membership: AHIMA membership category for members who are 65 years old or older.

Employee engagement: Refers to the level of commitment employees demonstrate, their willingness to continue working for the organization, and to go above and beyond the minimum expectations

Employee relations: Broad term referencing the general management and planning of activities related to developing and improving employee relationships through communication and fair handling of disputes

Employee Retirement Income Security Act (ERISA): An act that sets minimum standards for most voluntarily established pension and health plans in private industry to provide protection for individuals in these plans (Public Law 93-406 1974)

Employment at will: Concept that employees can be fired at any time and for almost any reason based on the idea that employees can quit at any time and for any reason

Encoder: Specialty software used to facilitate the assignment of diagnostic and procedural codes according to the rules of the coding system

Encounter: The face-to-face contact between a patient and a provider who has primary responsibility for assessing and treating the condition of the patient at a given contact and exercises independent judgment in the care of the patient

Encryption: The process of transforming text into an unintelligible string of characters that can be transmitted via communications media with a high degree of security and then decrypted when it reaches a secure destination

End user: Persons who will use the system for their daily processes

Engage: A virtual network of AHIMA members who communicate via a web-based program managed by AHIMA

Enterprise information management: The set of function created by an organization to plan, organize, and coordinate the people, processes, technology, and content needed to manage information for the purposes of data quality, patient safety, and ease of use

Enterprise master patient index: An index that provides access to multiple repositories of information from overlapping patient populations that are maintained in separate systems and databases

Episode-of-care reimbursement: Reimbursement methods that include a period of continuous medical care performed by healthcare professionals in relation to a particular clinical problem or situation, and one or more healthcare services given by a provider during a specific period of relatively continuous care in relation to a particular health or medical problem or situation

e-Prescribing (e-Rx): When a prescription is written from the personal digital assistant and an electronic fax or an actual electronic data interchange transaction is generated that transmits the prescription directly to the retail pharmacy's information system

Equal employment opportunity law: Government efforts to ensure equal access to and fairness in employment without regard to race, religion, age, disability, gender, or other characteristics not related to a job

Equal Pay Act: The federal legislation that requires equal pay for men and women who perform substantially the same work (Public Law 88-38 1963)

Ethical principles: Concepts such as altruism, beneficence, consequentialism, deontology, egoism, least harm, and utilitarianism, upon which ethical decisions are made

Ethics: A field of study that deals with moral principles, theories, and values; in healthcare, a formal decision-making process for dealing with the competing perspectives and obligations of the people who have an interest in a common problem

Ethics committee: A committee tasked with reviewing clinical ethics violations to determine the course of action required to remedy the violations

Ethnography: A method of observational research that investigates culture in naturalistic settings using both qualitative and quantitative approaches

Evidence-based medicine: Healthcare services based on clinical methods that have been thoroughly tested through controlled, peer-reviewed biomedical studies

e-visits: Non-face-to-face interaction between patient and provider

Exclusive provider organizations (EPO): Hybrid managed care organization that provides benefits to subscribers only when healthcare services are performed by network providers; sponsored by self-insured (self-funded) employers or associations and exhibits characteristics of both health maintenance organizations and preferred provider organizations

Executive information system: A system that facilitates and supports senior managerial decisions

Executive management: The senior management of a healthcare organization, the people who oversee a broad functional area or group of departments or services; this level of management sets the organization's future direction and monitors the organization's operations in those areas

Exempt employees: Specific groups of employees who are identified as not being covered by some or all of the provisions of the Fair Labor Standards Act

Expenses: Amounts that are charged as costs by an organization to the current year's activities of operation

Experimental study: Study that strives to establish cause and effect; it entails exposing participants to different interventions in order to compare the result of these interventions with the outcome

Expert power: Refers to leaders who are experts in their field or have knowledge or skills that are in short supply

Explanation of benefits: A statement issued to the insured and the healthcare provider by an insurer to explain the services provided, amounts billed, and payments made by a health plan

Exploitive autocracy: The leader wields absolute power and uses the team to serve his or her own personal interests

Express contract: Agreement between physician and patient that is specifically articulated

Expressed consent: The spoken or written permission granted by a patient to a healthcare provider that allows the provider to perform medical or surgical services

Extended care facility: A healthcare facility licensed by applicable state or local law to offer room and board, skilled nursing by a full-time registered nurse, intermediate care, or a combination of levels on a 24-hour basis over a long period of time

External analysis: Development of the market assessment to determine opportunities and threats to the future of the organization

External audit: Audit conducted by an outside organization hired to validate the compliance activities of the organization

External customers: Individuals from outside the organization who receive products or services from within the organization

External threats: Threats that originate outside an organization

F

Facility-based registry: A registry that includes only cases from a particular type of healthcare facility, such as a hospital or clinic

Facility directory: A directory of patients being treated in a healthcare facility

Fair and Accurate Credit Transactions Act: Law passed in 2003 that contains provisions and requirements to reduce identity theft (Public Law 108-159 2003)

Fair Labor Standards Act (FLSA): The federal legislation that sets the minimum wage and overtime payment regulations (52 Stat. 1060 1938)

False Claims Act: Legislation passed during the Civil War, amended in 1986, that prohibits contractors from making a false claim to a governmental program; used to reinforce the prevention of healthcare fraud and abuse (Public Law 99-562 1986)

Family and Medical Leave Act (FMLA): The federal legislation that allows full-time employees time off from work (up to 12 weeks) to care for themselves or their family members with the assurance of an equivalent position upon return to work (Public Law 103-3 1993)

Federal Health IT Strategic Plan 2015-2020: Issued by the Office of the National Coordinator for Health Information Technology (ONC), this plan describes a vision of high-quality care, lower costs, healthy population, and engaged people and mission to improve the health and well-being of individuals and communities through the use of technology and health information that is accessible when and where it matters most

Federal poverty level: The income qualification threshold established by the federal government for certain government entitlement programs

Federal Rules of Civil Procedure (FRCP): Rules established by the US Supreme Court setting the "rules of the road" and procedures for federal court cases. FRCP include electronic records and continue to be very important as benchmarks in how these records can be used in courts, not only federal, but state and other courts as well (Public Law 97-462 1983)

Federal Rules of Evidence (FRE): Rules established by the US Supreme Court guiding the introduction and use of evidence in federal court proceedings that are an important benchmark for state and other courts. FRE governs what and how electronic records may be used, and the roles of record custodianship

Federal Trade Commission (FTC): An independent federal agency tasked with dealing with two areas of economics in the United States: consumer protection and issues having to do with competition in business

Fee-for-service reimbursement: A method of reimbursement through which providers retrospectively receive payment based on either billed charges for services provided or on annually updated fee schedules

Fee schedule: A complete listing of fees used by health plans to pay doctors or other providers

Fellowship program: Program of earned recognition for AHIMA members who have made significant and sustained contributions to the HIM profession through meritorious service, excellence in professional practice, education, and advancement of the profession through innovation and knowledge sharing

Fetal autopsy rate: The number of autopsies performed on intermediate and late fetal deaths for a given time period divided by the total number of intermediate and late fetal deaths for the same time period

Fetal death (stillborn): The death of a product of human conception before its complete expulsion or extraction from the mother regardless of the duration of the pregnancy

Fetal death rate: A proportion that compares the number of intermediate or late fetal deaths to the total number of live births and intermediate or late fetal deaths during the same period of time

Financial indicators: A set of measures designed to routinely monitor the current financial status of a healthcare organization or of one of its constituent parts

Financial management: The mechanism that all organizations and businesses use to fully comprehend and communicate their financial activities and status

Firewall: A computer system or a combination of systems that provides a security barrier or supports an access control policy between two networks or between a network and any other traffic outside the network

Fishbone diagram: A performance improvement tool used to identify or classify the root causes of a problem or condition and to display the root causes graphically

Flextime: A work schedule that gives employees some choice in the pattern of their work hours, usually around a core of midday hours

Flow charts: A graphic tool that uses standard symbols to visually display detailed information, including time and distance, of the sequential flow of work of an individual or a product as it progresses through a process

Force-field analysis: A performance improvement tool used to identify specific drivers of, and barriers to, an organizational change so that positive factors can be reinforced and negative factors reduced

Forced distribution: Ranking method similar to grading on a curve, where managers place subordinates into predetermined performance categories

Fraud: The intentional deception or misrepresentation that an individual knows (or should know) to be false, or does not believe to be true, and makes, knowing the deception could result in some unauthorized benefit to himself or some other person(s)

Free-text data: Data that are narrative in nature

Frequency: The number of times something occurs in a particular population or sample over a specific period of time

Frequency polygon: A type of line graph that represents a frequency distribution

Full-time equivalent (FTE): A statistic representing the number of full-time employees as calculated by the reported number of hours worked by all employees, including part-time and temporary, during a specific time period

Fully specified name (FSN): In SNOMED CT, the unique text assigned to a concept that completely describes that concept

Functioning: In International Classification of Functioning, Disability and Health, the umbrella term for body functions, body structures, activities, and participation

Fundraising: In these activities that benefit the covered entity, the covered entity may use or disclose to a BA or an institutionally related foundation, without authorization, demographic information and dates of healthcare provided to an individual

G

Gantt chart: A graphic tool used to plot tasks in project management that shows the duration of project tasks and overlapping tasks

General consent: Explicit consent for routine treatment given to by the patient to the healthcare provider or organization

Genetic Nondiscrimination Act (GINA): Legislation that prohibits genetic discrimination by health insurers and employers

Global payment: A form of reimbursement used for radiological and other procedures that combines the professional and technical components of the procedures and disperses payments as lump sums to be distributed between the physician and the healthcare facility

Go-live: First use of the system in actual practice

Granularity: Consisting of small components or details

Graph: A graphic tool used to show numerical data in a pictorial representation

Graphic rating scale: A checklist is used to numerically rate employees on general traits related to job performance, like teamwork

Great Person Theory: The belief that some people have natural (innate) leadership skills

Grievance: A formal, written description of a complaint or disagreement

Gross autopsy rate: The number of inpatient autopsies conducted during a given time period divided by the total number of inpatient deaths for the same time period

Gross death rate: The number of inpatient deaths that occurred during a given time period divided by the total number of inpatient discharges, including deaths, for the same time period

Grounded theory: A theory about what is actually going on instead of what should go on

Group membership: Allows multiple individuals from an organization to join AHIMA at one time; student and business groups are eligible for this membership type

Grouper: 1. Computer program that uses specific data elements to assign patients, clients, or residents to groups, categories, or classes 2. A computer software program that automatically assigns prospective payment groups on the basis of clinical codes

Guidelines: In forms control, provides general direction about the design of the form

H

Halo-horns effect: Occurs when an employee is strong or weak in one rated area and the supervisor unfairly generalizes that performance to rate the employee high or low across all other areas on the performance appraisal

Harassment: The act of bothering or annoying someone repeatedly

Health Care Fraud Prevention and Enforcement Action Team (HEAT): Created by HHS and the Department of Justice, this team's mission is to: prevent waste, fraud, and abuse; identify those who participate in fraud and abuse; reduce healthcare costs; improve the quality of care provided to Medicare and Medicaid patients; provide best practices in combating fraud and abuse; and expand partnership between HHS and the Department of Justice

Health Care Quality Improvement Act of 1986: A 1986 act that requires facilities to report professional review actions on physicians, dentists, and other facility-based practitioners to the National Practitioner Data Bank (NPDB) (Public Law 99-660 1986)

Health informatics: The field of information science concerned with the management of all aspects of health data and information through the application of computers and computer technologies

Health information exchange (HIE): The exchange of health information electronically between providers and others with the same level of interoperability, such as labs and pharmacies

Health information management (HIM): An allied health profession that is responsible for ensuring the availability, accuracy, and protection of the clinical information that is needed to deliver healthcare services and to make appropriate healthcare-related decisions

Health Information Management Systems Society (HIMSS): A cause-based, not-for-profit organization exclusively focused on providing global leadership for the optimal use of IT and management systems for the betterment of healthcare

Health information organization (HIO): An organization that supports, oversees, or governs the exchange of health-related information among organizations according to nationally recognized standards

Health Information Technology for Economic and Clinical Health (HITECH) Act: Legislation created to promote the adoption and meaningful use of health information technology in the United States. Subtitle D of the Act provides for additional privacy and security requirements that will develop and support electronic health information, facilitate information exchange, and strengthen monetary penalties. Signed into law on February 17, 2009, as part of ARRA (Public Law 111-5 2009)

Health insurance marketplace or exchange: Offers the purchase of federally regulated and subsidized health insurance to uninsured, eligible Americans based on their income

Health Insurance Portability and Accountability Act (HIPAA): The federal legislation enacted to provide continuity of health coverage, control fraud and abuse in healthcare, reduce healthcare costs, and guarantee the security and privacy of health information; limits exclusion for pre-existing medical conditions, prohibits discrimination against employees and dependents based on health status, guarantees availability of health insurance to small employers, and guarantees renewability of insurance to all employees regardless of size; requires covered entities (most healthcare providers and organizations) to transmit healthcare claims in a specific format and to develop, implement, and comply with the standards of the Privacy Rule and the Security Rule; and mandates that covered entities apply for and utilize national identifiers in HIPAA transactions (Public Law 104-191 1996)

Health IT: Under HITECH, hardware, software, integrated technologies or related licenses, intellectual property, upgrades, or packaged solutions sold as services that are designed for or support the use by health care entities or patients for the electronic creation, maintenance, access, or exchange of health information (Public Law 111-5 2009)

Health Level Seven (HL7): Founded in 1987, Health Level Seven International (HL7) is a not-for-profit, ANSI-accredited standards-developing organization dedicated to providing a comprehensive framework and related standards for the exchange, integration, sharing, and retrieval of electronic health information that supports clinical practice and the management, delivery, and evaluation of health services

Health maintenance organization: Entity that combines the provision of healthcare insurance and the delivery of healthcare services, characterized by: (1) an organized healthcare delivery system to a geographic area, (2) a set of basic and supplemental health maintenance and treatment services, (3) voluntarily enrolled members, and

(4) predetermined fixed, periodic prepayments for members' coverage

Health record: 1. Information relating to the physical or mental health or condition of an individual, as made by or on behalf of a health professional in connection with the care ascribed that individual 2. A medical record, health record, or medical chart that is a systematic documentation of a patient's medical history and care

Health reform: Steps taken to make major policy changes in how providers are reimbursed for healthcare services

Health Services Research: Research conducted on the subject of healthcare delivery that examines organizational structures and systems as well as the effectiveness and efficiency of healthcare services

Healthcare Cost and Utilization Project (HCUP): A family of databases and related software tools and products developed through a Federal-State-Industry partnership and sponsored by AHRQ. HCUP databases are derived from administrative data and contain encounter-level, clinical and nonclinical information including all-listed diagnoses and procedures, discharge status, patient demographics, and charges for all patients, regardless of payer (such as, Medicare, Medicaid, private insurance, uninsured), beginning in 1988

Healthcare data analytics: The practice of using data to make business decisions in healthcare

Healthcare insurance: Protection from having to pay the full cost of healthcare by prepaying for a plan for healthcare coverage

Healthcare research organizations: Organizations that conduct, promote, or support research across healthcare organizations

Hearsay: A written or oral statement made outside of court that is offered in court as evidence

High Reliability Organization (HRO): Organizations that focus on creating an environment that eliminates or minimizes error

HIPAA Security Rule: The federal regulations created to implement the security requirements of HIPAA

Histogram: A graphic technique used to display the frequency distribution of continuous data (interval or ratio data) as either numbers or percentages in a series of bars

History and physical (H&P): The pertinent information about the patient, including chief complaint, past and present illnesses, family history, social history, and review of body systems

Home health prospective payment system: The case mix reimbursement system developed by the Centers for Medicare and Medicaid Services in 2008, to cover home health services, including therapy visits and different resource costs provided to Medicare beneficiaries

Home healthcare: Limited part-time or intermittent skilled nursing care and home health aide services, physical therapy, occupational therapy, speech-language therapy, medical social services, durable medical equipment (such as wheelchairs, hospital beds, oxygen, and walkers), medical supplies, and other services

Hospice: An interdisciplinary program of palliative care and supportive services that addresses the physical, spiritual, social, and economic needs of terminally ill patients and their families

Hospital: A healthcare entity that has an organized medical staff and permanent facilities that include inpatient beds and continuous medical or nursing services and that provides diagnostic and therapeutic services for patients as well as overnight accommodations and nutritional services

Hospital-acquired condition (HAC): CMS identified eight hospital-acquired conditions (not present on admission) as "reasonably preventable," and hospitals will not receive additional payment for cases in which one of the eight selected conditions was not present on admission; the eight originally selected conditions include: foreign object retained after surgery, air embolism, blood incompatibility, stage III and IV pressure ulcers, falls and trauma, catheter-associated urinary tract infection, vascular catheter-associated infection, and surgical site infection—mediastinitis after coronary artery bypass graft; additional conditions were added in 2010 and remain in effect: surgical site infections following certain orthopedic procedures and bariatric surgery, manifestations of poor glycemic control, and deep vein thrombosis (DVT)/pulmonary embolism (PE) following certain orthopedic procedures

Hospital-acquired (nosocomial) infection rate: The number of hospital-acquired infections for a given time period divided by the total number of inpatient discharges for the same time period

Hospital autopsy: A postmortem (after death) examination performed on the body of a person who has at some time been a hospital patient by a hospital pathologist or a physician of the medical staff who has been delegated the responsibility

Hospital autopsy rate: The total number of autopsies performed by a hospital pathologist for a given time period divided by the number of deaths of hospital patients (inpatients and outpatients) whose bodies were available for autopsy for the same time period

Hospital death rate: The number of inpatient deaths for a given period of time divided by the total number of live discharges and deaths for the same time period

Hospital information system (HIS): The comprehensive database containing all the clinical, administrative, financial, and demographic information about each patient served by a hospital

Hospital inpatient: A patient who is provided with room, board, and continuous general nursing services in an area of an acute care facility where patients generally stay at least overnight

Hospital inpatient autopsy: A postmortem (after death) examination performed on the body of a patient who died during an inpatient hospitalization by a hospital pathologist or a physician of the medical staff who has been delegated the responsibility

Hospital newborn inpatient: A patient born in the hospital at the beginning of the current inpatient hospitalization

Hospital outpatient: A hospital patient who receives services in one or more of a hospital's facilities when he or she is not currently an inpatient or a home care patient

Hospital Standardization Program: An early 20th-century survey mechanism instituted by the American College of Surgeons and aimed at identifying quality-of-care problems and improving patient care; precursor to the survey program offered by the Joint Commission

Hostile work environment: A setting in which intimidating and abusive conduct takes place that interferes with an employee's job performance

House of Delegates: An important component of the volunteer structure of the American Health Information Management Association that conducts the official business of the organization and functions as its legislative body

Human capital: The sum of the knowledge, skills, and abilities of an organization's workforce

Human resources management (HRM): The process of acquiring, training, appraising, and compensating employees, and of attending to their labor relations, health and safety, and fairness concerns

Hybrid health record: A combination of paper and electronic records; a health record that includes both paper and electronic elements; *also known as hybrid record*

I

Identity management: Provides security functionality, including determining who (or what information system) is authorized to access information, authentication services, audit logging, encryption, and transmission controls

Identity matching algorithm: Rules established in an information system that predicts the probability that two or more patients in the database are the same patient

Identity proofing: Authentication credentials used to electronically sign prescriptions

Impact analysis: A collective term used to refer to any study that determines the benefit of a proposed project, including cost-benefit analysis, return on investment, benefits realization study, or qualitative benefit study

Implementation: Refers to technology having been installed, configured to meet the basic requirements of the healthcare organization, and demonstrated to users

Implementation specifications: As amended by HITECH, specific requirements or instructions for implementing a privacy or security standard

Implied consent: The type of permission that is inferred when a patient voluntarily submits to treatment

Implied contract: Type of agreement between physician and patient that is created by actions

Incidence rate: A computation that compares the number of new cases of a specific disease for a given time period to the population at risk for the disease during the same time period

Incident: An occurrence in a medical facility that is inconsistent with accepted standards of care

Incident detection: Methods used to identify both accidental and malicious events; detection programs monitor the information systems for abnormalities or a series of events that might indicate that a security breach is occurring or has occurred

Incident or occurrence report: A quality or performance management tool used to collect data and information about potentially compensable events (events that may result in death or serious injury)

Independent variable: The factors in experimental research that researchers manipulate directly.

Index: An organized (usually alphabetical) list of specific data that serves to guide, indicate, or otherwise facilitate reference to the data

Indian Health Service: The federal agency within the Department of Health and Human Services that is responsible for providing federal healthcare services to American Indians and Alaska natives

Individual: The person who is the subject of the protected health information

Individual data: Healthcare data that is housed within the electronic health record, data collected from a case study, a focus group of individuals, or during an interview or survey

Individually identifiable health information: As amended by HITECH, information that is a subset of health information, including demographic information collected from an individual, and: (1) is created or received by a health care provider, health plan, employer, or health care clearinghouse; and (2) relates to the past, present, or future physical or mental health or condition of an individual; the provision of health care to an individual; or the past, present, or future payment for the provision of health care to an individual; and (i) that identifies the individual; or (ii) with respect to which there is a reasonable basis to believe the information can be used to identify the individual (45 CFR 160.103 2013)

Infant mortality rate: The number of deaths of individuals under one year of age during a given time period divided by the number of live births reported for the same time period

Inferential statistics: 1. Statistics that are used to make inferences from a smaller group of data to a large one 2. A set of statistical techniques that allows researchers to make generalizations about a population's characteristics (parameters) on the basis of a sample's characteristics

Information: Data processed into usable form

Information governance: The accountability framework and decision rights to achieve enterprise information management (EIM). IG is the responsibility of executive leadership for developing and driving the IG strategy throughout the organization. IG encompasses both data governance (DG) and information technology governance (ITG)

Information Technology Asset Disposition (ITAD): Policy that identifies how all data storage devices are destroyed and purged of data prior to repurposing or disposal

Informed consent: 1. A legal term referring to a patient's right to make his or her own treatment decisions based on the knowledge of the treatment to be administered or the procedure to be performed 2. An individual's voluntary agreement to participate in research or to undergo a diagnostic, therapeutic, or preventive medical procedure

Injury (harm): In a negligence lawsuit, one of four elements, which may be economic (hospital expenses and loss of wages) and noneconomic (pain and suffering), that must be proved to be successful

Injury Severity Score (ISS): An overall severity measurement maintained in the trauma registry and calculated from the abbreviated injury scores for the three most severe injuries of each patient

Information: Refers to data elements that have been combined and then manipulated into something meaningful regarding a patient or a group of patients

Information assets: Information that has value for an organization

Information governance: The accountability framework and decision rights to achieve enterprise information management (EIM). IG is the responsibility of executive leadership for developing and driving the IG strategy throughout the organization. IG encompasses both data governance (DG) and information technology governance (ITG)

Informed consent: 1. A legal term referring to a patient's right to make his or her own treatment decisions based on the knowledge of the treatment to be administered or the procedure to be performed 2. An individual's voluntary agreement to participate in research or to undergo a diagnostic, therapeutic, or preventive medical procedure

Inpatient admission: An acute care facility's formal acceptance of a patient who is to be provided with room, board, and continuous nursing service in an area of the facility where patients generally stay at least overnight

Inpatient bed occupancy rate (percentage of occupancy): The total number of inpatient service days for a given time period divided by the total number of inpatient bed count days for the same time period

Inpatient discharge: The termination of hospitalization through the formal release of an inpatient from a hospital

Inpatient hospitalization: The period during an individual's life when he or she is a patient in a single hospital without interruption except by possible intervening leaves of absence

Inpatient prospective payment system: A system of payment for the operating costs of acute-care hospital inpatient stays under Medicare Part A based on prospectively expressed in the Social Security Act

Inpatient service day (IPSD): A unit of measure that reflects the services received by one inpatient during a 24-hour period

Inputs: Data entered into a hospital system (for example, the patient's knowledge of his or her condition, the admitting clerk's knowledge of the admission process, and the computer with its admitting template are all inputs for the hospital's admitting system)

Institutional Review Board (IRB): An administrative body that provides review, oversight, guidance, and approval for research projects carried out by employees serving as researchers, regardless of the location of the research (such as a university or private research agency); responsible for protecting the rights and welfare of the human subjects involved in the research. IRB oversight is mandatory for federally funded research projects

Integrated delivery network (IDN): Comprises a group of hospitals, physicians, other providers, insurers, or community agencies that work together to deliver health services

Integrated delivery system (IDS): A system that combines the financial and clinical aspects of healthcare and uses a group of healthcare providers, selected on the basis of quality and cost management criteria, to furnish comprehensive health services across the continuum of care

Integrated health record: A system of health record organization in which all the paper forms are arranged in strict chronological order and mixed with forms created by different departments

Integrity: 1. The state of being whole or unimpaired 2. The ability of data to maintain its structure and attributes, including protection against modification or corruption during transmission, storage, or at rest. Maintenance of data integrity is a key aspect of data quality management and security

Intentional tort: A circumstance where a healthcare provider purposely commits a wrongful act that results in injury

Interface: The zone between different computer systems across which users want to pass information (for example, a computer program written to exchange information between systems or the graphic display of an application program designed to make the program easier to use)

Internal analysis: Reviewing the inner working of the healthcare organization to determine strengths and weaknesses of the business practice and process

Internal audit: Audit conducted by employees within the organization to identify problems, concerns, and risks involving the operations, compliance, financial, and clinical areas of a healthcare organization

Internal customers: Customers within an organization, such as employees

Internal threats: Threats that originate within an organization

International Classification of Functioning, Disability, and Health (ICF): Classification of health and health-related domains that describe body functions and structures, activities, and participation

Interoperability: The capability of different information systems and software applications to communicate and exchange data

Interrogatories: Discovery devices consisting of a set of written questions given to a party, witness, or other person who has information needed in a legal case

Interval-level data: Data with a defined unit of measure, no true zero point, and equal intervals between successive values

Interval variables: Variables that have equal units with an arbitrary zero point

Intrusion detection: The process of identifying attempts or actions to penetrate a system and gain unauthorized access

Intrusion detection system (IDS): A system that performs automated intrusion detection; procedures should be outlined in the organization's data security plan to determine what actions should be taken in response to a probable intrusion

ISO 9000 certification: The ISO 9000 family addresses various aspects of quality management and contains some of ISO's best known standards. The standards provide guidance and tools for companies and organizations who want to ensure that their products and services consistently meet customers' requirements, and that quality is consistently improved

Issues management: Any issues that arise during the implementation are documented, brought to the attention of the vendor, and hopefully resolved, or escalated so that resolution is accomplished

J

Job analysis: Collecting and analyzing information about a job in order to better understand the significant component duties of the job, and to identify the skills and characteristics required of an employee who can successfully perform the job

Job classification: 1. A method of job evaluation that compares a written position description with the written descriptions of various classification grades 2. A method used by the federal government to grade jobs

Job description: A detailed list of a job's duties, reporting relationships, working conditions, and responsibilities

Job evaluation: The process of applying predefined compensable factors to jobs to determine their relative worth

Job interview: A conversation in which a hiring manager and a job applicant exchange information

Job sharing: A work schedule in which two or more individuals share the tasks of one full-time or one full-time-equivalent position

Job specifications: A list of a job's required education, skills, knowledge, abilities, personal qualifications, and physical requirements

Joinder: A complaint against a third party

Joint Commission: An independent, not-for-profit organization, the Joint Commission accredits and certifies more than 20,000 healthcare organizations and programs in the United States. Joint Commission accreditation and certification is recognized nationwide as a symbol of quality that reflects an organization's commitment to meeting certain performance standards

Judicial law: The body of law created as a result of court (judicial) decisions

Jurisdiction: The power and authority of a court to hear, interpret, and apply the law to and decide specific types of cases

Justice: Principle that recognizes the importance of treating people fairly, of applying rules consistently, and of fairly distributing cost and risk

K

Key indicator: A quantifiable measure used over time to determine whether some structure, process, or outcome in the provision of care to a patient supports high-quality performance measured against best practice criteria

Kiosk: Special form of input device geared more to people less familiar with computers

Knowledge: The information, understanding, and experience that give individuals the power to make informed decisions

L

Laboratory information system (LIS): Health information system that includes hardware; software; communications and network technologies; operational and cultural adaptations that people must make to use the technologies in performing diagnostic studies on various specimens collected from patients and to apply professional judgment in evaluating the quality of the data representing the results; policies and standards from the local organization in which the system is housed as well as accrediting and licensing bodies that must be followed for design of the technology and its use; and workflow and process designs assure the most efficient and effective use of the technology

Laissez-faire leadership: Delegative leadership style that reflects a leader who holds a title and responsibility, but has everyone else perform the work

Layoff: A temporary dismissal where employees are told there is no work available now, but that they may be recalled; there is no guarantee of being recalled

Leader–member relations: Group atmosphere much like social orientation; includes the subordinates' acceptance of, and confidence in, the leader as well as the loyalty and commitment they show toward the leader

Leadership: Visionary thinking, decisions responsive to membership and mission, and accountability for actions and outcomes

Leadership criteria: Division of leadership traits that includes leader emergence, leader effectiveness, and leader advancement and promotion

Leadership grid: Blake and Mouton's grid that marked off degrees of emphasis toward orientation using a nine-point scale and finally separated the grid into five styles of management based on the combined people and production emphasis

Leading: One of the four management functions in which people are directed and motivated to achieve goals

Leading by example: The leader is in a role model position and team members follow or emulate the leader's behavior

Lean: A process improvement methodology focused on eliminating waste and improving the flow of work processes

Lean Six Sigma: Methodology that utilizes elements of elimination of waste from Lean and critical process quality characteristics from Six Sigma

Learning health system: The alignment of science, informatics, incentives, and culture for continuous improvement and innovation, with best practices seamlessly embedded in the delivery process and new knowledge captured as an integral by-product of the delivery experience

Legal health record: Documents and data elements that a healthcare provider may include in response to legally permissible requests for patient information

Legal hold: A communication issued because of current or anticipated litigation, audit, government investigation, or other such matters that suspend the normal disposition or processing of records. Legal holds can encompass business procedures affecting active data, including, but not limited to, backup tape recycling. The specific communication to business or IT organizations may also be called a "hold," "preservation order," "suspension order," "freeze notice," "hold order," or "hold notice"

Legitimate power: Power derived from your position or status within the organization

Length of stay (LOS): The total number of patient days for an inpatient episode, calculated by subtracting the date of admission from the date of discharge

Licensure: The legal authority or formal permission from authorities to carry on certain activities that by law or regulation require such permission (applicable to institutions as well as individuals)

Likelihood determination: An estimate of the probability of threats occurring

Line authority: The authority to manage subordinates and to have them report back, based on relationships illustrated in an organizational chart

Line graph: A graphic technique used to illustrate the relationship between continuous measurements; consists of a line drawn to connect a series of points on an arithmetic scale; often used to display time trends

Litigation: A civil lawsuit or contest in court

Living will: A legal document, also known as a medical directive, that states a patient's wishes regarding life support in certain circumstances, usually when death is imminent

Logical Observations, Identifiers, Names and Codes (LOINC): A database protocol developed by the Regenstrief Institute for Health Care aimed at standardizing laboratory and clinical codes for use in clinical care, outcomes management, and research that enable exchange and aggregation of electronic health data from many independent systems

Loose material: Documentation that needs to be filed in the health record

M

Malfeasance: A wrong or improper act

Malware: Software applications that can take over partial or full control of a computer and can compromise data security and corrupt both data and hard drives

Managed care: 1. Payment method in which the third-party payer has implemented some provisions to control the costs of healthcare while maintaining quality care 2. Systematic merger of clinical, financial, and administrative processes to manage access, cost, and quality of healthcare

Managed care organization (MCO): A type of healthcare organization that delivers medical care and manages all aspects of the care or the payment for care by limiting providers of care, discounting payment to providers of care, or limiting access to care

Management: The process of planning, organizing, leading and controlling organizational activities

Mandatory eligibility groups: Children, pregnant women, elderly adults, people with disabilities and low-income adults that qualify for Medicaid

Market assessment: Determining the number of positions on the market and the eligible workforce looking for work

Marketing: As amended by HITECH, means to make a communication about a product or service that encourages recipients of the communication to purchase or use the product or service, or where the covered entity receives financial remuneration in exchange for making communication (45 CFR 164.501 2013)

Master patient index: A patient-identifying directory referencing all patients related to an organization and which also serves as a link to the patient record or information, facilitates patient identification, and assists in maintaining a longitudinal patient record from birth to death

Maternal death rate (hospital based): For a hospital, the total number of maternal deaths directly related to pregnancy for a given time period divided by the total number of obstetrical discharges for the same time period; for a community, the total number of deaths attributed to maternal conditions during a given time period in a specific geographic area divided by the total number of live births for the same time period in the same area

Maternal mortality rate (community-based): A rate that measures the deaths associated with pregnancy for a specific community for a specific period of time

Mean: A measure of central tendency that is determined by calculating the arithmetic average of the observations in a frequency distribution

Meaningful Use: A regulation that was issued by CMS on July 28, 2010, outlining an incentive program for professionals (EPs), eligible hospitals, and CAHs participating in Medicare and Medicaid programs that adopt and successfully demonstrate meaningful use of certified EHR technology

Measurement: The systematic process of data collection, repeated over time or at a single point in time

Measures of central tendency: The typical or average numbers that are descriptive of the entire collection of data for a specific population

Measures of variability: Examination of the spread of different values around the measures of central tendency; these include the range, variance, and standard deviation.

Median: A measure of central tendency that shows the midpoint of a frequency distribution when the observations have been arranged in order from lowest to highest

Mediation: In law, when a dispute is submitted to a third party to facilitate agreement between the disputing parties

Medicaid: A joint federal and state program that helps with medical costs for some people with low incomes and limited resources. Medicaid programs vary from state to state, but most healthcare costs are covered if a patient qualifies for both Medicare and Medicaid

Medicaid Fraud Control Units (MFCU): Groups that investigate and prosecute Medicaid fraud as well as patient abuse and neglect in healthcare facilities

Medical device integration: Connecting medical devices to the EHR

Medical identity theft: The fraudulent use of an individual's identifying information in a healthcare setting

Medical necessity: 1. The likelihood that a proposed healthcare service will have a reasonable beneficial effect on the patient's physical condition and quality of life at a specific point in his or her illness

or lifetime 2. As amended by HITECH, a covered entity or business associate may not use or disclose protected health information, except as permitted or required (45 CFR 164.502 2013) 3. The concept that procedures are only eligible for reimbursement as a covered benefit when they are performed for a specific diagnosis or specified frequency (42 CFR 405.500 1995)

Medical examiner: Usually an appointed official who is a physician, commonly holding a specialty in pathology or forensic medicine with duties similar to coroner

Medical history: Portion of clinical data that addresses the patient's current complaints and symptoms and lists his or her past medical, personal, and family history

Medical identity theft: A type of healthcare fraud that includes both financial fraud and identity theft, it involves either (a) the inappropriate or unauthorized misrepresentation of one's identity (for example, the use of one's name and Social Security number) to obtain medical services or goods, or (b) the falsifying of claims for medical services in an attempt to obtain money

Medical Literature, Analysis, and Retrieval System Online (MEDLINE): Medline is the US National Library of Medicine's (NLM) premier bibliographic database that contains over 19 million references to journal articles in life sciences with a concentration on biomedicine

Medical malpractice: A type of action in which the plaintiff must demonstrate that a healthcare provider-patient relationship existed at the time of the alleged wrongful act

Medical staff: The staff members of a healthcare organization who are governed by medical staff bylaws; may or may not be employed by the healthcare organization

Medical staff bylaws: Standards governing the practice of medical staff members; typically voted upon by the organized medical staff and the medical staff executive committee and approved by the facility's board; governs the business conduct, rights, and responsibilities of the medical staff; medical staff members must abide by these bylaws in order to continue practice in the healthcare facility

Medical staff classification: Refers to the organization of physicians according to clinical assignment

Medical staff privileges: Categories of clinical practice privileges assigned to individual practitioners on the basis of their qualifications

Medicare: A federally funded health program established in 1965 to assist with the medical care costs of Americans 65 years of age and older as well as other individuals entitled to Social Security benefits owing to their disabilities

Medicare administrative contractors: Required by section 911 of the Medicare Prescription Drug, Improvement and Modernization Act of 2003, CMS is completing the process of awarding Medicare claims processing contracts through competitive procedures resulting in replacing its current claims payment contractors, fiscal intermediaries and carriers, with new contract entities called MACs. Initially 19 MACs were expected through three procurement cycles. Currently there are 15 A/B MAC jurisdictions that have served as the foundation for CMS's initial series of A/B MAC procurements. CMS will continue to consolidate to 10 A/B MAC jurisdictions

Medicare Advantage: A type of Medicare health plan offered by a private company that contracts with Medicare to provide the beneficiary with all Part A and Part B benefits. These plans include Health Maintenance Organizations, Preferred Provider Organizations, Private Fee-for-Service Plans, Special Needs Plans, and Medicare Medical Savings Account Plans. Enrollees in Medicare Advantage Plans have their services are covered through the plan are not paid for under original Medicare

Medicare Fraud Strike Force: The result of the Health Care Fraud Prevention and Enforcement Action Team, this group uses data analytics to look for evidence of fraud and abuse

Medicare Part A: Insurance that assists in covering inpatient care in hospitals, including critical access hospitals, and skilled nursing facilities (not custodial or long-term care). It also assists in covering hospice care and some home healthcare. Beneficiaries must meet certain conditions to get these benefits

Medicare Part B: An optional and supplemental portion of Medicare that beneficiaries pay a monthly premium for. Part B assists coverage with doctors' services and outpatient care. It also covers some other medical services that Part A does not cover, such as some of the services of physical and occupational therapists, and some home healthcare. Part B pays for these covered services and supplies when they are medically necessary

Medicare Part D: Medicare drug benefit created by the Medicare Modernization Act of 2003 (MMA) that offers outpatient drug coverage to beneficiaries for an additional premium. Starting January 1, 2006, new Medicare prescription drug coverage became available to everyone with Medicare. This coverage assists in lowering prescription drug costs and protect against higher costs in the future

Medicare Provider Analysis and Review (MEDPAR) File: A database containing information submitted by fiscal intermediaries that is used by the Office of the Inspector General to identity suspicious billing and charge practices

Medicare severity diagnosis-related groups (MS-DRGs): The US government's 2007 revision of the DRG system, the MS-DRG system better accounts for severity of illness and resource consumption

Medication five rights: The right drug, in the right dose, through the right route, at the right time, and to the right patient

Medication reconciliation: Process that monitors and confirms that the patient receives consistent dosing across all facility transfers, such as on admission, from nursing unit to surgery, and from surgery to ICU

Mentoring: A type of coaching and training in which an individual is matched with a more experienced individual who serves as an advisor or counselor

Merger: A business situation where two or more companies combine, but one of them continues to exist as a legal business entity while the others cease to exist legally and their assets and liabilities become part of the continuing company

Message format standards: Protocols that help ensure that data transmitted from one system to another remain comparable

Metadata: Descriptive data that characterize other data to create a clearer understanding of their meaning and to achieve greater reliability and quality of information. Metadata consist of both indexing terms and attributes. Data about data: for example, creation date, date sent, date received, last access date, last modification date

Middle management: The management level in an organization that is concerned primarily with facilitating the work performed by supervisory- and staff-level personnel as well as by executive leaders

Minimum Data Set (MDS) for Long-Term Care: A federally mandated standard assessment form that Medicare- and Medicaid-certified nursing facilities must use to collect demographic and clinical data on nursing home residents; includes screening, clinical, and functional status elements

Minimum necessary standard: Requires that uses, disclosures, and requests must be limited to only the amount needed to accomplish an intended purpose

Misfeasance: Relating to negligence or improper performance during an otherwise correct act

Mission: A written statement that sets forth the core purpose and philosophies of an organization or group; defines the organization or group's general purpose for existing

Mixed-methodology: Research study approach that includes using both quantitative and qualitative data

Mode: A measure of central tendency that consists of the most frequent observation in a frequency distribution

Moral values: A system of principles by which one guides one's life, usually with regard to right or wrong

Morbidity: The state of being diseased (including illness, injury, or deviation from normal health); the number of sick persons or cases of disease in relation to a specific population

Multivoting technique: A decision-making method for determining group consensus on the prioritization of issues or solutions

N

National Cancer Registrars Association (NCRA): A not-for-profit association representing cancer registry professionals and Certified Tumor Registrars (CTR). The primary focus is education and certification with the goal to ensure all cancer registry professionals have the required knowledge to be superior in their field

National Center for Health Statistics (NCHS): The federal agency responsible for collecting and disseminating information on health services utilization and the health status of the population in the United States; developed the clinical modification to the International Classification of Diseases, Ninth Revision (ICD-10) and is responsible for updating the diagnosis portion of the ICD-10-CM

National Council for Prescription Drug Programs (NCPDP): A not-for-profit ANSI-accredited standards development organization founded in 1977 that develops standards for exchanging prescription and payment information

National Committee for Quality Assurance (NCQA): A private not-for-profit organization dedicated to improving healthcare quality. Since its founding in 1990, NCQA has been a central figure in driving improvement throughout the healthcare system, helping to elevate the issue of healthcare quality to the top of the national agenda

National Drug Codes (NDC): Codes that serve as product identifiers for human drugs, currently limited to prescription drugs and a few selected over-the-counter products

National Fraud Prevention Partnership: A voluntary program designed to reduce healthcare fraud by pooling resources with the private sector and using data analysis techniques to sort through claims data

National Labor Relations Act (NLRA): Federal pro-union legislation that provides, among other things, procedures for union representation and prohibits unfair labor practices by unions, such as coercing nonstriking employees, and by employers, such as interference with the union selection process and discrimination against employees who support a union

National Labor Relations Board (NLRB): US government agency that holds elections for labor union representation and that reviews and looks into unfair labor practices

National Library of Medicine: The world's largest medical library and a branch of the National Institutes of Health

National patient safety goals (NPSGs): Goals issued by the Joint Commission to improve patient safety in healthcare organizations nationwide

National Practitioner Data Bank (NPDB): A confidential information clearinghouse created by Congress with the primary goals of improving healthcare quality, protecting the public, and reducing healthcare fraud and abuse in the United States. The NPDB is primarily an alert or flagging system intended to facilitate comprehensive review of the professional credentials of healthcare practitioners, healthcare entities, providers, and supplies

National Vital Statistics System (NVSS): The oldest and most successful example of intergovernmental data sharing in public health, and the shared relationships, standards, and procedures that form the mechanism by which NCHS collects and disseminates the nation's official vital statistics. These data are provided through contracts between NCHS and vital registration systems operated in the various jurisdictions and legally responsible for the registration of vital events—births, deaths, marriages, divorces, and fetal deaths

Natural language processing (NLP): A technology that converts human language (structured or unstructured) into data that can be translated then manipulated by computer systems; branch of artificial intelligence

Need-to-know principle: The release-of-information principle based on the minimum necessary standard

Negligence: A legal term that refers to the result of an action by an individual who does not act the way a reasonably prudent person would act under the same circumstances

Negligent hiring: Occurs when employees with prior criminal records were not subjected to thorough pre-employment screening

Neonatal mortality rate: The number of deaths of infants under 28 days of age during a given time period divided by the total number of births for the same time period

Net autopsy rate: The ratio of inpatient autopsies compared to inpatient deaths calculated by dividing the total number of inpatient autopsies performed by the hospital pathologist for a given time period by the total number of inpatient deaths minus unautopsied coroners' or medical examiners' cases for the same time period

Net death rate: The total number of inpatient deaths minus the number of deaths that occurred less than 48 hours after admission for a given time period divided by the total number of inpatient discharges minus the number of deaths that occurred less than 48 hours after admission for the same time period

Network control: A method of protecting data from unauthorized change and corruption at rest and during transmission among information systems

New employee orientation: A group of activities that welcome new employees and introduce them to the organization, to the assigned department, unit or workgroup and to the specific job to be performed

New graduate membership: AHIMA membership level for student members who are recent graduates of accredited associate, bachelor's, and master's degree programs as well as AHIMA-approved coding programs

Newborn (NB): An inpatient who was born in a hospital at the beginning of the current inpatient hospitalization

Newborn autopsy rate: The number of autopsies performed on newborns who died during a given time period divided by the total number of newborns who died during the same time period

Newborn death rate: The number of newborns who died divided by the total number of newborns, both alive and dead

Nomenclature: A recognized system of terms that follows pre-established naming conventions; a disease nomenclature is a listing of the proper name for each disease entity with its specific code number

Nominal group technique: A group process technique that involves the steps of silent listing, recording each participant's list, discussing, and rank ordering the priority or importance of items; allows groups to narrow the focus of discussion or to make decisions without becoming involved in extended, circular discussions

Nominal-level data: Data that fall into groups or categories that are mutually exclusive and with no specific order (for example, patient demographics such as third-party payer, race, and sex)

Nominal variables: Variables in which a number is assigned to a specific category; such as a 1= male and 2 = female

Noncovered services: Services not reimbursable under a managed care plan

Nonexempt employees: All groups of employees covered by the provisions of the Fair Labor Standards Act

Nonfeasance: A type of negligence meaning failure to act

Nonmaleficence: A legal principle that means "first do no harm"

Normal distribution: A theoretical family of continuous frequency distributions characterized by a symmetric bell-shaped curve, with an equal mean, median, and mode; any standard deviation; and with half of the observations above the mean and half below it

North American Association of Central Cancer Registries (NAACCR): Organization that has a certification program for state population-based registries; Certification is based on the quality of data collected and reported by the state registry; NAACCR has developed standards for data quality and format and works with other cancer organizations to align their various standards

Nosocomial (hospital-acquired) infection: An infection acquired by a patient while receiving care or services in a healthcare organization

Notice of privacy practices: As amended by HITECH, a statement (mandated by the HIPAA Privacy Rule) issued by a healthcare organization that informs individuals of the uses and disclosures of patient-identifiable health information that may be made by the organization, as well as the individual's rights and the organization's legal duties with respect to that information (45 CFR 164.520 2013)

Notifiable disease: A disease that must be reported to a government agency so that regular, frequent, and timely information on individual cases can be used to prevent and control future cases of the disease

Numeric filing system: A system of health record identification and storage in which records are arranged consecutively in ascending numerical order according to the health record number

Nursing information system: System that manages the nursing department, including staffing, credentialing, training, budgeting, and other managerial functions

O

Object-oriented database: A type of database that uses commands that act as small, self-contained instructional units (objects) that may be combined in various ways

Occasion of service: A specified identifiable service involved in the care of a patient that is not an encounter (for example, a lab test ordered during an encounter)

Occupational Safety and Health Act: The federal legislation that established comprehensive safety and health guidelines for employers (Public Law 91-596 1970)

Office of Inspector General (OIG): Mandated by Public Law 95-452 (as amended) to protect the integrity of HHS programs, as well as the health and welfare of the beneficiaries of those programs. The OIG has a responsibility to report both to the Secretary and to the Congress program and management problems and recommendations to correct them. The OIG's duties are carried out through a nationwide network of audits, investigations, inspections, and other mission-related functions performed by OIG components

Office of the National Coordinator for Health Information Technology (ONC): The principal federal entity charged with coordination of nationwide efforts to implement and use the most advanced health information technology and the electronic exchange of health information. The position of National Coordinator was created in 2004, through an Executive Order, and legislatively mandated in the HITECH Act of 2009

Offshoring: Outsourcing jobs to countries overseas, wherein local employees abroad perform jobs that domestic employees previously performed

Onboarding: Socialization into the values and culture of an organization

Online analytical processing (OLAP): A data access architecture that allows the user to retrieve specific information from a large volume of data

Online learning: Broad term referring to the use of electronic media instead of classroom-based learning to deliver training

Online transaction processing (OLTP): The real-time processing of day-to-day business transactions from a database

On-the-job training: A method of training in which an employee learns necessary skills and processes by performing the functions of his or her position

Operating rules: Rules that further explain the business requirements so their use is consistent across health plans

Operation index: A list of the operations and surgical procedures performed in a healthcare facility, which is sequenced according to the code numbers of the classification system in use

Operational planning: The specific day-to-day tasks that are required in operating a healthcare organization or an HIM department

Operative report: A formal document that describes the events surrounding a surgical procedure or operation and identifies the principal participants in the surgery

Opportunity for improvement: A healthcare structure, product, service, process, or outcome that does not meet its customers' expectations and, therefore, could be improved

Opt in/opt out: A type of HIE model that sets the default for health information of patients to be included automatically, but the patient can opt out completely

Optimization: Reflects not only good adoption for all routine operations, but also an understanding and appropriate use of the technology's features

Ordinal-level data: Data where the order of the numbers is meaningful, not the number itself

Ordinal variables: Ranked variables in which a number is assigned to rank a category in an ordered series but does not indicate the magnitude of the difference between any two data points

Organization: The planned coordination of the activities of multiple people to achieve a common purpose or goal

Organizational chart: A visual graphic or diagram showing the structure and reporting relationships between positions, departments, and employees of an organization

Organizational structure: The framework of authority and supervision for the employees within the healthcare organization

Out of pocket: Paying for the services provided with one's own funds

Outcome indicators: An indicator that assesses what happens or does not happen to a patient following a process; agreed upon desired patient characteristics to be achieved; undesired patient conditions to be avoided

Outcome measures: 1. The process of systematically tracking a patient's clinical treatment and responses to that treatment, including measures of morbidity and functional status, for the purpose of improving care 2. A measure that indicates the result of the performance (or nonperformance) of a function or process

Outguide: A device used in paper-based health record systems to track the location of records removed from the file storage area

Outlier providers: Those whose coding or billing practices are significantly outside the norm

Outpatient: A patient who receives ambulatory care services in a hospital-based clinic or department

Outpatient prospective payment system: The Medicare prospective payment system used for hospital-based outpatient services and procedures that is predicated on the assignment of ambulatory payment classifications

Outpatient visit: A patient's visit to one or more units located in the ambulatory services area (clinic or physician's office) of an acute care hospital in which an overnight stay does not occur

Outputs: The outcomes of inputs into a system (for example, the output of the admitting process is the patient's admission to the hospital)

Outsourcing: The hiring of an individual or a company external to an organization to perform a function either on site or off site

Overcoding: The practice of assigning more codes than needed to describe a patient's condition. Some instances of overcoding may be contrary to the guidance provided in the Official Coding Guidelines

Overlap: Situation in which a patient is issued more than one medical record number from an organization with multiple facilities

Overlay: Situation in which a patient is issued a medical record number that has been previously issued to a different patient

Overpayment: A higher reimbursement than deserved

P

Paper health record: Health record that is completely available in paper media

Parallel work division: A type of concurrent work design in which one employee does several tasks and takes the job from beginning to end

Pareto chart: A bar graph that includes bars arranged in order of descending size to show decisions on the prioritization of issues, problems, or solutions

Part-time employee: An employee who works less than the full-time standard of 40 hours per week, 80 hours per two-week period, or 8 hours per day

Participative leadership: Plans and decisions are made by the team and the leader is there to provide advice and assistance

Password: A series of characters that must be entered to authenticate user identity and gain access to a computer or specified portions of a database

Pathology report: A type of health record or documentation that describes the results of a microscopic and macroscopic evaluation of a specimen removed or expelled during a surgical procedure

Patient account number: A number assigned by a healthcare facility for billing purposes that is unique to a particular episode of care; a new account number is assigned each time the patient receives care or services at the facility

Patient acuity staffing: The number of nurses and other care providers is based on how sick the patient is

Patient advocacy: A healthcare organization program where an employee speaks on a patient's behalf and helps get any information or services needed

Patient assessment instrument (PAI): A standardized tool used to evaluate the patient's condition after admission to, and at discharge from, the healthcare facility

Patient financial system (PFS): Information system that manages patient accounts

Patient-identifiable data: Personal information that can be linked to a specific patient, such as age, gender, date of birth, and address

Patient portal: Information system that allows patient to log in to obtain information, register, and perform other functions

Patient safety: Preventing harm to patients, learning from errors, and building a culture of safety

Pay for performance: 1. A type of incentive to improve clinical performance using the electronic health record that could result in additional reimbursement or eligibility for grants or other subsidies to support further HIT efforts 2. The Integrated Healthcare Association initiative in California based on the concept that physician groups would be paid for documented performance

Peer review organization (PRO): Until 2002, a medical organization that performed a professional review of medical necessity, quality, and appropriateness of healthcare services provided to Medicare beneficiaries

Percentile: A measure used in descriptive statistics that shows the value below which a given percentage of scores in a given group of scores fall

Performance appraisal: Refers to the formal system of review and evaluation methods used to assess employee and team performance

Performance improvement (PI): The continuous study and adaptation of a healthcare organization's functions and processes to increase the likelihood of achieving desired outcomes

Performance indicators: A measure used by healthcare facilities to assess the quality, effectiveness, and efficiency of their services

Performance management: An ongoing, goal-oriented process focused on productivity and continuous improvement of employees and teams

Performance measurement: The process of comparing the outcomes of an organization, work unit, or employee against pre-established performance plans and standards; results are typically expressed in quantifiable terms

Personal health record (PHR): An electronic or paper health record maintained and updated by an individual for himself or herself; a tool that individuals can use to collect, track, and share past and current information about their health or the health of someone in their care

Personal representative: Person with legal authority to act on a patient's behalf

Pharmacy information system: This system receives an order for a drug in a hospital, aids the hospital's pharmacist in checking for contraindications, directs staff in compounding any drugs requiring special preparation, aids in dispensing the drug in the appropriate dose and for the appropriate route of administration, maintains inventory (documenting medications in stock using the National Drug Code, the terminology maintained by the Food and Drug Administration [FDA] for use in identifying FDA-approved drugs), supports staffing and budgeting, and performs other departmental operations

Physician champion: An individual who assists in communicating and educating medical staff in areas such as documentation procedures for accurate billing and appropriate EHR processes

Physician query process: The process by which questions are posed to a provider to obtain additional, clarifying documentation to improve the specificity and completeness of the data used to assign diagnosis and procedure codes in the patient's health record

Physician Self-Referral Law: Originally a part of the Omnibus Budget Reconciliation Act of 1989, it is a law that prohibits physicians from ordering designated health services for Medicare (and to some extent Medicaid) patients from entities with which the physician, or an immediate family member, has a financial relationship

Physical examination: The physician's assessment of the patient's current health status after evaluating the patient's physical condition

Physical safeguards: As amended by HITECH, security rule measures such as locking doors to safeguard data and various media from unauthorized access and exposures; includes facility access controls, workstation use, workstation security, and device and media controls

Physician index: A list of patients and their physicians usually arranged according to the physician code numbers assigned by the healthcare facility

Physician Quality Reporting System (PQRS): An incentive payment system for eligible professionals who satisfactorily report data on quality measures for covered professional services furnished to Medicare beneficiaries; formerly known as the Physician Quality Reporting Initiative (PQRI)

Physician orders: A physician's written or verbal instructions to the other caregivers involved in a patient's care

Picture archiving and communications system (PACS): An integrated computer system that obtains, stores, retrieves, and displays digital images (in healthcare, radiological images)

Pie chart: A graphic technique in which the proportions of a category are displayed as portions of a circle (like pieces of a pie); used to show the relationship of individual parts to the whole

Plaintiff: The group or person who initiates a civil lawsuit

Planning: 1. Governing principles that describe how a department or an organization is supposed to handle a specific situation or execute a specific process 2. Binding contracts issued by a healthcare insurance company to an individual or group in which the company promises to pay for healthcare to treat illness or injury; such contracts may also be referred to as health plan agreements and evidence of coverage

Point of care (POC): The place or location where the physician administers services to the patient

Point-of-care charting: A system whereby information is entered into the health record at the time and location of service

Point of service plans: A type of managed care plan in which enrollees are encouraged to select healthcare providers from a network of providers under contract with the plan but are also allowed to select providers outside the network and pay a larger share of the cost

Policies: 1. Governing principles that describe how a department or an organization is supposed to handle a specific situation or execute a specific process 2. Binding contracts issued by a healthcare insurance company to an individual or group in which the company promises to pay for healthcare to treat illness or injury; such contracts may also be referred to as health plan agreements and evidence of coverage

Policyholder: An individual or entity that purchases healthcare insurance coverage

Population-based registry: A type of registry that includes information from more than one facility in a specific geopolitical area, such as a state or region

Population-based statistics: Statistics based on a defined population rather than on a sample drawn from the same population

Portals: Windows into information systems

Postneonatal mortality rate: The number of deaths of persons aged 28 days up to, but not including, one year during a given time period divided by the number of live births for the same time period

Postoperative infection rate: The number of infections that occur in clean surgical cases for a given time period divided by the total number of operations within the same time period

Potentially compensable event: An event (for example, an injury, accident, or medical error) that may result in financial liability for a healthcare organization, for example, an injury, accident, or medical error

Power and influence theory: Leadership theory noting there are various ways that leaders use authority, control, and their impact to get things done

Power user: Users who are able to use technology to significantly improve their productivity

Precertification: Process of obtaining approval from a healthcare insurance company before receiving healthcare services

Preemption: In law, the principle that a statute at one level supersedes or is applied over the same or similar statute at a lower level (for example, the federal HIPAA privacy provisions trump the same or similar state law except when state law is more stringent)

Preferred provider organization: A managed care contract coordinated care plan that: (a) has a network of providers that have agreed to a contractually specified reimbursement for covered benefits with the organization offering the plan; (b) provides for reimbursement for all covered benefits regardless of whether the benefits are provided with the network of providers; and (c) is offered by an organization that is not licenses or organized under state law as an HMO

Preferred term (PT): In SNOMED CT, the description or name assigned to a concept that is used most commonly; in the UMNDS classification system, a representation of the generic product category, which is a list of preferred concepts that name devices

Pregnancy Discrimination Act: The federal legislation that prohibits discrimination against women affected by pregnancy, childbirth, or related medical conditions by requiring that affected women be treated the same as all other employees for employment-related purposes, including benefits (Public Law 95-555)

Prejudice: Occurs when a person is judged solely based on cultural factors such as ethnicity, religion, age, gender, sexual orientation, or such

Premium: Amount of money that a policyholder or certificate holder must periodically pay an insurer in return for healthcare coverage

Presentation software: Software used to build slides when presenting a specific topic, idea, research data or any type of information

Present on admission (POA): A condition present at the time of inpatient admission

Prevalence rate: The proportion of people in a population who have a particular disease at a specific point in time or over a specified period of time

Preventive service: Healthcare services to prevent illness or early detection tests and diagnostic tools, when treatment is most likely to be effective

Primary care physician (PCP): 1. Physician who provides, supervises, and coordinates the healthcare of a member and who manages referrals to other healthcare providers and utilization of healthcare services both inside and outside a managed care plan. Family and general practitioners, internists, pediatricians, and obstetricians and gynecologists are primary care physicians 2. The physician who makes the initial diagnosis of a patient's medical condition

Primary data source: The health record is this type of source because it contains information about a patient that has been documented by the professionals who provided care or services to that patient

Principles of organization: Principles that include specialization, functional definition, span of control, hierarchical chain, and unity of command used by managers at all levels

Prior approval (authorization): Process of obtaining approval from a healthcare insurance company before receiving healthcare services

Privacy: The quality or state of being hidden from, or undisturbed by, the observation or activities of other persons, or freedom from unauthorized intrusion; in healthcare-related contexts, the right of a patient to control disclosure of protected health information

Private healthcare insurance: Commercial insurance purchased by individuals, self-employed business people, and groups of people (such as associations and religious organizations), for themselves and for their dependents; typically these plans have high deductibles or limited covered services; a premium for coverage is paid each month to the third-party payer and those funds are used to help pay for the healthcare services

Privacy officer: A position mandated under the HIPAA Privacy Rule—covered entities must designate an individual to be responsible for developing and implementing privacy policies and procedures

Privacy Rule: The federal regulations created to implement the privacy requirements of the simplification subtitle of the Health Insurance Portability and Accountability Act of 1996; effective in 2002; afforded patients certain rights to and about their protected health information

Private key infrastructure: Two or more computers share the same secret key and that key is used to both encrypt and decrypt a message; however, the key must be kept secret and if it is compromised in any way, the security of the data is likely to be eliminated; *see also single-key encryption*

Private law: The collective rules and principles that define the rights and duties of people and private businesses

Privileged communication: The protection afforded to the recipients of professional services that prohibits medical practitioners, lawyers, and other professionals from disclosing the confidential information that they learn in their capacity as professional service providers

Probabilistic algorithm: Algorithm that uses mathematical probabilities to determine the possibility that two patients are the same

Problem list: A list of illnesses, injuries, and other factors that affect the health of an individual patient, usually identifying the time of occurrence or identification and resolution

Problem-oriented health record: A patient record in which clinical problems are defined and documented individually

Procedure: 1. A document that describes the steps involved in performing a specific function 2. An action of a medical professional for treatment or diagnosis of a medical condition 3. The steps taken to implement a policy

Process indicators: Specific measures that enable the assessment of the steps taken in rendering a service

Process redesign: The steps in which focused data are collected and analyzed, the process is changed to incorporate the knowledge gained from the data collected, the new process is implemented, and the staff is educated about the new process

Productivity indicators: A set of measures designed to routinely monitor the output and quality of products or services provided by an individual, an organization, or one of its constituent parts; used to help determine status of a productivity bonus

Professional component: 1. The portion of a healthcare procedure performed by a physician 2. A term generally used in reference to the elements of radiological procedures performed by a physician

Program evaluation and review technique (PERT) chart: A project management tool that diagrams a project's time lines and tasks as well as their interdependencies

Progress notes: The documentation of a patient's care, treatment, and therapeutic response, which is entered into the health record by each of the clinical professionals involved in a patient's care, including nurses, physicians, therapists, and social workers

Progressive penalties: Ensures that the minimum penalty appropriate to the level of offense is applied

Project management: A formal set of principles and procedures that help control the activities associated with implementing a usually large undertaking to achieve a specific goal, such as an information system project

Project management life cycle: The period in which the processes involved in carrying out a project are completed, including project definition, project planning and organization, project tracking and analysis, project revisions, change control, and communication

Proportion: The relation of one part to another or to the whole with respect to magnitude, quantity, or degree

Proportionate mortality rate (PMR): The total number of deaths due to a specific cause during a given time period divided by the total number of deaths due to all causes

Prospective payment system: A type of reimbursement system that is based on preset payment levels rather than actual charges billed after the service has been provided; specifically, one of several Medicare reimbursement systems based on predetermined payment rates or periods and linked to the anticipated intensity of services delivered as well as the beneficiary's condition

Prospective review: A review of a patient's health records before admission to determine the necessity of admission to an acute care facility and to determine or satisfy benefit coverage requirements

Prospective study: A study designed to observe outcomes or events that occur after the identification of a group of subjects to be studied

Protected class: Identified groups, such as racial minorities and women, that are protected by law based on past employment discrimination

Protected health information (PHI): As amended by HITECH, individually identifiable health information: (1) Except as provided in paragraph (2) of this definition, that is: (i) transmitted by electronic media; (ii) maintained in electronic media; or (iii) transmitted or maintained in any other form or medium. (2) Protected health information excludes individually identifiable health information: (i) in education records covered by the Family Educational Rights and Privacy Act, as amended, 20 USC 1232g; (ii) in records described at 20 USC 1232g(a)(4)(B)(iv); (iii) in employment records held by a covered entity in its role as employer; and (iv) regarding a person who has been deceased for more than 50 years (45 CFR 160.103 2013)

Protocol: In healthcare, a detailed plan of care for a specific medical condition based on investigative studies; in medical research, a rule or procedure to be followed in a clinical trial; in a computer network, a rule or procedure used to address and ensure delivery of data

Provider: Physician, clinic, hospital, nursing home, or other healthcare entity (second party) that delivers healthcare services

Proximal attributes: Division of leadership traits that includes problem-solving skills, social appraisal skills, and expertise and tacit knowledge derived from the distal attributes and are part of a leader's operating environment

Public health: An area of healthcare that deals with the health of populations in geopolitical areas, such as states and counties

Public key infrastructure (PKI): In cryptography, an asymmetric algorithm made publicly available to unlock a coded message

Public law: A type of legislation that involves the government and its relations with individuals and business organizations

Q

Qualitative analysis: A review of the health record to ensure that standards are met and to determine the adequacy of entries documenting the quality of care

Qualitative research: Research design that collects types of data that includes a participant's perceptions, attitudes, feelings or attitudes about a certain subject; methods used to collect qualitative data can include observations, focus groups, case studies, informal conversational interviews, and in-depth interviews

Qualitative variables: Categorical variables; all are discrete and include both nominal and ordinal variables

Quality: The degree or grade of excellence of goods or services, including, in healthcare, meeting expectations for outcomes of care

Quality improvement organization (QIO): An organization that performs medical peer review of Medicare and Medicaid claims, including review of validity of hospital diagnosis and procedure coding information; completeness, adequacy, and quality of care; and appropriateness of prospective payments for outlier cases and nonemergent use of the emergency room. Until 2002, called peer review organization

Quality indicator: A standard against which actual care may be measured to identify a level of performance for that standard

Quantitative analysis: A review of the health record to determine its completeness and accuracy

Quantitative study: Data collected for research studies that are collated numerically with descriptive, inferential, or predictive statistics

Quantitative variables: Numerical variables; can be broken down into interval and ratio variables

Quasi-experimental study: Similar to the experimental study except that randomization of participants is not included in a quasi-experimental study, the independent variable may not be manipulated by the researcher, and there may be no control or comparison group; these studies can be performed over time and may not include individual participants but whole healthcare systems

Query: Communication tool for CDI staff to communicate with providers to obtain clinical clarification, provide a documentation alert, get documentation clarification, or ask additional questions regarding documentation

Qui tam: The "whistleblower" provisions of the False Claims Act which provides that private persons, known as relators, may enforce the Act by filing a complaint, under seal, alleging fraud committed against the government

Quid pro quo: A favor or advantage given for something expected in return; often in sexual harassment instances, sexual favors are requested in exchange for a job benefit or continued employment

R

Radio-frequency identification (RFID): An automatic recognition technology that uses a device attached to an object to transmit data to a receiver and does not require direct contact

Radiology information system (RIS): Performs functions similar to LIS, receiving an order for a procedure, scheduling it, notifying hospital personnel or the patient if performed as an outpatient, tracking the performance of the procedure and its output, tracking preparation of the report, performing quality control, maintaining an inventory of equipment and supplies, and managing departmental staffing and budget

Randomization: The assignment of subjects to experimental or control groups based on chance

Range: A measure of variability between the smallest and largest observations in a frequency distribution

Ranking method: Appraiser ranks all employees in a group or unit from highest to lowest based on overall performance

Rate: A measure used to compare an event over time; a comparison of the number of times an event did happen (numerator) with the number of times an event could have happened (denominator)

Ratio: 1. A calculation found by dividing one quantity by another 2. A general term that can include a number of specific measures such as proportion, percentage, and rate

Ratio-level data: Data where there is a defined unit of measure, a real zero point, and the intervals between successive values are equal

Ratio variables: The most common quantitative variables used in healthcare; these variables include numbers that can be compared meaningfully with one another; zero is truly zero on the ratio scale

Reasonable cause: As amended by HITECH, an act or omission in which a covered entity or business associate knew, or by exercising reasonable diligence would have known, that the act or omission violated an administrative simplification provision, but in which the covered entity or business associated did not act with willful neglect (45 CFR 160.401 2013)

Reasonable diligence: As amended by HITECH, means the business care and prudence expected from a person seeking to satisfy a legal requirement under similar circumstances (45 CFR 160.401 2013)

Record locator service (RLS): A process that seeks information about where a patient, once identified, may have a health record available to the HIO

Record reconciliation: The process of assuring that all the records of discharged patients have been received by the HIM department for processing

Recovery audit contractor (RAC): A governmental program whose goal is to identify improper payments made on claims of healthcare services provided to Medicare beneficiaries. Improper payments may be overpayments or underpayments

Recovery room report: A type of health record documentation used by nurses to document the patient's reaction to anesthesia and condition after surgery

Recruitment: The process of finding, soliciting, and attracting employees

Red Flags Rule: Consists of five categories of red flags that are used as triggers to alert the organization to a potential identity theft; the categories are: (1) alerts, notifications, or warnings from a consumer reporting agency; (2) suspicious documents; (3) suspicious personally identifying information such as a suspicious address; (4) unusual use of, or suspicious activity relating to, a covered account; (5) Notices from customers, victims of identity theft, law enforcement authorities, or other businesses about possible identity theft in connection with an account

Referent power: The ability of the team members to identify with leaders who have desirable resources or personal traits

Referred outpatient: An outpatient who is provided special diagnostic or therapeutic services by a hospital on an ambulatory basis but whose medical care remains the responsibility of the referring physician

Registered health information administrator (RHIA): A type of certification granted after completion of an AHIMA-accredited four-year program in health information management and a credentialing examination

Registered health information technician (RHIT): A type of certification granted after completion of an AHIMA-accredited two-year program in health information management and a credentialing examination

Registration: The act of enrolling

Registration-Admission, Discharge, Transfer (R-ADT): A type of administrative information system that stores demographic information and performs functionality related to registration, admission, discharge, and transfer of patients within the organization

Registry: A collection of care information related to a specific disease, condition, or procedure that makes health record information available for analysis and comparison

Reimbursement: Compensation or repayment for healthcare services

Relationship: A type of connection between two terms

Relational database: A type of database that stores data in predefined tables made up of rows and columns

Release of information: The process of disclosing patient-identifiable information from the health record to another party

Reliability: A measure of consistency of data items based on their reproducibility and an estimation of their error of measurement

Remittance advice: An explanation of payments (for example, claim denials) made by third-party payers

Requirements specification: Determining and documenting the detailed features and functions desired in the system in order to meet the organization's specific goals

Requisition: Request for the health record

Research methodologies: Research studies that can range from exploratory or descriptive studies that strive to generate new hypotheses based on data collected to experimental studies that provide interventions or treatments that can reduce the spread of an existing disease

Resident assessment instrument (RAI): In skilled nursing facilities, the care plan is based on a format required by federal regulations

Resource allocation: A process and strategy of deciding where resources should be used in the accomplishment of the mission, values, and goals of the organization

Resource-based relative value scale: A scale of national uniform relative values for all physicians' services. The relative value of each service must be the sum of relative value units representing the physicians' work, practice expenses net of malpractice insurance expenses, and the cost of professional liability insurance

Respect: Appreciation of the value of differing perspectives, enjoyable experiences, courteous interaction, and celebration of achievements that advance our common cause

Results management: An EHR application that enables diagnostic study results (primarily lab results) to be both reviewed in a report format and the data within the reports to be processed

Retrospective documentation: Healthcare providers add documentation after care has been given, possibly for the purpose of increasing reimbursement or avoiding a medical legal action

Retrospective review: The part of the utilization review process that concentrates on a review of clinical information following patient discharge

Retrospective study: A type of research conducted by reviewing records from the past (for example, birth and death certificates or health records) or by obtaining information about past events through surveys or interviews

Revenue: The recognition of income earned and the use of appropriated capital from the rendering of services during the current period

Revenue cycle: 1. The process of how patient financial and health information moves into, through, and out of the healthcare facility, culminating with the facility receiving reimbursement for services provided 2. The regularly repeating set of events that produces revenue

Revenue cycle management (RCM): Refers to the entire process of creating, submitting, analyzing, and obtaining payment for healthcare services

Reward power: Power based on the leader's ability to give rewards to team members for commendable work, such as letters of recommendation, compliments, additional training or responsibilities, and additional compensation for working on the team

Right of access: Allows an individual to inspect and obtain a copy of his or her own PHI contained within a designated record set, such as a health record

Right to request accounting of disclosures: An individual has the right to receive an accounting of certain disclosures made by a covered entity

Right to request amendment: One may request that a covered entity amend PHI or a record about the individual in a designated record set

Right to request confidential communications: Healthcare providers and health plans must give individuals the opportunity to request that communications of PHI be routed to an alternative location or by an alternative method

Right to request restrictions of PHI: An individual can request that a covered entity restrict the uses and disclosures of PHI to carry out treatment, payment, or healthcare operations

Right-to-work laws: Federal legislation dealing with labor rights (examples include workers' compensation, child labor, and minimum wage laws)

Risk: 1. The probability of incurring injury or loss 2. The probable amount of loss foreseen by an insurer in issuing a contract 3. A formal insurance term denoting liability to compensate individuals for injuries sustained in a healthcare facility

Risk analysis: The process of identifying possible security threats to the organization's data and identifying which risks should be proactively addressed and which risks are lower in priority

Risk management: A comprehensive program of activities intended to minimize the potential for injuries to occur in a facility and to anticipate and respond to ensuring liabilities for those injuries that do occur. The processes in place to identify, evaluate, and control risk, defined as the organization's risk of accidental financial liability

Risk management program: A comprehensive program of activities intended to minimize the potential for injuries to occur in a facility and to anticipate and respond to ensuring liabilities for those injuries that do occur. The processes in place to identify, evaluate, and control risk, defined as the organization's risk of accidental financial liability

Risk of mortality: The likelihood of an inpatient death for a patient

Role-based access control (RBAC): A control system in which access decisions are based on the roles of individual users as part of an organization

Root-cause analysis: A technique used in performance improvement initiatives to discover the underlying causes of a problem. Analysis of a sentinel event from all aspects (human, procedural, machinery, material) to identify how each contributed to the occurrence of the event and to develop new systems that will prevent recurrence

Rules and regulations: Operating documents that describe the rules and regulations under which a healthcare organization operates

Rules-based algorithm: Algorithm that assigns weights to specific data elements and uses those weights to compare one record to another

Run chart: A type of graph that shows data points collected over time and identifies emerging trends or patterns

RxNorm: A clinical drug nomenclature developed by the Food and Drug Administration, the Department of Veterans Affairs, and HL7 to provide standard names for clinical drugs and administered dose forms

RxNorm concept unique identifier (RXCUI): The drug name and all of its synonyms, which represent a single concept

S

Sale of information: Addressed specifically by ARRA, which prohibits a covered entity or BA from selling (receiving direct or indirect compensation) in exchange for an individual's PHI without that individual's authorization; the authorization must also state whether the individual permits the recipient of the PHI to further exchange the PHI for compensation

Scales of measurement: A reference standard for data collection and classification

Scatter charts: A graph that visually displays the linear relationships among factors

Scorecards: Reports of outcomes measures to help leaders know what they have accomplished

SCRIPT: The NCPDP standard developed for electronically transmitting a prescription

Secondary data source: Data derived from the primary patient record, such as an index or a database

Security: 1. The means to control access and protect information from accidental or intentional disclosure to unauthorized persons and from unauthorized alteration, destruction, or loss 2. The physical protection of facilities and equipment from theft, damage, or unauthorized access; collectively, the policies, procedures, and safeguards designed to protect the confidentiality of information, maintain the integrity and availability of information systems, and control access to the content of these systems

Security breach: Unauthorized data or system access

Security program: A plan outlining the policies and procedures created to protect healthcare information

Security threat: A situation that has the potential to damage a healthcare organization's information system

Selection: The act or process of choosing

Selection test: Assessment that identifies job skills, abilities, or job-related attitudes that may not surface in an interview

Self-directed learning: An instructional method that allows students to control their learning and progress at their own pace

Semantic interoperability: Mutual understanding of the meaning of data exchanged between information systems

Semi-automated review: Reviews that start with an automated review but also incorporate health record documents analyzed by humans

Sentinel event: According to the Joint Commission, an unexpected occurrence involving death or serious physical or psychological injury, or the risk thereof. Serious injury specifically includes loss of limb or function. The phrase "or risk thereof" includes any process variation for which a recurrence would carry a significant chance of serious adverse outcome. Such events are called "sentinel" because they signal the need for immediate investigation and response

Serial numbering system: System where a patient is issued a unique numerical identifier for every encounter at the healthcare facility; if a patient is admitted to the healthcare facility five times he or she will have five different health record numbers

Serial-unit number system: A combination of the serial and unit numbering systems; the patient is issued a new health record number with each encounter but all of the documentation is moved from the last number to the new number

Serial work division: Tasks or steps in a process are handled separately in sequence by individual workers, as with a factory assembly line, to complete a process

Severity of illness (SOI): A type of supportive documentation reflecting objective clinical indicators of a patient illness (essentially the patient is sick enough to be at an identified level of care) and referring to the extent of physiologic decompensation or organ system loss of function

Sexual harassment: A type of harassment that may include verbal comments, unwanted physical contact, sexual advances or requests for sexual favors

Shared Nationwide Interoperability Roadmap: ONC's three stage vision for interoperability; 2015 – 2017: Nationwide ability to send, receive, find, and use a common clinical data set; 2018 – 2020: Expand interoperable data, users, sophistication, and scale; 2021 – 2024: Broad-scale learning health system

Simulation: A training technique for experimenting with real-world situations by means of a computerized model that represents the actual situation

Single-key encryption: Two or more computers share the same secret key and that key is used to both encrypt and decrypt a message; however, the key must be kept secret and if it is compromised in any way, the security of the data is likely to be eliminated; *see also private key infrastructure*

Single sign-on: A type of technology that allows a user access to all disparate applications through one authentication procedure, thus reducing the number and variety of passwords a user must remember and enforcing and centralizing access control

Six Sigma: Disciplined and data-driven methodology for getting rid of defects in any process

Skilled nursing facility (SNF): A facility which primarily provides inpatient skilled nursing care and related services to patients who require medical, nursing, rehabilitative services but does not provide the level of care or treatment available in a hospital

Skilled nursing facility prospective payment system: A per-diem reimbursement system implemented in July 1998 for costs (routine, ancillary, and capital) associated with covered skilled nursing facility services furnished to Medicare Part A beneficiaries

SMART goals: Statements that identify results that are: Specific, Measurable, Attainable, Relevant, and Time-based

Sniffers: A software security product that runs in the background of a network, examining and logging packet traffic and serving as an early warning device against crackers

SNOMED CT identifier: A unique integer assigned to each SNOMED CT component

Software as a Service (SaaS): Arrangement similar to an application service provider with generally less custom configuration ability and that offers a pay as you go model, where there is payment for only the actual time using the system; may be delivered via dedicated communications technology or cloud computing

Source data: The location from which the data originates such as a database or a data set

Source-oriented health record: A system of health record organization in which information is arranged according to the patient care department that provided the care

Source systems: 1. A system in which data was originally created 2. Independent information system application that contributes data to an EHR, including departmental clinical applications (for example, laboratory information system, clinical pharmacy information system) and specialty clinical applications (for example, intensive care, cardiology, labor and delivery)

Special-cause variation: An unusual source of variation that occurs outside a process but affects it

Speech dictation: Method of collecting information in an information system through spoken word

Spoliation: The act of destroying, changing, or hiding evidence intentionally

Staffing: Decisions about the types of employees needed, how many employees are needed, how work will be organized, and how employees are scheduled

Stage of the neoplasm: Pathological data characterizing the cancer, specifically the amount of metastasis, if any.

Standard: 1. A scientifically based statement of expected behavior against which structures, processes, and outcomes can be measured 2. A model or example established by authority, custom, or general consent or a rule established by an authority as a measure of quantity, weight, extent, value, or quality 3. Under HITECH, a technical, functional, or performance-based rule, condition, requirement, or specification that stipulates instructions, fields, codes, data, material, characteristics or actions (45 CFR 170.102 2012) 4. As amended by HITECH at section 160.103, a rule, condition, or requirement: (1) describing the following information for products, systems, services, or practices: (i) classification of components; (ii) specification of materials, performance, or operations; or (iii) delineation of procedures; or (2) with respect to the privacy of protected health information (45 CFR 160.103 2013)

Standard deviation: A measure of variability that describes the deviation from the mean of a frequency distribution in the original units of measurement; the square root of the variance

Standard of care: An established set of clinical decisions and actions taken by clinicians and other representatives of healthcare organizations in accordance with state and federal laws, regulations, and guidelines; codes of ethics published by professional associations or societies; regulations for accreditation published by accreditation agencies; usual and common practice of equivalent clinicians or organizations in a geographical region

Standards development organization: A private or government agency involved in the development of healthcare informatics standards at a national or international level

Standing orders: Orders the medical staff or an individual physician has established as routine care for a specific diagnosis or procedure

Stark law: Originally a part of the Omnibus Budget Reconciliation Act of 1989, it is a law that prohibits physicians from ordering designated health services for Medicare (and to some extent Medicaid) patients from entities with which the physician, or an immediate family member, has a financial relationship

Statistical packages: Software that can be used to facilitate the data collection and analysis process; these packages simplify the statistical analysis of data and are often used in addition to spreadsheet software

Statistical process control chart: A type of run chart that includes both upper and lower control limits and indicates whether a process is stable or unstable

Statistics-based modeling: The use of analytical and graphical techniques to assist in the display and interpretation of raw data

Statute: A piece of legislation written and approved by a state or federal legislature and then signed into law by the state's governor or the president

Statute of limitations: A specific time frame allowed by a statute or law for bringing litigation

Statutory law: Written law established by federal and state legislatures

Steering committee: An overarching committee comprised of key stakeholders to health information systems in general, or, less commonly, a steering committee will be convened for each specific health information system project and include only stakeholders associated with that project

Stem and leaf plots: A visual display that organizes data to show its shape and distribution, using two columns with the stem in the left-hand column and all leaves associated with that stem in the right-hand column; the "leaf" is the ones digit of the number, and the other digits form the "stem"

Stereotyping: An assumption that everyone within a certain group are the same

Storage management: The process of determining on what type of media to store data, how rapidly data must be accessible, arranging for replication of storage for back up and disaster recovery, and where storage systems should be maintained

Straight numeric filing system: A health record filing system in which health records are arranged in ascending numerical order

Strategic information systems planning: The process of identifying and prioritizing various upgrades and changes that might be made in an organizations information systems

Strategic plan: The document in which the leadership of a healthcare organization identifies the organization's overall mission, vision, and goals to help set the long-term direction of the organization as a business entity

Strategic planning: Involves how the organization will react to changes in the external environment in the foreseeable future

Strategy: A course of action designed to produce a desired (business) outcome

Strike: A temporary work stoppage called in an effort to express an employment contract negotiation demand

Structure indicators: Indicators that measure the attributes of the setting, such as number and qualifications of the staff, adequacy of equipment and facilities, and adequacy of organizational policies and procedures

Structured brainstorming: A group problem-solving technique wherein the team leader asks each participant to generate a list of ideas for the topic under discussion and then report them to the group in a nonjudgmental manner

Structured data: Binary, machine-readable data in discrete fields; data able to be processed by the computer

Student membership: AHIMA membership level that includes any student who does not have an AHIMA credential, has not previously been an active member of AHIMA, and who is formally enrolled in a Professional Certificate Approval Program or Approved Committee for Certificate Programs, or in a CAHIIM-accredited HIM program

Subacute care: Offers patients access to constant nursing care while recovering at home

Subjective, objective, assessment, plan (SOAP): Documentation method that refers to how each progress note contains documentation relative to subjective observations, objective observations, assessments, and plans

Subpoena: A command to appear at a certain time and place to give testimony on a certain matter

Subpoena ad testificandum: A subpoena that seeks testimony

Subpoena duces tecum: A written order commanding a person to appear, give testimony, and bring all documents, papers, books, and records described in the subpoena. The devices are used to obtain documents during pretrial discovery and to obtain testimony during trial

Summons: An instrument used to begin a civil action or special proceeding and is a means of acquiring jurisdiction over a party

Sunsetting: No longer selling or supporting a product

Supervisory management: Management level that oversees the organization's efforts at the staff level and monitors the effectiveness of everyday operations and individual performance against preestablished standards

Supply management: Management and control of the supplies used within an organization

Supreme courts: The highest courts in a system, which hear final appeals from intermediate courts of appeal

Surgical operation: One or more surgical procedures performed at one time for one patient via a common approach or for a common purpose

Surgical procedure: Any single, separate, systematic process upon or within the body that can be complete in itself; is normally performed by a physician, dentist, or other licensed practitioner; can be performed either with or without instruments; and is performed to restore disunited or deficient parts, remove diseased or injured tissues, extract foreign matter, assist in obstetrical delivery, or aid in diagnosis

SWOT analysis: Analysis tool used to outline the organization's strengths (S) and weaknesses (W), which are internal to the organization, and the opportunities (O) and threats (T) external to the organization

Synchronous: Occurring at the same time

System: Refers to all the components (technology, standards, people, policy, and process) that must work together to achieve a desired goal (interoperability)

System build: The creation of data dictionaries, tables, decision support rules, templates for data entry, screen layouts, and reports used in a system; also known as *system configuration*

System characterization: The process of creating an inventory of all systems that contain data, including documenting where the data are stored, what type of data are created or stored, how they are managed, with what hardware and software they interact, and providing basic security measures for the systems

System configuration: The creation of data dictionaries, tables, decision support rules, templates for data entry, screen layouts, and reports used in a system; also known as *system build*

System integration: A translation process that hardwires the applications together in order to be able to interoperate and exchange data seamlessly across the different applications

Systems development life cycle (SDLC): A model used to represent the ongoing process of developing (or purchasing) information systems

Systems thinking: An objective way of looking at work-related ideas and processes with the goal of allowing people to uncover ineffective patterns of behavior and thinking and then finding ways to make lasting improvements

T

Table: An organized arrangement of data, usually in columns and rows

Taft-Hartley Act: Federal legislation passed in 1947 that imposed certain restrictions on unions while upholding their right to organize and bargain collectively

Target data: The location from which the data is mapped or to where it is sent

Team building: The process of organizing and acquainting a team and building skills for dealing with later team processes

Team charter: A document that explains the issues the team was initiated to address, describes the team's goal or vision, and lists the initial members of the team and their respective departments

Team leader: A performance improvement team role responsible for championing the effectiveness of performance improvement activities in meeting customers' needs and for the content of a team's work

Team member: A performance improvement team role responsible for participating in team decision making and plan development; identifying opportunities for improvement; gathering, prioritizing, and analyzing data; and sharing knowledge, information, and data that pertain to the process under study

Team norms: The rules, both explicit and implied, that determine both acceptable and unacceptable behavior for a group

Technical component: The portion of radiological and other procedures that is facility based or nonphysician based (for example, radiology films, equipment, overhead, endoscopic suites, and so on)

Technical safeguards: As amended by HITECH, the Security Rule means the technology and the policy and procedures for its use that protect electronic protected health information and control access to it

Telecommuting: A work arrangement in which at least a portion of the employee's work hours is spent outside the office (usually in the home) and the work is transmitted back to the employer via electronic means

Telehealth: A telecommunications system that links healthcare organizations and patients from diverse geographic locations and transmits text and images for (medical) consultation and treatment

Template: A pattern used in computer-based patient records to capture data in a structured manner

Terminal-digit filing system: A system of health record identification and filing in which the last digit or group of digits (terminal digits) in the health record number determines file placement

Termination: The act of ending something (for example, a job)

Theory X and Y: A management theory developed by McGregor that describes pessimistic and optimistic assumptions about people and their work potential

Third-party administrator: 1. An entity required to make or responsible for making payment on behalf of a group health plan 2. A business associate that performs claims administration and related business functions for a self-insured entity

Third-party payer: An insurance company (for example, Blue Cross/Blue Shield) or healthcare program (for example, Medicare) that pays or reimburses healthcare providers (second party) or patients (first party) for the delivery of medical services

Time ladders: Tools that support the collection of data that must be oriented by time; they specify intervals of time necessary to address the problem under consideration listed down the right side of one, two, or three columns; then, as the data collector observes, he or she records them next to the time of occurrence

Timekeeper: A performance improvement team role responsible for notifying the team during meetings of time remaining on each agenda item in an effort to keep the team moving forward on its performance improvement project

Title VII of the Civil Rights Act of 1964: The federal legislation that prohibits discrimination in employment on the basis of race, religion, color, sex, or national origin (Public Law 88-352 1964)

Tort: An action brought when one party believes that another party caused harm through wrongful conduct and seeks compensation for that harm

Total length of stay (discharge days): The sum of length of stay for all patients discharged for a given period of time

Traditional fee-for-service reimbursement: A reimbursement method involving third-party payers who compensate providers after the healthcare services have been delivered; payment is based on specific services provided to subscribers

Training: A set of activities and materials that provide the opportunity to acquire job-related skills, knowledge, and abilities

Trait theory: Proposes that leaders possess a collection of traits or qualities that distinguish them from nonleaders

Transaction: As amended by HITECH, under HIPAA, the transmission of information between two parties to carry out financial or administrative activities related to health care. It includes the following types of information transmissions: (1) Health care claims or equivalent encounter information; (2) Health care payment and remittance advice; (3) Coordination of benefits; (4) Health care claim status; (5) Enrollment and disenrollment in a health plan; (6) Eligibility for a health plan; (7) Health plan premium payments; (8) Referral certification and authorization; (9) First report of injury; (10) Health claims attachments; (11) Health care electronic funds transfers (EFT) and remittance advice; (12) Other transactions that the secretary may prescribe by regulation (45 CFR 160.103 2013)

Transactional leadership: Refers to the role of the manager who strives to create an efficient workplace by balancing task accomplishment with interpersonal satisfaction

Transfer record: A review of the patient's acute stay along with current status, discharge and transfer orders, and any additional instructions that accompanies the patient when he or she is transferred to another facility

Transformational leadership: The leadership of a visionary who strives to change an organization

Transitional model: Model created by William Bridges that defines three stages: (1) ending, losing, and letting go; (2) a neutral zone; and (3) new beginnings; each stage identifies the different emotions employees have as their daily work is either changed or replaced

Traumatic injury: A wound or other injury caused by an external physical force such as an automobile accident, a shooting, a stabbing, or a fall

Treatment, payment, and operations (TPO): The Privacy Rule provides a number of exceptions for PHI that is being used or disclosed for TPO purposes; *treatment* means providing, coordinating, or managing healthcare or healthcare-related services by one or more healthcare providers; *payment* includes activities by a health plan to obtain premiums, billing by healthcare providers or health plans to obtain reimbursement, claims management, claims collection, review of the medical necessity of care, and utilization review; the Privacy Rule provides a broad list of activities that are healthcare *operations* that includes quality assessment and improvement, case management, review of healthcare professionals' qualifications, insurance contracting, legal and auditing functions, and general business management functions such as providing customer service and conducting due diligence

Trial court: The lowest tier of state court, usually divided into two courts: the court of limited jurisdiction, which hears cases pertaining to a particular subject matter or involving crimes of lesser severity or civil matters of lower dollar amounts; and the court of general jurisdiction, which hears more serious criminal cases or civil cases that involve large amounts of money

TRICARE: The federal healthcare program that provides coverage for the dependents of armed forces personnel and for retirees receiving care outside military treatment facilities in which the federal government pays a percentage of the cost; formerly known as Civilian Health and Medical Program of the Uniformed Services

Trigger events: Review of access logs, audit trails, failed logins, and other reports generated to monitor compliance with the policies and procedures

Turnaround time: In an ROI system, the time between receipt of request and when the request is sent to requester

Turnover: The rate at which employees leave a firm and have to be replaced

Two-factor authentication: A signature type that includes at least two of the following three elements: something known, such as a password; something held, such as a token or digital certificate; and something that is personal, such as a biometric in the form of a fingerprint, retinal scan, or other

U

Unbundling: The practice of using multiple codes to bill for the various individual steps in a single procedure rather than using a single code that includes all of the steps of the comprehensive procedure

Undercoding: A form of incomplete documentation that results when diagnoses or procedures that should be coded are not assigned

Unified Medical Language System (UMLS): A program initiated by the National Library of Medicine to build an intelligent, automated system that can understand biomedical concepts, words, and expressions and their interrelationships; includes concepts and terms from many different source vocabularies

Unintended consequence: An unanticipated and undesired effect of implementing

Union: An organization formed by employees for the purpose of acting as a unit when dealing with management regarding work issues

Unit numbering system: A health record identification system in which the patient receives a unique medical record number at the time of the first encounter that is used for all subsequent encounters

Universal chart order: A system in which the health record is maintained in the same format while the patient is in the facility and after discharge

Unsecured electronic protected health information (e-PHI): e-PHI that has not been made unusable, unreadable, or indecipherable to unauthorized persons

Unstructured brainstorming method: A group problem-solving technique wherein the team leader solicits spontaneous ideas for the topic under discussion from members of the team in a free-flowing and nonjudgmental manner

Unstructured data: Nonbinary, human-readable data

Upcoding: The practice of assigning diagnostic or procedural codes that represent higher payment rates than the codes that actually reflect the services provided to patients

Use: As amended by HITECH, with respect to individually identifiable health information, the sharing, employment, application, utilization, examination, or analysis of such information within an entity that maintains such information (45 CFR 160.103 2013)

Use case: A technique that develops scenarios based on how users will use information to assist in developing information systems that support the information requirements

User-based access control (UBAC): A security mechanism used to grant users of a system access based on identity

Usual, customary, and reasonable charges: Type of retrospective fee-for-service payment method in which the third-party payer pays for fees that are usual, customary, and reasonable, wherein "usual" is usual for the individual provider's practice; "customary" means customary for the community; and "reasonable" is reasonable for the situation

Utilization management (UM): 1. A collection of systems and processes to ensure that facilities and resources, both human and nonhuman, are used maximally and are consistent with patient care needs 2. A program that evaluates the healthcare facility's efficiency in providing necessary care to patients in the most effective manner

Utilization review: The process of determining whether the medical care provided to a specific patient is necessary according to preestablished objective screening criteria at time frames specified in the organization's utilization management plan

Utilization Review Act: Legislation in 1977 that made it a requirement for hospitals to conduct continued-stay reviews for Medicare and Medicaid patients

V

Validity: 1. The extent to which data correspond to the actual state of affairs or that an instrument measures what it purports to measure 2. A term referring to a test's ability to accurately and consistently measure what it purports to measure

Value: Refers to the combination of quality and cost

Value-based purchasing (VBP): CMS incentive plan that links payments more directly to the quality of care provided and rewards providers for delivering high-quality and efficient clinical care. It incorporates clinical process-of-care measures as well as measures from the Hospital Consumer Assessment of Healthcare Providers and Systems (HCAHPS) survey on how patients view their care experiences

Values: The social and cultural belief system of a person or a healthcare organization

Variability: The dispersion of a set of measures around the population mean

Variable costs: Resources expended that vary with the activity of the organization, for example, medication expenses vary with patient volume

Variance: A disagreement between two parts; the square of the standard deviation; a measure of variability that gives the average of the squared deviations from the mean; in financial management, the difference between the budgeted amount and the actual amount of a line item; in project management, the difference between the original project plan and current estimates

Vendor selection: Formal process by a healthcare organization that is just starting to acquire health information systems or replacing entire set of components with new components; steps in the process include needs identification, requirements specification, request for proposal (RFP), analysis of RFP responses, due diligence, and contract negotiation.

Veteran's Health Administration: The nation's largest integrated healthcare system with more than 1,700 hospitals, clinics, community living centers, domiciliaries, readjustment counseling centers, and other facilities operated by the US Department of Veterans Affairs

Virtual private network (VPN): An encrypted tunnel through the Internet that enables secure transmission of data

Virtuoso teams: Group of experts brought together to address an issue or situation

Vital statistics: Data related to births, deaths, marriages, and fetal deaths

Voice recognition technology: A method of encoding speech signals that do not require speaker pauses (but uses pauses when they are present) and of interpreting at least some of the signals' content as words or the intent of the speaker; *Also called* continuous speech recognition; continuous speech technology

Voir dire: Process of jury selection

W

Warrant: A judge's order that authorizes law enforcement to seize evidence and conduct a search

Waste: The overutilization or inappropriate utilization of services and misuse of resources, and typically is not a criminal or intentional act

Web services architecture (WSA): An architecture that utilizes web-based tools to permit communication among different software applications

Willful neglect: As amended by HITECH, conscious, intentional failure or reckless indifference to the obligation to comply with the administrative simplification provision violated (45 CFR 160.401 2013)

Workers' compensation: Insurance that employers are required to have to cover employees who get sick or injured on the job

Workstations on wheels (WOWs): Notebook computers mounted on carts that can be moved through the facility by users

Work analysis: The process of gathering information about what it takes to get a job done

Work measurement: Assessment of internal data collected on actual work performed within the organization and the calculation of time it takes to do the work

Workflow: Any work process that must be handled by more than one person

Workflow analysis: A technique used to study the flow of operations for automation

Workforce: As amended by HITECH, employees, volunteers, trainees, and other persons whose conduct, in the performance of work for a covered entity or business associate, is under the direct control of such covered entity or business associate, whether or not they are paid by the covered entity or business associate (45 CFR 160.103 2013)

Workforce planning: Reviewing national demographic, social, and economic data and trends and relating these to an organization's local staffing needs

World Health Organization (WHO): The United Nations specialized agency created to ensure the attainment by all peoples of the highest possible levels of health; responsible for a number of international classifications, including ICD-10 and ICF

Wrongful discharge: Unfair dismissal of employment due to failure of the employer to comply with law, organizational policy, or a contract

Index